Oral and Maxillofacial Surgery, Medicine, and Pathology for the Clinician

Oral and Maxillofacial Surgery, Medicine, and Pathology for the Clinician

Edited by

Harry Dym, DDS
Chairman, Department of Dentistry and Oral and Maxillofacial Surgery
Brooklyn Hospital Center
Brooklyn, NY, USA

Clinical Professor, Oral and Maxillofacial Surgery
Columbia University College of Dental Medicine
New York, USA

Leslie R. Halpern, DDS, MD, PHD, MPH, FACS, FICD
Professor and Section Chief of Oral and Maxillofacial Surgery
New York Medical College/NYCHHC
New York, USA

Orrett E. Ogle, DDS
Former Chief and Residency Program Director Oral and Maxillofacial Surgery
Woodhull Hospital Center
Brooklyn, NY, USA

Former Associate Clinical Professor of Oral Surgery
Columbia University College of Dental Medicine
New York, USA

Lecturer, Mona Dental Program
Faculty of Medicine, University of the West Indies
Kingston, Jamaica

WILEY Blackwell

Published by John Wiley & Sons, Inc., Hoboken, New Jersey.
Published simultaneously in Canada.

Library of Congress Cataloging-in-Publication Data

Names: Dym, Harry, editor. | Halpern, Leslie R., editor. | Ogle, Orrett E., editor.
Title: Oral and maxillofacial surgery, medicine, and pathology for the clinician / edited by Harry Dym, Leslie R. Halpern, Orrett E. Ogle.
Description: Hoboken, NJ : Wiley-Blackwell, 2023. | Includes bibliographical references and index.
Identifiers: LCCN 2023000304 (print) | LCCN 2023000305 (ebook) | ISBN 9781119361497 (hardback) | ISBN 9781119362555 (adobe pdf) | ISBN 9781119362562 (epub)
Subjects: MESH: Oral Surgical Procedures | Dentistry, Operative
Classification: LCC RK501 (print) | LCC RK501 (ebook) | NLM WU 600 | DDC 617.6/05—dc23/eng/20230328
LC record available at https://lccn.loc.gov/2023000304
LC ebook record available at https://lccn.loc.gov/2023000305

Cover Design: Wiley
Cover Image: Courtesy of Harry Dym

Set in 9.5/12.5pt STIXTwoText by Straive, Chennai, India

SKY10046632_042723

Contents

Contributors

Shelly Abramowicz, DMD, MPH, FACS
Section Chief, Pediatric Oral and Maxillofacial Surgery
Children's Healthcare of Atlanta
Associate Professor and Director of Research, Oral and Maxillofacial Surgery and Pediatrics
Emory University School of Medicine
Atlanta, GA, USA

David R. Adams, DDS
Associate Professor (Clinical) Oral and Maxillofacial Surgery University of Utah School of Dentistry
Salt Lake City, UT, USA

Nathan Adams, MD, DMD, FACS
Assistant Professor
University of Utah School of Dentistry
Salt Lake City, UT, USA

Dina Amin, DDS, FACS
Clinical Associate Professor
Head and Neck Oncology and Microvascular Reconstructive Surgery
Department of Oral and Maxillofacial Surgery, School of Dentistry
Texas A & M University, TX, USA

Ricardo Boyce, DDS
Chief and Program Director, General Dentistry and Oral Medicine
The Brooklyn Hospital Center
New York, USA

Steven Caldroney, DDS, MD, FRCS
Private practice in oral and maxillofacial surgery
Framingham, MA, USA

Michael Chan, DDS
Director OMFS
Department of Veterans Affairs, New York Harbor Healthcare System
Senior Attending OMFS
The Brooklyn Hospital Center
New York, USA

Earl Clarkson, DDS
Chairman of Dentistry and Department of Oral and Maxillofacial Surgery
The Brooklyn Hospital Center
New York, USA

Prince Dhillon, DMD, MD
Assistant Attending Oral and Maxillofacial Surgeon
Department of Dentistry
St Barnabas Hospital
Bronx, NY, USA

Jonathan C. Elmore, DDS
Former Resident
Department of Oral and Maxillofacial Surgery
The Brooklyn Hospital Center
New York, USA

Yijiao Fan, DDS
Resident, Oral and Maxillofacial Surgery
The Brooklyn Hospital Center
New York, USA

Michael A. Gladwell, MD, DMD, FACS
Assistant Professor
University of Utah School of Dentistry
Salt Lake City, UT, USA

Tarun Kirpalani, DMD
Oral and Maxillofacial Surgeon Resident
The Brooklyn Hospital Center
New York, USA

Vivian Lim, DDS
Resident
NYC Health + Hospitals/Woodhull
New York, USA

Gary W. Lowder, DDS
Associate Professor (Clinical) TMD and DSM
University of Utah School of Dentistry
Salt Lake City, UT, USA

Pushkar Mehra, BDS, DMD, FACS
Professor and Chair
Department of Oral and Maxillofacial Surgery
Boston University
Boston, MA, USA

Justine S. Moe, DMD, MD
Clinical Assistant Professor, Residency Program Director, Oral and Maxillofacial Surgery, Associate Fellowship Director, Oral/Head and Neck Oncologic and Reconstructive Surgery
University of Michigan
Ann Arbor, MI, USA

Junaid Mundiya, DMD
OMS private practice, Suffolk Oral Surgery Associates
OMS Attending, St Barnabas Hospital
New York, USA

Mihai Radulescu, DMD, FRCD(C), FACS
Assistant Professor in Surgery
OMFS Residency Attending
Geisinger Commonwealth School of Medicine
Scranton, PA, USA

Andrew R. Rahn, DDS
Adjunct Instructor
University of Utah School of Dentistry
Salt Lake City, UT, USA

Arvind Babu Ravendra Santosh, BDS, MDS
Oral and Maxillofacial Pathologist
Senior Lecturer, School of Dentistry
Faculty of Medical Sciences, The University of the West Indies, Mona, Jamaica
Research Fellow, Faculty of Dental Medicine
Department of Oral Medicine
Universitas Airlangga, Surabaya, Indonesia

Feiyi Sun, DDS
Oral and Maxillofacial Surgeon Resident
The Brooklyn Hospital Center
New York, USA

Alexander Toth, DMD
Assistant Oral and Maxillofacial Surgeon
Windsor Dental Center
New Windsor, NY, USA

Bryan Trump, DDS, MS
Associate Professor
University of Utah School of Dentistry
Salt Lake City, UT, USA

Michael Turner, DDS, MD, MSc
Chief, Oral and Maxillofacial Surgery
Mount Sinai Hospital
Program Director
Mount Sinai/Jacobi Einstein
Residency in Oral and Maxillofacial Surgery
Associate Professor
Icahn School of Medicine at Mount Sinai
New York, USA

Dwight Williams, DDS, MPH
Assistant Director of Oral and Maxillofacial Surgery
Woodhull Medical Center
Brooklyn, NY, USA
Owner, Optimum Dental Care
Bronx, NY, USA

Lester Woo, DDS
Oral and Maxillofacial Surgeon
Lakewood, WA, USA

Preface

The successful practice of dentistry and oral surgery requires the serious practitioner to engage in a lifelong pursuit of continuous knowledge improvement and education, while failure to do so will ultimately lead to poor patient clinical outcomes along with a diminished sense of satisfaction with their chosen profession. Textbooks such as this are a valuable resource in assisting the dentist and oral surgeon in the pursuit of up-to-date clinical information that can assist them in their practice.

I am grateful to all our contributors for their well-written additions to this text. Despite their busy schedules, they have all provided valuable concise clinical information that should prove meaningful for our readers, including younger dentists as well as established dental and oral surgical practitioners.

I am indebted to my coeditor and colleague Dr Orrett E. Ogle who I have known and worked with for over four decades; he is a trusted friend and mentor. Dr Ogle is also an educator and a gifted clinician who has dedicated his entire professional career to the education of dental and oral and maxillofacial surgery residents.

Dr Leslie R. Halpern, my other coeditor, is also a dear friend who, like Dr Ogle, has spent her entire career involved in the education of dental students in the area of oral and maxillofacial surgery.

I have been privileged to spend my entire career working at the Brooklyn Hospital Center where I am Chairman of the Department of Dentistry and Oral and Maxillofacial Surgery. I am indebted to Ms Lizanne Fontaine, Chairperson of the Brooklyn Hospital Center Board of Trustees, and Mr Gary Terrinoni, President and CEO of the Brooklyn Hospital Center, for their continued support of my department.

Acknowledgment is due to my colleagues Dr Earl Clarkson and Dr Peter Sherman for their ongoing friendship; they have always been available for consultation and support.

Appreciation is due to all my past and present oral and maxillofacial surgical residents as they have been the impetus for my passion in teaching and writing.

Finally, all credit is due to my wife Freidy who has always stood by me these many decades.

Harry Dym

Part I

Basics

1

Patient Evaluation and Management of Medical Problems in the Oral Surgery Patient

Orrett E. Ogle

When a new patient presents for an oral surgical procedure, it is the responsibility of the surgeon to not only address the patient's dental issues but also to assess the patient's medical status to ensure that he/she can provide surgical services that is medically appropriate for each patient.

The first encounter with a new patient should always involve a medical history as part of the initial evaluation. The most efficient and commonly used method of obtaining the medical history is to use a medical questionnaire. There are several types of questionnaires available for both adults and children but it is best for the dentist to select one that is detailed and comprehensive. The more detailed the health questionnaire, the more information will be obtained and the dentist will be better able to make informed decisions. A detailed medical history will identify potential management problems (physiologic and pharmaceutical) and allow the oral surgeon to formulate a treatment plan in light of the medical status. On the questionnaire, all health questions must be answered. Pertinent positive answers must be addressed and certain negative answers, such as allergies or bleeding history, must be confirmed. The patient should be verbally questioned about the severity and control of their disease. All medications must be noted.

The purpose of taking the medical history is to achieve the following specific goals.

- The identification of potential management problems (physiologic and pharmaceutical) and referral for further medical evaluation if necessary.
- Assessment of risk potential.
- Formulation of a dental/oral and maxillofacial surgery (OMFS) treatment plan to minimize risk in light of the medical status.
- Avoidance of drug interactions.

Once the dentist has obtained the full medical history, a useful step in patient assessment based solely on the history is to assign an American Society of Anesthesiologists (ASA) physical status classification (Box 1.1). This will inform the dental team of the degree of risk the patient's physical ailments constitute and simplify decision making (Figure 1.1).

Risk Assessment

Risk (the probability that an adverse event will occur during dental treatment due to an existing underlying disease) assessment will allow the dentist to make treatment decisions, which will act as a framework to avoid complications during or after the oral surgical intervention and produce an optimal outcome. Some quick risk assessments that should be made from the medical history include the following.

- The patient's physiologic reserves: cardiovascular disease (CV) assessment.
- Risks of infection: diabetes mellitus, immune deficiencies.
- Current medications: bleeding risks, drug interactions, medications that need to be modified before dental treatment.
- Control of chronic diseases: diabetes, hypertension, heart problems, arthritis, other chronic diseases which may cause modification to routine surgical care.

Oral and Maxillofacial Surgery, Medicine, and Pathology for the Clinician, First Edition. Edited by Harry Dym, Leslie R. Halpern, and Orrett E. Ogle.

Box 1.1 Modified ASA classification

- **ASA 1**: Normal healthy patient
- **ASA 2**: Patient with mild systemic disease. Patient with one systemic disease that is controlled
- **ASA 3**: Patient with severe systemic disease. Two or more systemic diseases – controlled or uncontrolled. One systemic disease that is not controlled
- **ASA 4**: Patient with severe systemic disease that is a constant threat to life
- **ASA 5**: Moribund patient who is not expected to survive without surgical intervention.
- **ASA 6**: Declared brain-dead patient whose organs are being removed for donor purposes

Factors not listed in the ASA classification but that must be regarded as an additional risk are extreme age (more than 80 years), increased body mass index, and pregnancy that is close to the estimated date of delivery.

Source: Modified from [1].

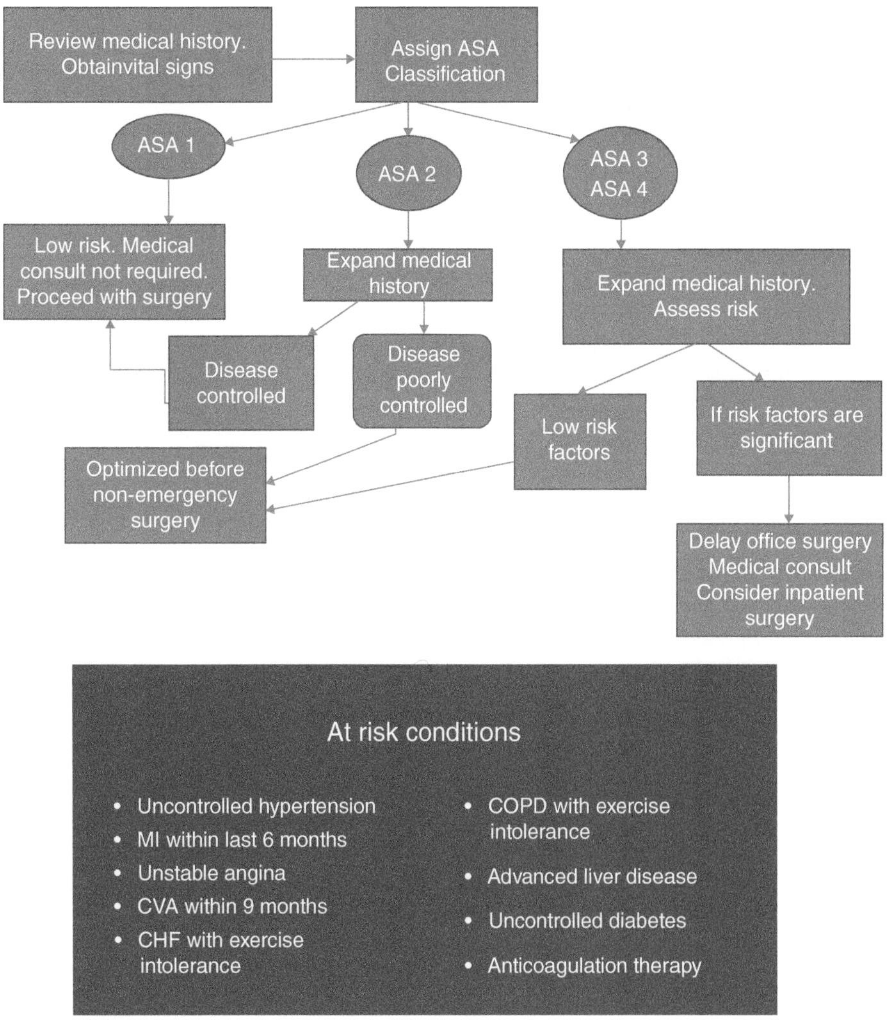

Figure 1.1 After determining the ASA classification, follow the algorithm to decide how the patient should be managed.

Documentation

Medical/dental notes are important to any clinical practice, and the dental practitioner is urged to keep accurate records and adequately document all encounters with patients. Chart notes should be written immediately after seeing each patient and it is good practice to write notes in full sentences that are well organized and include the pertinent data from the encounter. Acceptable medical abbreviations can be used. Good clinical notes will be very useful to the practitioner if ever having to defend a legal claim of clinical negligence. Most importantly, billing documents should not be included anywhere within the clinical notes.

As a part of the documentation, the history form must be dated and signed by the patient or parent/guardian and by the dentist. Failure of the dentist to sign the form may imply that he/she did not review it. Any medical condition that could affect dental treatment or that could be affected by dental treatment should be noted on the record treatment page under a section for past medical history. If the condition is critical (e.g., allergies or heart conditions), the external portion of the chart should be flagged with a sticker for medical alerts or annotated in red ink. Electronic records should also be flagged using the method available in the software system. For individuals with a serious illness, the name and telephone number of the primary care physician should also be obtained. Oral surgery practice will often not have multiple office visits, but if there are serious medical issues, the health history should be updated at every procedural visit (e.g., two-stage implant surgery or serial extractions) and any changes in the condition should be noted in the record.

The patient's medical record should also list all drugs that the patient is currently taking – both prescribed and over-the-counter medications. The oral surgeon should know what each drug (particularly recently introduced ones) is and why it is being used. Medications are a useful indication of conditions for which the patient is being treated. Special attention should be paid to side-effects associated with the medications, because some side-effects may affect dental treatment. For example, heart medications, blood pressure drugs, muscle relaxants, and other medications may contribute to bladder control problems. Patients taking these drugs may need to urinate frequently and will not be able to tolerate long appointments. Thiazides, all diuretics, alpha-blockers, and carbonic anhydrase inhibitors are examples of drugs that will cause frequent urination and urgency [2].

Management of Patients with Medical Problems

Patients will present to the dentist with one or multiple established diagnoses which will be garnered from the medical history. These conditions may alter how dental care is delivered. Medical illness may predispose the patient to acute physiologic decompensation under stress or failure to do well post treatment. Drugs prescribed by a dentist may lead to a drug interaction which may negatively compromise the medical therapy. The job of the clinician is to know how these medical problems will impact dental care or how dental care may affect the medical care. The dentist must therefore be aware of potential outcomes and what precautions must be taken to minimize risks. They must identify issues that should be addressed prior to treatment (e.g., insulin, warfarin, or aspirin use), illnesses that may cause physiologic decompensation during treatment (e.g., angina, seizure disorders, or asthma), and conditions that may affect the posttreatment phase (e.g., diabetes [infection and delayed wound healing] or aspirin use [impaired hemostasis]) [1].

Approximately one in seven Americans is over the age of 65. People 65+ represented 14.5% of the population (46.2 million) in 2014 but are expected to grow to be 21.7% of the population by 2040 [3]. This aging population will produce millions of people with systemic medical conditions that will present for dental care and they will undoubtedly become a numerically significant part of oral surgical practice in the upcoming years. It is imperative, therefore, that the dental practitioner has a full understand of the potential complications that can occur as a consequence of dental treatment of a medically compromised patient and how office management may need to be modified to prevent potential complications. Each systemic disease will affect dental care in its own unique way and there is no generalized protocol that will be applicable in all situations.

This chapter will review some of the more common medical problems that oral surgeons may encounter in their daily practice and present suggested methods for managing individuals with existing disease. There is a long list of diseases (Box 1.2) that can impact dental care, but only the more commonly seen ones can be discussed in this chapter.

A starting point for the oral surgeon preparing to treat a patient with a preexisting disease should be the determination of disease status. Is the patient in optimal condition despite the underlying disease; where in the continuum of disease is the patient; and, lastly, is it possible to reverse the disease? A disease that is poorly controlled, deterioration in symptoms or changes in the condition of the patient will warrant medical evaluation and appropriate referral should be made. An individual with moderate disease who has frequent exacerbations should be reevaluated at each visit. Always remember that unless it is a true dental emergency (infection, trauma, severe pain), the surgery can be delayed and the first responsibility of the clinician is to ensure that the patient is in as good a medical condition as possible. For patients whose disease is stabilized, routine office surgery will generally not present a problem.

Box 1.2 Diseases that may affect dental treatment

- Cardiovascular disease: hypertension, coronary artery disease, stroke, heart failure, certain congenital heart diseases
- Endocrine disorders: diabetes, parathyroid and thyroid diseases, adrenal gland alterations
- Hepatic disease
- Renal disease
- Pulmonary disease: asthma, chronic obstructive pulmonary disease (COPD)
- Pregnancy
- Bleeding disorders: drug induced, congenital
- Malignancies: chemotherapy, radiation therapy
- Allergies (drugs, latex, others)
- Medical conditions associated with geriatric patients
- Eating disorders: bulimia, anorexia
- Leukemia
- Anemia
- Blood-borne pathogens: HIV, hepatitis B and C
- Poor nutrition
- Obstructive sleep apnea

The management of specific diseases is described below.

Cardiovascular Disease

Cardiovascular (CV) disease is America's leading health problem, and the leading cause of death. Cardiovascular problems that may cause modification of dental treatment plans and will be discussed here include hypertension, ischemic heart disease (coronary artery disease [CAD]), myocardial infarction (MI), strokes, cardiac arrhythmias, and heart failure.

Hypertension

Hypertension is a highly prevalent cardiovascular disease, with a steep increase with aging, that is frequently encountered in the dental setting. Table 1.1 summarizes the classification of hypertension from the Joint National Committee on Prevention, Detection, Evaluation, and Treatment of High Blood Pressure [4].

Patients with stage 2 or 3 hypertension are at increased risk because the stress from surgery may further increase blood pressure and trigger a devastating complication such as stroke or cardiac arrest. To date, there are no randomized clinical trials that set a limit on the maximum blood pressure for elective oral surgical treatment. Long years of clinical practice, however, have indicated that oral surgery would only be deferred at blood pressure readings of systolic >160 mmHg or diastolic >100 mmHg [5]. Without obvious target organ disease, there are no grounds for postponing oral surgery, nor is one isolated reading of a high blood pressure immediately before surgery a reason not to do the surgery. Emergency dental procedures could be performed for stage 2 patients but should be avoided in patients with a blood pressure of greater than 180/110 mmHg. These individuals should be referred for immediate medical attention and the dental emergency managed in the hospital if severe, e.g., Ludwig angina. Hypertension is associated with several comorbidities such as ischemic heart disease, cardiac failure, strokes, and kidney disease and, as a result, the surgeon should rule out these diseases or make sure that they are stable before sedation or in-office general anesthesia.

The most important aspect of treating hypertensive patients is effective control of pain and anxiety. Endogenous catecholamines triggered by pain and stress may increase blood pressure and cardiac output. The dental surgeon should aim at good pain control and decreased anxiety. One of the easiest and most effective methods of controlling anxiety is the use of nitrous oxide, which has excellent sedative, analgesic, and antihypertensive properties, or, preferably, IV sedation with midazolam with or without supplemental nitrous oxide/oxygen. When administering N_2O to patients using beta-blockers, hypotension may occur and the blood pressure should be monitored.

In many patients, local anesthesia (LA) is often the method of pain control and local anesthetics with epinephrine are widely used because they produce longer and more effective anesthesia. Small doses of local vasoconstrictor produce minimal change in blood pressure readings [6, 7]. The maximum recommended dose of epinephrine in a patient with cardiac risk is 0.04 mg, which is equal to what is contained in about two cartridges of LA with 1:100 000 epinephrine, or four cartridges with 1:200 000 epinephrine [8]. If adequate anesthesia is not achieved with the

Table 1.1 Classification of hypertension.

Classification	Systolic	Diastolic
Normal	<120	<80
Pre-hypertension	121–139	81–89
Stage 1	140–159	90–99
Stage 2	160–179	100–109
Stage 3	≥180	≥110

two cartridges containing the vasoconstrictor then the anesthesia may be supplemented with a nonvasoconstrictor-containing agents such as mepivacaine 3%. Again, IV sedation is always an option.

The question of using local anesthetic with epinephrine in patients taking nonselective beta-blockers (propranolol and nadolol) has been raised. The small amounts of epinephrine combined with LA used in routine dental procedures are unlikely to be a problem in patients on nonselective beta-blockers [9]. The use of vasoconstrictors in hypertensive individuals still remains controversial. There are no absolute contraindications to the use of vasoconstrictors in dental local anesthetics, since epinephrine is an endogenously produced neurotransmitter [10]. In addition, the release of endogenous epinephrine from inadequate pain control would be far greater than the injected exogenous epinephrine. The American Heart Association and the American Dental Association issued a joint statement in 1964 stating that "the typical concentrations of vasoconstrictors contained in local anesthetics are not contraindicated with cardiovascular disease so long as preliminary aspiration is practiced, the agent is injected slowly, and the smallest effective dose is administered" [11].

Antihypertensive drugs can have several oral manifestations such as xerostomia, oral lichenoid reactions, and gingival hyperplasia but these expressions will not alter the actual clinical management of the hypertensive patient. These drugs, however, have side-effects that may be consequential. Angiotensin-converting enzyme (ACE) inhibitors are associated with cough and loss of taste (ageusia) or taste alteration (dysgeusia). Patients taking enalapril, for example, may have a dry cough and may have to cough frequently. This coughing will be disruptive when it is necessary for the patient to keep their mouth open or blood is in their mouth. Diuretics may cause frequent urination or even urinary incontinence. Patients may have to make more frequent bathroom visits, making them intolerant to long dental procedures. With elderly patients, in rare cases they may need to be excused during the procedure. The antihypertensive medication should not be stopped or altered.

Other groups of patients who are not necessarily hypertensive but whose blood pressure should be monitored are: (i) diabetic patients; (ii) elderly patients in whom orthostatic hypotension is a common problem due to altered blood pressure regulatory mechanisms and autonomic dysfunction; and (iii) pregnant women, because pregnancy may alter the patient's BP values and more than 10% of pregnant women have relevant hypertension [12].

Angina Pectoris

Angina pectoris is chest pain that occurs when an area of the heart muscle is not receiving an adequate oxygen supply. It is the primary symptom of CAD, the most common type of heart disease. Angina attacks which could lead to infarction and cardiac arrest may be precipitated by dental treatment.

The risk in patients with a history of angina is that they may have an attack during dental treatment secondary to stress. The risk increases with increase in classification (Tables 1.2 and 1.3). The most dangerous complication to be concerned about with angina is a heart attack. Totally elective surgical procedures in patients with unstable angina should be delayed until they can be stabilized. Emergencies – infections, severe pain, trauma – should be treated as an inpatient in a hospital setting with monitoring of cardiac status with ECG by an anesthesiologist. Frequently, patients with unstable angina will be given anticoagulants, which will need to be addressed.

The angina patient should be scheduled for short appointments, preferably in the morning [13]. Local anesthetic with epinephrine (1:100 000) should be injected slowly after aspiration and when possible nitrous oxide-oxygen sedation or IV sedation provided. The patient with mild or moderate angina should be advised to bring their nitroglycerin tablets to the scheduled surgical visit in case of an attack during treatment. Persons with a history of frequent attacks, or with attacks often triggered by situational anxiety should be given sublingual nitroglycerin prophylactically 5–10 minutes before injection of LA. Although not absolutely contraindicated, epinephrine should be avoided in this group as the transient tachycardia may stress the myocardium and provoke an attack. Mepivacaine would be a reasonable substitute. Angina may also be avoided by delivery of oxygen via nasal cannula at 3 L/min during the dental procedure.

If the patient develops chest pain during treatment:

- loosen tight clothing around the waist to facilitate breathing
- administer nitroglycerin (best to use the patient's own nitroglycerin tablets), one tablet sublingually. Positive drug action is hastened by sitting the patient upright in the dental chair and asking them to inhale deeply. Relief should follow within 1–3 minutes and reach a peak at 5 minutes [14]
- if the first tablet does not relieve the pain, wait 5 minutes and administer another tablet. Up to three tablets may be given with 5 minute intervals between each tablet
- blood pressure readings should be taken after each tablet since nitroglycerin can lower the blood pressure. If the systolic pressure falls by more than 20–30 mmHG, do not administer another dose. If the chest pain is unresolved, give aspirin and call the local EMS (911) service.

Table 1.2 Classification of angina pectoris.

Stable angina	Unstable angina
• Chest pain/discomfort that occurs with a predictable, reliable amount of exertion or stress, and when that pattern has been present for more than 4 weeks • It is triggered by activities that increase cardiac demand – physical and emotional exertion or stress • The pain or discomfort is similar to past episodes of angina with similar amounts of exertion and usually resolves in less than 5 minutes • The chest pain usually stops after medication is taken or at rest • Stable angina can become unstable	• Chest pain occurring for the first time, or has been happening for less than 2 weeks • If there is a change in the usual pattern of angina that occurs with exertion • Unstable angina can occur without exertion • If the symptoms stop, they usually return in a short period of time • The pain is often more severe and lasts longer than stable angina – more than a few minutes • The pain may not go away with rest or use of angina medication

For all angina patients, the dosage of epinephrine should be limited to that contained in two 1.8 mL cartridges of anesthetic containing epinephrine 1:100 000.

Myocardial Infarction

Myocardial infarction (heart attack) is the irreversible death (necrosis) of heart muscle secondary to prolonged lack of oxygen supply (ischemia) [15]. It is unlikely that a dental patient will suffer a MI without having a history of ischemic heart disease. Based on the medical history of heart disease, the dentist should be able to fairly accurately recognize an MI and take appropriate actions. When there is a suspicion of a MI, the oral surgery should attach an ECG machine as soon as possible, and monitor vital signs.

As previously mentioned, the patient's history is critical and sometimes may provide the only clue that the person could be having a MI. Patients with typical acute MI usually present with retrosternal chest pain on the left side that is intense and continuous for 30–60 minutes. The pain often radiates up to the shoulder, down to the left arm, and up to the neck and jaws. They may also complain of lightheadedness, shortness of breath, and nausea.

Physical examination findings may vary but typical clinical findings include:

- profuse sweating
- increased pulse which may be irregular

Table 1.3 Symptomatic classification of angina pectoris.

Class	Description
Class I	Angina only with strenuous exertion
Class II	Angina with moderate exertion
Class III	Angina with mild exertion. Difficulties walking one or two stores or climbing one flight of stairs at normal pace
Class IV	Angina at rest

- blood pressure is initially elevated (because of peripheral arterial vasoconstriction resulting from an adrenergic response to pain, anxiety, and ventricular dysfunction) [15]
- increased respiratory rate
- peripheral cyanosis.

Not all patients will experience the same symptoms or experience them to the same degree. However, the more signs and symptoms that are present, the greater the probability that the individual may be having a heart attack. If the patient develops chest pain, administer nitroglycerin and take the blood pressure. If nitroglycerin does not decrease the pain or the pain persist for longer than 15 minutes, then suspect that the patient is having a MI. A MI will not respond to nitroglycerin.

When it is believed that the person is having a MI, have them chew a 325 mg tablet of chewable aspirin. If the chewable form is unavailable, then use regular aspirin. (Aspirin has a bitter taste, thus may be difficult to chew and may cause nausea.) Aspirin will work within 15 minutes to prevent the progression of clots in the coronary arteries and allow oxygen-rich blood to get to the damaged heart muscle.

MONA is the classic mnemonic for the treatment of an acute MI (morphine, oxygen, nitroglycerin, aspirin). Although the mnemonic is MONA, this does not describe the order in which the drugs are used, it is only a memory guide. Treatment steps are as follows.

- Stop dental procedure.
- Give sublingual nitroglycerin until it is proven that the chest pain is not angina.
- Take vital signs.
- Call EMS.
- Administer MONA (oxygen, 325 mg aspirin chewed for 30 seconds then swallowed, nitroglycerin and morphine for pain control if necessary). In addition to morphine, nitrous oxide/oxygen via a nasal cannula may be used until EMS arrives if the chest pain is severe and the morphine is not adequately controlling the pain.
- Monitor vital signs every 5 minutes.

The practitioner should be prepared to start basic life support (BLS) if the patient goes on to have a cardiac arrest. The use of an AED (automatic external defibrillator) may be necessary since most deaths caused by MI occur early and are attributable to primary ventricular fibrillation (VF)

For patients who have had a heart attack, elective oral surgery should NOT be done within the first 6 months after the MI. If patient needs extraction before 6 months, consult with the cardiologist as there may still be cardiac irritability with an increased risk of a secondary cardiac event. Patients are generally placed on antiplatelet medications (usually clopidogrel in combination with aspirin) for 12 months after a MI. When there is a need for tooth extraction, these medications should not be stopped. Try to limit extractions to a single tooth, but no more than three teeth. Limited amounts of LA with vasoconstrictor should be used and bleeding controlled with local hemostatic measures – hemostatic agents, sutures, and extended pressure.

Stroke/Cerebrovascular Accident

A stroke, or cerebrovascular accident (CVA), is the rapid loss of brain function(s) due to disturbance in the blood supply to the brain. This can be due to ischemia caused by blockage (thrombosis, arterial embolism) or a hemorrhage (bursting a blood vessel). Stroke survivors are always at risk for a recurrent stroke, therefore the dentist must be diligent about ways to prevent another stroke. Researchers have reported that patients who had an ischemic stroke within 3 months before undergoing elective surgical/dental procedure were at relatively high risk for cardiovascular events and mortality but that the risks stabilized after 9 months. These results suggest that patients who have sustained a stroke should wait 9 months before having elective procedures [16, 17]. After 9 months, surgical procedures may be provided with the use of LA containing epinephrine 1:100 000 alone or in conjunction with IV sedation.

Since CAD and stroke share many of the same risk factors, several types of cardiovascular diseases may be present in stroke patients. If the stroke patient has associated cardiovascular problems, the dosage of epinephrine in LA should be reduced to conform to recommendations for the specific cardiovascular disease.

Patients who have had a stroke are often on antiplatelet agents – usually aspirin, clopidogrel or aspirin plus clopidogrel. The dentist should question the patient regarding their antiplatelet regimen. For simple exodontia, local hemostatic measures should be used.

On average, someone in the US suffers a stroke every 40 seconds and every 4 minutes, someone dies of stroke [18]. When an individual has a stroke, it occurs quickly and the symptoms often appear without warning. The main symptoms of stroke are as follows [19].

- Confusion, including trouble with speaking and understanding.
- Headache, possibly with altered consciousness or vomiting.
- Numbness of the face, arm or leg, particularly on one side of the body.
- Trouble with seeing, in one or both eyes.
- Trouble with walking, including dizziness and lack of coordination.

Management of suspected stroke patient includes the following measures.

- Stop dental procedure.
- Give oxygen.
- Take vital signs.
- Recognize stroke: using the F.A.S.T. acronym can help identify the onset of stroke more quickly [19].
  - *Face drooping*: if the person tries to smile, does one side of the face droop?
  - *Arm weakness*: if the person tries to raise both their arms, does one arm drift downward?
  - *Speech difficulty*: if the person tries to repeat a simple phrase, is their speech slurred or strange?
  - *Time to call 911*: if any of the above signs are observed, contact the local EMS.
- Call EMS – 911. Alert the 911 operator that you are calling about a suspected stroke patient. Stroke patients should be transported rapidly to the closest available certified stroke center. If no stroke centers exist, the patient should be transported to the nearest hospital that provides emergency stroke care. In order for a stroke patient to have the best prognosis, they will need to be treated at a hospital within 3 hours of their symptoms first appearing.
- Continue to monitor vital signs until EMS arrive.
- If cardiopulmonary resuscitation is necessary, place the patient in a supine position and initiate cardiopulmonary resuscitation.
- Elevate the patient's head slightly, if the blood pressure is elevated.
- Continue cardiopulmonary resuscitation or other supportive care until EMS arrive to transport the patient to an emergency facility.

Cardiac Arrhythmias

An arrhythmia is simply a disorder of the heart rate (pulse) or in the regularity with which the heart beats. Some arrhythmias may be harmless while others may cause cardiovascular collapse and sudden death. It is very unlikely that a person with a healthy heart would experience any momentous cardiac arrhythmia during dental treatment. An increase in heart rate and transient irregular beats are common reactions to the injection of epinephrine in LA and generally should not be disturbing.

In patients with preexisting heart disease, however, the circumstances may be different. Individuals with underlying heart disease are at increased risk for developing harmful arrhythmias from the stress of dental care. This risk is significantly increased in patients with cardiomyopathies, heart failure, and valvular disease. Such patients should therefore be evaluated by their physician and fully optimized, if necessary, before nonurgent surgical procedures. Pain and multispace infections may necessitate hospital admission and inpatient surgery. The oral surgeon should keep their advanced cardiovascular life support (ACLS) certification current and be prepared to manage dangerous arrhythmias. It is important that the oral surgeon confirms at the procedural visit that patients with heart disease have been taking their medications regularly.

Patients who have been identified from their history as disposed to developing harmful arrhythmias should be managed by a stress and anxiety reduction protocol. IV sedation with midazolam or propofol (propofol has antiarrhythmic and proarrhythmic effects) may be ideal. Local anesthetic with epinephrine should be used to obtain adequate pain control. The total dose of epinephrine should be limited to no more than two 1.8 mL cartridges. The use of periodontal ligament or intraosseous injections using a vasoconstrictor-containing LA is not recommended in these patients [20].

If a high-risk cardiac patient with severe heart disease is suspected of having an arrhythmia during treatment, the dentist should discontinue treatment or rapidly complete the surgery, give supplemental oxygen and closely monitor the rhythm with an ECG machine along with the overall condition. While monitoring the cardiac rhythm, a sample strip in lead 2 should be recorded and placed in the chart. When in doubt, the patient should be referred to a physician for medical evaluation. With any loss of consciousness, even if brief, EMS should be called to transport the patient to a hospital emergency department.

Atrial fibrillation is the most common chronic arrhythmia. These patients are usually under medical care and the main issue regarding surgical treatment will be the anticoagulant which is used in patients with atrial fibrillation.

Heart Failure

Congestive heart failure (CHF) is defined as inability of the heart to pump oxygenated blood to meet the metabolic needs of the body [21]. Patients often may not be aware that they are in heart failure as this disease develops over a prolonged period of time and patients often fail to notify their physician of changes in symptoms. Even patients who are aware that they have CHF will often not inform their dentist. The treating dentist may have to determine if the patient is in heart failure based on their symptoms and should question patients with history of hypertension, CAD, cardiomyopathy, valvular heart disease, and diabetes about symptoms of CHF. Box 1.3 lists some common symptoms of CHF. A good method to assess risk in the patient with heart failure is to use the New York Heart Association classification of heart failure (Table 1.4).

Treatment Guidelines

- *Class 1 and 2: Low risk.* Oral surgery can be performed without additional work-up or medical evaluation. The dentist should verify that the patient has been taking their medication as prescribed. Appointments should be short (20 minutes) and office procedures simple. Dental chair position is generally not a problem in this class of patients [23].

Box 1.3 Common signs of heart failure

Shortness of breath during activity (most commonly), at rest, or while sleeping, which may come on suddenly and wake the individual

- Chronic fatigue and difficulty with activities of daily living, such as shopping, climbing stairs, carrying groceries, or walking
- Persistent cough that produces white or pink blood-tinged mucus
- Swelling in the feet, ankles, legs, or abdomen
- Increased heart rate and heart palpitation
- Confusion, impaired thinking, memory loss, and feelings of disorientation

Source: Adapted from American Heart Association. Heart failure signs and symptoms. www.heart.org/HEARTORG/Conditions/HeartFailure/WarningSignsforHeartFailure/Warning-Signs-of-Heart-Failure_UCM_002045_Article.jsp#.WKEtgzsrLIU

Table 1.4 New York heart association classification of heart failure.

NYHA class	Symptoms
Class 1	Patients with cardiac disease but with no limitations in physical activity
Class 2	Slight limitation of physical activity. Fatigue, palpitations, and dyspnea with ordinary physical activity, but no symptoms at rest
Class 3	Comfortable at rest. Less than ordinary activity causes fatigue, palpitation, dyspnea, or anginal pain
Class 4	Inability to carry on any physical activity without discomfort. Symptoms may be present even at rest. Any physical activity results in increased discomfort

Source: Adapted from NYHA [22].

- *Class 3: Moderate risk.* Obtain medical consultation before treatment. Optimize patient if possible. No extensive treatment. Avoid the use of epinephrine or levonordefrin. Short visits. Keep chair in semi-supine or upright position during treatment.
- *Class 4: High risk.* Not candidates for elective oral surgery. For pain and infection, treat in hospital with monitoring by an anesthesiologist.

Endocrine Disorders

Diabetes Mellitus

Diabetes is a major US public health issue and both the CDC [24] and the American Diabetes Association [25] reported that in 2012, 9.3% (approximately 29.1 million) of the US population had diabetes. Because of the number of people with diabetes in society, practicing dentists are likely to encounter it frequently. Patients with diabetes mellitus are at risk for a multitude of complications that are directly related to the disease itself and it is imperative that the surgeon look for complications of the diabetes. Patients with significant complications related to the disease are at increased risk for bad outcomes during or after oral surgery. Individuals with significant complications of their diabetes should be referred to a diabetic specialist for evaluation and to obtain a glycemic control that is as good as it could be.

Common complications of diabetes are listed in Box 1.4 and risks in Box 1.5.

In the uncontrolled or brittle diabetic patient, only acute dental infection should be treated on an outpatient basis. Local anesthesia with epinephrine is not contraindicated as the small amounts of epinephrine in dental local anesthetics at 1:100 000 concentration will have no significant effect on blood glucose levels. Antibiotics should be prescribed following treatment and monitored carefully for sensitivity and efficacy [26, 27]. Patients with controlled diabetes require no alterations to their delivery of dental care.

In general, morning appointments are advisable for patients with diabetes since endogenous cortisol levels are typically higher at this time. Because cortisol increases

Box 1.4 Complications of diabetes mellitus

Hypertension
- Polyuria: may reflect glycosuria or chronic kidney disease
- History of poor/slow wound healing
- Peripheral arterial disease: problems with lower limb ischemia – pain and/or cramping in the lower leg due to inadequate blood flow to the muscles
- Chronic kidney disease (diabetic nephropathy)
- Cardiovascular disease: evidence of angina, postural hypotension (a late indication of autonomic neuropathy)
- Neuropathies: numbness, pain, paresthesia, leg ulcers; symptoms/history of transient ischemic attacks

Box 1.5 Risks in diabetic patients

Postoperative wound infection
Poor vascularization: slow wound healing
Increased frequency of MI which may be silent (no obvious symptoms)
Cardiac arrest as a consequence of autonomic neuropathy
Stroke: generally increased risk in diabetes mellitus

blood sugar levels, the risk of hypoglycemia is less [26]. The most serious event that can occur while treating diabetic patients is the development of hypoglycemia (blood sugar below 70 mg/dL). This complication is most often a result of lack of coordination between the use of hypoglycemic medications and food intake. It is the current belief of many physicians who treat diabetes that management with intensive glycemic control will limit, delay or prevent the chronic complications of diabetes. Because of this intensive diabetes treatment, oral surgeons may encounter patients with an increased risk of hypoglycemia which is a true medical emergency requiring prompt recognition and treatment. Insulin and sulfonylureas are the drugs that are responsible for most of the hypoglycemia seen in diabetic subjects.

Except in elderly or chronically ill individuals or in association with prolonged fasting, severe hypoglycemia is unlikely to occur when appropriate doses of oral glucose-lowering agents are used to manage blood glucose. Mild hypoglycemia may occur and can be managed very easily with sugary drinks. Sulfonylureas, which stimulate the pancreas to release more insulin both right after a meal and then over several hours, can cause hypoglycemia. Combination pills may cause hypoglycemia if one of the medications contained in the combination has this effect. (See Table 1.5 for medications which may cause hypoglycemia.)

The dentist should use the medication guide to schedule and management patients. Patients taking medication that can cause severe hypoglycemia should be given morning appointments, take their medication, and be sure to have a good morning meal. Hypoglycemia with metformin, miglitol, pioglitazone, and similar drugs is uncommon and patients taking these medications can be scheduled at any time of day but should be advised to maintain their usual eating regimen.

For patients using short- and/or long-acting insulin therapy, their appointments should be scheduled so they do not coincide with peak insulin activity, which would increase the risk of hypoglycemia. Check the patient's injection times and type of insulin and schedule appropriately. Box 1.6 lists various types of insulin. These patients should take their medication and maintain their eating regimen if being treated under local anesthesia. For patients scheduled for sedation, the dose of insulin should be modified. A widely used regimen is for the patient to take half of the normal dose of insulin preoperatively and the remaining half after surgery when food is consumed. Some oral surgeons doing IV sedation prefer to use normal saline as fluids rather than dextrose 5% in water (D5W); however, for the small amounts of fluids used during IV sedation in oral surgery, D5W should not produce wide fluctuations in blood glucose levels in most patients.

For example, the greatest risk of hypoglycemia would be about 45–90 minutes after injecting lispro insulin, 3–5 hours after glargine and 4–8 hours after NPH.

The risk for head and neck cancer is almost 50% higher in patients with diabetes than in individuals without diabetes. It is recommended that dental patients with diabetes be screened annually for oral cancer [28].

Table 1.5 Oral antiglycemic medications.

Can cause hypoglycemia	Hypoglycemia is rare
Glimepiride (Amaryl®)	Metformin (Glucophage®)
Glyburide (Diabeta®, Micronase®)	Repaglinide (Prandin®)
Glipizide (Glucotrol®, Glucotrol XL®)	Nateglinide (Starlix®)
Micronized glyburide (Glynase®)	Pioglitazone (Actos®)
Combination drugs	Acarbose (Precose®)
Glyburide + metformin (Glucovance®)	Miglitol (Glyset®)
Glipizide + metformin (Metaglip®)	

Thyroid Disease

Thyroid disease is relatively common with an increased prevalence in women and the elderly [29]. Patients who have well-compensated thyroid disease (euthyroid) do not need special consideration prior to oral surgery as long as it can be documented that the patient is on a stable dose of

Box 1.6 Types of insulin and peak activity

- *Short-acting insulins*: aspart, lispro, and glulisine. Onset of action of approximately 15 minutes, *peak at 1–1.5 hours* and last 3–4 hours.
- *Intermediate-acting insulins*: isophane insulin, also known as neutral protamine Hagedorn (NPH). These have an onset of action of 2–4 hours, *peak at 6–7 hours* and last 20 hours.
- *Long-acting insulin analogs*: detemir and glargine. They have an onset of action at 1–3 hours, *peak at 5 hours*, then plateau and last for 20–24 hours. They are used once or twice daily, and achieve a steady state to produce a constant level of insulin.

Source: Information from www.diabetesnet.com/about-diabetes/insulin/insulin-action-time and Slagle M. Medication Update. South Med J. 2002;95.

medication and has been euthyroid for the past 6 months. Monitoring of thyroid function on an annual basis is customarily a part of routine care. Patients who have recently been diagnosed with a thyroid disorder, those who have not seen their endocrinologist in over a year, do not take their medications regularly or with vague history of a thyroid disorder should be seen by their physician before nonurgent oral surgical procedures. Every attempt should be made to get these individuals euthyroid before extensive nonurgent dental treatment. (Methimazole is the preferred drug to quickly reverse hyperthyroidism but it will require an average of 6 weeks to lower T4 levels back to normal) [30]. Table 1.6 outlines the risk of uncontrolled thyroid disease to the surgeon. For emergency situations, pulse, blood pressure, and temperature should be assessed and a decision made based on the clinical picture. Local anesthesia without epinephrine should be used.

Patients with poorly controlled hyperthyroidism, oral surgical procedures or the injection of exogenous epinephrine can precipitate thyroid storm – a potentially life-threatening condition. For patients with hypothyroidism, the risk is less and clinical decisions should be made on the severity of hypothyroidism. Their cardiovascular status should be checked.

Analgesics containing acetylsalicylic acid are contraindicated in patients with hyperthyroidism because acetylsalicylic acid interferes with the protein binding of T4 and T3, thereby increasing their free form. This may worsen the symptoms of thyrotoxicosis [31]. NSAIDs should also be used with caution.

Some medications used to treat thyroid disease may have an effect on surgical treatment. Propylthiouracil (PTU) has antivitamin K activity and can cause hypoprothrombinemia that could pose a risk for hemorrhage. Thus, patients taking PTU must be carefully evaluated before oral surgery [32]. Thionamides can result in oral infections and inadequate wound healing and methimazole, like PTU, can increase the risk of bleeding and can lower white blood cell count, effects which tend to develop rapidly and precipitously, and not gradually. This will increase the risk of infections. Patients should have a CBC done before extensive oral surgery.

Table 1.6 Risks with poorly controlled thyroid disease.

Hypothyroidism	Hyperthyroidism
• Increased bleeding from small vessels in mucosa and skin • Delayed wound healing and susceptibility to infection • Cardiovascular disease from arteriosclerosis and elevated low-density lipoproteins. Poor cardiac output, angina • Exaggerated responses to local anesthetics	• Elevated blood pressure and heart rate • Increased levels of anxiety, and stress or surgery can trigger a thyroid storm • Arrhythmias • Epinephrine is contraindicated

Adrenal Insufficiency

Adrenal insufficiency (AI) is an endocrine disorder caused by the inadequate production of mineralocorticoids and glucocorticoids by the adrenal cortex.

The vast majority of patients with AI that oral surgeons will encounter are on chronic glucocorticoids which can suppress the HPA axis, resulting in the patient not being able to produce sufficient levels of ACTH and cortisol to meet physiologic demands during stressful events. Physiologically, the result is a selective glucocorticoid deficiency. Adrenal crisis with hypotension and shock may occur if these individuals are subjected to physiologic stress from surgery and/or general anesthesia. However, adrenal crisis is rare in dental patients, with only six reports having been published in the past 66 years [33].

In reality, the evidence that adrenal crisis does in fact occur is mainly anecdotal. There are only a few case studies that show confirmed clinical and biochemical evidence of intraoperative AI in patients who did not receive perioperative glucocorticoids after stopping them shortly before surgery [34].

To prevent the potential life-threatening complication of adrenal crisis, it is recommended that supplemental glucocorticoid (steroid prep) be given to those patients with presumed HPA axis suppression. Any patient who has been taking more than 10 mg of prednisone or its equivalent per day for more than 3 weeks, who has received corticosteroids 10 mg daily within the 3 months preceding the current dental encounter, or is on high-dose inhaled corticosteroids (for example, beclometasone 1.5 mg a day) probably has HPA axis suppression and should be considered for supplemental steroid. Most anesthesia and endocrine texts recommend perioperative supplemental glucocorticoids in patients who have had HPA axis suppressive doses of glucocorticoids within 1 year of major surgery [34].

Steroid supplementation for dental procedures is listed in Table 1.7.

Hepatic Disease

Liver disease is important to the dentist due to potential bleeding problems, effects on the metabolism of drugs, and the possibility of being exposed to serious viral infections. The most frequently encountered liver disease in clinical practice is hepatitis, with hepatitis C (HCV) being the most

Table 1.7 Steroid recommendations for dental procedures.

	Routine dentistry LA	Minor oral surgery LA	Minor surgery GA	Major surgery GA
Long-term steroid usage	No supplement	Supplement	Supplement	Supplement
Supplemental action	None	Double the usual dose on the day of surgery	100 mg hydrocortisone intramuscular	100 mg hydrocortisone as a bolus preop and 50 mg q8h for 48 h

GA, general anesthesia; LA, local anesthesia.
No alteration of local anesthetic use is required for patients with adrenal insufficiency. *Source:* Adapted partially from Gibson N, Ferguson JW. Steroid cover for dental patients on long-term steroid medication: proposed clinical guidelines based upon a critical review of the literature. Br. Dent. J. 2004;197:681–685.

problematic. This poses the risk of the dentist contracting HCV and of cross-infection in the office. Other significant risks are bleeding in patients with advanced liver disease and alterations in the metabolism of certain drugs.

For patients with active hepatitis, strict sterilization measures are required. Needles that have been used to penetrate tissues should be covered immediately after use and discarded in special containers. Instruments used in any surgical procedures should be isolated and sterilized after each use. Sterilization should be done with steam under pressure (autoclaving), dry heat, or heat/chemical vapor (gas). Deficient sterilization can expose other patients to hepatitis infection. The dentist and clinical staff should utilize standard universal protective measures and barrier techniques.

The risk of bleeding during oral surgery is related to the severity of the liver disease. Surgery is contraindicated in patients with acute hepatitis, acute liver failure, end-stage liver disease, or alcoholic hepatitis [35]. For patients with stable chronic liver disease, the bleeding during minor oral surgery can generally be controlled with careful, nontraumatic surgical technique, pressure and using hemostatic agents such as oxidized cellulose (Surgicel®), absorbable gelatin (Gelfoam®), or chitosan hemostatic oral wound dressing (HemCon® Dental Dressing). For major oral surgical procedures, international normalized ratio (INR) results should be obtained. Abnormal results should be discussed with a gastroenterologist and surgery preferably performed in a hospital setting.

The liver is responsible for the metabolism and excretion of the majority of drugs introduced into the human body. Liver disease can alter the metabolism of certain drugs to produce an undesirable effect. The common analgesics, antibiotics, and local anesthetics used in dentistry are generally not a problem in patients with mild-to-moderate liver disease. However, modifications will be necessary in patients with advanced liver disease [36].

All drugs prescribed should be selected with reference to possible hepatotoxicity. Local anesthesia is preferred to IV sedation or general anesthetic as anesthetic agents are mostly metabolized in liver and may be poorly tolerated. For pain control, avoid acetaminophen; NSAIDs are the best choice although they affect platelets and may increase bleeding. The dosage of local anesthetics should be reduced. In these cases, initial injection with rapid-onset anesthetics such as lidocaine or mepivacaine followed by injection with a long-acting anesthetic like etidocaine or bupivacaine may be the best protocol for limiting total anesthetic dosage while achieving an adequate duration of pain control [37]. For antibiotic selection see Table 1.8.

Table 1.8 Guidelines for selection of antibiotics in patients with liver disease.

Good	Use with extreme caution or avoid	Avoid
All penicillins and derivatives	Metronidazole	Erythromycin
All cephalosporins		Clindomycin
Tetracycline/doxycyline		Azithromycin
Ciprofloxacin		Amoxicillin/clavulanate
Moxifloxacin		Tetracycline – high dose
		Metronidazole
		Ketoconazole
		Fluconazole

Source: Data from Andrade RJ, Tulkens PM. Hepatic safety of antibiotics used in primary care. J. Antimicrob. Chemother. 2011;66(7):1431–1446.

Renal Disease

Patients with renal disease will be of two types: those with advanced kidney disease who are not on dialysis and those who are on dialysis. Kidney disease usually gets worse slowly over time and symptoms may not appear until the kidneys are badly damaged or no longer functioning. The most frequent causes of chronic renal failure (CRF) are diabetes mellitus (40–60% of all patients with CRF), arterial hypertension (15–30%), and glomerulonephritis (less than 10%) [38].

There is no uniform treatment plan for the patient with kidney disease, and management will depend on the stage of the disease. These patients should be evaluated by a nephrologist and oral surgery provided in consultation with the renal specialist.

Dialyzed Patients

Patients on peritoneal dialysis require no special measures with regard to oral surgery. Patients undergoing hemodialysis will have their blood anticoagulated with heparin to facilitate blood transit through the dialysis machine. To minimize bleeding due to heparinization, oral surgical procedures should be delayed for 4–6 hours after dialysis. To minimize the risk of bleeding and other uremic complications, patients on hemodialysis should preferably have oral surgical procedures on a nondialysis day.

For procedures that will cause bleeding, antibiotic prophylaxis is recommended for the first several months after the placement of synthetic vascular access grafts. The purpose is to avoid bacterial seeding of the grafts before epithelialization occurs [39]. Vancomycin has been routinely used for this purpose, but bacteria have been developing resistance to this drug. Hence, a first-generation cephalosporin in a dosage appropriate for renal function would be a better choice for empiric therapy [39]. The role of antibiotic prophylaxis for invasive dental procedures in patients on long-term dialysis who have a synthetic arteriovenous fistula is unclear. In a review article, 53% of oral surgeons would consider antibiotic prophylaxis if the patient had a synthetic arteriovenous fistula. The recommended regimen is a single dose of 2 g amoxicillin orally or 600 mg clindamycin orally (if patients are allergic to penicillin) 1 hour preoperatively [40].

Drug choices should be selected by the route of primary elimination, with preference given to drugs that have hepatic clearance. Drugs whose elimination will be altered in renal failure should have dose adjustment or modification of the dosing frequency (Table 1.9).

Pulmonary Disease

Asthma

Dental management of asthmatic patients is primarily aimed at prevention of an acute asthma attack in the dental office. Patients with asthmatic symptoms such as coughing and wheezing should not be treated until their symptoms have been relieved. General guidelines for managing the asthmatic patient are listed in Box 1.7 and emergency management of an acute asthmas attack in Box 1.8.

Chronic Obstructive Pulmonary Disease

Chronic obstructive pulmonary disease refers to a group of diseases that cause airflow blockage and breathing-related problems. It includes emphysema, chronic bronchitis, and in some cases asthma. Chronic bronchitis, emphysema or most often combinations of these two conditions are the two most common diseases classified as COPD. Chronic bronchitis results in excessive tracheobronchial mucus

Table 1.9 Drug use in patients with kidney disease (creatinine clearance <50 ml/min or blood creatinine >2.5 mg/dl).

Drugs that require no dose adjustments	Drugs that require dose adjustments	Drugs to avoid
Clindamycin	Amoxicillin (I)	Tetracycline
Doxycycline	Ampicillin (I)	Aspirin
Azithromycin	Amoxicillin/clavulanate (I)	Ibuprofen
Acetaminophen	Metronidazole (I)	Naproxen
Codeine	Aciclovir (I)	
Lidocaine		
Mepivacaine		
Diazepam		
Prednisone		

I, increase dosing interval. *Source:* Data from: Plantinga L, Grubbs V, Sarkar U et al. Nonsteroidal anti-inflammatory drug use among persons with chronic kidney disease in the United States. Ann. Fam. Med. 2011;9:423-430; Cerveró AJ, Bagán JV, Soriano YJ, Roda RP. Dental management in renal failure: patients on dialysis. Med. Oral Patol. Oral Cir. Bucal. 2008;13:419–426; Álamo SL, Esteve CG, Pérez GS. Dental considerations for the patient with renal disease J. Clin. Exp. Dent. 2011;3(2):112–119.

Box 1.7 General guidelines for managing the asthmatic patient

- Ascertain the frequency and severity of acute episodes.
- Determine how the patient routinely manages their asthma and necessity for past emergency care.
- Review the patient's medications. The more medications needed to control the asthma, the more severe the asthma.
- Schedule appointments from late morning to late afternoon.
- At each visit, confirm that they have taken their most recent scheduled dose of asthma medication.
- Have the patient or parent bring the patient's own metered-dose inhaler bronchodilator to each appointment.
- Patients with moderate to severe persistent asthma should be given a prophylactic dose of beta-2 agonist bronchodilator using their own inhaler before being seated in the dental chair.
- Provide a stress-free environment.
- During treatment, use pulse oximeter for patients with moderate-to-severe persistent asthma.
- Local anesthesia with epinephrine is recommended.
- Avoid aspirin, NSAIDs, and narcotics for pain management. The analgesic of choice is acetaminophen.
- Be able to recognize signs of an asthma attack

Box 1.8 Emergency management of an acute asthmatic attack

- Stop the dental procedure and remove dental materials and/or instruments from the patient's mouth.
- Sit the patient upright.
- Administer a bronchodilator supplied by the patient or from the office emergency kit.
- If there is no improvement, the bronchodilator can be repeated two more times.
- If after three doses of the bronchodilator there is no improvement, take additional measures.
  - *Administer oxygen*: it is very important to keep a satisfactory oxygen saturation level until the patient is free of wheezing or until EMS arrives to transport the patient to an emergency room.
  - *Call for medical assistance*: document the episode in detail and report to the child's primary care physician or to the emergency room physician.
  - *Administer epinephrine* 1:1000 concentration for an adult, 1:2000 concentration for a child.
- If the attack is resolved quickly, the patient may be discharged on their own.
- If the administration of epinephrine was necessary, the patient should be discharged to EMS for transport to the hospital.

Source: Modified and adopted from: Schwartz S. Management of Pediatric Medical Emergencies in the Dental Office: Acute Asthmatic Attack. www.dentalcare.com/en-us/professional-education/ce-courses/ce391/acute-asthmatic-attack; Zhu JF, Hidalgo HA, Holmgreen C et al. Dental management of children with asthma. Pediatric Dentistry 1996;18(5):363–370.

production with symptoms ranging from chronic cough and sputum production, severe disabling shortness of breath and cyanosis – the so-called "blue bloater." Emphysema refers to distention of the air spaces distal to the terminal bronchioles due to erosion of the lining between air sacs. This leads to large air pockets in the lungs, which trap air rather than allowing the absorption of oxygen before exhalation. The most frequent symptom of emphysema is shortness of breath. Patients are barrel chested with pursing of lips upon exhalation.

Patients with COPD need special attention during surgical care to avoid procedures that can limit breathing to avoid further respiratory depression, including the use of adequate pain control and shortened visits. Patients who are under good medical management and have no recent history of lung infections, severe shortness of breath at rest, arrhythmia or CHF may have any indicated oral surgery. Local anesthesia with epinephrine is acceptable, if there is no concomitant cardiac disease. Patients with mild-to-moderate COPD can undergo conscious sedation with midazolam and propofol.

General guidelines for managing the patient with COPD are listed in Box 1.9.

Pregnancy

Pregnancy produces many changes in the physiology of the cardiovascular, respiratory, hematologic, endocrine, genitourinary, gastrointestinal and orofacial systems of the female patient. All elective dental/oral surgical procedures should be postponed until post partum as treatment of the pregnant patient can seriously affect the lives of the mother and unborn fetus.

Box 1.9 Guidelines for management of patients with COPD

- Avoid treatment if upper respiratory infection is present: common cold, sinusitis, laryngitis, bronchitis, epiglottitis
- Schedule short appointments (20 minutes)
- Use upright chair position
- Use stress reduction techniques
- Do not obstruct breathing
- Use pulse oximeter
- Do not use nitrous oxide-oxygen sedation in cases of severe emphysema
- Avoid narcotics
- Outpatient general anesthesia contraindicated. Sedation with low-dose midazolam or propofol [41, 42] is acceptable but avoid barbiturates and narcotics

Box 1.10 General guidelines for managing the gravid patient

- For pregnant women with hyperemesis, morning appointments should be avoided.
- Short dental appointments should be scheduled during the third trimester.
- Check the blood pressure at each visit. If the blood pressure is elevated, the patient should be referred to her obstetrician to be evaluated for possible development of preeclampsia.
- In the second and third trimesters, ask the patient to empty her bladder just prior to starting the dental procedure.
- During dental procedures, the pregnant patient should be seated in a semi-supine or otherwise comfortable position. The right hip should be elevated 4–5 in. or place the patient in a 5–15% tilt on her left side to relieve pressure on the inferior vena cava [45].
- If the patient becomes nauseous, stop the procedure immediately and reposition the chair upright.

During dental treatment, the supine position of the pregnant female in the dental chair should be avoided for a variety of reasons.

- To avoid the possible development of the "supine hypotensive syndrome of pregnancy." Approximately 8–10% of women in the second and third trimesters of pregnancy [43] when placed in the supine position may manifest symptoms of pallor, sweating, dizziness, nausea, hypotension, and tachycardia. The supine hypotensive syndrome is caused by the gravid uterus compressing the inferior vena cava when a pregnant woman is in a supine position, leading to decreased venous return centrally [43]. There will be a decrease in cardiac output resulting in hypotension, syncope, and decreased uteroplacental perfusion which could be damaging to the fetus. If a woman develops symptoms, she should be turned on her left side which should rapidly resolve the symptoms.
- To avoid the potential decrease in arterial oxygen tension (PaO_2).
- To minimize the risk of dyspepsia from gastroesophageal reflux secondary to an incompetent lower esophageal sphincter. Reflux occurs as a result of increased intragastric pressure due to the enlarging fetus.
- To decrease the risk of developing deep vein thrombosis, due to compression of the inferior vena cava, leading to venous stasis and clot formation [44].

General guidelines for managing the pregnant female are listed in Box 1.10.

A radiation dose of 10 Gy (5 Gy in the first trimester, when organogenesis is initiated) causes congenital fetal

Table 1.10 Common drugs used in dentistry.

Drugs that are safe to be used	Drugs to avoid or use with caution	Drugs to be avoided
Amoxicillin	Oxycodone	Tetracycline
Penicillin	Hydrocodon	Aspirin[a]
Clindamycin	Mepivacaine[b]	Ibuprofen[a]
Metronidazole	Bupivacaine[b]	Naproxen[a]
Cephalosporin		Nitrous oxide[c]
Nystatin		
Acetaminophen		
Lidocaine		

[a] Avoid in third trimester.
[b] Fetal bradycardia.
[c] Associated with spontaneous abortions.

abnormalities. It has been estimated that the dose to the fetus is approximately 1/50 000 of that to the mother's head in any exposure ranging from full-mouth X-ray to CT images of head and neck. The exposure of any radiographic films required for management of the pregnant patient in most situations should not place the fetus at increased risk. Adequate shielding and protective equipment must be used at all times [44].

Medications should be prescribed by the dentist that will minimize adverse outcomes. Table 1.10 lists the risks of drugs commonly prescribed in dentistry.

Conclusion

Oral and maxillofacial surgeons are hospital trained and qualified to manage patients with coexisting medical problems. As the years go by, however, and practice becomes totally office based, some of the medical training may fade. This chapter has reviewed the management of the more frequently encountered medical problems seen in the office setting. The diseases discussed should also serve as a reservoir for people in training and for nonoral and maxillofacial surgeons.

References

1 Petranker, S., Nikoyan, L., and Ogle, O.E. (2012). Preoperative evaluation of the surgical patient. *Dent. Clin. North Am.* 56 (1): 163–181.
2 Ogle, O. (2015). Pretreatment evaluation of the dental patient. In: *Medical Emergencies in Dental Practice* (ed. O. Ogle, H. Dym and R. Weinstock), 1–8. Hanover Park, IL: Quintessence Publishing Company.
3 Department of Health and Human Services. (2015) A Profile of Older Americans. https://acl.gov/sites/default/files/Aging%20and%20Disability%20in%20America/2015-Profile.pdf
4 Chobanian, A.V., Bakris, G.L., Black, H.R. et al. (2003). The seventh report of the joint national committee on prevention, detection, evaluation, and treatment of high blood pressure: the JNC 7 report. *JAMA* 289: 2560–2571.
5 Weinstock, R. (2015). Hypertension and hypotensin. In: *Medical Emergencies in Dental Practice* (ed. O. Ogle, H. Dym and R. Weinstock), 112–118. Hanover Park, IL: Quintessence Publishing Company.
6 Cioffi, G.A., Chernow, B., Glahn, R.P. et al. (1985). The hemodynamic and plasma catecholamine responses to routine restorative dental care. *J. Am. Dent. Assoc.* 111: 67–70.
7 Tolas, A.G., Pflug, A.E., and Halter, J.B. (1982). Arterial plasma epinephrine concentrations and emodynamic responses after dental injection of local anesthetic with epinephrine. *J. Am. Dent. Assoc.* 104: 41–43.
8 Malamed, S.F. (1997). *Handbook of Local Anesthesia*, 4e. St Louis, MO: Mosby-Year Book.
9 Horn JR, Hansten PD. The dangers of beta-blockers and epinephrine. 2009. www.pharmacytimes.com/publications/issue/2009/2009-05/druginteractionsbetablockers-0509
10 Pallasch, T.J. (1998). Vasoconstrictors and the heart. *J. Calif. Dent. Assoc.* 26: 668–676.
11 Working Conference of ADA and AHA (1964). Management of dental problems in patients with cardiovascular disease. *J. Am. Dent. Assoc.* 68: 333–342.
12 Perloff, D., Grim, C., Flack, J. et al. (1993). Human blood pressure: determination by sphygmomanometry. *Circulation* 88 (5(Part 1)): 2460–2470.
13 Waters, B.G. (1995). Providing dental treatment for patients with cardiovascular disease. *Ont. Dent.* 72 (6): 24–32.
14 Nitrostat. Product Information. Parke-Davis Div of Pfizer Inc.
15 Zafari AM and Abdou MH. Myocardial infarction https://emedicine.medscape.com/article/155919-overview
16 Jørgensen, M.E., Torp-Pedersen, C., Gislason, G.H. et al. (2014). Time elapsed after ischemic stroke and risk of adverse cardiovascular events and mortality following elective noncardiac surgery. *JAMA* 312 (3): 269–277.
17 Anderson P. Wait on elective surgery after stroke. www.medscape.com/viewarticle/828447
18 Mozzafarian, D., Benjamin, E.J., Go, A.S. et al. (2016). on behalf of the American Heart Association Statistics Committee and Stroke Statistics Subcommittee. Heart disease and stroke statistics – 2016 update: a report from the American Heart Association. *Circulation* 133 (4): e38–e360.
19 McIntosh J. Everything you need to know about stroke. www.medicalnewstoday.com/articles/7624.php
20 Muzyka, B.C. (1999). Atrial fibrillation and its relationship to dental care. *J. Am. Dent. Assoc.* 130 (7): 1080–1085.
21 (2002). Academy Report. Periodontal management of patients with cardiovascular diseases. *J. Periodontol.* 73 (8): 954–968.
22 Criteria Committee of the New York Heart Association (1994). *Nomenclature and Criteria for Diagnosis of*

Diseases of the Heart and Great Vessels, 9e, 253–256. Boston, MA: Little, Brown.

23 Little, J.W., Falace, D., Miller, C., and Rhodus, N.L. (ed.) (2013). Heart failure. In: *Dental Management of the Medically Compromised Patient*, 8e, 90. Philadelphia, PA: Elsevier.

24 Centers for Disease Control and Prevention (2014). *National Diabetes Statistics Report: Estimates of Diabetes and Its Burden in the United States, 2014*. Atlanta, GA: US Department of Health and Human Services.

25 American Diabetes Association. Statistics about diabetes. www.diabetes.org/diabetes-basics/statistics

26 Lalla, R.V. and D'Ambrosio, J.A. (2001). Dental management considerations for the patient with diabetes mellitus. *J. Am. Dent. Assoc.* 132 (10): 1425–1432.

27 Burgess J and Meyers AD. Dental management in the medically compromised patient. : http://emedicine.medscape.com/article/2066164-overview#a2

28 Tseng, K.S., Lin, C., Lin, Y.S., and Weng, S.F. (2014). Risk of head and neck cancer in patients with diabetes mellitus: a retrospective cohort study in Taiwan. *JAMA Otolaryngol. Head Neck Surg.* 140 (8): 746–753.

29 Canaris, G.J., Manowitz, N.R., Mayor, G., and Ridgway, E.C. (2000). The Colorado thyroid disease prevalence study. *Arch. Intern. Med.* 160 (4): 526–534.

30 Ross DS. Antithyroid drugs (beyond the basics). www.uptodate.com/contents/antithyroid-drugs-beyond-the-basics

31 Huber, M.A. and Terezhalmy, G.T. (2008). Risk stratification and dental management of the patient with thyroid dysfunction. *Quintessence Int.* 39 (2): 139–150.

32 Pinto, A. and Glick, M. (2002). Management of patients with the thyroid disease: oral health considerations. *J. Am. Dent. Assoc.* 133 (7): 849–858.

33 Khalaf, M.W., Khader, R., Cobetto, G. et al. (2013). Risk of adrenal crisis in dental patients. *J. Am. Dent. Assoc.* 144 (2): 152–160.

34 Schiff, R.L. and Welsh, G.A. (2003). Perioperative evaluation and management of the patient with endocrine dysfunction. *Med. Clin. North Am.* 87 (1): 175–192.

35 Friedman, L.S. (2010). Surgery in the patient with liver disease. *Trans. Am. Clin. Climatol. Assoc.* 121: 192–204.

36 Demas, P.N. and McClain, J.R. (1999). Hepatitis: implications for dental care. *Oral Surg. Oral Med. Oral Pathol. Oral Radiol. Endod.* 88 (1): 2–4.

37 Budenz, A.W. (2000). Local anesthetics and medically complex patients. *J. Calif. Dent. Assoc.* 28 (8): 611–619.

38 Snyder, S. and Pendergraph, B. (2005). Detection and evaluation of chronic kidney disease. *Am. Fam. Physician* 72 (9): 1723–1732.

39 Krishnan, M. (2002). Preoperative care of patients with kidney disease. *Am. Fam. Physician* 66 (8): 1471–1477.

40 Tong, D.C. and Walker, R.J. (2004). Antibiotic prophylaxis in dialysis patients undergoing invasive dental treatment. *Nephrology* 9 (3): 167–170.

41 Stolz, D., Grendelmeier, P., Jahn, K., and Tamm, M. (2014). Propofol sedation for flexible bronchoscopy in patients with and without chronic obstructive pulmonary disease. *Eur. Respir. J.* 43 (2): 591–560.

42 Conti, G., Dell'Utri, D., Vilardi, V. et al. (1993). Propofol induces bronchodilation in mechanically ventilated chronic obstructive pulmonary disease (COPD) patients. *Acta Anaesthesiol. Scand.* 37 (1): 105–109.

43 Lanni, S.M., Tillinghast, J., and Silver, H.M. (2002). Hemodynamic changes and baroreflex gain in the supine hypotensive syndrome. *Am. J. Obstet. Gynecol.* 187 (6): 1636–1641.

44 Kurien, S., Kattimani, V.S., Sriram, R.R. et al. (2013). Management of pregnant patient in dentistry. *J. Int. Oral Health* 5 (1): 88–97.

45 Duvekot, J.J. and Peeters, L.L. (1994). Maternal cardiovascular hemodynamic adaptation to pregnancy. *Obstet. Gynecol. Surv.* 49 (Suppl): S1–S14.

2

Risk Reduction Strategies

Harry Dym

Medical malpractice has unfortunately been a part of a practitioner's clinical experience for hundreds of years, with the first reported case in the United States occurring in 1700 in the State of Connecticut [1]. Clinicians must be aware of the real concerns of a possible malpractice claim as it will most likely affect every practitioner in the course of his/her clinical life time. Poor or unexpected outcomes following surgical procedures are not at all unusual or rare and can occur even if perfect technique is executed. Poor outcome is itself not an indication of any failure to follow the standard of care; nevertheless, an outcome less than perfect can sometimes result in a malpractice suit. A clinician can focus on certain risk reduction strategies to help mitigate the chances of a lawsuit ever being initiated and if one is brought to trial, to help his/her chances to achieve a favorable jury decision.

Methods of Risk Reduction

Malpractice claims often revolve around three areas of practice: poor communications/rapport, lack of informed consent, and faulty record keeping. It is the patient's perception of the quality of care received that is the most critical factor in their initiating and possibly winning a malpractice lawsuit.

The patient's perception of the doctor often begins with their initial phone call to the office. A friendly, helpful, and courteous voice on the other end of the line can set the tone for the patient's overall perception. The staff must be trained to help put patients at ease and respond to questions in a polite manner. The practitioner should make every effort to gain a patient's trust. This is often hard to do if the patient is only coming for one or two visits, but it can be accomplished if the clinician establishes good communication with the patient. Techniques for improving patient communication can be learned (Box 2.1) and will enhance the patient–doctor relationship if put into practice. Communication breakdown which can precipitate a lawsuit can occur if the doctor:

- fails to return patient calls relating to postclinical procedures
- ignores questions or concerns
- fails to explain or if staff fail to explain and answer patient questions regarding procedures and follow-up protocols.

Faulty Record Keeping

Patient records are not only vital to good patient care but a requirement of most state dental boards as well. Although what is legally required to be contained in the dental record is fairly basic (Box 2.2), it may be best for the doctor if he/she can be more expansive as lawsuits take years to develop and memories fade, and the medical record may become the critical basis for a solid defense in the face of a potential lawsuit.

Informed Consent

Prior to any oral surgical procedures, the patient must be informed of the planned procedure and possible results of poor outcomes. This protocol has been established for well over 100 years, dating back to a landmark 1914 court case – Schloendorff vs Society of New York Hospitals. The court ruled that "Every human being of adult years and sound mind has a right to determine what shall be done with his or her own body ... and a surgeon who operates

Oral and Maxillofacial Surgery, Medicine, and Pathology for the Clinician, First Edition. Edited by Harry Dym, Leslie R. Halpern, and Orrett E. Ogle.

Box 2.1 Improving interaction and communications with patients during examinations/consultations and after hours

Once the examination or consultation begins, the dentist or oral surgeon should keep in mind these suggestions for more successful communication.

- Greet the patient by name and use the patient's name during the conversation.
- Sit down so that you are at eye level with the patient and maintain eye contact.
- Scan the problem list for what you perceive as the most important problem and let the patient know that you will address that one first because you want to make sure it is discussed before you run out of time.
- It is always a good idea to call the patient following complex office surgical procedure (24–48 hours).
- If the patient does develop postoperative complications, it is a good idea to see that patient or to stay in touch frequently.
- You may need to ask the patient to make another appointment if time does not allow an evaluation of all the problems on the patient's list, which indicates that even though all problems may not be addressed at this visit, they will not be dismissed.
- Once the patient begins to discuss his/her problems, practice listening for at least 2–3minutes before you say anything. Show that you are listening by leaning forward and reacting to the patient's body language.
- If you need to turn away from a patient who is in the chair or you have to leave the room, explain where you are going and when you will return. Do not just leave the room.
- Try to become acquainted with the patient on a personal level, asking questions about their work or hobbies during the initial visit. Keep a sheet with this information on the inside cover of the chart or in another easily accessible section and glance at it before meeting with the patient. Discussing personal details while addressing the patient's problems indicates your interest in the whole person.
- Facilitate patient interaction and information exchange by using probing, open-ended questions, such as "What do you think caused this problem to happen?"
- Give the patient your after-hours contact number, especially following surgery.
- Assure the patient that the office is always available and ready to deal with postprocedure complications.

Box 2.2 Essentials of good record keeping

- Required patient information
- Completed and signed patient medical history form
- Radiographs (label and dated)
- Patient name, address, telephone number, date of birth, and age
- Physician's name and telephone number, if applicable
- Emergency contact information

Patient visit note

- Date of each entry
- Note of review of medical and allergic history (initial encounter)
- Drugs administered to patient
- Prescription given to patient
- Referrals made and referrals or instructions not followed
- Telephone conversation with patient and physician
- Cancelation/new appointment
- Laboratory tests ordered
- Results of laboratory tests or consultant's report
- Type of implant used
- Cases have been lost due to poor legibility of records so try to write clearly
- Always remember that your chart can be your friend or your worst enemy even though your records truly do not reflect the quality of care given

without the patient's consent commits an assault for which he/she is liable for damage." Though most oral surgeons have a preprinted consent form listing many of the possible postsurgical complications, in many communities dentists and some oral surgeons may only take a verbal consent. If a written consent is not obtained, it would be beneficial if the consent discussion held with the patient was referenced in the body of the patient records.

Conclusion

Practitioners may practice outstanding oral surgery with strict attention to detail but still have a poor outcome. The decision on a medical malpractice suit will often be made on the basis of the patient's or the jury's perception of what they feel is or is not a deviation from the standard of care. Risk reduction strategies should be part of every clinician's clinical practice.

Reference

1 Dym, H. and Ogle, E. (2009). *Handbook of Dental Practice*. Philadelphia, PA: Saunders.

3

Preparing the Dental Office for Medical Emergencies: Essentials of an Emergency Kit

Harry Dym and Yijiao Fan

Dentistry is thought of as a rather benign field of practice. Most morbidities that can happen to a dental patient are functional or cosmetic issues that can be improved or reversed completely with additional dental procedures. However, serious and medical emergencies can and do happen in the dental office. This is compounded by advances in medicine, patients having longer lifespans, and patients taking multiple medications for chronic health issues [1, 2]. When a medical emergency happens to a dental patient, there can be serious and irreversible consequences, especially if the response to the emergency is inappropriate.

Although 90% of dentists have encountered at least one medical emergency in a 10-year period [1], many dental offices, especially those in private practice, are lacking in the necessary preparation for a medical emergency. Failure to respond appropriately when a medical emergency occurs in the dental office can lead to patient morbidity and mortality, as well as legal and financial responsibilities detrimental to the dental office and the dentist. The American Dental Association's position is that all dentists should have an emergency drug kit, equipment, and knowledge to properly use all items [3]. Therefore, it is imperative that the dental office is prepared for the common and serious medical emergencies that can occur.

Just about any medical emergency can occur, but certain medical emergencies the dental office must be well rehearsed because they are common and/or pose greater threat to life. The most common medical emergencies in order of prevalence are altered consciousness, cardiovascular events, allergy, respiratory events, seizures, and diabetes-related events [1]. The ability to respond to myriad situations naturally varies from practice to practice but a minimum level of preparedness is expected of any dental office treating patients. This includes having the appropriate equipment, rescue/reversal drugs, and staff who are trained to implement your medical emergency plan.

Staff

Everyone in the dental office team is expected to be able to contribute to the response effort in a medical emergency [4]. The core of the emergency plan is having the dental office team certified and prepared to provide basic life support (BLS) and to able to seek emergency medical services in an efficient and timely manner. The dentist should be the head of the team, but other members of the staff should also have distinct responsibilities. The dentist should be able to diagnose and treat common emergent problems. The front office staff should have emergency telephone numbers on hand. In an unconscious patient, definitive treatment of the underlying etiology must wait until the patient is stabilized.

Everyone in the office should be familiar with the basic rescue algorithms to maintain compressions, protect the airway, and give rescue breaths (CAB). Continuing education courses or advanced rescue courses can be used to supplement BLS. Establishing a code and having regular mock drills help to keep the office coordinated and ready to respond. Drugs and emergency equipment are necessary but having the personnel with the knowledge to use them is a prerequisite (Box 3.1) [1, 2, 4].

Oral and Maxillofacial Surgery, Medicine, and Pathology for the Clinician, First Edition. Edited by Harry Dym, Leslie R. Halpern, and Orrett E. Ogle.

Box 3.1 Emergency Preparedness Checklist

- Staff have assigned duties
- Contingency plan if a staff member is absent or unavailable
- Regular training and BLS recertification
- Mock drills
- Emergency phone numbers current and readily accessible
- Emergency equipment appropriately stocked and accessible
- Oxygen tanks and delivery systems checked regularly
- Emergency equipment and drugs checked for stock regularly and after each use

Equipment

Oxygen

Oxygen is of the utmost importance in emergency preparedness [1, 2, 4]. The basic tenant of life support is maintaining oxygen delivery to vital systems and organs. Oxygen is indicated when a patient is breathing on their own but not well or if not breathing. A portable E cylinder (660 L at 1900 psi) (Figure 3.1) is recommended as the office oxygen source. It should be easily accessible and transportable. It should be regularly checked to see that it is adequately full. Supplemental oxygen delivery can be done with nasal cannula, masks, or nasal hoods. An Ambu-bag (a proprietary name for a bag-valve-mask device, abbreviated as BVM) is good to provide positive pressure manually, but a variety of sources can provide dependable oxygenation in emergencies.

Airway Adjuncts

When the patient fails to maintain airway on their own, oropharyngeal airways (Figure 3.1a) are needed. For adults, size 7–9 cm airways should be stocked [1, 4]. Nasopharyngeal airways should be available for cases when an oropharyngeal airway cannot be established. Magill forceps are (Figure 3.1b) useful in retrieving foreign bodies from the oropharynx. Laryngoscopes and endotracheal tubes are necessary for those providers who offer in-office sedation procedures in case there is a respiratory arrest event requiring intubation.

Automated External Defibrillators (Figure 3.2)

Automated external defibrillators (AEDs) adhering to AHA guidelines are an integral part of the BLS and advanced cardiovascular life support (ACLS) chain of survival when the heart needs to be shocked [4]. AEDs are mandated in many states. They are used to restore the heart to a normal rhythm in lethal situations such as ventricular fibrillation [4].

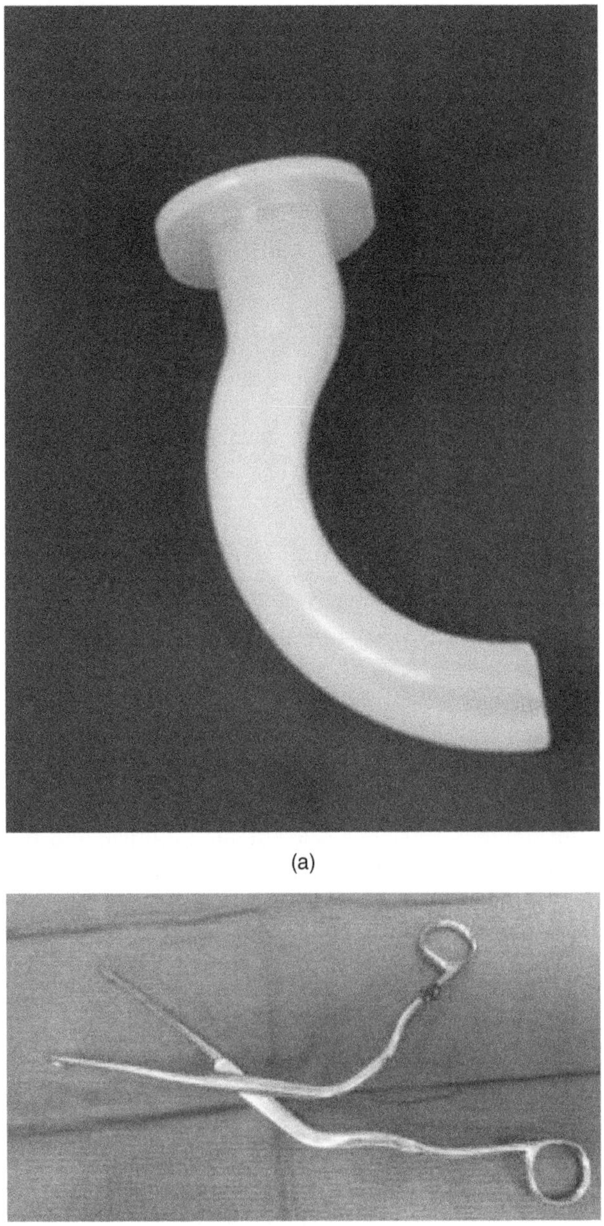

(a)

(b)

Figure 3.1 (a, b) Oropharyngeal airway and Magill forceps.

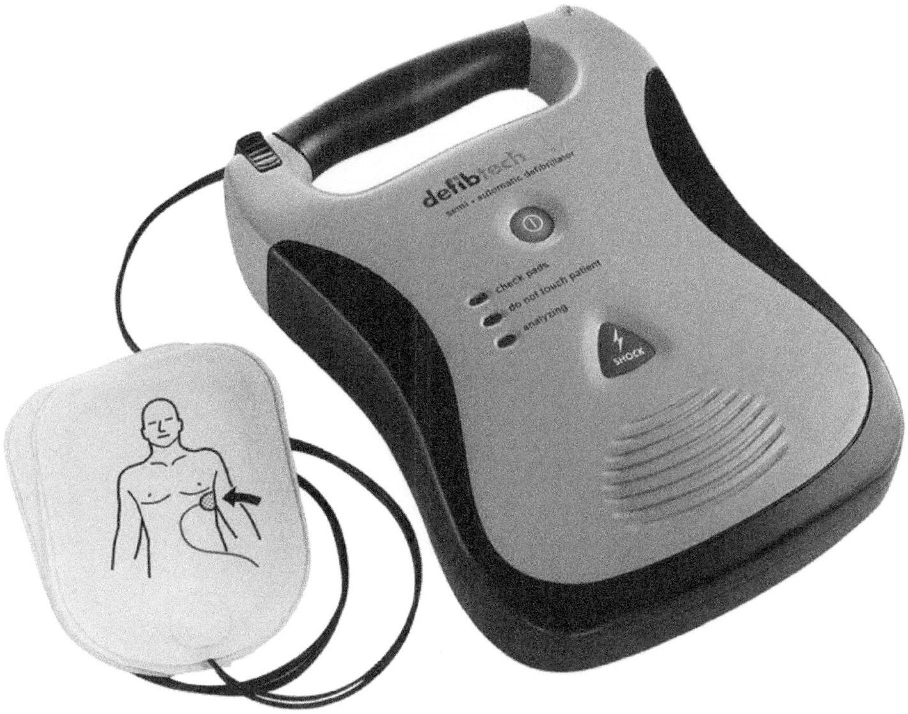

Figure 3.2 Automated external defibrillator (Defibtech LLC).

Vitals Monitoring

Automated vitals monitors are useful in constant monitoring of all the patient's basic vital signs, including blood pressure, pulse rate, oxygen saturation, temperature, and, if needed, ECG tracings. Manual monitoring devices including stethoscope and sphygomomanometer with adult and child cuffs should also be available to supplement or confirm automated monitors.

Intravenous Kits

Fluids and medications are extremely useful in medical emergencies. IV fluids should be given when the patient is in hypotension. IV kits should have tourniquets, alcohol gauze, syringes, angiocatheters, and fluids (normal saline or D5 half normal saline), and personnel should know when to start an IV (Figure 3.3).

Emergency Drug Kit

Every dental office should have a basic emergency drug kit whether the office does in-house IV sedations or not. Those offices that administer sedation anesthesia should have additional rescue medications related to sedation medications. Emergency drugs should be checked regularly for stock and expiry dates. Emergency drugs can be noninjectable or administered via subcutaneous, intramuscular, sublingual, intraosseous, or intravenous routes.

Oxygen

As mentioned earlier, oxygen and respiratory support is of the utmost importance in medical emergencies. Hypoxemia can develop from acute disturbances involving the cardiovascular, respiratory, and nervous systems. The end goal of providing enriched oxygen is to deliver oxygen to hypoxic tissues. Enriched oxygen can be given via a variety of routes such as nasal cannulas and Ambu-bags. A variety of delivery systems will help to ensure effective oxygen delivery depending on the specific rescuer and patient [1, 2, 4].

Aromatic Ammonia

This is a medicine used to treat or prevent fainting. Syncope is the most common presentation of a medical emergency in the dental office. The drug is crushed and inhaled. It works by stimulating the body's respiratory center to increase ventilation. When coupled with supplemental oxygen, aromatic ammonia can bring many patients back to consciousness. The drug should be kept at room temperature and away from heat as it is flammable [1].

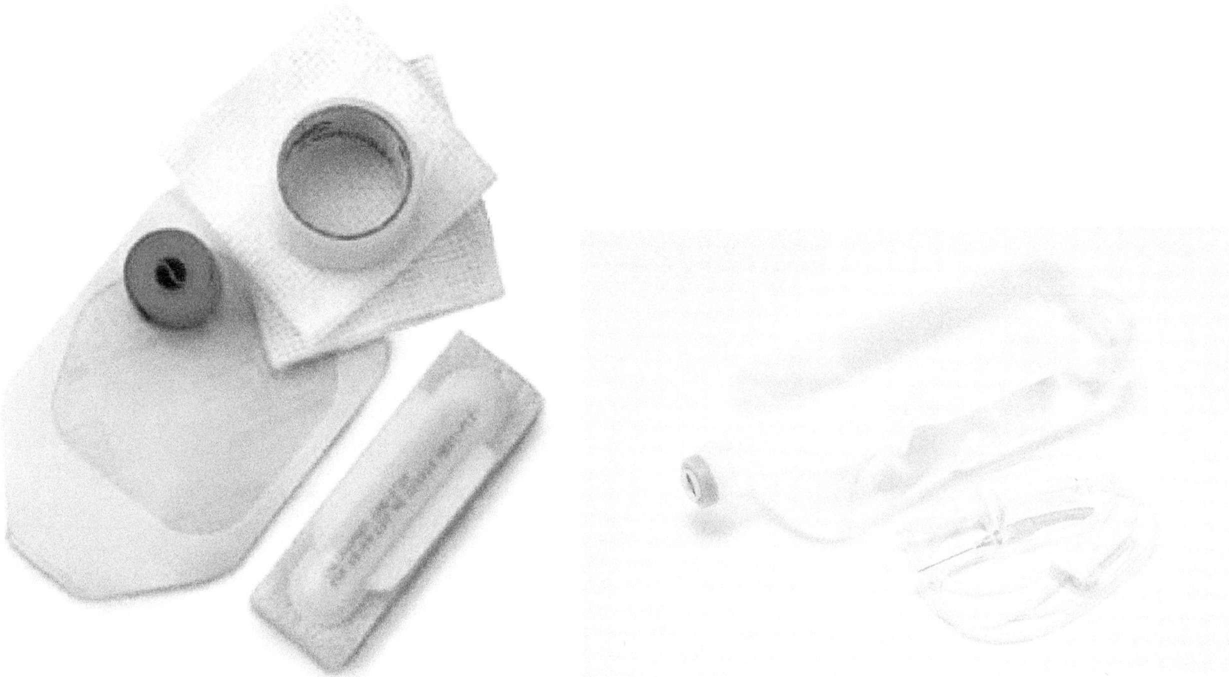

Figure 3.3 D5 1/2NS IV fluid with tourniquets, alcohol gauze, syringes, and angiocatheters.

Aspirin

In a patient experiencing chest pain, radiating pain to jaw and shoulder, suspected of having a heart attack or ischemic event, aspirin is the treatment of choice. Aspirin is antiplatelet, or anticlotting, and prevents progression to full-scale heart attack by keeping the vessels feeding the heart muscles patent. Chewed aspirin has been shown to work the fastest, taking approximately 5 minutes to reduce thromboxane B2, a marker of platelet aggregation, concentration in the blood by 50%. A standard 325 mg dose should be used in rescue first aid [1].

Albuterol

Asthma is common in the dental chair. The aerosols and stress of being in the dental chair can provoke an asthma attack in an otherwise controlled patient. Albuterol is a quick-acting selective B2 agonist that promotes bronchial smooth muscle relaxation, thus increasing airway diameter to promote breathing. Asthmatic patients should bring their own inhaler with them before any dental work is initiated, but the dental office should also keep an emergency inhaler on hand in case the patient's own is not available or functional [1].

Glucose

There is a myth that patients should not eat prior to going to the dentist. The dental office sees many hypoglycemic patients who can present with altered mental status and fainting. Routine blood glucose testing in diabetic patients is useful but sometimes patients still have hypoglycemic events in the dental chair. The conscious patient should receive fast-absorbing oral glucose such as glucose paste or juice. The unconscious patient can receive glucose by IM glucagon injections or IV infusion of D5W (dextrose 5% in water) fluids. The unconscious patient should not receive glucose by mouth due to risk of aspiration [1, 4].

Nitroglycerin

In cases of angina, especially in patients with a history of cardiovascular disease, nitroglycerin can be administered for rapid chest pain relief and can potentially prevent a mycardial infarction. It is a potent vasodilator and smooth muscle relaxant that increases coronary perfusion and decreases systemic vascular resistance. Nitroglycerin is administered as 0.4 mg aerosol or sublingual tablet. The aerosol form has a longer shelf-life. The dentist can repeat the dose every 5 minutes up to a total of three doses. If symptoms are refractory to treatment, consider that the patient may be having a myocardial infarction. Side-effects are related to its vasodilatory effects and include headache, dizziness, and flushing. Therefore nitroglycerin is contraindicated in patients with hypotension [1].

Diphenhydramine

For mild allergic reactions, diphenhydramine is a good choice in both oral and parenteral forms. It is an antagonist of histamine receptors and is readily available under the trade name Benadryl® [1].

Epinephrine

For severe allergic reactions, including anaphylaxis, epinephrine is the drug of choice. It is an endogenous catecholamine alpha- and beta-adrenergic receptor stimulator and acts to increase the patient's blood pressure to maintain perfusion of vital organs. It is administered immediately after recognition of the acute allergic event subcutaneously 0.3–0.5 mg in 1:1000 solution or intramuscularly 0.4–0.6 mg in 1:1000 solution for more serious events. Epinephrine is available as preloaded syringes known as EpiPens®. Epinephrine is also administered in severe asthma attacks by the same mechanism [1, 3, 4].

Sedation-Specific Emergencies

Dentists with advanced training may offer intravenous sedation in their offices. The knowledge and expertise required to safely sedate and monitor these patients are beyond the scope of this chapter.

The IV sedation drug kit can include medicine for analgesia, anticholinergics, anticonvulsants, antihypertensives, antihypoglycemics, corticosteroids, vasopressors, etc. Naloxone and flumazenil must be available for reversal of opioid- and benzodiazepine-related airway depression and sedation. Dantrolene should be stocked for treatment of muscle spasms and malignant hyperthermia. Advanced airway management and ACLS should also be part of the sedation provider's repertoire. Simply having the rescue medications in stock does not substitute for the advanced training these providers must undertake in order to safely provide sedation anesthesia [1, 4].

Summary

Medical emergencies can and do happen in the dental office. Providers and office staff need to be keenly aware of how to recognize and manage medical emergencies. A prepared staff as well as an arsenal of appropriate medical emergency drugs and equipment is the best way to be ready in case a medical emergency occurs.

References

1 Dym, H. (2001). Stocking the oral surgery office emergency cart. *Oral Maxillofac. Surg. Clin. North Am.* 13: 103–118.
2 Dym, H. (2008). Preparing the dental office for medical emergencies. *Dent. Clin. North Am.* 52: 605–608.
3 Roberson, J.B. (2012). Emergency drug kit. www.dentistrytoday.com/news/todays-dental-news/ item/2816-dental-offi ces-need-medical-emergencypreparedness-standards
4 Rosenberg, M. (2010). Preparing for medical emergencies. *J. Am. Dent. Assoc.* 141: 14–19.

Part II

Dentoalveolar Surgery

4

Surgical Management of the Impacted Canine

Harry Dym and Yijiao Fan

The impacted permanent canine tooth is a frequently encountered phenomenon in dental settings, second only to the third molar. The incidence of impacted maxillary canine is estimated to be 1–3.5% [1–4]. Impacted mandibular canines occur less frequently at an estimated rate of 0.3% [3]. As such, the majority of literature and clinical focus is on maxillary impacted canines. This chapter will also focus on maxillary canines unless explicitly stated otherwise. There is a 2:1–3:1 female predilection over males in both maxillary and mandibular canine impactions [1–3].

An impacted canine is defined as one that cannot erupt into its final position in the dental arches. Unlike impacted third molars, impacted canines can cause prominent deficits in occlusion, functional excursive movements, and esthetics (Figure 4.1). Cysts, adenomatoid odontogenic tumor, and other pathology can develop in association with the impacted canine (Figure 4.2) [3]. Partially erupted canines can be a nidus for recurrent infections. In addition, impacted canines can adversely affect the adjacent dentition, contributing to malposition, periodontal compromise, and/or resorption of adjacent teeth. Orthodontic challenges often arise because of loss of arch space.

When an impacted permanent canine tooth is present, there should be an interdisciplinary management that involves the oral and maxillofacial surgeon, the orthodontist, and the general or pediatric dentist. The latter are often the first or only providers a patient sees, and are responsible for timely and appropriate referral when an impaction is suspected. The diagnostic and treatment planning work is usually assumed by the orthodontist. The surgeon is finally consulted for surgical planning and treatment. If there is a lack of coordination between members of the interdisciplinary team, inappropriate treatment can be requested or performed, which can cause delays or irreversible consequences. Therefore, appropriate dialog between providers is of paramount importance in managing patients who present with impacted permanent canines.

Etiology

The exact etiology of why impactions of permanent canines occur is speculative. Two schools of thought exist: impactions occur either by gene mediation or local factors affecting the guided migration/eruption of the canine. Although no locus of significance has been identified, proponents of the gene mediation theory argue for a genetically driven mechanism for impaction due to increased coincidence with other dental anomalies, increased familial occurrence, and differences in gender and population. Proponents of the local factor theory, such as Bishara [5], proposed multiple factors that could influence canine impaction: tooth size arch length discrepancy, prolonged retention or early loss of the primary canine, abnormal tooth bud position, presence of clefts, ankylosis, cystic or neoplastic formations, dilacerations of roots, iatrogenic causes or trauma, and idiopathic factors. Labially impacted canines in particular have been correlated with loss of arch length such as in the case of early loss of the primary canine. No such relationship exists for palatally impacted canines, which account for 40–85% of maxillary canine impactions [3]. In reality, there is likely a combination of genetic and environmental factors contributing to canine impactions.

Diagnosis

Timely diagnosis of an impaction is key to a successful outcome. Early diagnosis leads to early intervention,

Oral and Maxillofacial Surgery, Medicine, and Pathology for the Clinician, First Edition. Edited by Harry Dym, Leslie R. Halpern, and Orrett E. Ogle.

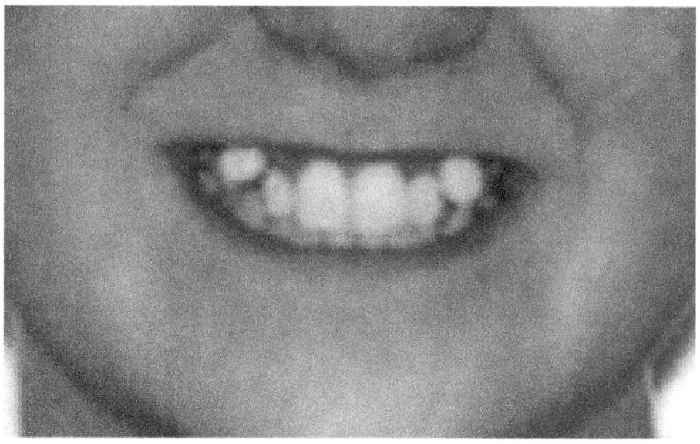

Figure 4.1 Impacted canines can be prominent when smiling.

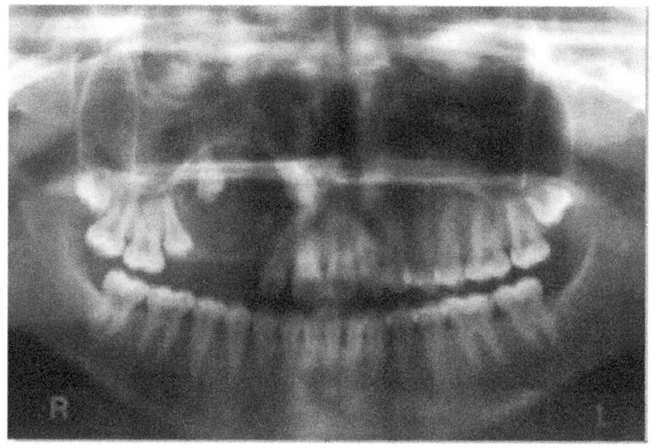

Figure 4.2 Impacted canine associated with pathology (dentigerous cyst).

which leads to reduced treatment time, complexity, and complications. Diagnosis can be made at ages 9–10 years old. Normally, the canines erupt at 10–12 years of age, and a prominent facial bulge can be appreciated clinically 1 year before this [3]. Clinical signs that point a provider to a possible impaction include absence of canine budge (as in palatal impactions), presence of palatal bulge (Figure 4.3), overretained primary canine, asymmetry of primary canine, asymmetry of canine bulge, malpositioned, peg-shaped, or missing lateral incisors, and constricted maxilla with dental crowding [3, 6–10].

Radiographic exam can be accomplished with plain films or cone beam CT. Plain films include panographic, periapical, occlusal, and lateral cephalometric films. Clark's rule can assist in determining the facial-palatal/lingual position of the impacted tooth [3, 10]. (Clark's rule is the use of two slightly different angled radiographs to assess the buccal lingual relationship of an object. If an object or the impacted canine in the film moves in the same direction as the tube head in the second radiograph then the object is lingual. If it moves opposite the movement of the tube head then it is buccal.) Radiographic signs of possible impaction include lateral or central incisor overlapped by erupting canine, enlarged follicular sac of the erupting canine, lack of resorption of the root of the primary canine, and presence of impacted mandibular bicuspids.

A variety of methods and classifications have been proposed to predict canine impactions based on plain film findings. Sajnani and King [11] proposed that impactions are related to the angulation of the erupting canine to the midline and distance from the occlusal plane on panographs. Erikson and Warford [cited in 3] separately advocated that the erupting canine's cusp tip position with respect to the root of the lateral incision mesial-distally is the best predictor for future impaction. Warford's [3] findings showed that canines with cusp tips completely distal to the lateral incisor root on a panograph have a predictive value of 0.06 for future impaction. Canines that overlap the distal half of the lateral incisor root have a predictive value of 0.38. Canines that overlap the mesial half of the lateral incisor root have a predictive value of 0.87. And canines with cusp tips on the mesial of the lateral incisor have a predictive value of 0.99 for future impaction. Overall, there is a 82% chance for future impaction if there is any overlap of the eruption canine cusp tip with the lateral incisor on a panograph film. If this is seen, a prudent dental provider should evaluate or refer the patient for possible canine impaction so that intervention can be initiated at the earliest possible time.

One of the sequelae of untreated canine impactions is resorption of the roots of the adjoined incisors. Cone beam CT is especially useful in this application as it has been shown to be 63% better at detecting root resorptions [12]. Cone beam CT provides a three-dimensional view of the erupting canine and surrounding structures. It is unambiguous in establishing the facial-palatal/lingual relationship of the impacted tooth which is a major determinant of surgical approach. It can detect and visualize vital structures and pathology with better spatial clarity. Disadvantages of its use include increased exposure to radiation and associated cost/time of operation. At this

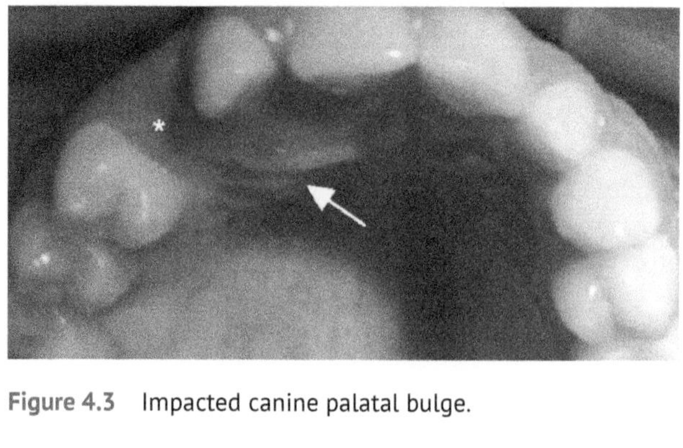

Figure 4.3 Impacted canine palatal bulge.

time, cone beam CT is not the consensus standard of care, but it is agreed that it is a valuable tool in both diagnosis and presurgical planning in cases of impacted canines.

Treatment and Management of the Impacted Canine

Goals

- Eruption of the canine tooth into proper arch position with functional occlusion.
- Satisfactory dentofacial and gingival esthetics.
- Maintain adequate zone of attached soft (in labial impactions).
- Minimize or avoid damage to adjacent dentition and periodontium.

Interceptive Treatment to Prevent Impactions

If an ectopic canine is caught early, some studies have shown that extraction of the overlying primary canine can aid in the proper eruption of the permanent canine. Erikson [3] showed that deciduous canine extraction before the age of 11 will normalize the position of the ectopically erupting permanent canine 91% of the time if the canine crown is distal to the midline of the lateral incisor. There is no agreed mechanism for this observation. Some orthodontists have taken to the regional acceleratory phenomena theory which suggests that the trauma and healing of the extraction triggers localized inflammatory response and remodeling, which in turn aids in the guided eruption of the permanent canine in the vicinity.

Surgical Management of the Impacted Canine

Once a diagnosis of impaction has been made, it is necessary to evaluate the prognosis of the impacted tooth. If the prognosis is favorable, a combination of surgery and orthodontics can be used to bring the impacted canine to its proper arch position. If the prognosis is unfavorable, extraction may be indicated. Extraction may be considered if there is evidence of ankylosis, internal or external root resorption, severely dilacerated root, severe impaction with high risk to adjacent dentition if orthodontics is attempted, functional occlusion with first premolar already in place of the unerupted canine, and if there is associated pathology. In lieu of the crown of the erupted canine in the dental arch, extraction of the impacted canine may be accompanied by:

- retention of primary canine
- orthodontic closure of space substituting the first premolar for the extracted canine (aka bicuspid substitution)
- single-unit implant-supported crown
- autotransplantation of extracted canine into its proper anatomic position [3, 13].

Due to the importance of the permanent canine in the dental arch and the availability of highly predictive surgical exposure techniques with guided orthodontics, extraction of the impacted canine is rarely employed. A variety of surgical techniques exist under the umbrella term "exposure and bond" of the impacted canine. All operate under the basic tenet of gaining access to the impacted tooth, removing pericoronal soft and hard tissue without violating the periodontium, and fixating the exposed canine crown to appliances the orthodontist can use to bring the tooth into the dental arch. In the past, circumcoronal wires and even coronal preps were used to gain leverage to the canine crown [8]. But these techniques were difficult and excessively invasive by modern standards. Currently, most surgeons use resin bond-retained orthodontic brackets attached to gold chains that can be manipulated by the orthodontist.

Open vs Closed Surgery

Two general approaches exist to expose an impacted canine. In open surgery (Figure 4.4), a variety of soft tissue approaches exist to access the impacted tooth, but always the tooth is left exposed through the soft tissue for the orthodontist to manipulate directly. A periodontal dressing is applied over the access to the tooth so that a soft tissue fistula may develop and guide the erupting canine. In closed surgery (Figure 4.5), a flap is raised over the impacted tooth, the tooth is exposed, the orthodontic bracket is placed, and the flap is sutured back to its original position. Only the gold eruption chain attached to the

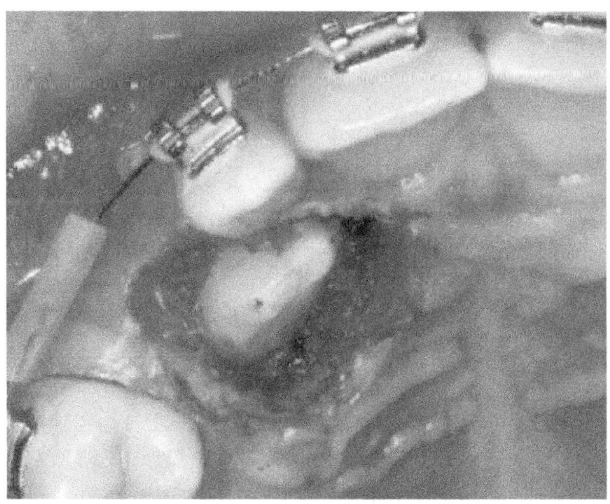

Figure 4.4 Open passive eruption.

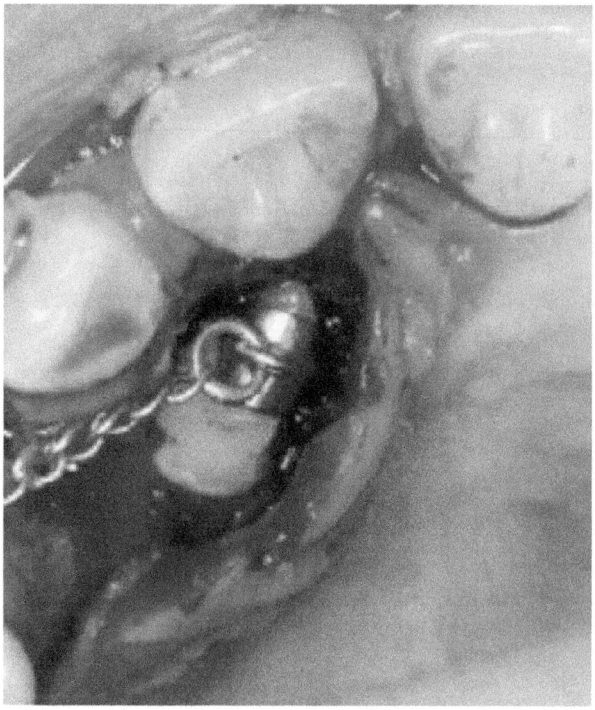

Figure 4.5 Closed guided eruption.

orthodontic bracket is exposed for the orthodontist to manipulate the tooth.

Before the widespread use of bonded resin, surgeons used open techniques exclusively and allowed the tooth to migrate passively into occlusion. Some surgeons advocate to always attempt passive eruption to allow the body a chance to heal itself. However, most patients would still benefit from postsurgical orthodontics as often there is some facial-palatal malposition even if the axial position is corrected [3]. This is why most surgeons now advocate to place bonded orthodontic brackets either during or shortly after open surgery so that the orthodontist can guide the eruption of the canine after it is exposed.

The choice between closed and open surgery is mostly up to surgeon and orthodontist preference in the case of palatally and facially impacted canines. Literature comparing the two approaches shows no evidence to support one over the other in terms of dental health, esthetics, economics, and patient factors [3]. In the case of midalveolar impactions, the opportunity to tunnel the eruption chain within the alveolus to exit via the socket of the extracted primary canine makes closed eruption the preferred management technique most of the time.

Palatal Maxillary Impactions

The specifics of the surgical approach are dictated by the location or spatial considerations of the impacted tooth. Up to 85% of impacted maxillary canines are palatally impacted [6]. In this case, both closed and open approaches are viable.

In the closed approach, a sulcular incision is made from the palatal spanning the first or second bicuspid to the midline, depending on amount of exposure needed. It is rarely necessary to cross the midline. A vertical release may be utilized if needed. The incision is crestal if the canine area is edentulous. A full-thickness mucoperiosteal flap is raised to gain access to the impacted canine. The primary canine is extracted if it has not already been extracted. Soft tissue and bone are removed from the crown of the tooth without violating the cementoenamel junction (CEJ). The field is irrigated and isolated with cotton pellets. Etch and bond may be applied according to the manufacturer's instructions. The orthodontic bracket attached to the gold eruption chain is then placed and secured on the canine's crown using resin. The orthodontist prefers the bracket close to the incisal edge [3]. However, this must be balanced clinically with a flat sound surface on which the bracket can be secured. The flap is then reapproximated and sutured back to its original position. The gold chain exits the tissue intraosseously through the extraction socket of the primary canine, or under the soft tissue flap, or through a fenestration made through the soft tissue, and is secured to existing orthodontic appliances with silk sutures.

If an open technique is used, all steps are the same as the above except a soft tissue opening is made after reapproximating the flap so that the crown of the impacted canine can be clinically visualized through soft tissue. Orthodontic bracket may be applied now or later if a guided open eruption approach is desired. Periodontal packing (typically 0.25 in. gauze strip) is placed and sutured in place over the exposed crown so that a fenestration may form.

Labial Maxillary Impactions

With labial impactions, there is the added nuance of preserving keratinized soft tissue around the erupted canine's final position. This is not a concern with palatal impactions as the hard palate is entirely keratinized soft tissue. Both closed and open techniques are used in labially impacted canines. The closed eruption technique used for labial maxillary impactions is identical to that used in palatal maxillary impactions. A sulcular incision is made on the labial and a full-thickness flap is raised appropriate for the depth of impaction. The crown of the impacted canine is located and exposed by removing pericoronal bone without violating areas apical to the CEJ. The orthodontic bracket and chain is bonded onto the crown and the flap is sutured back to its original position. The gold eruption chain is left exposed for the orthodontist to manipulate.

Open surgery for labial impactions generally uses one of two approaches. If the depth of impaction is low and there is at least 3 mm of keratinized tissue that can be maintained after exposure, the gingivectomy procedure can be used to simply remove the overlying soft and hard tissue covering the unerupted canine [3]. Such a mild impaction is, however, rarely the case. More often, the open procedure of choice is the apically positioned flap (AFP) where crestal attached gingiva can be preserved rather than excised. Mesial and distal vertical releases are made appropriate to the depth of impaction on either side of the impacted canine. A horizontal crestal incision is made to connect the two releasing incisions and a full-thickness flap can be raised. After exposing and bonding the impacted canine, the flap is repositioned apical to its original position and apical to the crown of the exposed canine, and is then secured with resorbable sutures. With this technique, the keratinized crestal tissue is moved apically to support the exposed canine. If the tooth is impacted high in the alveolus, a closed approach is less challenging to execute.

Mandibular Impactions

Mandibular canine impactions (Figure 4.6) are much rarer than maxillary canine impactions [3, 14]. Orthodontic eruption is also less predictable due to their higher tendency to be horizontally impacted and the dense bone of the alveolus. Recoverable mandibular impacted canines tend to be facially impacted as opposed to lingually impacted. Management of these recoverable teeth in the mandible is the same as for facially impacted teeth in the maxilla. Closed procedures are more common as there is less available keratinized tissue to preserve.

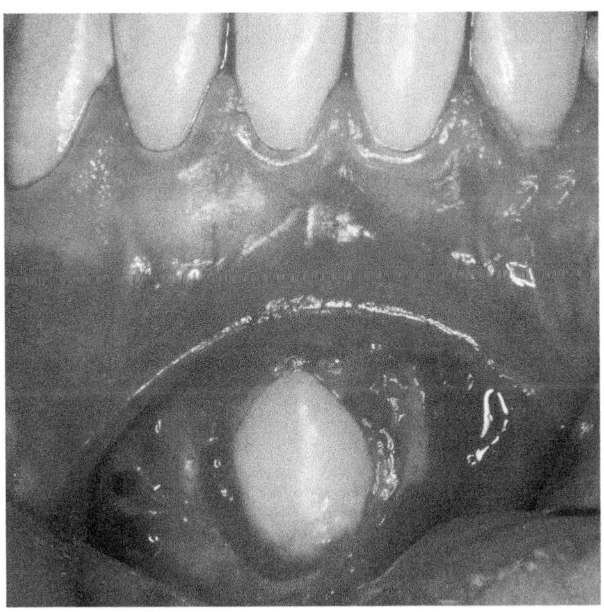

Figure 4.6 Mandibular impaction. *Source:* Coronation Dental Specialty Group/Wikimedia Commons/CC BY 3.0.

Complications

Potential complications include the following.

- Bleeding
- Swelling
- Pain
- Infection
- Paresthesia
- Damage to adjacent structures
- Noneruption
- Inadequate attached gingiva
- Devitalization of the pulp

Bleeding occurs often, especially in patients taking anticoagulants or antiplatelets. Minimal manipulation of the soft tissue reduces the risks of bleeding and swelling. Infection is a risk common to all surgical procedures. Proper sterile techniques minimize postoperative infection. Postoperative antibiotics are not strictly indicated as infection is rare, and they are typically prescribed by the surgeon on a case-by-case basis.

Paresthesia is more of a concern for impacted mandibular canines due to the proximity of the mental nerve and its branches. Surgery in the midsymphyseal area is often accompanied by paresthesia of the lower incisors and gingiva. There may be paresthesia also to the chin and lower lip if the mental nerve is compromised. Palatal surgery can sometimes damage the nasopalatine nerve though patients rarely complain even if paresthesia develops in this region. There can be damage to adjacent structures such as dental roots, walls of the maxillary sinus or nasal cavity into which the impacted tooth may also become dislodged. Rarely, the soft tissue lining of the sinus and piriform may also be compromised.

If a tooth fails to erupt despite surgical and orthodontic intervention, consider ankylosis, blocked eruption, cystic degeneration, and inadequate space for eruption. The area must be reexplored for the above. Ankylosed teeth have an extremely poor prognosis. Some authors advocate mild luxation of the tooth but the merits of this are controversial. Before the advent of implants, cases of localized dentoalveolar osteotomies and distraction procedures were described in literature with some success [15].

Keratinized tissue is integral to a healthy periodontium. In labially impacted canines, often this keratinized tissue is lost. Flap design such as the AFP can help reduce this loss. If loss of keratinized tissue does develop, connective tissue grafting or pedicle/rotation flaps can be considered.

Finally, manipulation of an impacted tooth often results in pulpitis or devitalization with or without symptoms. Endodontic therapy should be considered when possible or the tooth may ultimately require extraction [11].

References

1 Bedoya, M. and Park, J. (2009). A review of the diagnosis and management of impacted maxillary canines. *J. Am. Dent. Assoc.* 140 (12): 1485–1493.

2 Sherwood, K. (2013). Evidence-based surgical-orthodontic management of impacted teeth. *Atlas Oral Maxillofac. Surg. Clin. North Am.* 21 (2): 199–210.

3 Beadnell, S.W. (2012). Management of the impacted canine. In: *Current Therapy in Oral and Maxillofacial Surgery* (ed. S.C. Bagheri, R.B. Bell and H.A. Khan), 135–145. St Louis, MO: Saunders.

4 Tiwana, P.S. and Kushner, G.M. (2005). Management of impacted teeth in children. *Oral Maxillofac. Surg. Clin.* 17 (4): 365–373.

5 Bishara, S.E. (1998). Impacted maxillary canines: a review. *Am. J. Orthod. Dentofac. Orthop.* 101 (2): 159–171.

6 Ferneini, E.M. and Bennett, J.D. (2010). Oral surgery for the pediatric patient. In: *McDonald and Avery Dentistry's for the Child and Adolescent*, 9e (ed. J.A. Dean, D.R. Avery and M.D. RE), 627–644. St Louis, MO: Mosby.

7 Chawla, S., Goyal, M., Marya, K. et al. (2011). Impacted canines: our clinical experience. *Int. J. Clin. Pediatr. Dent.* 4 (3): 207–212.

8 Andreasen, G.F. (1971). A review of the approaches to treatment of impacted maxillary cuspids. *Oral Surg.* 31 (4): 479–484.

9 Suri, L., Gagari, E., and Vastardis, H. (2004). Delayed tooth eruption: pathogenesis, diagnosis, and treatment. A literature review. *Am. J. Orthod. Dentofac. Orthop.* 126 (4): 431–445.

10 Alberto, P.L. (2007). Management of the impacted canine and second molar. *Oral Maxillofac. Surg. Clin.* 19 (1): 59–68.

11 Sajnani, A.K. and King, N.M. (2014). Complications associated with the occurrence and treatment of impacted maxillary canines. *Singapore Dent. J.* 35: 53–57.

12 Jawad, Z., Carmichael, F., Houghton, N., and Bates, C. (2016). A review of cone beam computed tomography for the diagnosis of root resorption associated with impacted canines, introducing an innovative root resorption scale. *Oral Surg. Oral Med. Oral Pathol. Oral Radiol.* 122 (6): 765–771.

13 Bagheri, S.C. and Khan, H.A. (2013). Dentoalveolar surgery. In: *Clinical Review of Oral and Maxillofacial Surgery: A Case-Based Approach*, 2e (ed. S.C. Bagheri), 81–105. St Louis, MO: Mosby.

14 Diaz-Sanchez, R., Castillo-de-Oyague, R., Serrera-Figallo, M. et al. (2016). Transmigration of mandibular cuspids: review of published reports and description of nine new cases. *Br. J. Oral Maxillofac. Surg.* 54 (3): 241–246.

15 Puricelli, E., Morganti, M., Azambuja, H. et al. (2012). Partial maxillary osteotomy following an unsuccessful forced eruption of an impacted maxillary canine – 10 year follow up. Review and case report. *J. Appl. Oral Sci.* 20 (6): 667–672.

5

Crown Lengthening

Tarun Kirpalani

D.W. Cohen first introduced the crown lengthening procedure in 1962. The procedure involves some combination of soft tissue reduction, osseous surgery, and/or orthodontics for a greater amount of tooth exposure in the oral cavity [1].

Crown lengthening may be functional or esthetically driven. From a functional standpoint, the amount of tooth structure exposed above the osseous crest must be enough to provide for a stable dentogingival complex and biological width to permit proper tooth preparation with adequate marginal placement. Esthetically driven crown lengthening follows the same biologic requirement as the functional exposure of sound tooth structure. Esthetic expectations require an increased emphasis on the appropriate diagnosis of hard and soft tissue relationships, as well as the definitive restorative parameters to be achieved. The objective is to enhance the appearance of the restorations placed in the esthetic zone [2].

Biologic Width

The concept of biologic width is utilized as a clinical guideline during the evaluation of periodontal restorative relationships. The concept is the existence of a vertical height of approximately 2 mm from the bottom of the gingival sulcus to the alveolar crest, composed of a junctional epithelium and a connective tissue attachment (Figure 5.1). A distance of 3 mm from the alveolar crest to the future reconstruction margin has been shown to be periodontally stable. Impingement on the biologic width may result in bone loss, gingival recession, or gingival inflammation in an attempt to reestablish its original dimension [1]. Thicker periodontium tends to demonstrate chronic inflammation, whereas thinner periodontium tends to demonstrate bone resorption and recession.

It is understood that the biologic width will reestablish itself during healing of the periodontal tissues following a crown lengthening procedure [3]. One of the theories proposed is that there is insufficient space for a "normal" length of junctional epithelium to develop. Furthermore, the area is easily damaged by mechanical oral hygiene practices causing chronic inflammation to persist or be easily induced. An alternative theory is that a deeply placed subgingival restorative margin impairs proper plaque control, promoting inflammatory changes not conducive to a healthy periodontal environment

Indications for Crown Lengthening [3]

- Increasing clinical crown height lost due to caries/fracture/wear.
- Meeting restorative requirements (esthetics, function and form, retention, and a good marginal seal).
- Accessing a perforation in the coronal third of root/external root resorption.
- Accessing subgingival caries.
- Producing a "ferrule" for restorations.
- Relocating margins of restorations impinging on biologic width.
- Uneven gingival contour.
- Treatment of a "gummy smile"/esthetics/short teeth.
- Altered passive eruption.

Oral and Maxillofacial Surgery, Medicine, and Pathology for the Clinician, First Edition. Edited by Harry Dym, Leslie R. Halpern, and Orrett E. Ogle.

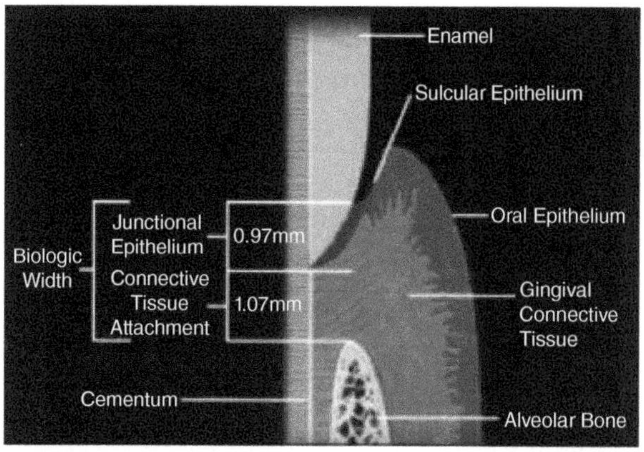

Figure 5.1 Schematic drawing of the structures comprising the periodontium and the biologic width.

Contraindications for Crown Lengthening [1]

- Inadequate crown-to-root ratio.
- Nonrestorability of caries/root fracture.
- Esthetic compromise.
- High furcation.
- Inadequate predictability.
- Tooth–arch relationship inadequacy.
- Compromise of adjacent periodontium or esthetics.
- Insufficient restorative space.
- Nonmaintainability.

Note: Orthodontic extrusion may be able to overcome some factors.

Procedures Carried Out Prior to Crown Lengthening [4]

- Full clinical and radiographic analysis.
  - Determine the finish line prior to surgery. If one cannot determine this, it should be anticipated.
  - Bone sounding of tooth and adjacent teeth.
  - Tooth structure topography, anatomy, and curvature.
  - Gingival form and osseous scallop.
- Caries control.
- Removal of defective restorations.
- Placement of provisional restoration (control inflammation, better assessment of crown lengthening required, improved surgical access, enhanced predictability of margin placement).
- Endodontic therapy (precedes surgery; if this is not possible then it is done 4–6 weeks post surgery).
- Control of gingival inflammation (plaque control, scaling, root planing).
- Reevaluate for orthodontic treatment vs surgical therapy.
- Surgical crown lengthening if indicated.

Bone Sounding [2]

Before any crown-lengthening procedure, especially in the esthetic region, one must determine the level of the alveolar crest. This is done by bone sounding where a periodontal probe is inserted into the sulcus until contact is made with underlying bone to determine the level of the bone on the labial aspect and the interproximal aspects (Figure 5.2). In this way, one can also assess the thickness of the soft tissue and, more importantly, assess if any osseous recontouring/hard tissue removal is needed as part of the crown-lengthening procedure.

Note: The total amount of tooth structure for exposure is determined by the biologic width and prosthetic requirements of the case [3].

Sequence of Treatment for Crown Lengthening

Please refer to Tables 5.1 and 5.2 for treatment options and classifications for crown lengthening.

External Bevel Gingivectomy

Only soft tissue removal using a scalpel, laser, or electrocautery. This technique is performed when there is sufficient sulcular depth and keratinized tissue so that the incision does not violate the biologic width or expose the alveolar bone. Incisions are started apical to the point where the tissue is to be removed and directed coronally, beveled approximately 45° to the tooth surface. The excised tissue should be removed.

Internal Bevel Gingivectomy

This technique also involves the removal of only soft tissue. In this technique, the blade is directed apically, in the opposite direction to the external bevel.

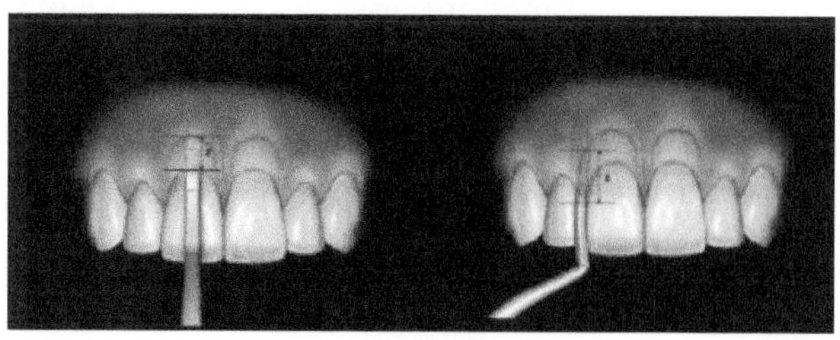

Figure 5.2 Bone sounding.

Table 5.1 Treatment options for crown-lengthening procedures.

	Soft tissue evaluation and management	Hard tissue evaluation and management (bone sounding)
Option 1	Adequate keratinized tissue (>3 mm) – external or internal bevel gingivectomy	Bone crest more apical/ biologic width not violated with soft tissue removal – no bone removal indicated
Option 2	Inadequate keratinized tissue (<3 mm) – apically position flap	Bone crest more coronal/ biologic width violated with soft tissue removal – bone removal indicated

Flap Surgery with Osseous Surgery

This is the most common procedure used for functional crown lengthening.

Step 1: A scalloped incision is made around the teeth with removal of the col to access the interproximal bone. The flap is extended at least one tooth anterior and posterior for adequate osseous surgery to be performed. The scalloping of the flap should reflect the patient's own anticipated healthy gingival architecture.

Step 2: Osseous surgery/bone reduction circumferentially around the tooth. Osteoplasty is completed before ostectomy. This procedure is carried out using a combination of rotary instruments and chisels. A high speed with a

Table 5.2 Classification system for esthetic crown lengthening.

Classification	Characteristics	Advantages	Disadvantages
Type I	Sufficient soft tissue allows gingival exposure of the alveolar crest or violation of the biologic width	May be performed by the restorative dentist	
		Provisional restorations of the desired length may be placed immediately	
Type II	Sufficient soft tissue allows gingival excision without exposure of the alveolar crest but in violation of the biologic width	Will tolerate a temporary violation of the biologic width	Requires osseous contouring
		Allows staging of the gingivectomy and osseous contouring procedures	May require a surgical referral
		Provisional restorations of the desired length may be placed immediately	
Type III	Gingival excision to the desired clinical crown length will exposure the alveolar crest	Staging of the procedures and alternative treatment sequence may minimize display of exposed subgingival structures	Requires osseous contouring
		Provisional restorations of desired length may be placed at second-stage gingivectomy	May require a surgical referral Limited flexibility
Type IV	Gingival excision will result in inadequate band of attached gingiva		Limited surgical options
			No flexibility
			A staged approach is not advantageous
			May require a surgical referral

Source: [2], Table 1 (p.772)/Lee E.

diamond bur can be used for initial bone reduction with the final removal of bone adjacent to the tooth done with hand instrumentation. Interproximal bone reduction can be completed with Brasseler end-cutting burs to avoid damage to adjacent teeth and should be done carefully to maintain the anatomic structures so that the interproximal tissues are allowed to coronally proliferate; the papilla should replace the distance from the bone crest to the base of the contact (5 mm or less) [5]. An adequate biologic width should be maintained with a minimum dimension of at least 4 mm of healthy tooth structure above the osseous crest.

Step 3: Suturing for flap positioning. The position postsurgically is determined by the quantity of keratinized tissue present.

- Wide (>4 mm): flap positioned 1 mm coronal to osseous crest
- Normal (3 mm): flap positioned at the osseous crest
- Narrow (<3 mm): apically positioned flap below the crest of the bone with a partial thickness flap or gingival augmentation or supragingival margin placement.

Apically Positioned Flap With or Without Osseous Surgery

As stated above, this procedure is indicated to preserve attached tissue. The technique involves an intrasulcular incision with vertical releases to apically position the flap with or without bone recontouring to expose sound tooth structure. This technique can be used to crown lengthen multiple teeth in a quadrant or sextant of dentition, but is contraindicated to surgically crown lengthen a single tooth in the esthetic zone.

Combined with Orthodontic Extrusion

Avoids excessive bone reduction around the affected tooth and adjacent teeth. This can be considered in the esthetic zone because it results in a better crown:root ratio and improved esthetics compared to surgical crown lengthening. The procedure is contraindicated if a tooth has a short root length or poor root form [3].

The extrusion can be performed in two ways.

- *Low orthodontic force* – tooth extruded slowly, bringing the bone and gingival tissue with it. The tooth is extruded until the bone has been carried coronal to the ideal level by the amount that will need to be removed surgically to correct the attachment violation. Surgical crown lengthening is then performed to correct hard and soft tissue levels.
- *Rapid orthodontic force* – tooth extruded rapidly during which a supercrestal fibrotomy is performed weekly in an effort to prevent the soft and hard tissue from following the tooth. Surgical crown lengthening may not be needed in such cases. The tooth is stabilized for 12 weeks at the desired level of extrusion.

Classification of Esthetic Crown Lengthening [2]

The decision on what treatment option to use is contingent on a correct diagnosis. Dr Ernesto Lee has proposed the following classification system for esthetic crown-lengthening cases. He also offers treatment sequences depending on the classification that will avoid a prolonged period of time from completion of crown lengthening to tooth restoration, an interim that is unacceptable to patients in the esthetic zone. In such cases, the whole periodontal condition of the patients and their hygiene habits should be evaluated. Furthermore, an accurate diagnostic and interdisciplinary approach is mandatory for obtaining predictable results [5].

- *Type 1*: only a gingivectomy procedure is needed to establish the desired gingival margin level. Since there is sufficient gingival tissue coronal to the alveolar crest, there is no violation of biologic width and no osseous reduction is needed. Teeth can get provisional restorations immediately (Figure 5.3).
- *Type 2*: surgical repositioning of gingiva without exposure of the osseous crest but with violation of biologic width. In such cases, the procedure can be staged. Stage 1 is a gingivectomy with immediate provisional restorations to desired length (knowingly violating the biologic width). Stage 2 follows soft tissue healing; a full-thickness flap is raised with papilla preservation, and osseous surgery completed with the provisional restorations serving as a surgical template (Figure 5.4).

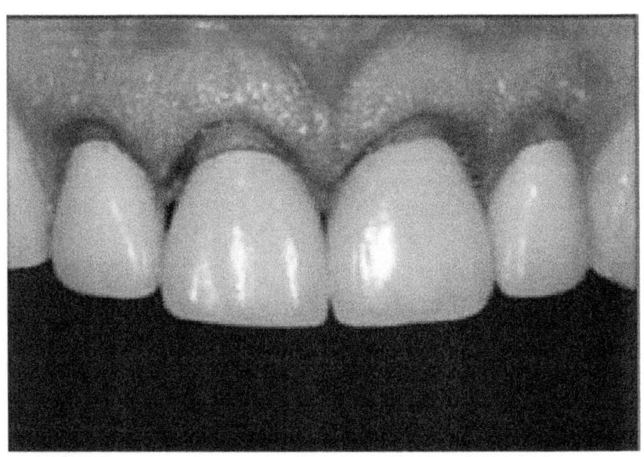

Figure 5.3 Gingivectomy for crown lengthening of a type 1 case.

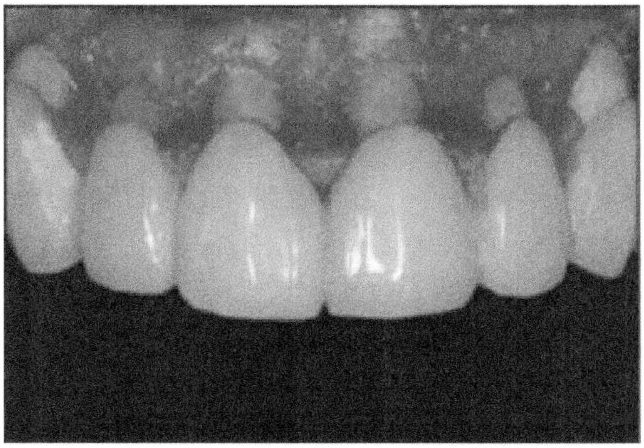

Figure 5.4 Stage 2 of type II case with provisional restorations serving as a guide for osseous recontouring and reestablishment of biologic width.

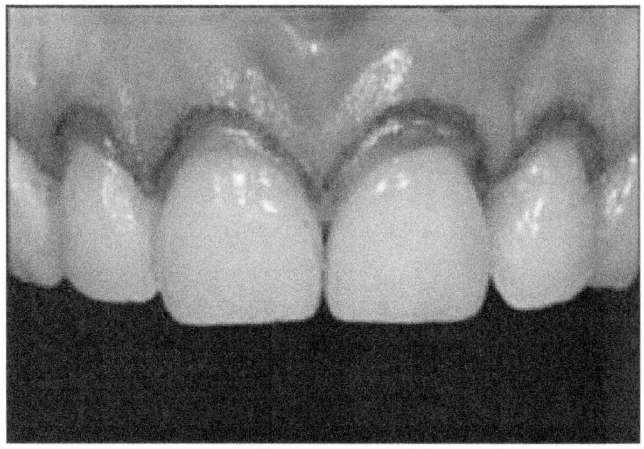

Figure 5.5 Stage 2 of type III case with gingivectomy being performed 4–6 weeks after osseous surgery.

- *Type 3*: surgical repositioning of gingiva will expose the osseous crest. In this scenario, stage 1 is the osseous surgery with coronal reposition of the soft tissue flap to permit anticipated revisions to the gingival margin that will follow once the patient has healed from the osseous surgery. Four to six weeks later, a gingivectomy is performed at stage 2 to establish a definitive gingival margin while placing provisional restorations (Figure 5.5).
- *Type 4*: inadequate amount of attached gingiva, so one must use apically positioned flaps regardless of the need for osseous recontouring. In this scenario, definitive gingival margin placement and provisional fabrication may not be possible in the same appointment.

Postoperative Care [3]

- A periodontal dressing may be placed for patient comfort and to aid in maintaining flap adaptation.
- Gentle brushing and flossing can follow removal of dressing approximately 1 week after procedure.
- Peridex® rinses for 4–6 weeks.
- Definitive restorations to be delayed for 3–6 months following surgery (procedure can be staged for esthetic cases as explained above with provisional restorations).

References

1 Misch, C. (2007). Crown lengthening. In: *Atlas of Cosmetic and Reconstructive Periodontal Surgery*, 3e (ed. E. Cohen), 249–257. Hamilton, ON: BC Decker.

2 Lee, E. (2004). Aesthetic crown lengthening: classification, biologic rationale, and treatment planning considerations. *Pract. Proced. Aesthet. Dent.* 16 (10): 769–778.

3 Gupta, G., Gupta, R., Gupta, N., and Gupta, U. (2015). Crown lengthening procedures – a review article. *J. Dent. Med. Sci.* 14 (1): 27–37.

4 Allen, E.P. (1993). Surgical crown lengthening for function and esthetic. *Dent. Clin. North Am.* 37: 163–179.

5 Oliveira, P.S., Chiarelli, F., Rodrigues, J. et al. (2015). Case report: aesthetic surgical crown lengthening procedure. *Case Rep. Dent.* 2015: 437412.

Part III

Implantology

6

Bone-Grafting Techniques and Biomaterials for Alveolar Ridge Augmentation

Michael Chan

Bone Graft Materials and Healing Physiology

Introduction

With an aging population, better dental IQs, insurance reimbursement, and technological advances in implant dentistry, the application of a bone graft is increasingly sought. There are many factors to consider when clinicians prepare the alveolus ridge for optimal implant placement for form and function. From single tooth sites to full arch reconstruction, understanding bone and membrane properties, physiology of healing, and types of defects to reconstruct will allow clinicians to choose the proper regenerative technique. This chapter will discuss common commercially available materials and literature reviews to seek out the best current choice for each type of augmentation. Additionally, data on implant survival and success post bone grafting has been added to ensure clinicians perform each technique with confidence.

Bone Graft and Tissue Engineering Materials – Outline

Autogenous (Natural)

Intraoral sites:

- Ramus – corticocancellous
- Symphysis – corticocancellous
- Tuberosity – cancellous
- Other (e.g., scraper, bone suction traps)
- Ramus – cortical
- Exotosis – cortical

Allograft (Natural)

Demineralized freeze-dried bone allograft (DFDBA) = (resorbable)

- Cortical
- Cancellous
- Corticocancellous

1) Puros® (Zimmer Dental)
2) MinerOss® (BioHorizon)
3) Creos® (Nobel Biocare)

Demineralized bone matrix (DBM) = not as structurally strong (resorbable)

1) Puros (Zimmer Dental)
2) Grafton® (BioHorizon)
3) Creos allo.gain (Nobel Biocare)

Mineralized freeze-dried bone allograft (FDBA) = (resorbable)

- Cortical
- Cancellous
- Corticocancellous

1) Puros (Zimmer Dental)
2) MinerOss (BioHorizon)
3) Creos (Nobel Biocare)

Xenograft – Bovine, Porcine, Equine, Marine Coral, or Algal Sources

Natural hydroxyapatite (HA) – bovine

1. Bio-Oss® (Geistlich Biomaterials) = (resorbable)

Natural carbonate apatite – porcine

1. Zcore® (Osteogenic Biomedical) = (resorbable)

Natural HA – marine coral-derived calcium carbonate

1. Biocoral® (Biocoral Inc.) = (resorbable – limited)

Fluorohydroxyapatite (FHA) (natural marine algae)

1. Frios® Algipore® (Friadent GmbH) = (resorbable)

Alloplast

Bioactive ceramics

Oral and Maxillofacial Surgery, Medicine, and Pathology for the Clinician, First Edition. Edited by Harry Dym, Leslie R. Halpern, and Orrett E. Ogle.

Nonresorbable hydroxyapatite (synthetic HA)
Polycrystalline ceramic sintered HA

1. Calcitite® (Calcitek, Inc.) = (nonresorbable)
2. Osteograf®/D300 and Osteograf/D700 (CeraMed Corp.) = (nonresorbable)

Resorbable hydroxyapatite (synthetic HA)

1. Osteograf/LD-300 (CeraMed Corp) = (resorbable)

Calcium phosphate – nonceramic HA

1. OsteoGen® (Impladent®) = (resorbable)

Marine coral-derived source (HA) calcium carbonate – coralline porous hydroxyapatite (synthetic HA)

1. Interpore® 200 (Interpore International) = (resorbable)
2. Interpore 500 (Interpore International) = (resorbable)
3. Pro Osteon® 200 (Interpore Cross International) = (90% HA) (resorbs slowly)
4. Pro Osteon 500 (Interpore Cross International) (90% HA) = (resorbs slowly)
5. Pro Osteon 200 R (Interpore Cross International) (85% $CaCO_3$ and 15% HA) = (resorbs faster)
6. Pro Osteon 500 R (Interpore Cross International) (85% $CaCO_3$ and 15% HA) = (resorbs faster)

Nanocrystalline hydroxyapatite (synthetic HA)

1. Ostium® (Heraeus Kulzer) = (resorbable)

Tricalcium phosphate (TCP) (synthetic HA)

1. IngeniOs® (Zimmer Dental) = (resorbable)

Biphasic HA and B-TCP material (synthetic combination)

1. BoneCeramic™ (Straumann) = (resorbable)

Calcium sulfate (gypsum natural mineral)

1. Nanocrystalline calcium sulfate
    1. Nanogen® (Orthogen, LLC) = (resorbable)

Biphasic calcium sulfate (synthetic)

1. Bondbone® (MIS) = (resorbable)

Bioactive glass ceramics (synthetic)

1. PerioGlas® (NovaBone Company) = (resorbable)

Other Synthetic Sources (Engineered)

Recombinant bone morphogenetic protein (rhBMP) (synthetic)

1. rhBMP-2 Infuse® (Medtronic) = (resorbable)

Autologous Platelet Concentrate

Platelet-rich plasma (PRP) and growth factors (GF)
Platelet-derived growth factors (PDGFs)
Transforming growth factor-beta (TGF-beta)
Vascular endothelial growth factors (VEGFs)
Epithelial growth factor (EGF)
Fibroblast growth factor (FGF)
Insulin-like growth factor (IGF)
Platelet-rich fibrin (PRF)

Bone Graft and Tissue Engineering Materials

Autograft

Considered as the "gold standard" among all bone-grafting materials, this has osteocompetent cells available for bone regeneration capable of healing by osteogenesis, osteoinduction, and osteoconduction [1]. Advantages of autogenous bone include the ability to transfer viable cells for osteoblast proliferation for new bone formation, nonimmunogenic (no risk of disease transmission), non-antigenic (no rejections), and ability to harvest a variety of cancellous, cortical, or a combination thereof for desired reconstruction. The cancellous portion undergoes "rapid incorporation" when osteogenic cells are brought into the graft site while the host is able to provide cellular and vascular ingrowth support to help these cells survive during the initial period of healing. This transplanted graft, now somewhat in a necrotic state, will be removed and replaced by host bone during this concurrent neovascularization phase. After graft incorporation, the osteoid fabricated by osteoblasts will mineralize before maturing in 6–12 months [2].

While cortical graft is much denser and possesses more structural support, it also provides fewer osteogenic cells and resorbs much more slowly than cancellous bone. Despite these cellular deficiencies, it does contain bone morphogenetic protein (BMP) which stimulates host bone to release growth factors and osteoprogenitor cells for healing [3]. This process of resorption followed by vascular ingrowth and osteoblast for bony deposition is called "creeping substitution." With further mineralization and continual remodeling, osteoid will eventually become lamella bone in months to years.

Of the two, cortical grafts may have less overall bone formation than cancellous because of the difficulty osteoclasts have in penetrating the highly dense structure to effect complete revascularization [2]. Disadvantages include morbidity of the second surgical site and increased operative time.

Allograft

Obtained from genetically different persons within the same species (e.g., cadaveric bone). It comes in various morphologies: cortical (block), cancellous (particulate), corticocancellous, and putty. Preparations are fresh, frozen, or freeze-dried in either mineralized or demineralized state. Freeze-dried bone is the form most commonly utilized in dentistry due to its low immunogenicity when compared to fresh allograft. The degree of mineralization determines whether the bone will possess either osteoconductive or osteoinductive properties. By removing the inorganic mineral salts (Ca^{2+} and PO_4) from the mineralized matrix, BMP (TGF-beta) and other growth factors (IGF-I, BMP2, BMP7, parathyroid hormone, angiogenic factor) are exposed and available to stimulate bone formation derived from host cells [3, 4]. Moreover, the lack of calcium content makes demineralized bone structurally weaker.

An allograft undergoes a process of ethanol washing (disinfection and lipid removal) and terminal low-dose gamma irradiation (sterilization) while still maintaining a lattice structure; it is then freeze-dried for a longer shelf-life. Although small, the chance of HIV transmission from allogeneic bone is 1 in 1.6 million grafted patients [5].

Allograft is widely used for alveolar ridge augmentations alone or combined with autogenous bone with good success despite the known possible risk of disease transmission. Indications for allograft include sinus floor elevation, socket preservation, horizontal and vertical augmentation, and periodontal defects.

Advantages of allograft include abundant supply, lack of donor site morbidity, and possession of both primarily osteoconductive and lesser osteoinductive properties depending upon the preparation. Disadvantages include lack of available osteocompetent cells and minute chance of disease transmission.

Mineralized Freeze-Dried Bone Allograft

A host's cell-mediated conversion from mineralized to demineralized state is required in order to activate the inherently stored BMP and growth factors [3, 4]. In essence, mineralized bone acts like a scaffold and needs the host's cellular and angiogenic potential to initiate and maintain bone incorporation rendering only osteoconductive properties [6].

Demineralized Freeze-Dried Bone Allograft

Demineralized freeze-dried bone allograft goes through a process of acid treatment, leaving behind an organic collagen and BMP with other growth factors capable of activating osteoprogenitor cells from host bone formation, known as osteoinduction [4]. Because of the exposed BMP, DFDBA is traditionally regarded as having faster bone formation than FDBA [5]. However, Haggerty et al. have found the contrary, with particulate FDBA healing 2 months faster than DFDBA in small contained sites (e.g., extraction socket grafting) [7]. Moreover, recent investigations have revealed that osteoinductive potential from procured bone is age dependent, with younger individuals having more bioactivity than the older population, and not due to the demineralization condition as once thought by researchers [5].

Particulate Cortical, Cancellous, and Corticocancellous Allograft

When transplanted, cancellous allograft heals under a local inflammatory environment which triggers a fibrous encapsulation around the graft site, preventing much needed essential cellular and vascular nutrients from penetrating for proper healing, which may result in prolonged graft incorporation. Particulate cortical bone heals under a similar milieu with host osteoclasts paving the way for osteoblasts' osteoid deposit for eventual new bone formation [2]. The strength and density of cortical bone serve better as a space maintainer with slower resorption than the cancellous counterpart. Indications include socket preservation, ridge, and sinus augmentation.

Xenograft

A xenograft is defined as a graft from genetically different species other than human (e.g., bovine, porcine, equine, marine coral, sea algae).

Natural Hydroxyapatite

Bio-Oss – Bovine Derived

The process of purification is through deproteinization and deorganification and removal of any potential antigens for bovine-derived HA. Hence, without protein, it becomes an inorganic HA crystalline matrix with osteoconductive properties. Bio-Oss's matrix resembles bone's natural HA, making it very appealing to biomaterial researchers and the most studied bovine bone on the market for more than 20 years. Similar to allograft, disease transmission, specifically bovine spongiform encephalopathy, is also very negligible, making this a viable grafting option [8, 9]. Traditionally, xenograft is regarded to be inferior to allograft because of less initial bone formation, slow resorption (>6 months), and increased connective tissue (CT) formation [3, 7]. However, numerous successful outcomes support the use of xenografts for ridge augmentation [5].

Natural Hydroxyapatite – Marine Coral Derived

Calcium Carbonate – Biocoral

Natural marine coral is made up of calcium carbonate and has been used for dental applications since the 1970s. The attractiveness of this material is that it resembles human cancellous bone, being biocompatible and osteoconductive [10]. Biocoral has been used for periodontal defect and oral surgery applications. Thus far, long-term data is only available for correction of infrabony periodontal defects [11]. Limited biodegradability also hinders its usefulness for other alveolar bone-grafting procedures [11]. Currently, researchers are investigating a bioactive version by incorporating silicium ions that can biodegrade in a more predictable fashion along with host bone replacement [12].

Fluorohydroxyapatite (FHA) – Natural Sea Algae Derived

Frios Algipore is derived from marine algae with the calcified form having a pore size of 10–50 μm. It is nonimmunogenic and biocompatible with interconnecting pores enabling protein binding (growth factors) to engage for enhanced healing. Human study showed good bone regeneration with Algipore for sinus augmentation after 7 months of implantation [13].

Alloplast (Synthetic Sources)

A synthetic material possesses either bioactive or bioinert properties. Bioactive material has the ability to interact with host tissue whereas bioinert materials (e.g., stainless steel, alumina, zirconia, and ultra high molecular weight polyethylene) have minimal interactions [14]. These grafts can only heal by osteoconduction. An important aspect of using alloplastic material is to understand the ability for bone to be resorbed and replaced by host bone if regeneration of bone is desired for socket preservation and/or guided bone regeneration [GBR]); otherwise, it can only be used as filler (i.e., under a pontic space) and is not suitable for periimplant site development for future implant placement. Additionally, pore size and interconnecting pores are crucial bone properties essential for cellular and vascular ingrowth for graft success. Typical human pore size is 300–600 μm (cancellous) and 10–50 μm (cortical) while porosity is 75–85% (cancellous) and 5–10% (cortical) [15].

Bioactive ceramics represent the largest group of alloplastic materials used in dentistry. Furthermore, the composition of alloplastic materials has expanded based on their structural properties.

Hydroxyapatite Based (Synthetic HA)

Historically, calcium phosphate-derived synthetic HA has been used for repair of periodontal defects, alveolar and sinus augmentation, and grafting tumor defects after ablation. Synthetic HA has similar characteristics to the mineral composition of teeth and bone and is usually classified based on how well it resorbs *in vivo* [16]. Moreover, the temperature at which the HA is sintered will provide the material's characteristics. The higher the temperature at which the material is sintered, the more dense it is and less resorbable, with the inverse being true with lower temperature.

According to Misch, the rate of resorption for calcium phosphate (HA/TCP) is dependent upon four factors: pH, porosity, particle size, and volume. The lower the pH, higher porosity, smaller particle size and smaller volume, the more likely it will resorb [17].

Generally, synthetic HA utilized in oral surgery is regarded as nonresorbable and possessing poor mechanical strength, making it an unfavorable choice for load-bearing regions [16]. Currently, nonresorbable synthetic HA for alveolar ridge application is better used for coverage of fenestration associated with periimplant defects or under non-load-bearing pontic regions.

Marine Coral Derived (Hydroxyapatite)

Coralline HA is synthetically manufactured from marine coral. The conversion from calcium carbonate to HA lattice structure occurs via hydrothermal methods (900 °C) in the presence of diammonium phosphate. The endproduct, coralline HA granules, has all the organic materials removed (nonimmunogenic) and is similar to the porous structure of human bone. There are reports of human studies showing excellent results in the following applications: craniomaxillary defects, periodontal defects, ridge augmentation, and socket preservation [18]. Lack of immunogenic response is an advantage of coralline HA. Disadvantages are that it can only be used as a filler in a nonload-bearing or low load-bearing region and it has weak mechanical properties. Two examples of coralline HA are described below.

Coralline Porous Hydroxyapatite – Interpore (Synthetic HA)

Interpore is a coralline HA manufactured in two sizes, 200 and 500, with both available in granule or block forms. Mandibular ridge augmentation with new bone replacement has been achieved with 0.4–1.0 μm granules while 0.4–6.0 μm granules have been used for periodontal defects, both with Interpore 500 [18].

Coralline Porous Hydroxyapatite – Pro Osteon (Synthetic HA)

Pro Osteon is an osteoconductive matrix that comes in particulate and block forms, with particulate having two sizes: 200R (craniomaxillary) and 500R (orthopedic/spine), with the number representing the pore size; both are composed of 85% calcium carbonate and 15% HA. Calcium phosphate (outer layer) and calcium carbonate (inner layer) make up the lattice structure. Upon transplanting to the host site, the slower resorbing calcium phosphate biodegrades until it reaches the faster resorbing calcium carbonate layer where host bone is eventually incorporated with grafted bone.

Literature review of clinical studies has demonstrated the use of coralline porous hydroxyapatite for repair of periodontal defect, maxillary sinus augmentation, and craniofacial reconstruction with relatively good outcomes for bony regeneration [19].

Nanocrystalline Hydroxyapatite (Synthetic HA)

This is a synthetic HA with nano-sized particles embedded in the silica matrix through a sol–gel process in the presence of SiO_2. The concept of nanotechnology is to take advantage of the particle size ranging from 0 to 100 nm, with a conversion of 1 µm equal to 1000 nm. The smaller the particle size, the more surface area available for bone attachment and blood plasma infiltration while simultaneously preventing unwanted cells in the matrix [20].

Ostim® (Heraeus Kulzer) is a nanocrystalline HA that is prepared in a syringe. Indications include socket preservation, periodontal defects, and sinus lifts. This company reported a 12-week resorption period with subsequent host bony replacement. Despite these claims, one biomaterial researcher found limited biodegradability with nanocrystalline HA [11]. Currently, there are only two comparative human studies in the literature for infrabony periodontal defects with one study on autogenous bone and the other with resorbable HA, both having good outcomes against the control group [21, 22].

Tricalcium Phosphate (Synthetic)

Tricalcium phosphate has both alpha (A) and beta (B) preparations, with the B version being utilized more in oral surgery. Earlier B-TCP used in the 1970s had poor results because of the material's lack of purity, leading to degradation and inconsistent results [11]. However, over the last 10 years, researchers have found that highly pure B-TCP (>99%) can biodegrade in a more controlled setting with increased porosity as a major contributing factor resulting in good host bone replacement in human trials and even compatible to autogenous bone [11].

Biphasic HA and B-TCP Material (Synthetic Combination)

A blend of two alloplastic materials, BoneCeramic (Straumann) is formulated to control the biodegrading process. Synthetic HA is known for its slower resorption and B-TCP for being quicker. By adding 40% B-TCP to 60% HA, bone can resorb quicker than its original form and be replaced by host bone. Indications include socket preservation, GBR (horizontal), treatment of periimplant fenestration and dehiscence, and sinus augmentation [23].

Calcium Sulfate – Gypsum Based (Synthetic)

Calcium sulfate has been used in surgery and dentistry for the past century. It possesses many desirable properties as a grafting material: biocompatible, biodegradable, nontoxic, complete resorption with host bone replacement, very stable, ample supply, relatively inexpensive, and environmentally friendly. Gypsum, a hydrated calcium sulfate, is a naturally occurring mineral found abundantly worldwide. The most well-known calcium sulfate, plaster of Paris, is manufactured from gypsum in the hemihydrate form. While medical-grade calcium sulfate has limitations, with fast resorption and lack of bony replacement, dental-grade preparations are showing some promising clinical results with two examples listed below.

Calcium Sulfate – Nanocrystalline (Synthetic)

Nanogen is a relatively new nanocrystalline calcium sulfate-based product that undergoes a conversion to smaller sized particles, 200–900 nm, after which they get tightly compressed to form 400–1000 µm granules. A unique chemical transformation from calcium sulfate to calcium phosphate occurs as a result of implantation and through the interactions of calcium ions from the graft and phosphate ions from the host body. There is a controlled degradation process which leads to predictable bone resorption in approximately 12 weeks, with host bone replacement in 3–4 months resulting in calcium phosphate found in natural bone. On histopathology examination, 100% of the vital bone was noted after 4 months. Currently, this product is only FDA approved for socket preservation. Advantages include biodegradable, biocompatible, nontoxic, promotes growth factor release during controlled degradation, barrier membrane capability, and hemostatic properties [24].

Biphasic Calcium Sulfate (Synthetic)

Bondbone is a fully synthetic biphasic calcium sulfate with dihydrate and hemihydrate properties that demonstrates biocompatibility, easy handling, and fast setting when mixed with saline. Macroporosity (300–800 µm) and microporosity (1–50 µm) are characteristics which allow essential cellular ingrowth and growth factors respectively to the graft site, enabling osteoconduction. Bondbone can be used for socket preservation (10 mm maximum) with at least a four wall defect (Box 6.1) or combined with other grafting materials with a recommended 2:1 ratio to enhance graft volume. It is initially radiopaque and then becomes radiolucent (3 weeks) before reverting back to radiopacity upon complete host bone incorporation in 3 months. The use of membrane is optional as Bondbone when hydrated in its rigid form also serves as a membrane [25].

Bioactive Glass Ceramics (Synthetic)

PerioGlas is a bioactive glass ceramic alloplastic material capable of being utilized in many different dental applications: socket preservation, ridge augmentation, sinus lift, treatment of periodontal defects, and bone loss associated with periimplantitis. When this material is placed in a host environment, it forms a calcium phosphate layer in which an interface is chemically bonded to host bone. It is osteoconductive and undergoes complete resorption with complete replacement of host bone. Most bioactive glass materials require a longer healing period when compared to autograft, allograft, and xenograft. Since alloplastic material is manufactured, advantages include abundant amounts, and it is nonimmunogenic. One disadvantage is that bone quality is generally inferior to autograft, allograft, and xenograft although some animal studies report better early bone formation when compared to xenograft [26, 27].

Other Synthetic Sources – Recombinant Bone Morphogenetic Protein (rhBMP)

Bone morphogenetic protein is a group of 20 proteins found in the bone matrix. More specifically, they are part of the TGF-beta superfamily [28]. Both rhBMP-2 (Medtronic) and rhBMP-7 (OP-1 Stryker Biotech) are commercially available and are manufactured through molecular biology techniques. The process entails identifying a specific human protein (i.e., BMP-2) and introducing it to mammalian cells for "recombination" and through its incorporation, the cell is able to replicate a new batch called rhBMP-2. An absorbable collagen sponge (ACS) is a necessary vehicle for the recombinant protein to be delivered to the graft site and should be protected against external compression to prevent vertical or horizontal displacement (i.e., titanium-reinforced membrane or other graft containment device).

The specific action of rhBMP-2 and rh BMP-7 is cellular recruitment of mesenchymal cells, in particular osteoblasts, and angiogenesis capable of inducing *de novo* bone formation [28, 29]. Alveolar reconstruction and sinus augmentation are the only two FDA-approved procedures thus far but some clinicians use it "off label" for maxillofacial reconstruction.

Disadvantages include high material cost and it is likely used only for intraoral challenging and/or compromised cases. Edema secondary to chemotaxis and angiogenesis with increased fluid recruitment have been associated with this product so educating these patients will decrease their anxiety during the postoperative period.

Autologous Platelet Concentrates (See Table 6.1 for Complete Formulations)

Platelet-Rich Plasma

Platelet-derived growth factor, TGF-beta, VEGF, EGF, FGF, and IGF are essential for bone and soft tissue healing. Except for FGF and IGF, the concept of PRP is to extract these cells to be delivered locally for enhanced healing. A high concentration (1 000 000/μL) of platelets is needed to have any meaningful therapeutic effect, with clinical plateau in 6 months.

The process starts with drawing the patient's whole blood (average 20–60 mL) and combining it with an anticoagulant agent (e.g., citrate dextrox-A) for dental application and through a double centrifugation technique separating the red blood cells (RBCs), white blood cells (WBCs), and clotting factors from platelets. After the second centrifuge, there is a definite separation between the darker platelet-rich bottom portion and the lighter platelet-poor plasma (PPP; top portion). The action of PRP works when it is in clotted form in which 90% starts secreting these growth factors within the first 10 minutes and the remaining over 30 minutes [17]. PRP can be applied directly to the bone graft material or membrane used for GBR. PRP and autogenous bone graft have been shown to create more dense bone formation when compared to control groups [5].

Platelet-Rich Fibrin

Known as the "second generation of platelet concentrates," PRF has several properties that help accelerate hard and soft tissue healing. It has a fibrin meshwork which contains leukocytes, cytokines, and inherently stored growth factors within the alpha granules of platelets (i.e., PDGF, TGF-beta, and VEGF). These growth factors provide the following healing properties: PDGF provides mesenchymal cellular recruitment and differentiation, TGF-beta promotes cellular proliferation, and VEGF promotes angiogenesis. Additionally, platelets have hemostatic properties [31].

Blood collection is time sensitive, with the blood samples needing to be centrifuged *immediately* after collection before natural coagulation occurs. For Choukroun's

Table 6.1 Growth factors [2, 5, 17, 30].

Growth factors	Storage site	Cell source [30]	Cellular function on bone healing
Platelet-derived growth factor (PDGF) (early phase) [5]	Platelet and bone matrix [17]	Platelets Macrophage Monocyte Endothelial cells Osteoblast	Chemotaxis for mesenchymal cell proliferation [2, 17, 30] Chemotaxis for inflammatory cells [2] Osteoblast for bone formation [5, 17] Promotes angiogenesis [2, 17] Supports growth factors for repair [17] Chondroblast for cartilage formation [17]
Fibroblast growth factor (FGF) (early phase) [5]	Extracellular bone matrix [17]	Macrophage Monocyte Fibroblast Endothelial cell Osteoblast Chondroblast Bone marrow-derived stem cell (BMSC)	Proliferation of fibroblasts for wound healing [2, 5, 30] Promotes angiogenesis [2, 17, 31] Osteoblast proliferation for bone formation [17, 30] Chondrocyte maturation [32]
Insulin-like growth factor (IGF) (early phase) [5]	Bone matrix [17]	Hepatocyte Osteoblast Chondrocyte Endothelial cell	Chemotaxis for mesenchymal cell proliferation [17] Osteoblast for bone formation [2, 5, 30] Extracellular matrix deposition [5, 30]
Transforming growth factor (TGF)-beta (late phase) [5]	Bone matrix [17]	Platelet Fibroblast Macrophage Endothelial cell Osteoblast Chondroblast Bone marrow Stromal cell (BMSC)	Chemotaxis for mesenchymal cell proliferation [2, 17] Fibroblast for connective tissue repair [2, 17] Osteoblastic for bone formation [2, 17] Promotes angiogenesis [5] Extracellular matrix deposition [5, 17, 30] Chondrocyte differentiation [2, 30]
Bone morphogenetic protein (BMP) (late phase) [5]	Extracellular bone matrix [17]	Osteoblast Chondroblast Endothelial cell BMP-2	Chemotaxis for mesenchymal cell differentiation [2, 5, 17] Osteoblast for bone formation [17] Chondroblast for cartilage formation [17] Promotes angiogenesis [5, 31] Extracellular matrix deposition [30]
Vascular endothelial growth factor (VEGF)	Platelets [2]	Platelet Osteoblast	Promotes angiogenesis [2] Conversion of cartilage into bone, osteoblast proliferation and differentiation [30]

original leukocyte-platelet-rich fibrin (L-PRF) protocol, use 4–6 9 mL plain (without anticoagulants) red-top glass tubes with vacuum container to draw blood. It is imperative these tubes are placed in an equal distribution across from each other in the centrifuge compartment for a "balanced" spin; otherwise, they will not separate into the desired cell layers (platelets and leukocytes, from RBCs). After centrifuge at 2700 rpm for 12 minutes, there should be three distinct layers: (i) the top one-third layer contains acellular PPP, (ii) the middle one-third layer has PRF "fibrin clot," and (iii) the bottom one-third layer contains dense RBCs. The ability to concentrate fibrinogen in the top two-thirds is the most important process, mainly without any external anticoagulant additives. This fibrin matrix helps entrap circulating mesenchymal cells for cellular differentiation and proliferation for osteocytes, leukocytes for immune regulation, and supports angiogenesis via endothelial cell and fibroblast recruitment [31].

Since the development of L-PRF by Choukroun in 2001, there have been modifications by other researchers, notably Ghanaati, to develop a total of six protocols, of which five are relevant for dental applications. Advanced PRF Liquid (A-PRF Liquid) is used to make "sticky bone" while the Advanced Platelet-Rich Fibrin (A-PRF) is reserved for membrane and plug fabrication [33]. The Injectable Platelet-Rich Fibrin for females (i-PRF) and Injectable Platelet-Rich Fibrin for males (i-PRF M) are in liquid form and can be applied to bone graft material or directly on the surgical site for enhanced tissue healing (www.biofixt.be). A recent publication has shown that lowering the centrifuge rate and time will yield a higher concentration of leukocytes, platelets, and growth factors than Chroukroun's original version. This technique is known as the low-speed centrifuge concept (LSCC) [34]. Researchers are still methodically analyzing the ideal revolutions per minute (rpm) or, more appropriately, the "g-force" of the centrifuge machine and the amount of time required in order to optimize cell separation [34].

For A-PRF Liquid preparation, concentrated platelets are found at the bottom of the supernatant layer (clear plasma top layer). A 18 or 21 gauge needle with a syringe is used to aspirate this supernatant layer and apply it to the bone graft for "sticky bone" production. As the name implies, it provides bone with better handling quality. As for the A-PRF protocol for membrane and plug fabrication, spin the unused test tubes for additional 3 minutes and remove them to the test tube holder immediately and allow a gel to form in approximately 5 minutes while uncapped. There should be two distinct layers: the "white" top portion contains concentrated platelets and leukocytes within the fibrin clot and the "red" portion contains RBCs. Separate these two layers with a pair of scissors and retain the fibrin clot. If a membrane is desired, place this fibrin clot in the box and allow the fluid to be "squeezed" out for a few minutes with a crusher. However, if the clinician wants to make a fibrin plug for an extraction socket, place the "white" layer into a white Teflon cylinder inside the box and condense it with a metal piston.

The advantages of PRF over PRP are numerous: ease of preparation, no additives (i.e., bovine thrombin, anticoagulants), eliminating cell lysis, only one centrifuge required, platelets and leukocytes are entrapped in the fibrin matrix with a longer shelf-life for sustained cellular activity. Since PRF has inherent thrombin, it undergoes a slower polymerization process (conversion from fibrinogen to fibrin by thrombin), yielding an increased number of cytokines available for sustained cellular recruitment for wound healing. This is superior to the PRP's growth factors which disappear more quickly when these additives are mixed (thrombin and calcium), causing a faster fibrin polymerization and loss of vital cytokines [17, 31, 35].

Dental applications of PRF include periimplantitis, sinus augmentation, GBR, postextraction socket, gingival recession, and correction of three-wall infrabony or furcation Class II defect [35, 36].

Ridge Preservation

Ridge Preservation Indications

Numerous studies have shown that natural resorption occurs after tooth extraction with the following pattern: (buccal > lingual/palatal) (anterior > posterior regions) (maxilla > mandible) (horizontal > vertical). Specifically, average vertical height diminishes up to 1.5–2.0 mm and horizontal width up to 50% in the first 12 months, with the majority of the horizontal loss occurring within the first 3 months [6, 37]. Researchers have examined various grafting materials and techniques hoping to eliminate these dimensional changes [38, 39].

The idea of ridge preservation is simply placing bone-grafting material within the socket after tooth extraction. The clinician can utilize any resorbable bone material and graft containment to occlude the coronal portion (e.g., membrane, collagen, or connective tissue graft) or perform primary closure [40]. Additionally, a collagen plug can be used as a stand-alone technique without graft containment. Despite these procedures, sufficient evidence does show that grafted sites significantly slow the progression of ridge resorption but do not prevent it entirely [38, 39].

Misch developed an implant wall classification which categorizes the number of number of walls surrounding an implant. A five wall defect represents the presence of buccal, lingual, mesial, distal, and apical wall while a one wall defect usually denotes the existence of lingual/palatal wall. This classification includes an additional apical bone as the fifth floor which is not associated with the traditional periodontal defect classifications (Box 6.1, Figure 6.1) [17].

Ridge Preservation Algorithm

In 2014, Frost et al. suggested an algorithm to guide clinicians facing ridge preservation by posing two fundamental questions [41] (Figure 6.2). First, will there be sufficient

Box 6.1 Misch's implant wall classification [17]

Five wall defect – buccal, lingual, mesial, distal, and apical walls present
Four wall defect – usually the buccal wall is missing
Three wall defect – buccal wall missing and apical wall is usually missing or compromised
Two wall defect – usually buccal, mesial, and distal walls are missing or any combination of two walls existing
One wall defect – usually lingual/palatal present

native bone in the future to receive an implant after normal extraction healing? If the answer is "no," then ridge preservation and/or GBR will be required. However, if the answer is "yes," then what is the current biotype and buccal plate thickness? Generally speaking, gingival biotype correlates with buccal bone thickness, with thinner biotypes having thinner buccal plates [42].

Regardless of site, Spray et al. demonstrated that thinner buccal plates (<2 mm) have a tendency to resorb on the facial aspect, causing unsatisfactory periimplant support [43]. In fact, 85% of the maxillary buccal plate has <1 mm thickness [44, 45]. For these situations, ridge preservation coverage is vital. Additionally, CT graft is needed for the esthetic zone to enhance gingival architecture. Conversely, thicker molar sites (>2 mm) may be exempt from grafting, leaving the informed decision to the patient. Molar buccal plates are more resistant to resorption, especially in the mandible due to the dense cortical bone [17]. Nonmolar sites, however, will still require ridge preservation in order to optimize future implant site(s). As buccal bone resorbs, it causes a decrease in horizontal width, resulting in a "shift" of the future implant site to a more lingual/palatal position, creating a "nonideal tooth set-up." Frost et al. added that pneumatized maxillary sinus could be prevented by placement of bone graft supplements [41].

Ridge Preservation Surgical Technique

Care must be taken to perform the extraction as atraumatically as possible using either a flapless or flapped approach. After local anesthesia is delivered, a #15 blade is used to separate the soft tissue around the tooth (Figure 6.3). Some clinicians insert a periotome before placing a forceps for tooth removal to facilitate loosening, which helps preserve buccal bone (Figure 6.4). For severely decayed teeth or an anticipated difficult extraction, surgical sectioning is useful to avoid traumatizing the buccal bone, leading to higher resorption. Once the tooth is removed, the socket is curetted, all granulation tissue is removed, and the socket is thoroughly irrigated (Figure 6.5).

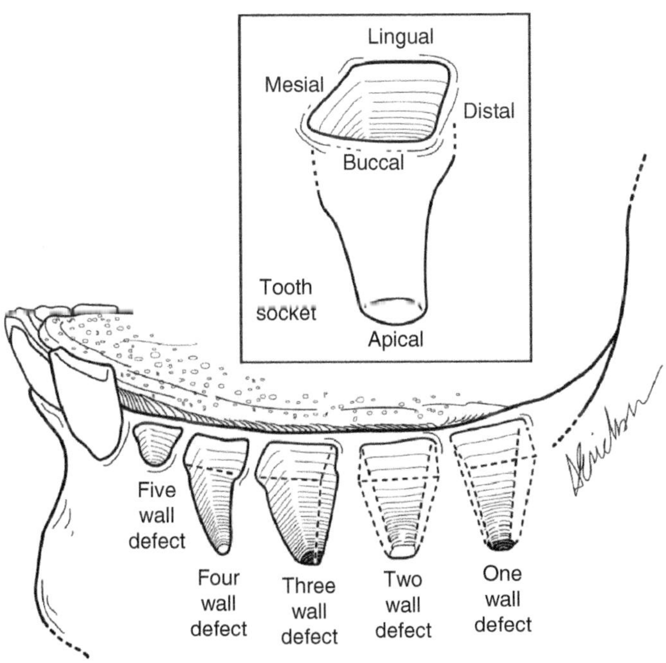

Figure 6.1 Implant wall classification. Tooth socket wall defect. Missing walls are indicated by dotted lines. *Source:* [17], with permission of Elsevier.

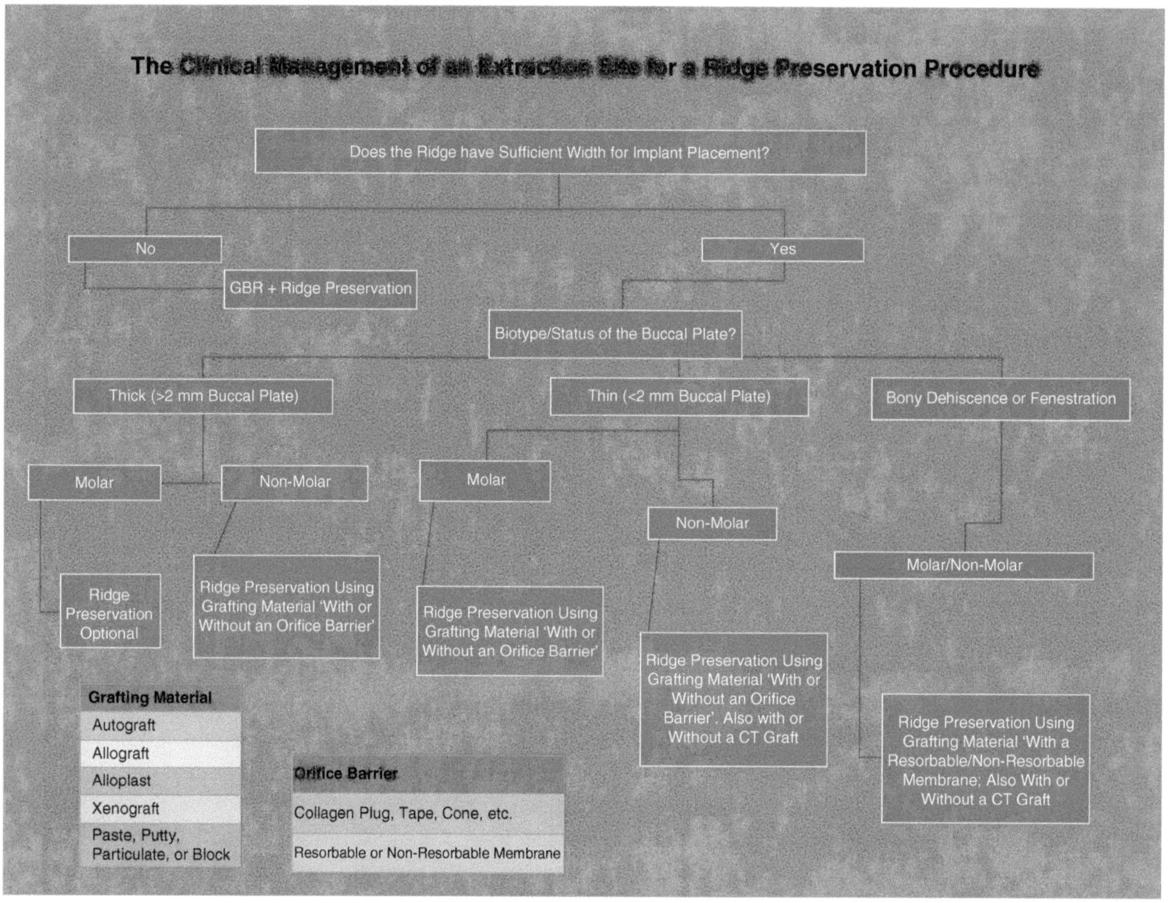

Figure 6.2 Decision tree selection of treatment strategy. Proper management of an extraction socket should be based on careful analysis of the clinical presentation and restorative treatment plan. Also, the clinician should consider intraoperative surgical findings, including thickness of the buccal plated clinical biotype, presence of buccal fenestrations or dehiscences, and molar versus nonmolar sites. Depending on the graft materials used, the clinician may choose to cover the graft with an orifice barrier in some cases. Adjunctive CT grafts may be indicated in areas with thin biotype, gingival recession, or other potential esthetic compromise. *Source:* [41], figure 4 (p.60)/With permission of John Wiley & Sons.

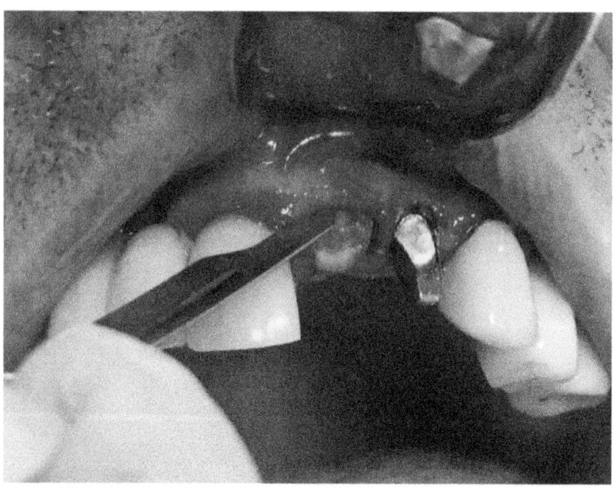

Figure 6.3 A #15 blade is used to separate the soft tissue from the tooth.

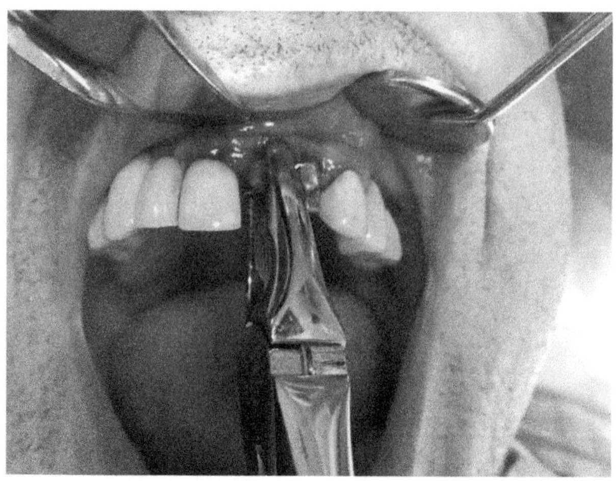

Figure 6.4 Atraumatic extraction using forceps.

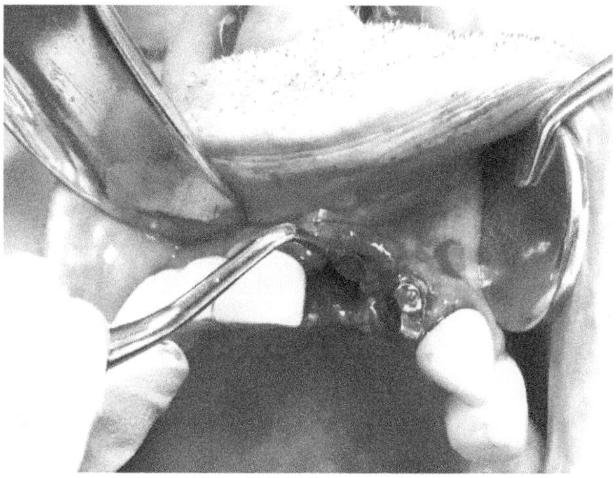

Figure 6.5 Removal of all granulation tissue with a curette.

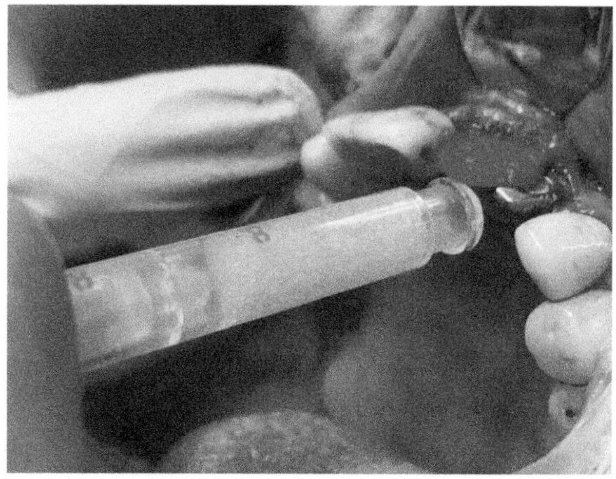

Figure 6.6 Apply bone graft material into the socket.

All types of resorbable bone are amenable to socket grafting when five walls are intact (Figure 6.6). The graft should be stabilized with sutures or horizontal mattress pattern with the following options: with or without a membrane, connective tissue or collagen plug, primary or partial closure each producing successful results (Figure 6.7). Most clinicians do not attempt primary closure for simple ridge preservation and most opt for graft containment to prevent bone material falling out. It is essential that no direct pressure is placed on the graft; a temporary prosthesis can be used (e.g., Essix retainer, fixed partial denture, or flipper).

Although Vignoletti et al. demonstrated that the combination of flapped procedure, membrane and primary closure produced better results, currently there is no clear consensus on which grafting material or technique is superior for ridge preservation [39]. Additional bone grafting for future implant placement may be needed despite the socket preservation procedure [41, 46].

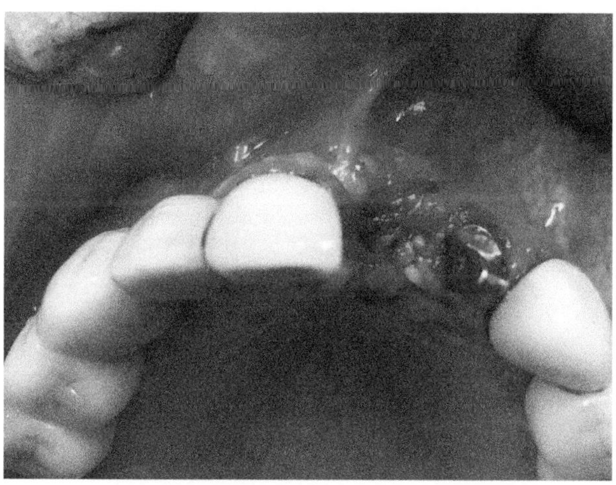

Figure 6.7 Closure performed with a figure-of-eight suture.

Ridge Preservation Surgical Complications

The main complication of ridge preservation is infection with frank purulent discharge. This will require complete graft removal with thorough irrigation and a postoperative course of antibiotics. Partial graft loss from spitting and rinsing to complete graft loss secondary to cigarette smoke have been noted by the author. Replacement of graft loss can only be performed with patient compliance by abstaining from smoking. Small partial graft loss can be addressed at the time of implant placement.

Ridge Preservation Implant Survival and Success Rates

"Survival" is defined as the presence of dental implant in the jaw while "success" as described by Karoussis et al. has the following criteria (Box 6.2) [referenced in 39]:

- absence of mobility
- absence of persistent subjective complaint
- no periodontal probing depth (PPD)>5 mm (normal PPD is 2–4 mm)
- no PPD with 5 mm and bleeding on probing (BOP)
- absence of continuous radiolucency around the implant
- annual bone loss after the first year does not exceed 0.2 mm.

Implant success studies after ridge preservation have been observed in three human trials. Norton and Wilson (2002) using alloplast (bioactive glass) showed a cumulative implant success rate of 90% while in 2013 Patel et al., using alloplast (BoneCeramic) and xenograft (Bio-Oss), demonstrated a similar success rate of around 80%. These observations were only for a 1-year period [referenced in 39]. A retrospective analysis by Apostolopoulos in 2016 showed a lower implant success rate of 51% (Bio-Oss with Bio-Guide) when compared to the control group with

Box 6.2 Karoussis et Al.'s criteria for implant success and survival – 2014 [referenced in 39]

1. Implant is present (survival criterion)
2. Absence of mobility (success criterion)
3. Absence of persistent subjective complaint (i.e., pain, dysesthesia) (success criterion)
4. No PPD >5 mm (normal PPD is 2–4 mm) (success criterion)
5. No PPD with 5 mm and BOP (success criterion)
6. Absence of continuous radiolucency around the implant (success criterion)
7. Annual bone loss after the first year does not exceed 0.2 mm (success criterion)

58% [40]. These percentages are lower than the previous two studies. It should be noted that the former two studies used Albrektsson et al.'s 1986 criteria for implant "success" and the latter used those of Karoussis et al . Direct comparison among these studies should be done with close scrutiny (Box 6.3) [47].

Ridge Preservation Conclusion (Box 6.4)

Socket preservation is a highly predictable procedure, making this a good procedure for all clinicians to perform, especially for periimplant site development. Various bone materials with or without tissue coverage have been reported to have good outcomes.

A systematic review conducted by Avila-Oritz et al. concluded that nonmolar ridge preservation had better clinical outcomes than a nongrafted group for both horizontal and vertical dimensions with statistically significant differences noted for the horizontal (buccal–lingual width) and vertical (midbuccal and midlingual) regions [48]. These were mean weighted differences based on six studies: buccal–lingual width = 1.89 mm, midbuccal = 2.07 mm, midlingual 1.18 mm. This represents the average difference between grafted and nongrafted sites at each particular surface and the amount of bone gained by utilizing the ridge preservation technique. This horizontal data was in agreement with findings reported by Vignoletti et al. [39] and Vittorini Orgeas et al. [referenced in 47]. However, vertical bone height could not be elicited because prior studies did not specify the vertical axis.

Despite these positive findings with grafting, dimensional loss still does occur and clinicians should still bear in mind that future grafting may be necessary during staged implant placement in order to avoid patient resentment for incurring additional expense [41, 46].

Box 6.3 Albrektsson et Al.'s criteria for implant success – 1986 [47]

1. Absence of mobility
2. Absence of periimplant radiolucency
3. Vertical bone loss after first year of function to be less than 0.2 mm
4. Absence of pain, infection or paresthesia
5. Implant success rate of 85% at end of 5 years and 80% at end of 10 years

Box 6.4 Key points for ridge preservation

1. Atraumatic extraction can help preserve native bone
2. Socket preservation limits dimensional socket loss (horizontal > vertical) [6, 39]
3. Anterior and bicuspid teeth benefit more than thicker molar sites (>2 mm buccal bone thickness) with socket preservation [41]
4. Thin biotype or buccal plate (<2 mm thickness) would benefit from socket preservation [41]
5. Currently, there is no consensus on the ideal combination of grafting materials or techniques [39]
6. All resorbable bone-grafting materials can be used for socket preservation in combination with the following graft containment (with or without membrane, collagen-based material, connective tissue, primary or partial closure) [6, 39]
7. Additional grafting may be required despite bone preservation technique [41, 46]
8. Time to implant placement with particulate FDBA = 3–4 months, DFDBA = 4–6 months and bovine bone = 6–8 months [7]

Guided Bone Regeneration (GBR)

Guided Bone Regeneration Indications

Guided bone regeneration can be performed simultaneously during implant placement (simultaneous approach), for ridge development (staged approach) or for treatment of periimplantitis. The concept of GBR is to provide an environment with or without bone graft material to heal under "ideal" conditions: (i) underneath a space maintainer with clot stabilization so growth factors can be released, (ii) able to prevent ingrowth of unwanted cells (epithelium and connective tissue) into the graft site, (iii) complete graft immobilization for undisturbed healing, (iv) primary closure to prevent oral contaminants [6].

Guided bone regeneration is a challenging procedure and attention to detail is required for surgical success. Of the two, horizontal augmentation is easier to perform, with 3–6 mm gain expected, than the more difficult and challenging 2–4 mm for vertical height [7]. Four wall defect (usually buccal wall missing) can be remedied with autogenous, allograft, or xenograft with membrane coverage [17]. Three wall defect (buccal wall missing and apical bone too narrowed or compromised) requires a combination of autogenous with either allogenic or xenograft, and a membrane with either titanium reinforcement or tenting screws support has been reported with good outcome [17]. Autogenous bone provides "viable" osteoprogenitor cells to the graft site while bone substitute supplies the volume and acts primarily as a scaffold. One to two wall defect will usually require more structural support (i.e., block graft) in order to replace missing walls, with usually lingual/palatal being still intact or compromised (see Box 6.1) [17]. A full arch titanium mesh tray along with 1:1 autogenous bone mixed with xenograft can reconstruct a large defect site [48].

In general, surgical difficulty increases as the number of walls to be reconstructed increases. This is also true for smaller site replacements (1–2 teeth) which would be more predictable than larger site defects (>4 teeth) [6, 17].

Various bone graft materials and membranes are commercially available; therefore, by understanding these biomaterials and the physiology of healing, clinicians can follow the basic principles of GBR and determine which combination of materials best works for them (Table 6.2).

Nonabsorbable Membrane

In general, nonabsorbable membranes require primary closure, unless specified by the manufacturer (e.g., Cytoplast®), and some require tacks or screws to ensure stabilization. Second-stage surgery for removal is often coordinated with implant insertion or healing abutment placement.

Nonabsorbable membranes include the following.

- Titanium mesh.
- Expanded polytetrafluoroethylene (e-PTFE) (e.g., Gore-Tex®).
- Nonexpanded highly dense polytetrafluoroethylene (d-PTFE) (e.g., Cytoplast).
- Titanium-reinforced PTFE (TR e-PTFE, TR d-PTFE).

Titanium Mesh

Titanium mesh has been widely used for surgical applications due to its adaptiveness, rigidity, biocompatibility, and high predictability, which make it a dependable substructure for bony augmentation, especially for moderate to large defects [50]. Macromesh and micromesh are available for the dental market. The key features of titanium mesh are porosity, allowing blood clot stabilization, and tissue ingrowth onto the mesh surface, thus improving stabilization [49, 50]. Additionally, when the mesh is prematurely exposed to the oral environment, graft success is not altered [49, 50]. Micromesh (0.2 mm) is an ideal thickness for flexibility, adaptiveness, and space-making capabilities [49, 50]. Disadvantages include fibrous ingrowth to the macroporous structure, which makes removal of mesh very challenging. Furthermore, fixation screws are required for stabilization. Micromesh design eliminates the adherent fibrous ingrowth associated with macromesh.

e-PTFE [51, 52]

Gore-Tex (e-PTFE) was considered the gold standard among all GBR membranes in the 1990s but is no longer utilized in dentistry primarily because of the difficulty of second-stage removal due to the adherent host–membrane interface and ability for bacterial invasion [6, 49, 50].

Nonexpanded d-PTFE (Osteogenics Biomedical) [6, 49–51, 53]

In 1993, d-PTFE was developed because of the shortcomings related to e-PTFE's properties: bacterial infiltration and adherent tissue ingrowth to the host–membrane interface. Cytoplast (d-PTFE) has unique preventive properties which make it an improved version of its predecessor. These membranes are treated with ethylene oxide for sterilization. The newly designed pore size of less than 0.3 μm prevents bacterial penetration into the graft site, primary closure is not mandatory when not possible, and removal during second-stage surgery is easier because of the nonadherent properties of the host–graft interface. The smaller pore size is impervious to fluid and the graft site is reliant on the host's vascular support through bony

Table 6.2 Membranes commercially available for GBR dental application.

Name of membrane	Types, pores, and/or thickness of membrane	Absorption time	Comments
Nonabsorbable membrane			
Ti-Micromesh (ACE)	Titanium mesh [49, 50] 1700 μm with 0.2 mm thickness	Nonapplicable	0.2 mm ideal thickness
Titanium mesh (KLS Martin)	Micromesh with 0.2 mm thickness	Nonapplicable	
Frios BoneShields (Dentsply)	0.03 mm with 0.1 mm thickness	Nonapplicable	
Tocksystem mesh	0.1–6.5 mm with 0.05–0.1 mm thickness	Nonapplicable	
Gore-Tex (e-PTFE) [51, 52]	Expanded polytetrafluoroethylene (e-PTFE) 0.5–20 μm pore size	Nonapplicable	Discontinued
Cytoplast (d-PTFE) [6, 49–51, 53] Cytoplast (TR d-PTFE) [53, 54]	Nonexpanded highly dense polytetrafluoroethylene (d-PTFE) Titanium-reinforced PTFE (TR d-PTFE) [53, 54] <0.3 μm pore size	Nonapplicable	Bacteria prevention with structural support, ease of removal, flap extender
Gore-Tex (TR e-PTFE) [54]	Titanium-reinforced PTFE (TR e-PTFE) 100–300 μm (outer); <0.8 μm (inner) pore size	Nonapplicable	Discontinued Gore-Tex [51, 52]
Absorbable membrane	*Origin: bovine, porcine, or human*		
BioMend [32]	Bovine – type I	8 wk	Use dry or hydrated
BioMend Extend [32]	Bovine – type I	18 wk	Use dry or hydrated
Bio-Gide [55]	Porcine – type I and III	24 wk	
Ossix Plus [56]	Porcine – type I	16–24 wk	Can tolerate exposure up to 3–5 wk
Alloderm [57]	Human dermis	12–16 wk	Flap extender
Puros Dermis [58]	Human dermis	16–24 wk	GTR, GBR, perio defect and soft tissue augmentation
Puros pericardium [58]	Human pericardium	16–24 wk	GBR, perio defect, block graft coverage, durable
Allo.Protect [59]	Human pericardium	16–24 wk	GBR, perio defect, ridge augmentation, durable
Absorbable membrane	*Origin: synthetic*		
Resolut Adapt [60]	Poly-D,L-lactide/Co-glycolide	20–24 wk	Good space maintainer
Resolut Adapt LT [60]	Poly-D,L-lactide/Co-glycolide	20–24 wk	Good space maintainer
Epi-Guide [61]	Poly-D,L-lactic acid	24–52 wk	
Guidor [62]	Poly-D,L-lactide and Poly-L-lactide	53 wk	Flap extender
Vivosorb [63]	Poly-D,L-lactide, e-caprolactone	104 wk	

GBR, guided bone regeneration; GTR, guided tissue regeneration.

perforations. Disadvantages include the need for stabilization methods (tacks, screw, sutures) and second-stage surgery for removal.

Titanium-reinforced PTFE [51, 54]

There are two classes of titanium-reinforced membranes: TR e-PTFE and TR d-PTFE. Cytoplast (TR d-PTFE) is "stiff" enough to be manipulated by hand and durable enough to prevent spontaneous collapse and regenerate bony defects ranging from single to multiple teeth sites. This membrane should be placed with stabilization methods. Be sure to place the dimple side toward the gingiva for correct positioning. Nonabsorbable monofilament sutures are recommended with two-layer closure [54].

Absorbable Membrane

Two basic types of absorbable membranes are commercially available for GBR: collagen (allogenic and xenograft) and polymer (synthetic) (Table 6.2). Collagen membranes are derived from tendon, dermis, skin, or pericardium from bovine, porcine, or human preparations. These membranes are further divided based on whether or not the collagen has been treated to become cross-linked. Noncross-linked membranes are absorbed more quickly by the host tissue than the cross-linked counterpart, with absorption times for all membranes ranging from 8 weeks to 6 months. Polymeric membranes are synthetically manufactured with the following availability for the dental market: polylactides (PLAs), polyglycolides (PGAs), polycaprolactone (PCL), and copolymers, with the combination of PLA and PGA being predominantly utilized. Advantages of absorbable membranes are that second surgery is not required, and collagen has minimum antigenicity while synthetic collagen is nonimmunogenic. One disadvantage is that most membranes require structural support (tenting screws or bone material) to prevent collapse. The reason for selecting an absorbable membrane is to ensure it outlasts the time required for the bone graft to completely heal.

Collagen Base (Bovine, Porcine, or Human Tendon, Dermis, Skin, or Pericardium)

BioMend® and BioMend Extend™ (Integra Life Sciences Corp.) are made from type I collagen derived from bovine deep flexor (Achilles) tendon. They are both semi-occlusive, enabling vital nutrients to pass through while preventing undesirable tissue (epithelium and connective tissue) from growing inward. BioMend absorbs in 8 weeks and BioMend Extend in 18 weeks. Indications are: (i) guided tissue regeneration (GTR) for periodontal defects, (ii) periimplant bone grafting reconstruction, and (iii) GBR. These products can be used either dry or hydrated and laid over the graft site with or without being sutured to the flap or use of absorbable tack [32].

Bio-Gide® (Geistlich Biomaterials) is derived from non-cross-linked type I and III porcine collagen with a unique bilayer structure. The smooth outer layer serves to prevent tissue ingrowth while the rougher inner porous lining provides a scaffold for osteoprogenitor cells and vascular ingrowth to enhance bone regeneration. Complete absorption occurs in 24 weeks based on animal studies [55].

Ossix® Plus (Datum Dental) is a porcine-derived collagen from a tendinous source that uses Glymatrix® technology, sugar, for cross-linking the membrane. It also has a dual-layer function that permits bony regeneration for up to 4–6 months before undergoing complete absorption. Upon premature exposure, this membrane can resist breakdown for 3–5 weeks [56].

Acellular dermal matrix (ADM) (human dermis, e.g., AlloDerm® regenerative tissue matrix, LifeCell Corp.) is intended for bone graft containment and as a bridge across the flap as an extender for primary closure. It has to be hydrated for 10–40 minutes prior to use. The dermal side has more blood adherence (hydrophilic) whereas the basement side will have a pink appearance (hydrophobic). ADM is a good alternative choice for absorbable membrane if primary closure is not achievable [57].

Puros® Dermis (human dermis) and Puros Processed Pericardium (human pericardium) (Integra) both undergo the unique Tutoplast® process with chemical sterilization and low-dose gamma radiation, resulting in low immunogenicity and leaving a 3-D collagen scaffold. This is indicated for soft tissue augmentation and GTR (dermis type only), periodontal defect repair (dermis and pericardium types), GBR (dermis and pericardium types), and block graft coverage (pericardium type only) [58].

Allo.Protect (human pericardium) (Nobel Biocare) membrane has been processed with antibiotics (polymyxin B and/or bacitracin) and sterilized with gamma radiation with cobalt 60. The membrane maintains a collagen matrix with both durability and adaptiveness. Indications include sinus augmentation, socket preservation, horizontal/vertical augmentation, and periodontal defects [59].

Polymeric Membrane (Manufactured Synthetic Membrane)

Polylactides (PLA), polyglycolides (PGA), polycaprolactone (PCL), and copolymers (combinations of two or more polymers) are examples of polymeric membranes. PLAs and PGAs are biodegradable through hydrolysis which is known to have a negative impact on bone formation because of the inflammatory response it triggers [6]. For these reasons, many clinicians are cautious in using these synthetic membranes. PCL, on the other hand, has not been shown to produce any local inflammatory reaction upon degradation; however, complete absorption takes 2–3 years and it is not applicable as a stand-alone material for GBR [51]. Vicryl®, a blend of PLA and PGA, has shown some promising results when compared to nonabsorbable membranes [50]. Additionally, for horizontal GBR augmentation, the use of synthetic membranes (PLA/PGA) has an equally successful outcome when compared to collagen, PTFE, and titanium mesh [64]. Below is a list of common synthetic membranes used for dental application.

- Vicryl Polyglactin 910 mesh (PLA and PGA) (Ethicon Inc.). This mesh comes in woven or knitted forms and in two sizes (15×15 cm or 30×30 cm). The 910 represents the ratio of 9 polylactide and 1 polyglycolide. It is uncoated and undyed similar to the Vicryl suture composition used commonly in dentistry and surgery. Complete absorption of the mesh can be seen between 8 and 12 weeks [65].

- Resolut Adapt® and Resolut Adapt LT (PLA and PGA) (W.L. Gore and Associates). A good space maintainer made from a combination of PLA and PGA that has an outer layer of randomly oriented fibers with microporous structure for tissue adhesion and stabilization while preventing ingrowth of epithelium. Resolute Adapt retains mechanical strength for 8–10 weeks and the LT version is extended to 16–24 weeks, with both having 5–6 months of complete absorption time [60].
- Epi-Guide® (PLA) (Curasan Inc.). A hydrophilic three-layer synthetic membrane that can be self-supportive without bone graft material. The outer layer allows fibroblast infiltration and cell attachment for stabilization, the middle layer allows collateral circulation while the inner layer aids in uptake of fluid and membrane adhesion to the graft site. Functioning time of Epi-Guide is 20 weeks with complete absorption taking 24–52 weeks [61].
- Guidor® (PLA) (Sunstar Americas, Inc.) is a bilayered synthetic membrane with an external layer that allows gingival and connective tissue ingrowth without further apical migration while the internal layer allows passage of vital nutrients to permeate through the graft site. It comes in two sizes for GBR application: 15 × 20 mm and 20 × 28 mm. The membrane becomes malleable under body temperature and is very adaptable. Primary closure is not necessary if not possible, and the product has 6 weeks of functioning time and complete membrane absorption in 13 months [62].
- Vivosorb® (PLA and PCL) (Polyganics). Vivosorb is a transparent absorbable synthetic membrane with 0.2 mm thickness that comes in four sizes ranging from 20 × 30 mm to 120 × 170 mm. The membrane separates the ingrowth of unwanted tissue and limits the adhesion to its surface. It retains mechanical strength for 10 weeks with complete absorption in 2 years [63].

Tuberosity Harvest Technique (Figures 6.9–6.11, Box 6.5)

Preoperative X-ray shows a good vertical bone source (Figure 6.9). A crestal incision is made from the second molar to the hamular notch with a relaxing incision, if needed, performed in a full-thickness fashion. Cancellous bone can be procured using a trephine bur without violating the sinus membrane (Figures 6.10 and 6.11). Alternatively, a rongeur can be used. Closure is done in a single layer after the harvest site is thoroughly irrigated and all sharp points removed. Complications include bleeding and sinus perforation. Small perforations can be treated conservatively with local measures and sinus precautions whereas those greater than 4 mm will require primary closure with either one or two layers [7].

Guided Bone Regeneration

Surgical Technique for Three Wall Defect (Figures 6.15–6.18)

The technique of GBR entails a full-thickness reflection of the alveolar site. A three wall defect is defined as having a buccal wall missing and an apical wall either missing or compromised. Decortication of the bone is preferred because of increased blood supply and growth factors allowed into the graft site. Allogenic bone graft is placed and shaped to the desired contour of the socket. A nonabsorbable titanium-reinforced membrane secured with fixation screws is placed over the grafted bone and primary closure is achieved. Reentry is performed in 6 months and dental implant insertion is completed with subsequent restoration.

Surgical Technique for Moderate-to-Severe Defect

For moderate-to-severe ridge defects, titanium mesh with a 1:1 ratio of autogenous and deproteinized bovine bone matrix (DBBM) is an option for a staged approach to reconstructing lost horizontal and vertical height [49]. A full-thickness mucoperiosteal flap is made with relaxed oblique incisions to expose the underlying native buccal and palatal

Box 6.5 Autogenous bone source (intraoral) (figure 6.8)

1. *Tuberosity*: if cancellous bone is desired, then maxillary tuberosity can provide up to 2 cc of uncompressed bone (Figures 6.9–6.11)
2. *Symphysis*: up to 5 cc of corticocancellous bone can be harvested through this site with a trephine bur. A 4 mm diameter burr can harvest up to 8–10 mm in length
3. *Lateral ramal shelf*: variable cortical bone amount using bone scrapers (e.g., MX Grafter) (Figure 6.12) or suction traps
4. *Exotosis*: variable cortical bone amount using bone shavings (e.g., MX Grafter) or suction traps
5. *Suction tip with internal suction trap*: various disposable suction traps are available to gather small amounts of bone to augment bank bone (Figures 6.13 and 6.14)

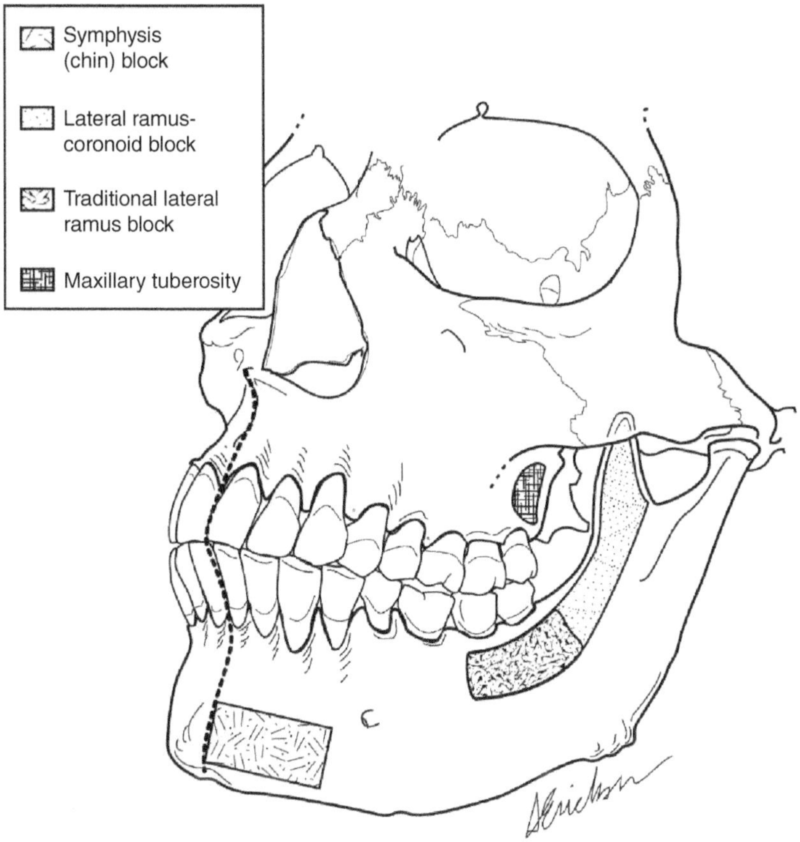

Figure 6.8 Intraoral bone harvest sites.

bone while avoiding the neuromuscular bundle [49]. Next, cortical perforations are made using a round surgical bur to facilitate blood supply from the host. Autogenous particulate bone source can be harvested from, e.g., mandibular symphysis, ramus, maxillary tuberosity, or iliac crest using a direct approach, trephines and/or scrapers. An adapted titanium mesh was performed with a 1:1 ratio of autogenous and DBBM placed inside the tray and fixed to the buccal and palatal bone with fixation screws [49]. Primary closure was performed with postoperative X-ray with and without mesh [49].

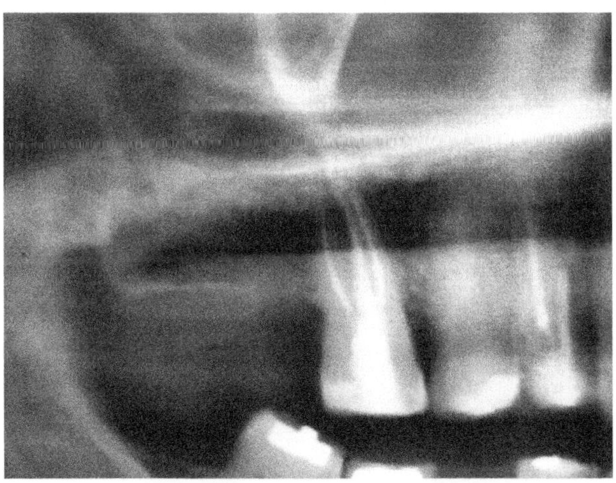

Figure 6.9 X-ray shows available cancellous bone in the maxillary tuberosity in vertical dimension. Note the relationship to the maxillary sinus floor.

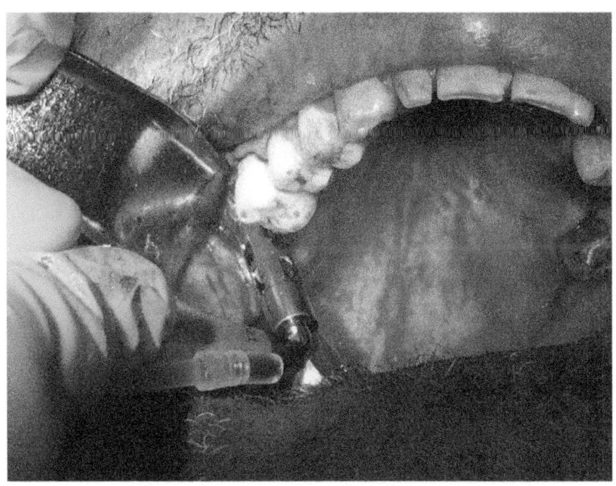

Figure 6.10 Tuberosity harvest technique using a trephine bur.

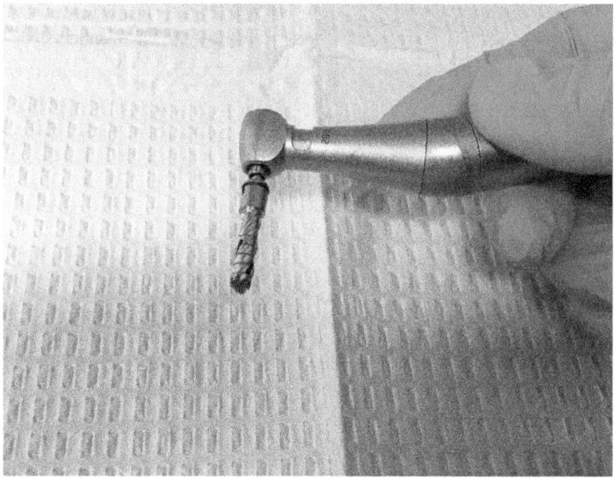

Figure 6.11 Bone collected with a trephine bur.

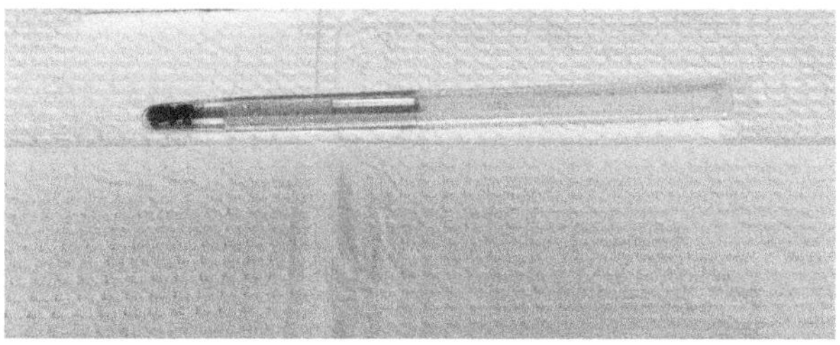

Figure 6.12 Bone scraper used to collect cortical bone.

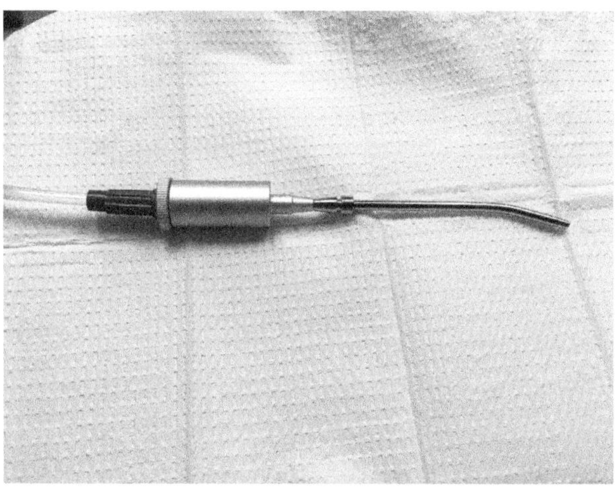

Figure 6.13 Bone-collecting suction with internal suction trap.

Particulate Graft Resorption Post Grafting

The range of horizontal bone resorption with particulate bone (allogenic, xenogeneic, or synthetic source) is from 0.7 ± 0.5 mm to 1.2 ± 0.9 mm with autogenous bone mixed with allograft and xenograft observed over 29.9 ± 30.6 months and 66.5 ± 37.2 months, respectively. There is no significant difference among material groups used. As for vertical bone resorption, 1.1 ± 0.6 mm with autogenous to 1.4 ± 1.0 mm

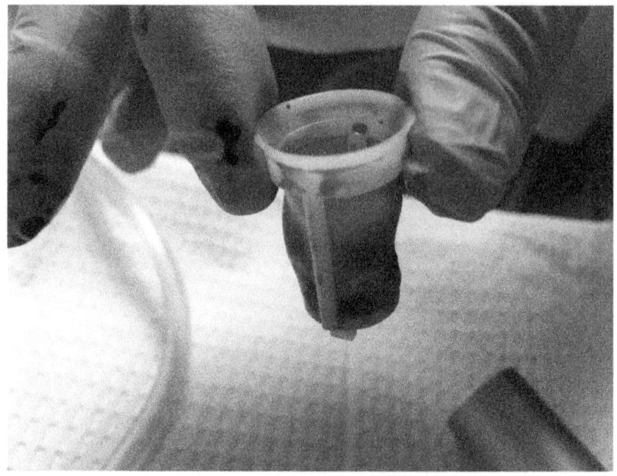

Figure 6.14 Suction trap with bone collected.

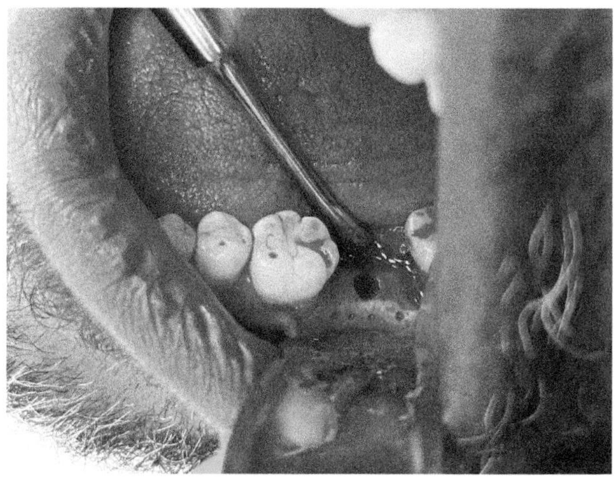

Figure 6.15 Buccal wall is decorticated to allow increased blood supply to the recipient site.

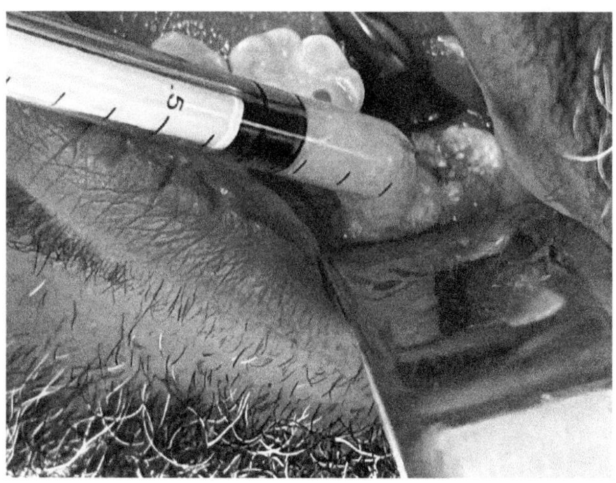

Figure 6.16 Allogeneic bone is placed on the buccal defect.

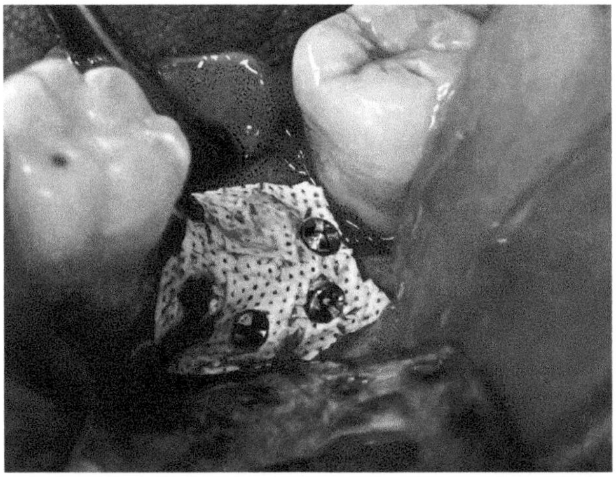

Figure 6.17 A nonabsorbable titanium-reinforced PTFE is placed with fixation screws stabilizing the bone graft.

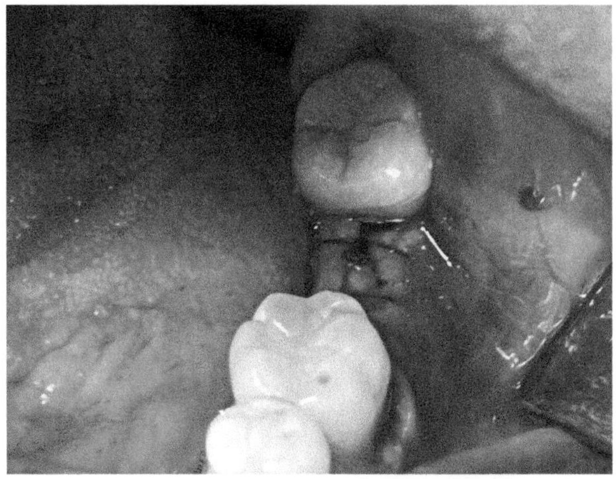

Figure 6.18 Primary closure was possible and obtained.

with allogenic bone has been observed over 28.3 ± 32.8 months and 22.9 ± 21.1 months, respectively. There is no significant difference among the material groups [64].

Guided Bone Regeneration Complications

The main complication associated with use of membranes is mucosal breakdown with possible graft infection. As stated previously, titanium mesh can tolerate premature exposure much better than other types of nonabsorbable and absorbable membrane without altering graft success [47]. When purulent discharge is present, removal of graft and membrane is mandatory regardless of membrane type. However, if late dehiscence is noted, chlorhexidine could be used until second-stage removal [7].

Guided Bone Regeneration Implant Survival and Success Rates

Troelzsch et al. reported that regardless of bone or membrane type, implant survival rate is 96.1–99.4%. Although they do not mention the observed period of implant survival, the bone graft preceding implant placements has been reported to be 9.1–80.8 months. Success rates were not included because of the extensive heterogeneous studies associated with this systematic review [64].

Guided Bone Regeneration Conclusion (Box 6.6)

Overall, GBR has been successfully performed using various bone materials alone or in combination: autogenous, allograft, xenograft, and resorbable allogenic material coupled with absorbable or nonabsorbable membranes. Particulate bone between 100 and 400 μm appears to be the ideal size for graft healing, allowing for better resorption and vascular ingrowth between pores for bone formation [6] while particular cortical bone provides space-making capabilities. Horizontal and vertical GBR augmentation could be performed in a predictable fashion, with a 3.7 mm overall weighted mean average gain in both directions expected [64]. The order of graft success for horizontal component is autogenous mixed with allograft or xenograft with 4.5 ± 1.0 mm > autogenous or allograft or xenograft alone > synthetic bone alone with 2.2 ± 1.2 mm without statistical significance [64] (Figure 6.19).

Box 6.6 Key points for GBR

1. GBR is a successful procedure, with smaller sites being more predictable than larger sites [6]
2. A mixture of autogenous and allograft or xenograft is preferred (1:1 ratio) if a moderate-to-large defect is to be reconstructed [49]
3. Particulate bone size between 100 and 400 μm is ideal for resorption and vascular ingrowth between pores for bone formation [6]
4. Horizontal GBR augmentation is amenable to various bone materials, with synthetic being the most inferior [64]. Mean weighted horizontal gain is 3.7 ± 1.2 mm [55], 3–6 mm horizontal potential gain [7]
5. There is no difference in membrane selection for horizontal augmentation [64]
6. Vertical GBR is more difficult to augment and would require titanium mesh for rigid protection which is more important than the bone materials being used [64]. Although synthetic bone was not included in a systematic review, mean weighted vertical gain is 3.7 ± 1.4 mm [64], 2–4 mm potential vertical gain [7]

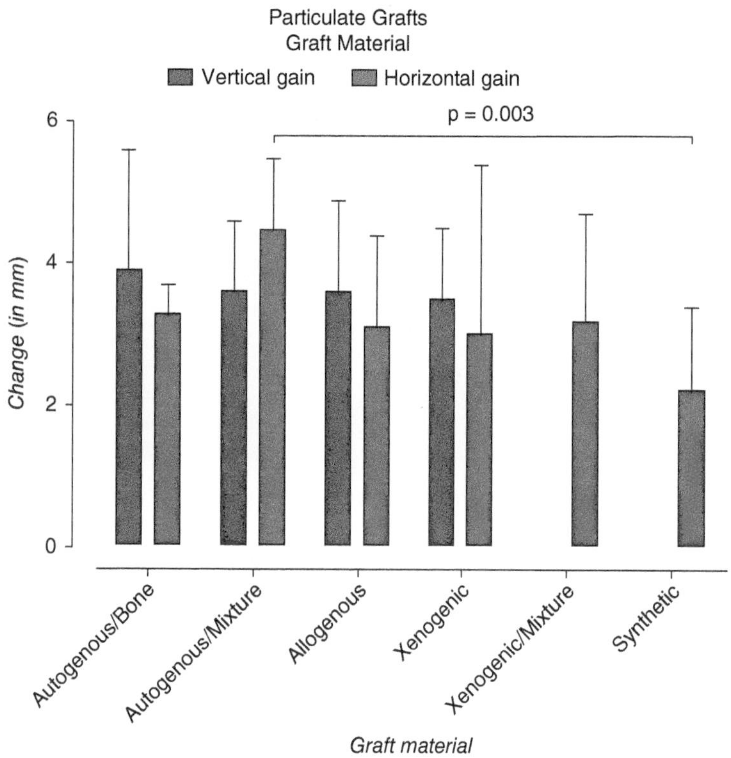

Figure 6.19 Particulate material: horizontal/vertical augmentation gains. *Source:* Troelzsch M, et al., 2016/With permission of Elsevier.

Based on Troeltzsch's findings, the author believes the best overall choice for horizontal bone augmentation is to use either allograft or xenograft material with the least amount of resorption (0.7 mm) without incurring a second surgical site. As for vertical augmentation, there is very little difference among materials tested, with all bone graft materials having similar gains: particulate autogenous mandibular bone reported at 3.9 ± 1.7 mm > autogenous/allograft/xenograft alone > autogenous with either allogenic or xenograft preparation at 3.6 ± 1.0 mm. Unfortunately, synthetic bone was not included in the vertical augmentation [64] (Figure 6.19). The author believes the best overall choice for vertical bone augmentation is using either allograft or xenograft with bone gain and resorption ratio relatively similar to other materials based on Troeltzsch's findings.

As for membrane selection, there is no significant difference for horizontal augmentation when compared among all membranes tested: collagen, PTFE, PLA/PGA, and titanium [64] (Figure 6.20). However, titanium mesh is the superior choice for vertical augmentation (6.0 ± 2.3 mm) owing to its rigid structure and graft protection when compared to others, despite having the highest overall complications [64] (Figure 6.20).

Generally speaking, smaller ridge augmentation sites enjoy a higher degree of success and can be treated with "bone off the shelf" such as allogenic, xenograft, or resorbable alloplastic materials [64]. Moderate-to-large defects will require autogenous bone mixed with allogenic or xenograft usually in a 1:1 ratio to achieve successful results [49]. The osteogenic potential from the autograft provides the live cells while bone substitutes act to increase volume and as a scaffold for eventual bone regeneration. This is very technique sensitive and should be reserved for experienced clinicians [6]. For those who are not ready for this reconstructive challenge, Esposito et al. have reported short implants to be a better alternative than vertical augmentation [referenced in 66].

Intraoral Onlay Graft

Indications (Particulate and Block Graft)

Whether the alveolus ridge lacks width and/or height, onlay grafts can be used to augment these deficiencies. Three to four wall defects with an inferior stop can be remedied with particulate onlay graft [7]. Lateral ridge augmentation using subperiosteal tunneling technique is amenable for correction of less than 4 mm width associated with saddle deformity [66] (Figure 6.21). For one to two wall defects, block grafts are needed for rigidity support for single to multiple compromised sites. The amount of bone that can be generated predictably for horizontal and vertical augmentation is

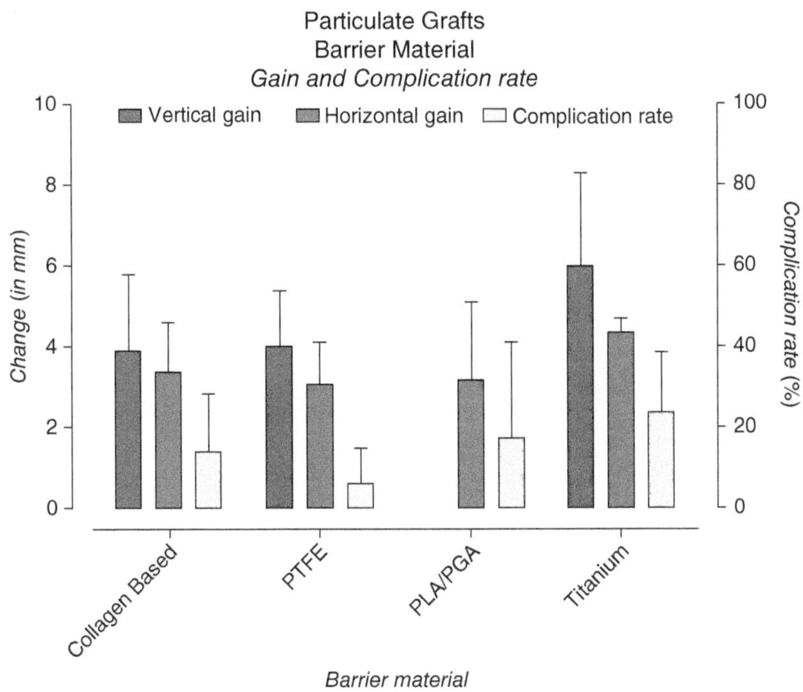

Figure 6.20 Particulate materials: barrier material – gain and complication rates. *Source:* Troelzsch M, et al., 2016/With permission of Elsevier.

3–4 mm from mandibular shelf and 4–6 mm from chin harvest respectively [7]. Allogenic and xenogeneic sources are alternatives to autogenous blocks.

Subperiosteal Tunneling Technique with Absorbable Membrane

After infiltrating with local anesthesia, a vertical incision is made one tooth mesial to the anticipated grafted site down to bone. A subperiosteal dissection is made with a periosteal elevator to help "tunnel" the necessary length to secure the graft area (Figure 6.22). In addition, the dissection is carried over to the lingual side subperiosteally 1–2 mm so the grafted bone can extend to the native bone. An absorbable collagen membrane is placed into the tunnel followed by bone graft material (Figure 6.23). Closure is done with chromic gut suture with healing in 4–6 months (Figure 6.24).

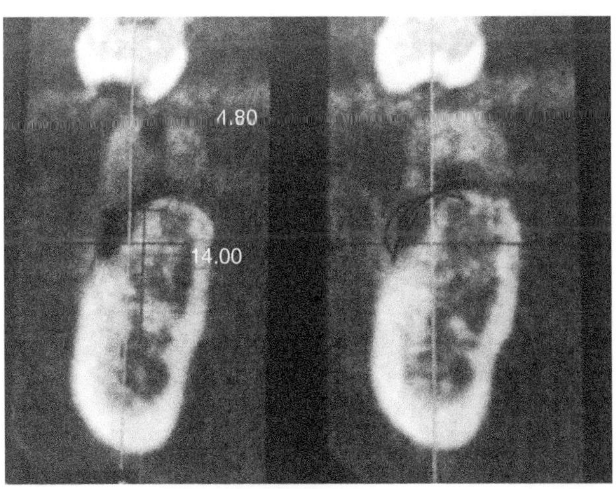

Figure 6.21 Saddle deformity with inferior stop. The buccal defect is shown with an outline.

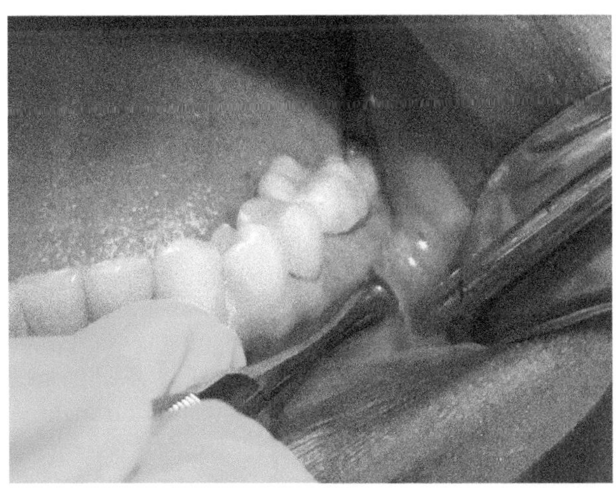

Figure 6.22 A subperiosteal dissection is performed to create a "tunnel" by using a periosteal elevator.

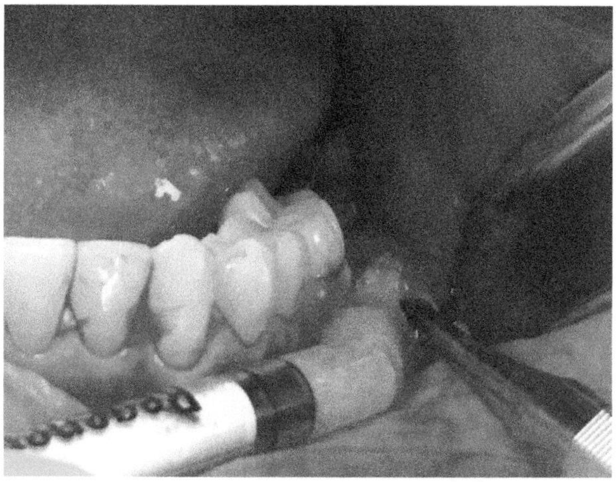

Figure 6.23 Bone graft material is inserted between the absorbable collagen membrane and the saddle deformity.

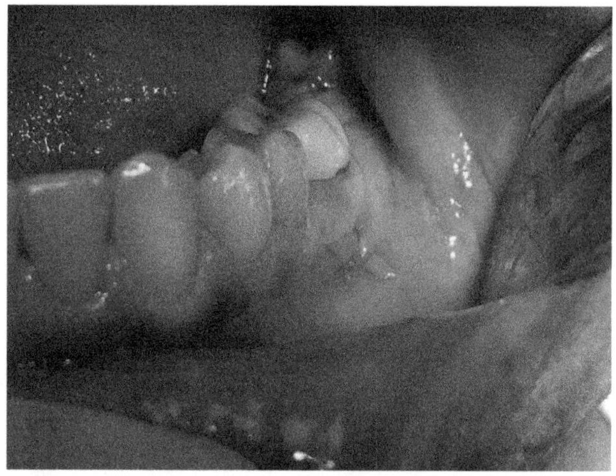

Figure 6.24 Closure is performed with simple interrupted chromic gut suture.

Autogenous Onlay Corticocancellous Grafts Healing

Two types of bone are responsible for the make-up of the human skeleton: intramembranous (skull, facial bones, clavicle) and endochondral (all other long bones). Corticocancellous bone of the jaw has dual properties, making onlay grafts an attractive option for alveolar reconstruction. The cancellous portion has the ability to revascularize faster owing to its porous characteristic while the thicker cortical component can withstand some resorption during physiologic healing. Block graft heals through a process called "creeping substitution" where osteoclasts pave the way for vascular ingrowth by resorbing the recipient bone before new osteoids (collagen matrix) are laid down by osteoblasts. These new osteoids will undergo mineralization and remodeling until complete graft incorporation which can be expected in 4–6 months.

Surgical Harvest Technique: Intraoral Lateral Ramal Shelf and Symphysis (Figure 6.8)

Lateral ramus and chin are two intraoral sites available to procure monocortical block grafts for horizontal and vertical ridge augmentation. Lateral ramus can provide up to 15 × 30 mm and chin 10 × 30 mm. If a larger amount of corticocancellous block graft is required, lateral ramus osteotomy can be extended to the sigmoid notch, creating a ramus-coronoid graft unit [7]. For the lateral ramus approach, a 45° hockey stick incision is used, similar to a mandibular third molar approach, with sulcular incision extending to the first molar region to expose the underlying lateral ramus and external oblique ridge.

Using a piezoelectric handpiece, start the outline 5 mm medial from the lateral cortex and make the osteotomy on the crestal alveolar ridge up to 30 mm in an anterior–posterior direction. For dentate patients, stay at least 2 mm away from the molars for this crestal osteotomy. Two separate vertical osteotomies are made just into bleeding bone on the lateral aspect connecting with the original osteotomy (Figure 6.25). An inferior cut is made in an incomplete

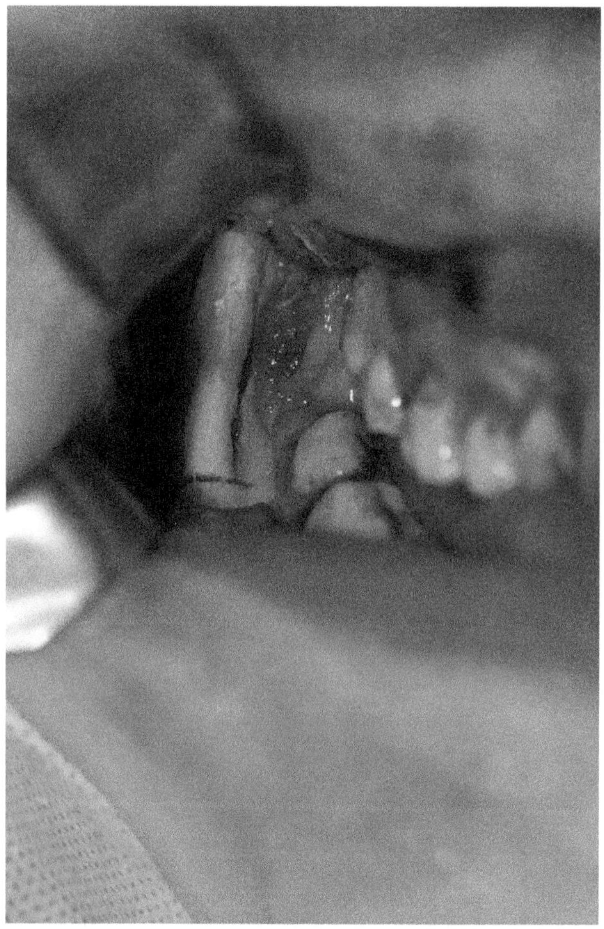

Figure 6.25 Superior view of the lateral ramus osteotomy outline. Note cuts are made down to the bleeding bone.

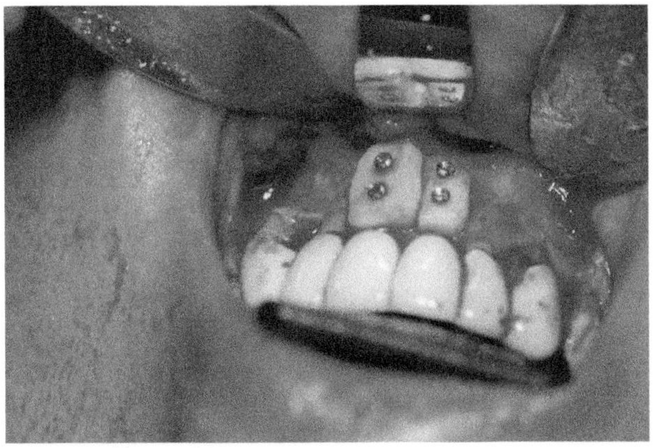

Figure 6.26 Block grafts are each secured with two fixation screws to prevent rotation.

fashion with at least 4 mm above the inferior alveolar neurovascular bundle. Graft is harvested using a small chisel with proper chin support and secured with two screws to prevent rotational movement (Figure 6.26). The addition of a particulate bone substitute and membrane to the block graft can reduce resorption by 0.25 mm or 5.5% [67, 68]. Hemostatic agent (bone wax) is usually placed in the harvest site before closure (Figures 6.27 and 6.28).

Symphyseal harvest can be performed with either sulcular or vestibular incision, with the sulcular approach reserved for patients with thick gingival biotype and sound periodontal conditions. This incision starts on the labial aspect of the lower anterior teeth with careful attention paid to preserving the mental nerves during the bilateral vertical releasing incision in the premolar region. Full-thickness dissection down to the symphysis should be performed. A vestibular incision is the alternative approach which is made 1 cm below the mucogingival line from the parasymphysis to the contralateral parasymphysis region in full-thickness fashion.

To avoid vital structures and harvest morbidity, the maximum outline of the osteotomy must be at least 5 mm from the apex of the lower teeth, 5 mm from the inferior border of the mandible, 5 mm anterior to the mental nerves and 5–6 mm in thickness. Again, an osteotomy can be used to outline the desired graft size and not to encroach on the above parameters, with graft harvest performed with a small chisel in the aforementioned manner. If there is a prominent bony midline protuberance, two separate block grafts can be removed on either side. Closure of the mentalis muscle and mucosa should be done in two separate layers and suspension tape placed to prevent postoperative chin ptosis or "witch's chin" [69] (Figure 6.29a–d).

Decorticating the recipient site will enhance blood supply between the graft–host interface. Harvested graft is shaped to the recipient site and fixated. Immobilization and primary closure are critical components to graft success because any disruption will significantly decrease the chance of integration. Generally, grafted sites can be reentered for implant insertion in 4 months (maxilla) and 6 months (mandible).

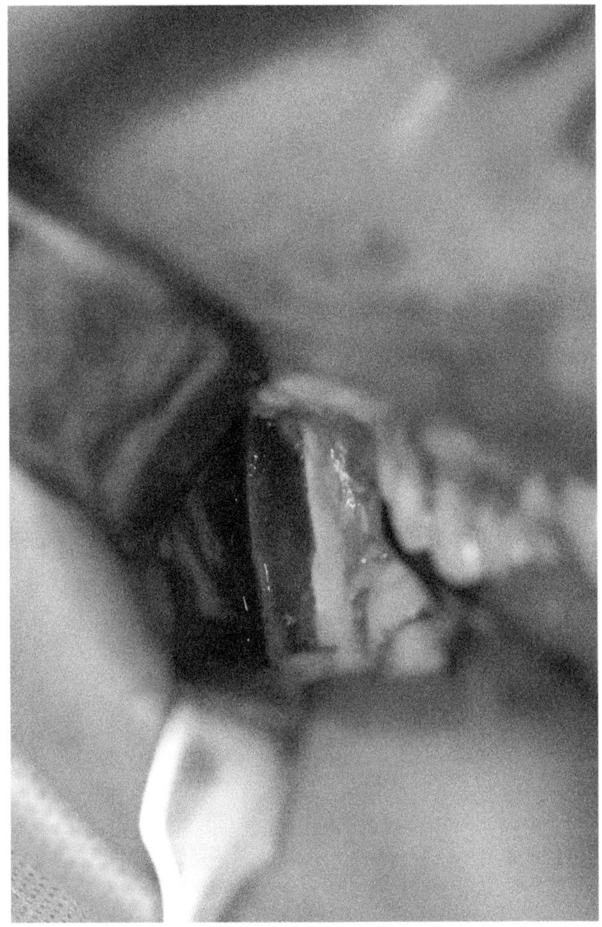

Figure 6.27 Hemostatic agent (i.e. bone wax) can be used to aid hemostasis.

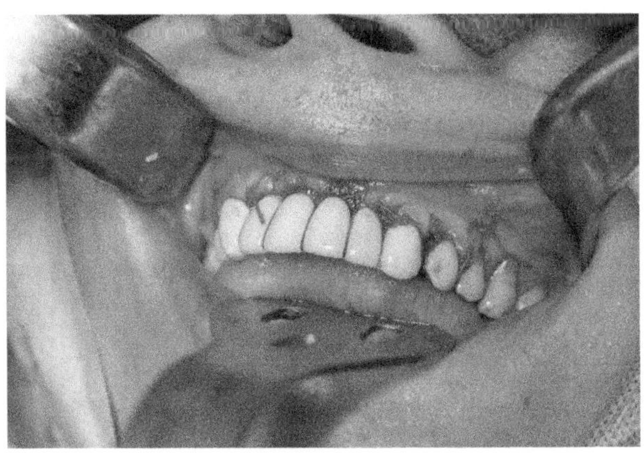

Figure 6.28 Surgical site is closed with chromic gut sutures.

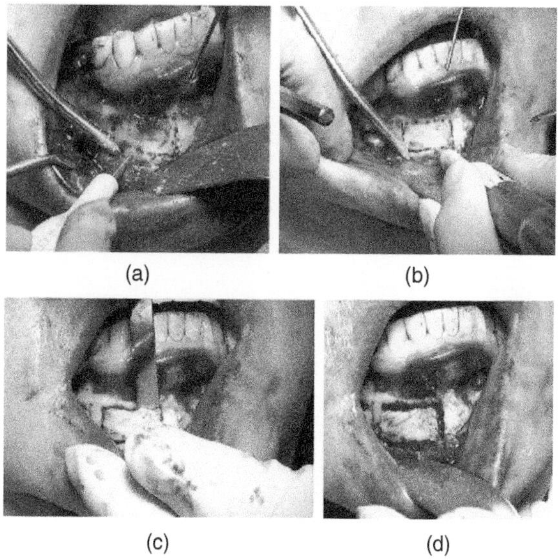

Figure 6.29 Osteotomies to outline the harvest are created with a small round bur and then fissure bur (a, b). A thin chisel is then used to complete the harvest (c, d). *Source:* Previously published with permission.

Autogenous Intraoral Block Grafts – Surgical Complications

Block graft harvest is relatively safe with few morbidities. Temporary paresthesia is one of the main complications associated with intraoral graft harvest, with chin harvest having a higher occurrence (10–50%) than lateral ramus (0–5%) [67]. Permanent paresthesia with symphysis approach has also been reported at 13–52% and lateral ramal harvest with 3–8.3% [70–72]. Other complications such as pain, swelling, infection, bleeding, devitalization of lower and molar teeth, dehiscence, trismus, and jaw fracture have also been implicated with this procedure. Overall, lateral ramus has less morbidity than chin owing largely to diminished paresthesia and pain experienced by patients.

Allogeneic Block Bone (Cadaver Bone)

Puros is an alternative to autogenous harvest used for alveolar reconstruction. The obvious advantages are lack of donor site morbidity and abundant supply. Sizes available for intraoral application are 10 and 15 mm (Figure 6.30). After 5–6 months of osteoconductive healing, implants can be placed into a grafted site with primary stability [69]. Multicenter studies have reported >90% success rate with the Puros block allograft technique, making it a viable alternative for horizontal alveolar reconstruction [73–75]. A systematic review reported by Troelzsch et al. has shown a mean gain of 4.6 mm for horizontal and 2.9 mm for vertical with 13% and 25% complications, respectively [64].

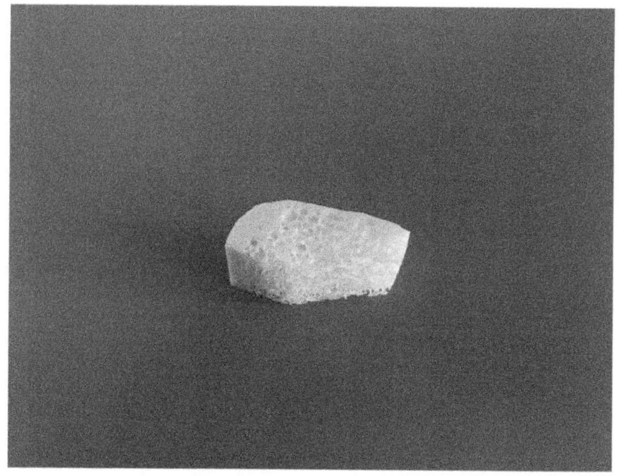

Figure 6.30 Allogeneic block graft.

Block Graft Implant Survival and Success Rate

In 2015, a literature review by Aloy-Prosper et al. concluded that overall lateral and vertical onlay augmentations had similar survival and success rates for implant osseointegration. Lateral augmentation enjoyed a 96.9–100% implant survival rate regardless of bone grafting technique used (block graft or GBR) within a 2-year period. However, results for vertical bone augmentation were slightly less (89.5–100%), in favor of the control group (distraction osteogenesis and short implants). The authors attributed the lower success rate to soft tissue pressure placed on vertical bone grafts causing a higher chance of resorption [67].

Montamedian et al. performed a systematic review for implant survival and success between autogenous and allogenic block bone and found 73.8–100% and 72.8–100%, respectively. Even though good success is reported widely for both techniques, a conclusion cannot be reached due to lack of controlled clinical trials in their systematic review, with long-term study still needed [76].

Block Graft Conclusion (Box 6.7)

Onlay block graft is a good technique for those who desire horizontal and vertical augmentation in a predictable fashion. For horizontal gain, there is no difference between iliac, calvarium, mandible, allogenic, and xenograft block graft, with an overall weighted mean of 4.5 ± 1.2 mm gain [64]. The decision to harvest for a second donor site should be discussed with the patient and most would harvest from the mandibular ramus on the ipsilateral side if needed, owing to lower morbidity compared to chin harvest. Tension-free primary closure along with particulate bone with membrane to the onlay graft has a higher success rate than block graft alone [67, 68]. While complications are the lowest with extraoral autogenous block graft

Box 6.7 Key points for intraoral onlay graft (particulate and block graft)

1. Particulate onlay graft can augment horizontally 1–4 mm. Best used for saddle depression with good apical stop and adequate lingual/palatal height, or exposed buccal threads. Time to implant placement is 3–4 months [7]
2. Autogenous ramus onlay block graft can augment horizontally and vertically 3–4 mm with fixation screws required for graft stabilization. Time to implant placement is 4–6 months [7]. Complications are lower with ramus harvest than chin [64]
3. Autogenous symphyseal onlay block graft can augment horizontally and vertically 4–6 mm. Time to implant placement is 4–6 months [7]
4. Allogeneic block graft can be an alternative to autogenous with mean weighted average gain for horizontal (4.6 mm) and vertical augmentation (2.9 mm) [64]. Highest complication is associated with vertical augmentation at 25% [64]
5. For horizontal gain using block grafts, there is no difference between block grafts (iliac, calvarium, mandibular, allogenic, or xenograft) with an overall mean weighted average of 4.5 ± 1.2 mm gain [64]. The addition of particulate bone with membrane can decrease block graft resorption [67, 68]
6. For vertical augmentation using block grafts, the best overall result is from hip or cranium (9.4 ± 3.1 mm) with statistical difference with overall mean average gain of 5.8 ± 2.8 mm among all graft materials. Complications are also higher with vertical augmentation, ranging from 14.4% (autogenous intraoral), with allogenic having the highest at 25% [64]

and highest with allogenic bone, the inverse is true with resorption [58].

For vertical augmentation, the best overall block graft comes from hip or cranium with statistical difference noted. This is followed by intraoral mandibular then allogeneic graft with an overall weighted mean of 5.8 ± 2.8 mm. Allogeneic grafts had the highest complication rate at 25% while mandibular graft was reported to be the lowest at 14.4% [64]. The pattern of resorption has been noted after 1–2 years with presumptive mucosal pressure as the cause of this phenomenon [67].

Ridge Split

Indications

Alveolar ridge split technique can only help to increase horizontal dimension to accept future implants and requires sufficient basal bone length, typically more than 10 mm from vital structures (inferior alveolar nerve or sinus cavities) [77]. The minimum crestal bone thickness should be 3 mm with at least 1 mm of cancellous bone in between two cortical plates where the osteotomy could be made. Ridge split can be performed either staged or with simultaneous implant placement along with various bone materials (autogenous, allogenic, xenograft, and alloplastic) with good success [77, 78]. Typically, maxilla is amenable to a one-stage approach [78] while mandible usually requires a two-stage approach because of the inelastic buccal cortices which make it susceptible to fracture [79]. Three to six months are needed for a staged approach before reentry for implant placement, with an average of 2–5 mm of horizontal gain expected [7, 77, 79, 80].

Advantages of the ridge split technique include no donor site morbidity or fixation required, and shorter time to completion of restoration (4 months) when simultaneous implant is performed for the maxillary arch [80]. Disadvantages include buccal plate fracture and the inability to lengthen height or correct a severely concave ridge [79].

Ridge Split Surgical Technique

A crestal incision is made with bilateral vertical releasing incisions on the buccal aspect in full-thickness manner to the defect site. A crestal osteotomy is then made with equal distance between the buccal and lingual cortices down to a depth of 10 mm and staying at least 1 mm away from neighboring teeth for the vertical osteotomies. A ridge expansion chisel is used to gently outfracture this segment to the desired width (Figure 6.31). Placement of grafting material in between the two cortices is performed (Figure 6.32). Graft healing is reliant on the lingual/palatal flap so maintenance of this blood supply is paramount for its success. For those who use the split-thickness flap apical to the mucogingival junction, a buccal flap can provide blood supply as well. Membrane coverage can be used as an extender if primary closure is unachievable (Figure 6.33).

Ridge Split Complications

The main complication associated with this technique is buccal plate fracture, followed by mild infection and temporary graft exposure, collectively cited at 14%. The

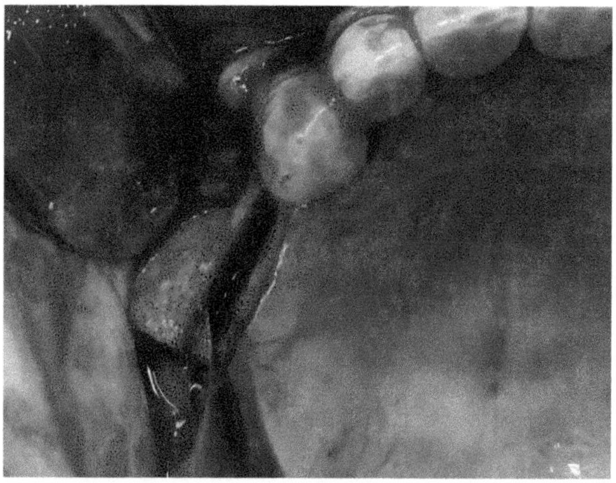

Figure 6.31 A chisel is used to gently outfracture the bony segment.

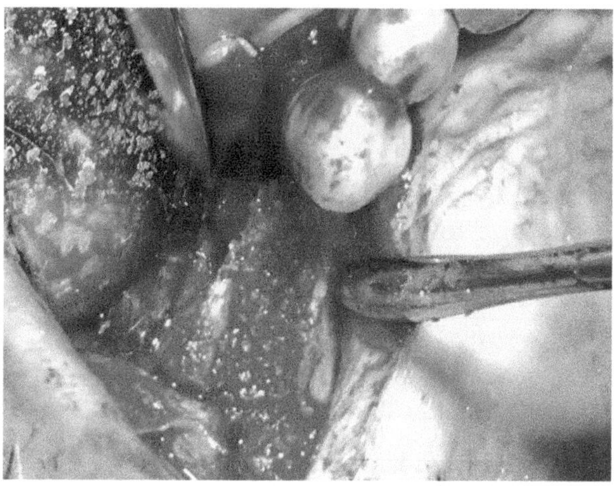

Figure 6.32 Bone graft material is placed into the ridge split site.

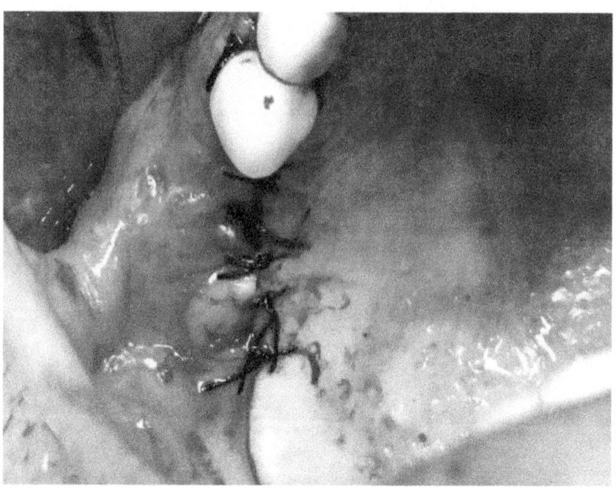

Figure 6.33 Primary closure is achieved.

incidence of a bad buccal plate split has been reported at 7.1%, in agreement with 6.8% reported by Milinkovic and Cordaro [81]. Large fractures require immediate fixation for corrective measures [7]. With a small bad split, the author has converted a buccal plate fracture into a GBR with tenting screws and nonabsorbable titanium-reinforced membrane for lateral augmentation as a salvage maneuver. In a comparative study between ridge split and autogenous onlay graft, the former had fewer significant complications, shortened surgical time, no donor site morbidity, and comparable success rate to onlay graft.

None of the above complications affects the eventual implant insertion and success rates [82].

Ridge Split Implant Survival and Success Rates

Simultaneous implant placement with ridge split survival rate has been reported to be 91.7–100% while the success rate was 88.2–100% during an observed 1–10-year period [81]. This is comparable to implants placed in pristine bone and with or without a GBR technique. The above data was based on 18 human and six animal studies in a systematic review which was regarded to have a high risk of bias. Furthermore, the lack of inclusion of randomized control groups and various implant success criteria which were used to interpret these results made this heterogeneous [83]. However, despite these limitations, ridge split with simultaneous implants does have a high degree of success. Future randomized trials with larger subject groups will be needed to truly assess the efficacy of this technique vs implants placed in either pristine bone or staged GBR.

Ridge Split Conclusion (Box 6.8)

Ridge split technique is an alternative to the established block graft and GBR for correction of horizontal deficiencies with 2–5 mm (average 3 mm) of expected gain [7, 77, 79, 80]. Block grafts have been used extensively to augment these deficiencies but at the expense of an additional harvest site with donor site morbidity. Additionally, fixation screws are required for graft security.

Ridge split can be performed as a staged procedure or simultaneously with implant placement which can reduce overall treatment time. Moreover, ridge split with bone graft and membrane showed significantly less post-graft bone resorption than ridge split alone [78]. Lastly, graft success is comparable to block grafts and GBR techniques [82].

Box 6.8 Key points for ridge split

1. Minimum of 3 mm width with at least 1 mm of cancellous bone in between the cortices [76]
2. Minimal of >10 mm vertical height to vital structures (i.e. inferior alveolar nerve and sinus cavities) [77]
3. 2–5 mm (average 3 mm) of horizontal gain can be expected [7, 77, 79, 80]
4. Cannot correct severe concave alveolar ridge (sagittal view) [77]
5. Can be done simultaneously with implant placement to shorten overall treatment time with prosthetics approximately 4 months for maxilla [82]
6. Mandible is usually treated as a staged approach because of thickness of the buccal plate and higher incidence of fracture [77]
7. Buccal plate fracture is the most common, with mean incidence of 6.8% [81]
8. Ridge split success is comparable to block graft and GBR [82]
9. Time to implant placement is 3–6 months [7]

Interpositional Bone Graft or "Sandwich Osteotomy"

Indications

The use of interposition bone graft or "sandwich osteotomy" is a good option for vertical bone augmentation, especially for the anterior maxilla or posterior mandible where most resorptions are associated with trauma, periodontal disease or tooth extraction(s) and long-term denture-bearing patients [84, 85]. Periodically, clinicians will have to reconstruct the anterior maxilla (1–4 teeth span) prior to implant placement. Augmenting the resorbed site enables the restorative dentist to convert a potential long clinical crown to a more favorable one, creating better esthetic results. Disuse atrophy and constant pressure from the denture can also result in severe bone loss in the posterior mandible, especially for the bilateral distal extension partial denture group.

In 2006, Jensen et al. described two techniques to help correct such deficiencies. Maximum vertical lengthening was limited to 5 mm for the anterior maxilla and 8 mm for the posterior mandible due to the allowable lingual/palatal soft tissue stretch. Blood supply may be compromised if these parameters are exceeded [85]. Anatomic requirement of 4–5 mm of native bone from the maxillary/nasal sinus cavity and inferior alveolar canal is required for safe osteotomies [7]. Second-stage surgery is sometimes required for hardware removal, and additional cost for materials is one of the negatives for this procedure.

Interpositional Bone Graft Surgical Technique

A vestibular incision is made in a full-thickness fashion to gain access to the desired site on the buccal aspect. The reason for this flap design is preservation of the lingual/palatal gingival tissue which is an important source of blood supply. For maxilla, a horizontal osteotomy is made with a piezotome handpiece at least 2 mm away from the sinus floor and with vertical osteotomies joining the horizontal segment. The movable "transport segment" is raised vertically with grafting materials placed in between. A combination of cortical, cancellous, and/or corticocancellous material such as autogenous, allograft, and xenograft can be used [7, 64, 85]. Jensen's technique utilized autogenous ramal graft and particulate material and in most cases did not use fixation devices to secure the graft and relied on tissue closure instead[85].

The mandibular segment is performed in the same manner with particular attention paid to staying at least 2 mm away from the inferior alveolar while identifying the mental nerve [84]. Again, it is vital not to cut through the lingual mucosa to maintain the blood supply (Figure 6.34). Autogenous graft harvest should be slightly larger than the anticipated graft site to allow for trimming and proper

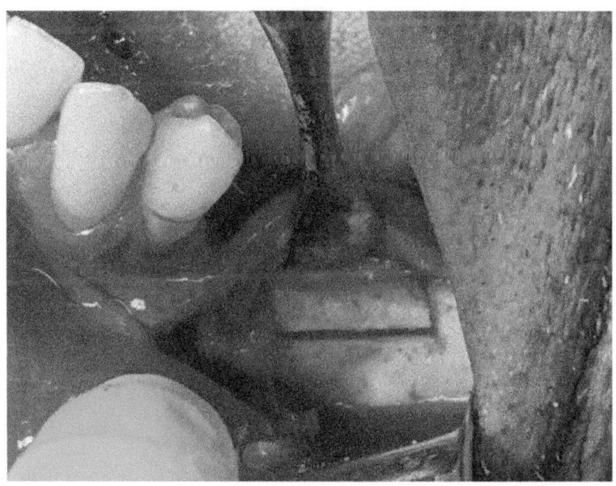

Figure 6.34 Sandwich osteotomy with mesial, distal, and inferior cuts. Preservation of lingual mucosa is very important. Additionally, stay at least 2 mm away from the mental and inferior alveolar nerves during the osteotomies.

contour (Figure 6.35). The autogenous bone is placed between the transported segment superiorly and the stationary native bone (Figure 6.36). Additional allogeneic grafting material is placed and the graft is secured with nonabsorbable titanium-reinforced membrane and fixation screws (Figure 6.37).

Primary closure is performed at the vestibular incision site (Figure 6.38). Alternatively, the corticocancellous autogenous block graft can be rigidly fixated with 1.2–1.5 mm monocortical screws. This is to prevent movement during graft healing and helps maintain vertical height. Average gains of 3–6 mm for the maxilla and 6 mm for mandible were reported with time to implant placement in approximately 3–4 months [84, 85].

Interpositional Bone Graft Complications

Complications with surgical site preparation have been associated with sinus perforation, violation of the inferior alveolar canal, and excessive stretching of the soft tissue which may compromise blood supply, resulting in potential loss of graft. Autogenous bone (ramus/symphysis) had a 7.8% complication rate while xenograft recorded the highest with 43.5% [64]. Bone resorption ranged from 0.5 to 2.3 mm without statistical difference [64].

Interpositional Bone Graft Implant Survival and Success Rates

Implant survival rates have been reported to be 92.5–100% without significant differences among all grafting materials used [64].

Interpositional Bone Graft Conclusion (Box 6.9)

Interpositional bone graft is an excellent technique to augment the resorbed maxilla and mandible in a vertical fashion as an alternative to onlay block or distraction osteogenesis. Periimplant site development is enhanced, especially in the esthetic zone. Troeltzsch et al. reported a mean gain of 4.4 mm with an intraoral autogenous source, with a range of 2.2 mm (allogenic) to 8.6 mm (iliac crest) [64]. This is in agreement with Jensen's findings (3–6 mm) for autogenous block and mineralized allograft combination [85]. One benefit of this technique is believed to be that "sandwiched" bone receives a better blood supply

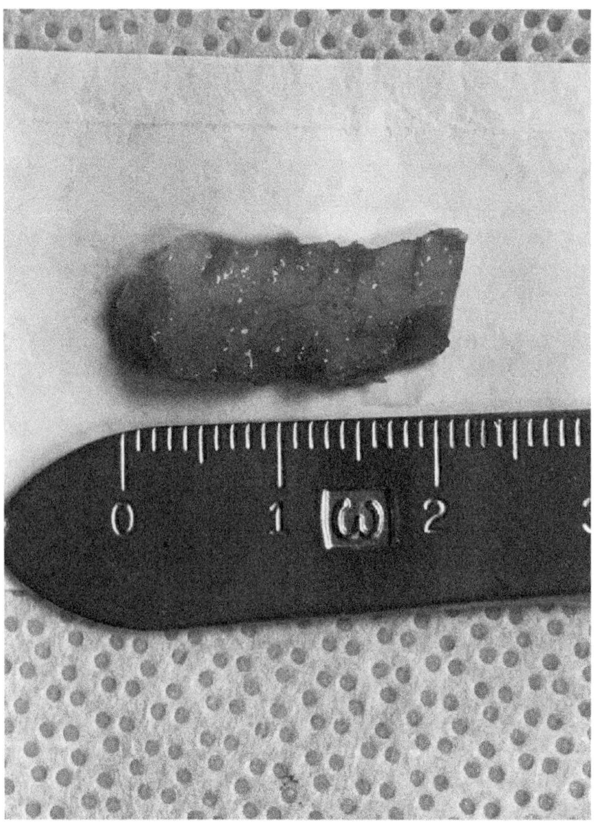

Figure 6.35 The size of the autogenous bone harvest should be slightly larger than the recipient site to allow for reshaping and adaptation.

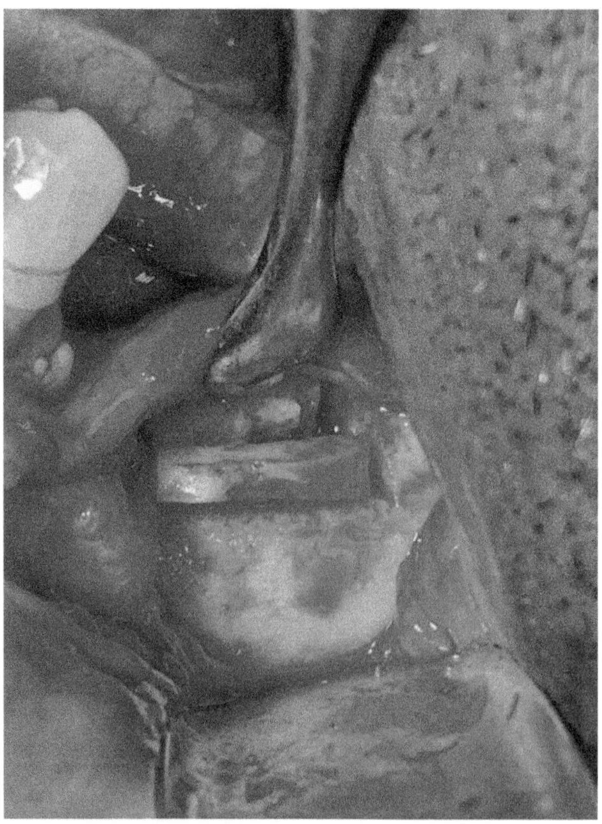

Figure 6.36 Autogenous bone placed between the previously prepared osteotomies.

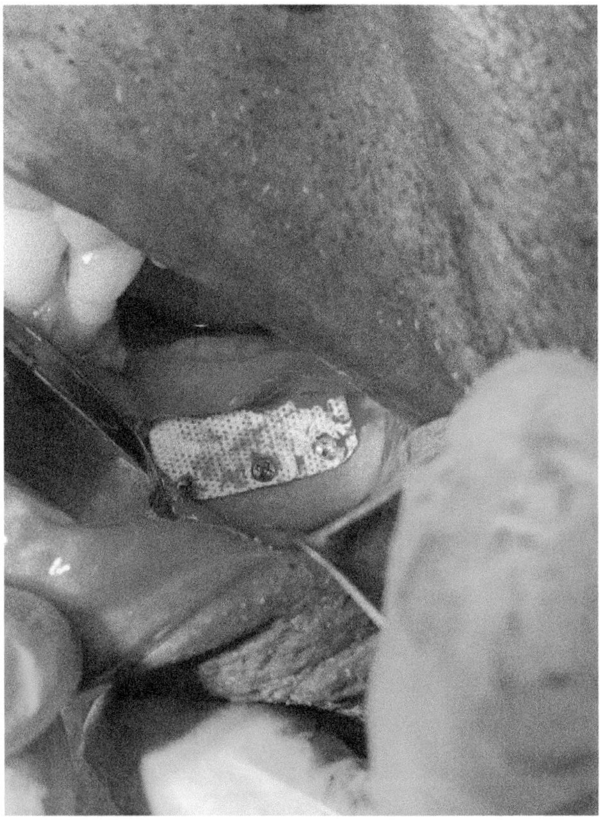

Figure 6.37 Additional allogeneic bone was added to the graft and secured with titanium-reinforced nonabsorbable membrane with fixation screws.

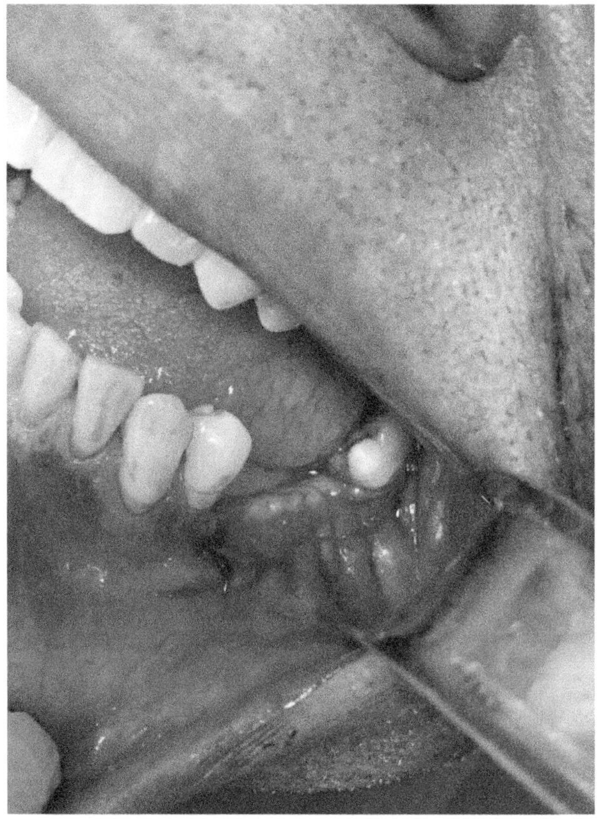

Figure 6.38 Primary closure achieved at the vestibular incision site.

from superior and inferior segments, surrounding periosteum and lingual/palatal tissue, resulting in less bone resorption when compared to onlay graft technique [86].

Distraction Osteogenesis

Indications

Distraction osteogenesis is a useful technique to increase concurrent moderate-to-severe alveolar hard and soft tissue deficiencies. Other maxillofacial applications include congenital birth defects (Pierre Robin syndrome, Treacher Collins syndrome, Goldenhar Syndrome, and hemifacial microsomia), and maxillary and mandibular hypoplasia. Devices are based on the vectors they can provide: vertical, horizontal, or bidirectional. These are further divided into intraosseous or extraosseous devices [87] (Table 6.3). An extraosseous vertical distractor for the alveolar ridge will be discussed here.

Four phases are identified with distraction osteogenesis (Box 6.10) [87]. After an intentional "osteotomy" is made,

Box 6.9 Key points for interpositional bone graft

1. Minimal native bone requirement is 4–5 mm from vital structures (maxillary/nasal sinus cavity and inferior alveolar nerve) [7]
2. Lingual/palatal tissue stretch of 5–8 mm (anterior and posterior region, respectively) limits the amount of vertical augmentation [85]
3. Potential gain is 3–6 mm for maxilla and 6 mm for mandible [84, 85]
4. Blood supply is from lingual/palatal flap, osteotomy segments, and periosteum [84, 85]
5. Autogenous (block) and alloplastic (cancellous) have predictable outcome and minimal bone resorption when implants are placed and loaded in a timely manner [84]
6. Rigid fixation may be needed in the majority of cases to stabilize the graft, with second-stage surgery for hardware removal [7, 84, 85]
7. Time to implant placement for maxilla is 4 months and mandible is 3–4 months [85]

Table 6.3 The spectrum of alveolar distraction systems.

Device	Manufacturer	Special feature
Vertical distraction Intra-osseous		
LEAD system	Stryker Leibinger, Germany	
ACE osteogenic distractor	ACE Surgical, USA	
Groningen Device Distractor (GDD)	KLS Martin, Germany	
Compact Alveolar Distractor (CAD)	Plan 1 Health Villanova, Italy	
Maastricht distraction screw	Medicon, Germany	
Mainz distractor	Medicon, Germany	
Extra-osseous		
TRACK system	KLS Martin, Germany	Variety of designs for different indications
Alveolar distractor	Synthes, Switzerland	Vector control mechanism
Modus	Medartis AG, Switzerland	Individual fixation of device component Vector control mechanism
Verona	Medicon, German	
Vertical distraction	Walter Lorenz, USA	Can be used with resorbable plate
Alveolar distractor device	CIBEI Medical, China	
Tooth-borne		
Multi-dimensional (Watzek et al.)	Prototype	Multi-dimensional
ROD-5	Oral Osteodistraction, USA	
Transverse distraction		
Crest widener	Surgi-Tec, Belgium	
Alveo-wider	OKD, Japan	Malleable mesh and screws
Horizontal alveolar distraction	KLS Martin, Germany	Single plate and screws
Bidirectional		
Bidirectional crest distractor (2D-CD)	Surgi-Tec, Belgium	
Multidimensional (Watzek et al.)	Prototype	
Alveolar distractor	Synthes, Switzerland	Vector control mechanism
Modus	Medartis AG, Switzerland	Individual fixation of device component Vector control mechanism
Implant distractor		
Veriplant	EverFab, USA	
Robinson Inter Os	Robinson, USA	
Distraction implant	SIS Trade Systems, Austria	
3i distraction device	Implant innovations, USA	
Dental Implant Distractor (DID)	Prototype, China	For jaw reconstruction

Source: Hariri F et al. (2013).

a "latency period" occurs within 5–7 days when hematoma and inflammatory cells enriched with pluripotent cells are recruited to form a soft callus. "Distraction phase" is the movement of the transport segment away from the basal bone with a typical recommended range of 0.5–1.0 mm/day along the bridging callus under the tension stress principle founded by Illizarov. Once the desired length is reached, the device can be maintained in the mouth for 12 weeks for the "consolidation phase" (bony remodeling) sufficient for implant placement. The disadvantage of this device is the inability to control the vector properly for bony elongation, primarily because of the lingual/palatal tissue torque on the segment. Patient cooperation and tolerance for this device are needed for a successful outcome.

Box 6.10 Key points for distraction osteogenesis

1. Indicated to augment moderate-to-severe hard and soft tissue defects [87]
2. Four phases of distraction osteogenesis [87]
   a. Osteotomy – bicortical cuts between the basal and transport segment with divergent vertical osteotomy toward the direction of desired distraction
   b. Latency phase (5–7 days) – awaiting bridging callus formation
   c. Distraction phase – 0.5–1.0 mm/day
   d. Consolidation phase – bone maturation for implant placement around 12 weeks
5. Buccal compensation of the transport segment may be needed to offset the lingual/palatal torque [81]
6. Vertical gain (3–20 mm) with mean 8.4 ± 2.6 mm has achieved long-term success in the region of 90% [7, 88, 89]

Distraction Osteogenesis Surgical Technique

A paracrestal incision is made in full-thickness fashion to gain access to the desired site on the buccal aspect, with vertical releasing incisions made two teeth away from the defect. The reason for this flap design is to preserve the lingual/palatal gingival tissue which is the major source of blood supply. After adapting the distraction device, an initial osteotomy is made between the transport and basal segments while maintaining at least 3 mm of existing bone from maxillary/nasal sinus floor and 2 mm from adjacent teeth. The device is removed and the vertical osteotomies join the horizontal segment in complete fashion. It is imperative that a divergent vertical osteotomy is created so the "path of draw" allows the transport segment to move unimpeded.

After placement of fixation screws, the device is checked for movement by turning it with a key in a clockwise fashion for 1 cm before returning it 1–2 mm to the original position. Any interference should be addressed prior to mucosal tissue closure.

The mandibular segment is performed in the same manner with particular attention paid to staying at least 3 mm away from the inferior alveolar canal. Three months are required for bony consolidation prior to implant placement.

Distraction Osteogenesis Complications

Complications associated with distraction osteogenesis include the inability to control the transport segment, resulting in a lingual/palatal torque (18–22%) [81]. Buccal compensation should offset this discrepancy. After device removal, 64% of the patients will still require some sort of bone grafting [81]. Infection and fistula formation have also been reported [87] (Table 6.4).

Distraction Osteogenesis Implant Survival and Success Rates

Kim et al. reported a 12-year long-term follow-up and implant survival and success rates for distraction osteogenesis were 97.3% and 92.7%, respectively [88]. These criteria are based on Albrektsson et al. (see Box 6.3).

Distraction Osteogenesis Conclusion (Box 6.10)

Distraction osteogenesis can vertically augment moderate-to-severe hard and soft tissue defects. It can also be used as an alternative to failed previous onlay block graft. Mean range of vertical distraction of 8.4 ± 2.6 mm (3–20 mm) has been reported [7, 88, 89]. Healing is based on an excellent pedicle lingual/palatal blood supply for osteogenesis, with a minimum of 3 months before implant placement. Graft resorption has been reported to be highest between time of graft placement and implant insertion so overcorrection of the graft is encouraged to anticipate some resorption [88]. Good long-term survival and success rates have been reported in the region of 90% [88].

Postoperative Instructions

Systemic antibiotics (e.g., amoxicillin 500 mg) for 1 week and chlorhexidine 0.12% for 2–4 weeks if the membrane is used as a flap extender. The potency of analgesia from nonsteroidal anti-inflammatory drugs (NSAIDs) to narcotics (hydrocodone or oxycodone), is based upon the anticipated level of postoperative pain. A Medrol dose pack can be used if significant postoperative edema is expected. The combination of steroids and NSAIDs has a fourfold increased risk of gastrointestinal bleed for those with an existing history [90]. Ice packs (10 minutes on and off) for the first 72 hours could be used to combat facial edema which typically lasts up to 7 days. Bruising on the face/neck can last up to 2 weeks, especially for those who resume their anticoagulants or are on NSAIDs. Educating these patients can alleviate their anxiety about the unattractive appearance.

Soft diet and avoidance of chewing on the operated side are preferred. Good oral hygiene during the healing period

Table 6.4 Preventive measures and management of common complications in alveolar distraction osteogenesis.

Phase	Complication	Prevention	Management
Intra-operative	Inadequate surgical excess	Determine suitable size of device Use previous extra-oral surgical scar if suitable	Adequate relieving incision without jeopardizing soft tissue vascularity
	Unfavorable fracture of basal or transport segment	3-Dimensional bone assessment Correct technique of osteotomy Use suitable cutting drills or saw Determine suitable device accordingly	Fixation of Fractured segment using mini or fracture plate
Post-operative	Infection	Compliance of patients Pre-surgical management of medical conditions Strict oral hygiene instruction Post-operative course of antibiotics Avoid habitual risks (e.g. smoking)	Debridement and irrigation Prescription of antibiotic Removal of source of infection (e.g. food particle) Strict oral hygiene measures OR Removal of device
	Intra-distraction bone fracture	Ensure adequate minimum bone available for fixation of device Rounding of any sharp angles Adjust rate of distraction accordingly	Fixation of fracture segment with mini or fracture plate Reduce rate of distraction accordingly
	Vector change or disturbance	Correct osteotomy technique to prevent bony hindrance Trial activation of transport segment before wound closure Fabrication of vector guidance prostheses Tooth-borne device or bi-directional device	Surgical exploration and removal of any bony hindrance
	Device failure	Trial activation before wound closure Avoid multiple bending of fixation plate	Removal of device an fixation of segment

Source: Hariri F et al. (2013).

should be reinforced. Warm salt water rinses should be used to remove debris after meals. Awareness of the temporary prosthesis not impinging on the surgical site is crucial to graft success.

Conclusion

Horizontal Augmentation Recap (Tables 6.5 and 6.6)

For horizontal augmentation, there is no difference among iliac crest, cranium, autogenous mandible, allogenic, or xenogeneic block graft with mean gain of 4.5 mm [64]. The use of block graft tends to average 1 mm gain more than the GBR technique [64]. Allogenic or xenogeneic block graft would be the most appealing choice as the "bone off the shelf" as long as patients are immunocompetent. Alternatively, autogenous mandibular ramal harvest is the preferred choice owing to lower morbidity compared to chin harvest. Tension-free primary closure along with particulate bone and membrane on the onlay graft have higher success rates than block graft alone. Ridge split graft has been shown to be as effective as block graft and GBR techniques, with 2–5 mm of gain expected. However, a minimum of 3 mm in thickness is recommended preoperatively. Additionally, absence of severe concavity and a minimum of 10 mm to vital structures are required for this procedure. This technique can be done with simultaneous implant placement thus shortening overall treatment time to as little as 4 months.

Lastly, there is no difference in the type of absorbable or nonabsorbable membrane used for horizontal GBR augmentation [64].

Horizontal Augmentation Complication Recap

A systematic review by Milinkovic and Cordaro have found complications to be the lowest for block graft with 6.3%, followed by ridge split with 6.8%, and staged GBR with

Table 6.5 Summary of horizontal and vertical augmentation [7].

Horizontal augmentation [7]		
Procedure	**Potential gain**	**Time to implant placement**
Socket preservation	Preventive	Mineralized graft = 3–4 mo
		Demineralized graft = 4–5 mo
		Bovine graft = 5–8 mo
Guided bone regeneration	3–6 mm	9–12 mo
Particulate onlay	1–4 mm	3–4 mo
Block grafts	Ramus = 3–4 mm	4–6 mo
	Chin = 4–6 mm	4–6 mo
Ridge split	2–5 mm (avg = 3 mm)	Immediate or 3–4 mo
Vertical augmentation [7]		
Procedure	**Potential gain**	**Time to implant placement**
Socket preservation	Preventive	Mineralized graft = 3–4 mo
		Demineralized graft = 4–5 mo
		Bovine graft = 5–8 mo
Guided bone regeneration	2–4 mm	9–12 mo
Block grafts	Ramus = 3–4 mm	4–6 mo
	Chin = 4–6 mm	4–6 mo
Interpositional bone graft	Anterior = 5 mm	3–4 mo
	Posterior = 8 mm	3–4 mo
Distraction osteogenesis	3–20 mm	3–4 mo

11.9%. Graft exposure, buccal plate fracture, and membrane exposures were the main problems associated with these procedures, respectively [81]. Troelzsch et al. reported extraoral autogenous bone sources had the lowest complications rate at 7.1% and allogenic bone with 13.1% among all block graft groups [64].

Vertical Augmentation Recap (Tables 6.5 and 6.6)

Vertical augmentation for the atrophied ridge allows the clinician to choose a variety of surgical options: GBR, onlay block graft, interpositional technique, distraction osteogenesis, or short implants. Each technique has its own inherent limitations.

Despite the best overall vertical gain being achieved with iliac crest/cranium source, most patients would not be amenable to distant harvest sites unless it is absolutely necessary because of second surgery morbidity, general anesthesia administration, and increased recovery time, with gait disturbance associated with hip harvest. Data suggests that the best risk:benefit ratio is the use of intraoral mandibular graft followed by interpositional technique with an average gain of 5.3 and 4.4 mm, respectively. A 6.0 mm gain was reported with GBR with titanium mesh, most likely in the hands of an experienced clinician, while allogeneic onlay block graft posted the worst results with the lowest gain and the highest complication rate [64].

For moderate-to-severe hard and soft tissue defects, distraction osteogenesis can help augment by 3–20 mm [7] with a mean of 8.4 mm [88]. Vector control is the most problematic issue with this technique, often leaving the device torqued to the lingual/palatal aspect [81, 88]. Moreover, additional bone grafting is required in 64% of cases after device removal [81]. These are the main reasons why distraction osteogenesis is not routinely used as the first choice for vertical augmentation.

Vertical augmentation remains the more difficult vector to perform predictably and has a steep learning curve. Mucosal pressure and poor blood supply have resulted in graft shrinkage and higher failure rates [67]. For those who are uncomfortable with the above procedures, some authors support the use of short implants (5–8 mm) because of its predictability, fewer complications and shortened surgical time and cost [91].

The future direction of bone grafting will certainly have biomedical researchers investigating synthetic bone as a

Table 6.6 Summary of horizontal and vertical augmentation. overall mean weighted average (mwa) and statistical difference * [64].

Procedure	Gains in mm	Main complication	Implant survival and success rate
Horizontal augmentation [52]			
Guided bone regeneration	3.7 ± 1.2 mm (mwa) [64]	Membrane exposure 11.9% [81]	Overall survival rate 96.1–99.4% [64]
Block grafts	4.5 ± 1.2 mm (mwa) [64]	Graft exposure 6.3% [81]	Undisclosed for mwa
Extraoral block	Undisclosed	7.1 ± 17% [64]	Undisclosed for extraoral
Intraoral block	Undisclosed	Undisclosed for intraoral	Survival and success rate 73.8–100% [76]
Allogenic block	4.6 ± 1.4 mm (mwa) [64]	13.3 ± 13.6% [64]	Survival and success rate 72.8–100% [76]
Xenograft block	3.7 mm (mwa) [64]	Undisclosed for xenograft	Undisclosed for xenograft
Ridge split	2–5 mm [7, 74, 79, 80]	Buccal plate fx 6.8% [81]	91.7–100% survival rate with simultaneous implants [83] 88.2–100% success rate with simultaneous implants [83]
Vertical augmentation [52]			
Procedure	**Gains in mm**	**Main complication**	**Implant survival and success rate**
Guided bone regeneration	3.7 ± 1.4 mm (mwa) [64]	Membrane exposure 11.9% [81]	Overall survival rate 96.1–99.4% [64]
Titanium mesh	6.0 ± 2.3 mm [64]		
Collagen membrane	3.9 ± 1.9 mm [64]		
Block grafts	5.8 ± 2.8 mm (mwa) [64]	Late graft resorption [67]	Undisclosed for mwa
*Iliac/cranium	9.4 ± 3.1 mm (mwa) [64]	20.1 ± 16.8% [64]	Undisclosed for iliac/cranium
Intraoral block	5.3± 1.6 mm (mwa) [64]	14.4 ± 14.5% [64]	Survival and success rate 73.8–100% [76]
Allogenic block	2.9 ± 1.3 mm (mwa) [64]	25 ± 20.3% [64]	Survival and success rate 72.8–100% [76]
Interpositional bone graft	See below for specific graft types	Vascular embarrassment with partial or complete graft loss [84, 85]	Overall survival rate 92.5–100% [64]
Iliac crest	8.6 mm (mwa) [64]	Undisclosed for iliac crest	
Xenograft	6.5 mm (mwa) [64]	43.5% [64]	
Intraoral mandible	4.4 mm (mwa) [64]	7.8% [64]	
Allogenic	2.2 mm (mwa) [64]	Undisclosed for allograft	
Distraction osteogenesis	8.4 ± 2.6 mm [88]	Vector control 18–22% [81] Future grafting needed 64% [81]	Overall survival rate 97.3% [88] Overall success rate 92.7% [88]

carrier for growth factors (i.e., BMP, PDGF, platelet gel, gene therapy, or autologous cell tissue engineering) to enhance bone formation similar to autogenous source. The ideal bone typography should emulate human pore size, porosity, biocompatible, and biodegradability in a predictable manner with eventual lamellar bone formation while still being cost-effective and easy to perform.

References

1 Sakkas, A., Wilde, F., Heufelder, M. et al. (2017). Autogenous bone grafts in oral implantology – is it still a "gold standard"? A consecutive review of 279 patients with 456 clinical procedures. *Int. J. Implant Dent.* 3 (1): 23.

2 Roberts, T. and Rosenbaum, A. (2012). Bone grafts, bone substitutes and orthobiololgics: the bridge between basic science and clinical advancement in fracture healing. *Organogenesis* 8 (4): 114–124.

3 Urist, M. (1965). Bone: formation by autoinduction. *Science* 150: 893–899.

4 Behnam K, Wei G, Beisser J, inventors; Warsaw Orthopedic Inc., assignee. Demineralized Bone Matrix Compositions and Methods. US Patent 8,202,539,B2. June 19, 2012.

5 Sheikh, Z., Sima, C., and Glogauer, M. (2015). Bone replacement materials and techniques used for achieving vertical alveolar bone augmentation. *Materials* 8: 2953–2993.

6 Lui, J. and Kerns, D. (2014). Mechanism of guided bone regeneration: a review. *Open Dent. J.* 8: 56–65.

7 Haggerty, C., Vogel, C., and Fisher, R. (2015). Simple bone augmentation for alveolar ridge defects. *Oral Maxillofacial. Surg. Clin. North Am.* 27: 203–226.

8 Sogal, A. and Tolefe, A.J. (1999). Risk assessment of bovine spongiform encephalopathy transmission through bone graft material derived from bovine bone used for dental applications. *J. Periodontol.* 70: 1053–1063.

9 Wenz, B., Oesch, B., and Horst, M. (2001). Analysis of the risk of transmitting bovine spongiform encephalopathy through bone grafts derived from bovine bone. *Biomaterials* 22: 1599–1606.

10 Kumar, P., Vinitha, B., and Ghousia, F. (2013). Bone grafts in dentistry. *J. Pharm. Bioallied Sci.* 5 (Suppl 1): S125–S127.

11 Knabe, C., Ducheyne, P., and Stiller, M. (2011). Dental graft materials. In: *Comprehensive Biomaterials*, vol. 6, 305–324. St Louis, MO: Elsevier.

12 Schwartz O, Binderman I, inventors; Ramot at Tel-Aviv University Ltd, Corebone Ltd, assignee. Coral Bone Graft Substitute. US Patent 836,638,B2. September 22, 2011.

13 Christian, S., Doris, M., Alexis, S. et al. (2003). The fluorohydroxyapatite (FHA) FRIOS, Algipore, is a suitable biomaterial for the reconstruction of severely atrophic human maxillae. *Clin. Oral Implants Res.* 14: 743–749.

14 Heness, G. and Ben-Nissan, B. (2004). Innovative bioceramics. *Materials Forum* 2: 104–114.

15 Lee S, Porter M, Was S, et al. (2012). Potential bone replacement materials prepared by two methods. Materials Research Society Symposium Proceedings. doi: 10.1557/opl.2012.671

16 Al-Sanabani, J.S., Madfa, A.A., and Al-Sanabani, F.A. (2013). Application of calcium phosphate materials in dentistry. *Int. J. Biomater.* 2013: 1–12.

17 Misch, C.E. (2008). *Contemporary Implant Dentistry*, 3e. St Louis, MO: Mosby/Elsevier.

18 Damien, E. and Revell, P. (2004). Coralline hydroxyapatite bone graft substitute: a review of experimental studies and biomedical application. *J. Appl. Biomater. Biomech.* 2: 65–73.

19 Pountos, I. and Giannoudis, P.V. (2016). Is there a role for coral bone substitutes in bone repair? *Injury* 47 (12): 2606–2613.

20 S, L. and Balasubramanian, D. (2013). Nanotechnology in dentistry – a review. *Int. J. Dent. Sci. Res.* 1 (2): 40–44.

21 Chitsazi, M., Shirmohammadi, A., Faramazie, P.R., and Rostamzadeh, A. (2011). A clinical comparison of nano crystalline hydroxyapatite (ostim) and autogenous bone graft in the treatment of periodontal intrabony defects. *Med. Oral Patol. Oral Cir. Bucal.* 16 (3): 448–453.

22 Kamboj, M., Arora, R., and Gupta, H. (2016). Comparative evaluation of the efficacy of synthetic nanocrystalline hydroxyapatite bone graft (Ostim) and synthetic microcrystalline hydroxyapatite bone graft (OsteoGen) in the treatment of human periodontal intramural defects: a clinical and dental scan study. *J. Indian Soc. Periodontol.* 20 (4): 423–428.

23 Straumann product catalog.

24 Jain, A., Chaturvedi, R., and Pahuja, B. (2012). Comparative evaluation of efficiency of calcium sulfate bone grafts in crystalline and nano-crystalline forms in fresh extraction sockets sites: a radiographic and histological pilot study. *Int. J. Oral Implants Clin. Res.* 3 (1): 58–61.

25 Bondbone product catalog.

26 Eschbach EJ, Montford MJ, Wheeler DL. Mechanical assessment of bovine and bioactive glass as cancellous bone graft. 45th Annual Meeting of the Orthopedic Research Society 1999.

27 NovaBone product catalog.

28 Chen, D., Zhao, M., and Mundy, G. (2004). Bone morphogenetic proteins. *Growth Factors* 22 (4): 233–241.

29 Sheikh, Z., Javaid, M.A., Hamdan, N., and Hashmi, R. (2015). Bone regeneration using bone morphogenetic proteins and various biomaterial carriers. *Materials* 8 (4): 1778–1816.

30 Devescovi, V., Leonardi, E., Ciapetti, G., and Cenni, E. (2008). Growth factors in bone repair. *Chir. Organi Mov.* 92 (3): 161–168.
31 Chandra, P. and Sivadas, A. (2014). Platelet-rich fibrin: its role in periodontal regeneration. *Saudi J. Dent. Res.* 5: 117–122.
32 BioMend product catalog, RTI Biologics.
33 Ghanaati, S., Booms, P., Orlowska, A. et al. (2014). Advanced platelet-rich fibrin: a new concept for cell-based tissue engineering by means of inflammatory cells. *J. Oral Implantol.* 40 (6): 679–689.
34 Choukroun, J. and Ghanaati, S. (2018). Reduction of relative centrifugation force within injectable platelet-rich-fibrin (PRF) concentrates advances patients' own inflammatory cells, platelets and growth factors: the first introduction to the low speed centrifugation concept. *Eur. J. Trauma Emerg. Surg.* 44: 87–95.
35 Alizade, F.L., Kazemi, M., Irani, S., and Sohrabi, M. (2016). Biologic characteristics of platelet rich plasma and platelet rich fibrin: a review. *Int. J. Contemp. Dent. Med. Rev.* 2016: 1–4.
36 Miron, R.J., Zucchelli, G., Pikos, M.A. et al. (2017). Use of platelet-rich fibrin in regenerative dentistry: a systematic review. *Clin. Oral Invest.* 21 (6): 2016: 1–4.
37 Schroop, L., Wenzel, A., Kostopoulous, L., and Karring, T. (2003). Bone healing and soft tissue contour changes following single-tooth extraction: a clinical and radiographic 12 month prospective study. *Int. J. Periodont. Restor. Dent.* 23: 313–323.
38 Araujo, M., Costa da Silva, J., Mendonca, A., and Lindhe, J. (2015). Ridge alteration following grafting of fresh extraction socket in man. A randomized clinical trial. *Clin. Oral Implants Res.* 26: 407–412.
39 Vignoletti, F., Matesanz, P., Rodrigo, D. et al. (2012). Surgical protocol for ridge preservation after tooth extraction. A systematic review. *Clin. Oral Implants Res.* 23: 22–38.
40 Apostolopoulos, P. and Darby, I. (2017). Retrospective success and survival rates of dental implants placed after a ridge preservation procedure. *Clin. Oral Implants Res.* 28: 461–468.
41 Frost, N., Banjar, A., Galloway, P. et al. (2014). The decision making process for ridge preservation procedure after tooth extraction. *Clin. Adv. Periodontics* 4: 56–63.
42 Cook, D., Mealy, B., Verrett, R. et al. (2011). Relationship between clinical periodontal biotype and labial plate thickness: an in vivo study. *Int. J. Periodont. Restor. Dent.* 31: 345–354.
43 Spray, J., Black, C., Morris, H., and Ochi, S. (2000). The influence of bone thickness on facial marginal bone response: stage 1 placement through stage 2 uncovering. *Ann. Periodontol.* 5: 119–128.
44 Januario, A., Duarte, W., Barriviera, M. et al. (2011). Dimensions of the facial bone wall in the anterior maxilla: a cone beam computed tomography study. *Clin. Oral Implants Res.* 22: 1168–1171.
45 Huynh-Ba, G., Pietursson, B., Sanz, M. et al. (2010). Analysis of the socket bone wall dimensions in the upper maxilla relation to immediate implant placement. *Clin. Oral Implants Res.* 21: 37–42.
46 Barone, A., Ricci, M., Tonelli, P. et al. (2013). Tissue change of extraction sockets in humans: a comparison of spontaneous healing vs. ridge preservation with secondary soft tissue healing. *Clin. Oral Implants Res.* 24: 1231–1237.
47 Albrektsson, T., Zarb, G., Worthington, P., and Eriksson, A.R. (1986). The long-term efficacy of currently used dental implants: a review and proposed criteria of success. *Int. J. Oral Maxillofac. Implants* 1 (1): 11–25.
48 Avila-Ortiz, G., Elangovan, S., Kramer, K.W.O. et al. (2014). Effects of alveolar ridge preservation after tooth extraction: a systematic review and meta-analysis. *J. Dent. Res.* 93 (10): 950–958.
49 Poli, P., Beretta, M., Cicciu, M., and Maiorana, C. (2014). Alveolar ridge augmentation with titanium mesh. A retrospective clinical study. *Open Dent. J.* 8: 148–158.
50 Rakhmatia, Y., Ayukawa, Y., Furushashi, A., and Koyano, K. (2012). Current barrier membrane: titanium mesh and other membranes for guided bone regeneration in dental applications. *J. Prosthodont. Res.* 57: 3–14.
51 Wang, J., Wang, L., Zhou, Z. et al. (2016). Biodegradable polymer membranes applied in guided bone/tissue regeneration: a review. *Polymers* 8: 1–20.
52 Malet, J., Mora, F., and Bouchard, P. (2012). *Implant Dentistry at a Glance.* Oxford: Wiley-Blackwell.
53 Osteogenics Biomedical's product catalog.
54 Ronda, M., Rebaudi, A., Torelli, L., and Stacchi, C. (2013). Expanded vs dense polytetrafluoroethylene membrane in vertical ridge augmentation around dental implants: a prospective randomized controlled clinical trials. *Clin. Oral Implants Res.* 25: 1–8.
55 Bio-Gide product catalog, Geistlich Company.
56 Ossix Plus product catalog, Datum Dental Company.
57 Alloderm product catalog, Biohorizon, Lifecell Corporation.
58 Puros Dermis & Puros processed pericardium product catalog, RTI/ Biologics.
59 Allo.Protect/Creos product catalog, Community Tissue Bank.
60 Resolut Adapt product catalog, W.L. Gore and Associate.
61 Epi-Guide product catalog, Curasan.
62 Guidor product catalog, Sunstar Americas, Inc.
63 Vivosorb product catalog, Polyganics.

64 Troelzsch, M., Troelzsch, M., Kauffmann, P. et al. (2016). Clinical efficacy of grafting materials in alveolar ridge augmentation: a systematic review. *J. Craniomaxillofac. Surg.* 44: 1618–1629.

65 Vicryl Polyglactin 910, Ethicon product catalog.

66 Block, M. and Kelly, B. (2013). Horizontal posterior ridge augmentation: the use of a collagen membrane over a bovine particulate graft: technique note. *J. Oral Maxillofac. Surg.* 71: 1513–1519.

67 Aloy-Prosper, A., Penarrocha-Oltra, D., Penarrocha-Diago, M., and Penarrocha-Diago, M. (2015). The outcome of intramural onlay bone block grafts on alveolar ridge augmentations: a systematic review. *Med. Oral Patol. Oral Cir. Bucal.* 20 (2): e251–e258.

68 Cordaro, L., Torsello, F., Morcavallo, S., and Di Torresanto, V.M. (2011). Effects of bovine bone and collagen membranes on healing of mandibular block graft: a prospective randomized controlled study. *Clin. Oral Implants Res.* 22: 1145–1150.

69 Dym, H., Huang, D., and Stern, A. (2012). Alveolar bone grafting and reconstruction procedure prior to implant placement. *Dent. Clin. North Am.* 56: 209–218.

70 Calvero, J. and Lundgren, S. (2003). Ramus or chin graft for maxillary sinus inlay and local onlay augmentation comparison of donor site morbidity and complications. *Clin. Implant Dent. Relat. Res.* 593: 154–160.

71 Chiapasco, M., Abati, S., Romero, E. et al. (1999). Clinical outcome of autogenous bone block or guided bone regeneration with e-PTFE membranes for the reconstruction of narrow edentulous ridge. *Clin. Oral Implants Res.* 10 (4): 278–288.

72 Silva, F.M., Cortex, A.L., Moreira, R.W. et al. (2006). Complications of intraoral donor site for bone grafting prior to implant placement. *Implant Dent.* 15 (4): 420–426.

73 Keith, J.D. Jr., Petrungaro, P., Leonetti, J.A. et al. (2006). Clinical and histological evaluation of a mineralized block allograft: results from development period (2001–2004). *Int. J. Periodont. Restor. Dent.* 26: 321–327.

74 Minichetti, J.C., D'Amore, J.C., Hong, A.Y.J., and Cleveland, D.B. (2004). Human histologic analysis of mineralized bone allograft (pros) before implant surgery. *J. Oral Implantol.* 30 (2): 74–82.

75 Leonetti, J.A. (2003). Localized maxillary ridge augmentation with a block allograft for dental implant placement: case reports. *Implant Dent.* 12 (3): 217–226.

76 Montamedian, S., Khojaste, M., and Khojasteh, A. (2016). Success rate of implants placed in autogeneous bone block versus allogenic bone blocks: a systematic literature review. *Ann. Maxillofac. Surg.* 6: 78–90.

77 Holtzclaw, D., Nicholas, T., and Rosen, P. (2010). Reconstruction of posterior mandibular alveolar ridge deficiencies with the piezoelectric hinge-assisted ridge split technique: a retrospective observational report. *J. Peridontol.* 81: 1580–1586.

78 Ella, B., Laurentjoye, M., Separate, C. et al. (2014). Mandibular ridge expansion using a horizontal bone-splitting technique and synthetic bone substitute: an alternative to bone block grafting? *Int. J. Maxillofac. Implants* 29: 135–140.

79 Koo, S., Dibart, S., and Weber, H. (2008). Ridge splitting technique with simultaneous implant placement. *Compend. Contin. Educ. Dent.* 29: 106–110.

80 Jensen, O. and Ellis, E. (2008). The book flap: a technique note. *J. Oral Maxillofac. Surg.* 66: 1010–1014.

81 Milinkovic, I. and Cordaro, L. (2014). Are there specific indications for the different alveolar bone augmentation procedures for implant placement? A systematic review. *Int. J. Oral. Maxillofac. Surg.* 43: 606–625.

82 Altiparmak, N., Akdeniz, S., Bayram, B. et al. (2017). Alveolar ridge splitting versus autogenous onlay bone grafting: complications and implant survival rates. *Implant Dent.* 26: 284–287.

83 Bassetti, M., Bassetti, R., and Bosshard, D. (2014). The alveolar ridge splitting/expansion technique: a systematic review. *Clin. Oral Implants Res.* 27: 310–324.

84 Block, M. (2011). *Color Atlas of Dental Implant Surgery*, 3e. Oxford: Elsevier.

85 Jensen, O., Kuhlke, L., Bedard, J.F., and White, D. (2006). Alveolar segmental sandwich osteotomy for anterior maxillary vertical augmentation prior to implant placement. *J. Oral Maxillofac. Surg.* 64: 290–296.

86 Schettler, D. and Holtermann, W. (1977). Clinical and experimental results of a sandwich-technique for mandibular alveolar ridge augmentation. *J. Maxillofac. Surg.* 5: 199–202.

87 Hariri, F., Chua, H.D.P., and Cheung, L.K. (2013). Distraction osteogenesis for the cranio-maxillofacial region (III): a compendium of devices for the dentoalveolus. *J. Oral Maxillofac. Surg. Med. Pathol.* 25 (2): 101–114.

88 Kim, J., Cho, M., Kim, S., and Kim, M. (2013). Alveolar distraction osteogenesis versus autogenous onlay bone graft for vertical augmentation of severely atrophic alveolar ridge after 12 years of long-term follow-up. *Oral Surg. Oral Med. Oral Pathol. Oral Radiol.* 116: 540–549.

89 Chiapasco, M., Consolo, U., Bianchi, A. et al. (2004). Alveolar distraction osteogenesis for the correction of vertically deficient edentulous ridges: a multicenter prospective study on humans. *Int. J. Oral Maxillofac. Implants* 19: 399–407.

90 Chan, M.H. (2022). Update on management of the oral and maxillofacial surgery patient on corticosteroids. *Oral Maxillofac. Surg. Clin. North Am.* 34 (1): 115–126.

91 Soldatos, N., Stylianou, P., Koidou, V. et al. (2016). Limitations and options using restorable versus nonresorbable membranes for successful guided bone regeneration. *Quintessence Int.* 48: 131–147.

7

Maxillary Sinus Augmentation

Jonathan C. Elmore and Harry Dym

Introduction

The maxillary sinus lift is a procedure that can be thought of as purely useful to facilitate placement of dental implants in an atrophic posterior maxilla. The goal of the procedure is to increase the vertical height of alveolar bone in the posterior maxilla. Tatum first proposed the sinus lift in 1976 at a conference in Alabama. It was Boyne and James, however, who first published the surgical technique in 1980 [1]. The procedure has now become a very predictable method for vertical augmentation allowing implant placement in the posterior maxilla.

Maxillary Sinus Anatomy

The maxillary sinus is an air-filled cavity of about 12–15 mL that occupies the midface bilaterally. It is believed that its purpose is to reduce the weight of the skull, regulate improve inhaled air humidity, and provide resonant function. It is pyramidal in shape and occupies the maxillary bone [2]. It is bound superiorly by the orbital floor, inferiorly by the alveolar process, medially by the lateral nasal wall, and laterally by the zygomatic process and buccal alveolus. This space in males is approximately 21–29 mm in width, 39–49 mm in height, and 36–43 mm in length. In females, these dimensions generally are slightly smaller, being 19–27 mm in width, 35–45 mm in height, and 33–41 mm in length.

The maxillary sinus is lined by a membrane, approximately 1.0 mm in thickness, known as the Schneiderian membrane. This membrane is made up of ciliated columnar epithelial cells that clear secretions to the ostia, which is located within the semilunar hiatus. The semilunar hiatus serves as the opening to connect the maxillary sinus to the nose and drains to the middle meatus. When evaluating the position of this passageway, it may be positioned anywhere from 18 to 35 mm above the nasal floor.

The maxillary artery provides the major blood supply for the maxillary sinus through its branches including the sphenopalatine, greater palatine, infraorbital, and alveolar arteries. Nerve innervation is supplied by branches of the maxillary nerve.

Indications, Contraindications, Limitations

Prior to treatment, a dental orthopantomogram should be taken to determine the appropriateness of implant placement in the posterior maxilla. It can also be determined whether the patient will require augmentation in the area. With advances in technology often available in the dental office, cone beam computed tomography (CT) may also be obtained to view the sinus and alveolar bone relationship in three dimensions.

Evaluation of the area for planning is very important. After extraction of a maxillary posterior tooth, the alveolar bone at the extraction socket resorbs and the maxillary sinus gradually expands to occupy the area. The combination of these two biologic activities results in limited vertical bone height for implant placement. The primary indication for a sinus lift procedure is pneumatization of the maxillary sinus preventing implant placement. Poor bone quality in the posterior mandible has been mentioned as an indication for sinus elevation in an attempt to increase the bone to implant contact area. Misch developed a

Oral and Maxillofacial Surgery, Medicine, and Pathology for the Clinician, First Edition. Edited by Harry Dym, Leslie R. Halpern, and Orrett E. Ogle.

Table 7.1 Grading of maxillary alveolar bone and possible need for sinus lift.

Misch grade	Remaining alveolar height (mm)
Grade I	>12 mm
Grade II	10–12 mm
Grade III	5–10 mm
Grade IV	<4 mm

grading system based on the remaining alveolar height in the posterior mandible (Table 7.1).

The overall concept for contraindications or limitations to a sinus lift pertains to any condition that blocks ventilation and/or clearance of the maxillary sinus. Before any medical procedures, a thorough history and physical examination should be completed. Factors that the surgeon may want to be aware of during the preoperative exam include patient's history of smoking, chronic sinusitis or nasal obstruction, previous treatment of head and neck cancer, or any other systemic diseases that could interfere with normal mucosal functioning.

Lateral Window Approach

The lateral window approach, commonly called the Caldwell–Luc approach, gains access to the maxillary sinus via its anterolateral wall (Figure 7.1). Local anesthesia is administered by a combination of local infiltration and regional blocks. A crestal incision is made along the alveolar crest which can be carried through the sulcus of teeth, if teeth are present, with anterior and posterior releasing incisions. Care must be taken to ensure a broad-based design so that the blood supply to the flap is not compromised. A full-thickness flap is elevated and the lateral wall of the maxillary sinus is exposed. The osteotomy is prepared using either a high-speed rotary instrument or a piezoelectric system. The inferior border of the window should be about 3 mm from the floor of the sinus. The posterior aspect of the tuberosity extends to the molar region while the anterior extension should be about 3 mm from the anterior wall of the sinus.

After completion of the osteotomy, the Schneiderian membrane is elevated. The elevation process begins at the inferior border of the window and is gently carried to the anterior and posterior aspects of the window. After the membrane has been mobilized anteriorly, posteriorly, and inferiorly, the window is luxated inward and upward into the maxillary sinus. The sinus lift instruments are used to continue the dissection laterally into the sinus as far as is needed. The bone graft material of choice is placed and the wound is closed with the operator's choice of suture.

Transalveolar (Crestal) Approach

An alternative to the lateral window approach is to elevate the sinus from a transalveolar approach, also referred to as an internal sinus lift, crestal approach, or Summer's approach. This approach attempts to access the maxillary sinus by creating an osteotomy through the alveolus and elevating the sinus membrane through this opening [3]. When this approach is chosen, immediate implant placement is often performed. This approach may be used with

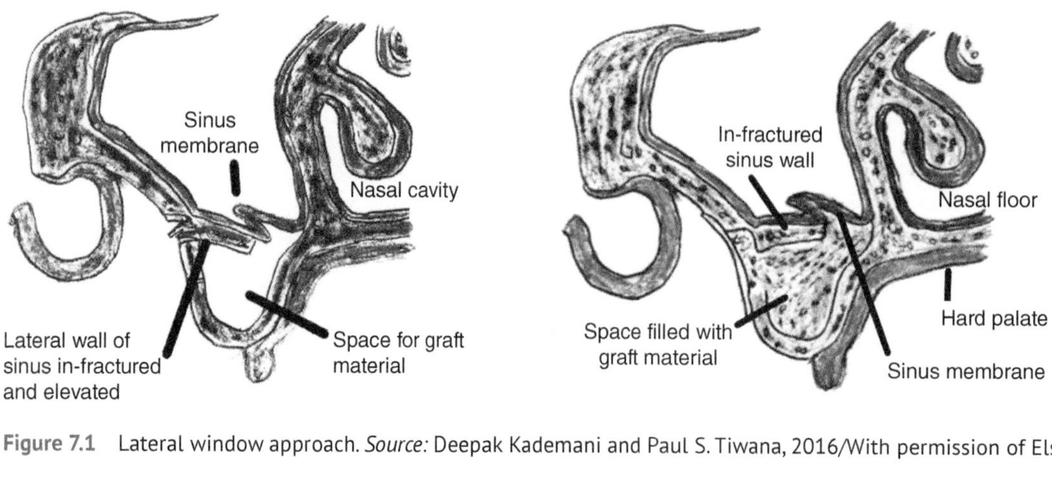

Figure 7.1 Lateral window approach. *Source:* Deepak Kademani and Paul S. Tiwana, 2016/With permission of Elsevier.

favorable outcomes in the atrophic maxilla with immediate implant placement when at least 4–5 mm of alveolar bone remains. Rosen and colleagues showed an implant survival rate of 96% when at least 4 mm of bone was present. That success rate decreased to 85.7% when less than 4 mm of alveolar bone was present [3].

The crestal approach was initially introduced as a less invasive option than removal of bone from the sinus wall. This technique is generally begun by raising a full-thickness mucoperiosteal flap and creating an osteotomy to a depth 1–2 mm less than the maxillary sinus floor (Figure 7.2). The osteotomy is then expanded to the appropriate size indicated for the implant to be placed in the area. Commonly, an osteotome is used to gently fracture the sinus floor. The operator will know the fracture has been completed based on the change in resistance to advancement of the osteotome or change in sound by tapping the osteotome. At this stage of the procedure, the operator prefers to insert a small collagen plug prior to the addition of grafting material. Grafting material is then advanced into the osteotomy site and the implant is placed (Figure 7.3).

Because the act of fracturing and elevating the sinus floor with the use of osteotomes can be uncomfortable for the patient, multiple systems have been developed to eliminate the need for osteotomes. These systems may utilize twist drills with noncutting ends or even hydraulic pressure to elevate the membrane.

Bone-Grafting Material

After access to the sinus has been achieved and the sinus membrane has been mobilized, the surgeon now has to make a decision on what materials, if any, will be placed prior to implant placement. Many materials have been described in the literature with high success rates. Autografts are still considered the gold standard for grafting. Additional materials include particulate allografts, xenografts, hydroxyapatite, and bone morphogenetic protein. Many surgeons will choose to mix different grafting materials together to benefit from each of their unique properties. Also of importance is a study by Lundgren et al. published in 2006 [4]. This demonstrated that with elevation of the membrane alone, without placement of graft material, it was possible to predictably grow bone. This phenomenon is likely due to the same principles of guided tissue regeneration. With many options available, the operating surgeon has numerous choices for graft materials to use during augmentation.

Complications

As with any surgical procedure, there are associated complications that may arise after treatment. The common complications include pain, bleeding, infection, sinus perforation, and vertigo. Pain can often be managed with nonsteroidal antiinflammatory medications, if the patient is able to tolerate the medication. If additional pain medication is needed, narcotics can be used as a second line of defense. A sinus lift generally does not generate a lot of bleeding. If bleeding is present, the first step is to apply direct pressure to the area. The area can also be packed with epinephrine-soaked gauze. Other local hemostatic agents may be used as well if needed.

Sinus perforations have been reported to range from 20% to 60%. The treatment goal of a perforated sinus membrane is to provide a secure barrier over the perforated region to

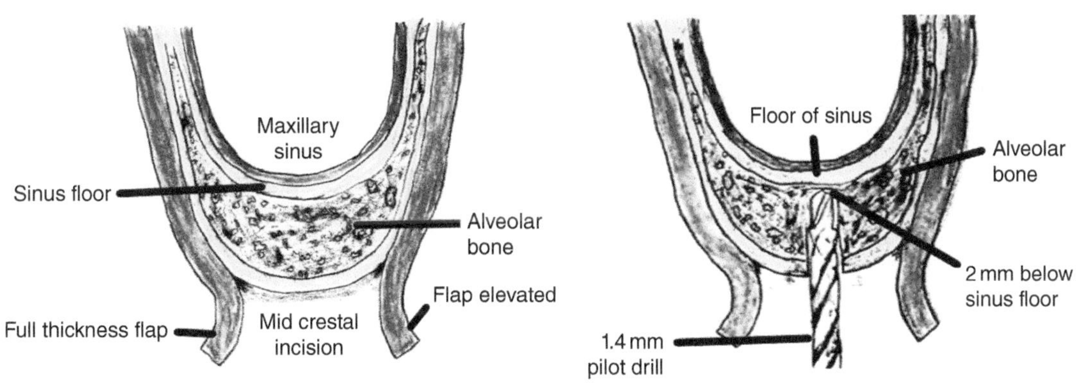

Figure 7.2 Crestal approach for sinus grafting (part 1). *Source:* Deepak Kademani and Paul S. Tiwana, 2016/With permission of Elsevier.

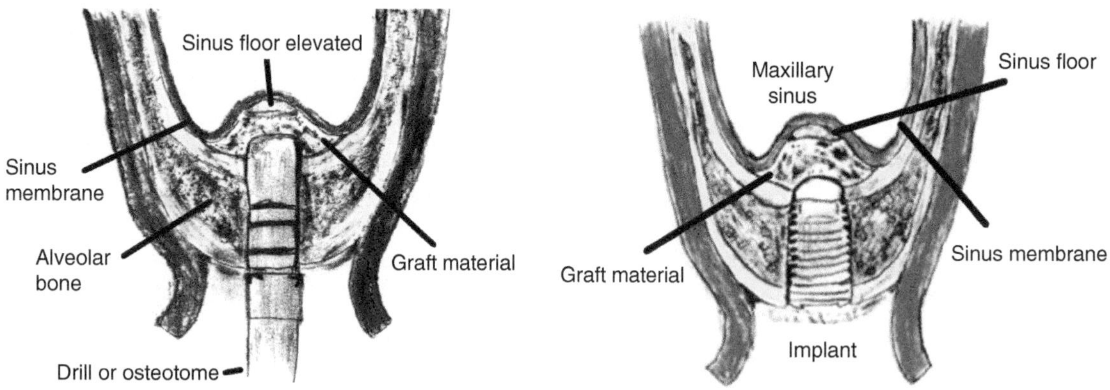

Figure 7.3 Crestal approach for sinus grafting (part 2). *Source:* Deepak Kademani and Paul S. Tiwana, 2016/With permission of Elsevier.

contain the grafting material. The treatment is guided by the extent of the membrane tear. There have been many attempts at classifying sinus membrane perforations based on size and location. In Table 7.2, the Valassis and Fugazzotto classification is given as an example of one scheme for membrane tear classifications [5].

No matter which classification scheme is used, a general step-wise process can be followed to aid in the treatment of membrane tears. The first step is to raise the surrounding membrane to reduce the tension in the region of the tear and prevent further tearing. At this point, if the tear is small, it will likely fold over on itself and no additional management is needed. If the tear is larger (~5 mm or more), it should be covered with a resorbable membrane prior to graft placement. Some tears are more extensive (>10 mm). In cases like these, a large, firm, resorbable membrane may be placed that extends beyond the lateral wall and is secured in place by mini screws or sutures. The graft can then be placed below the barrier.

Table 7.2 Valassis and fugazzotto classification of membrane tears.

Class	Comments
Class I	Adjacent to the osteotomy site. Often folding upon itself with further elevation
Class II	Located in the midsuperior aspect of the osteotomy, extending mesiodistally for two-thirds of the osteotomy site
Class III	Most common. Located at the inferior border of the osteotomy at its mesial or distal sixth
Class IV	Located in the central two-thirds of the osteotomy site
Class V	Preexisting area of exposure of the sinus membrane, possibly due to a combination of antral pneumatization and severe ridge resorption

When the sinus is manipulated and when grafting material is placed, there is always a chance of postoperative sinusitis. Studies have shown that one of the main predictors of postoperative sinusitis is preoperative chronic sinusitis. When infections exist, they can often be treated with antibiotics and nasal inflammatory spray [6]. The author will commonly suggest augmentin 875/125 mg every 12 hours for 10 days and fluticasone spray 50 µg 1–2 sprays once a day. When no improvement is seen, nasoendoscopic exploration with washout and drainage is recommended.

Another rare but possible occurrence after maxillary augmentation using the transalveolar approach is benign paroxysmal positional vertigo (BPPV) [7]. BPPV is a disorder involving the vestibulocochlear system. Systems commonly include brief periods of vertigo with sudden movements and may also include nausea. The underlying cause is a small calcified otolith, free floating within the inner ear. This small piece can become dislodged due to the trauma caused by the osteotome and mallet. Management of these patients includes referral to an otolaryngologist who may perform repositioning maneuvers (Epley maneuver, Semont maneuver).

References

1 Kademani, D. and Tiwana, P.S. (2016). *Atlas of Oral and Maxillofacial Surgery*, 199. St Louis, MO: Elsevier Saunders.

2 Danesh-Sani, S.A., Loomer, P.M., and Wallace, S.S. (2016). A comprehensive clinical review of maxillary sinus floor elevation: anatomy, techniques, biomaterials and complications. *Br. J. Oral Maxillofac. Surg.* 54 (7): 724–730.

3 Rosen, P.S., Summers, R., Mellado, J. et al. (1999). The bone-added osteotome sinus floor elevation technique: multicenter retrospective report of consecutively treated patients. *Int. J. Oral Maxillofac. Implants* 14: 853–858.

4 Lundgren, S., Andersson, S., Gualini, F., and Sennerby, L. (2004). Bone reformation with sinus membrane elevation: a new surgical technique for maxillary sinus floor augmentation. *Clin. Implant Dent. Relat. Res.* 6 (3): 165–173.

5 Ardekian, L., Oved-Peleg, E., Mactei, E., and Peled, M. (2006). The clinical significance of sinus membrane perforation during augmentation of the maxillary sinus. *J. Oral Maxillofac. Surg.* 64 (2): 277–282.

6 Moreno Vazquez, J.C., Gonzalez de Rivera, A., Serrano Gil, H., and Mifsut, R.S. (2014). Complication rate in 200 consecutive sinus lift procedures: guidelines for prevention and treatment. *J. Oral Maxillofac. Surg.* 72 (5): 892–901.

7 Saker, M. and Ogle, O. (2005). Benign paroxysmal positional vertigo subsequent to sinus lift via closed technique. *J. Oral Maxillofac. Surg.* 63 (9): 1385–1387.

8

Technologic, Material, and Procedural Advancements in Dental Implant Surgery

Alexander Toth and Dwight Williams

Introduction

Dental implant surgery has been a rapidly changing field since its modern inception in the 1950s, and continues to be the most advanced solution for the replacement of missing teeth. With advancements in computer-processing technology in recent decades, digital imaging and computer-based implant planning have come to represent a new frontier in dental implant treatment. Modern technology can reliably offer superior outcomes by eliminating many sources of human error and miscalculation, allowing for improved dental implant function and esthetics, improved speed and ease of procedure, increased patient and doctor satisfaction, and improved cost efficiency. Additionally, material advancements continue to contribute significantly to the progression of the field.

This chapter will discuss the various ways in which modern technology, novel materials, and surgical techniques are revolutionizing the field of implant dentistry. For a more in-depth review of the specific techniques and materials discussed, further reading should be pursued.

Three-Dimensional Imaging

Computed tomography (CT) revolutionized the medical world on its development in the early 1970s by Godfrey Hounsfield, utilizing mathematical origins dating back to the early twentieth century. CT is a digital imaging technique that creates tomographic sections of biologic tissue in which each section is not contaminated by blurred or overlaid structures from adjacent anatomy. These sections can then be digitally compiled into a three-dimensional representation of the subject, allowing for qualitative and quantitative analysis of the hard and soft tissues of the entire body. At the time of its invention, this provided extremely valuable medical diagnostic information that had previously been unattainable. Additionally, its usefulness for dental and maxillofacial diagnosis and treatment planning became clear, although concerns existed about the higher levels of radiation exposure associated with traditional fan beam medical-grade CTs.

To address this, a new type of CT, called cone beam computed tomography (CBCT), was developed specifically for dental and maxillofacial applications. The CBCT uses a cone beam X-ray emission source which reduces the radiation exposure to approximately 12.0 mSv, which is equivalent to about five D-speed dental X-rays, or 25% that of a panoramic X-ray. CBCTs also reduce scatter, are much faster, and can scan both arches simultaneously.

Cone beam CT produces axial images by utilizing an X-ray source which rotates 360° around the patient. The sensor converts received X-ray information into electronic data and, using mathematical algorithms, produces a three-dimensional image of the subject. It provides information as to the density of the subject, described in Hounsfield units, with −1000 representing air, 0 representing water, and +3000 representing enamel. Regarding implant therapy, CT imaging of the maxillofacial region can provide very useful information on the quality and quantity of alveolar bone, and the proximity of adjacent vital structures such as the inferior alveolar nerve canal and maxillary sinus (Figure 8.1).

Cone beam CT technology is not only highly valuable for diagnostic purposes in its own right, but its integration with other available technology expands its functionality considerably. It can be partnered with implant planning software to allow for the precise evaluation of implant width, length, angulation, relation to adjacent structures, and evaluation of restorative considerations. Further, with

Oral and Maxillofacial Surgery, Medicine, and Pathology for the Clinician, First Edition. Edited by Harry Dym, Leslie R. Halpern, and Orrett E. Ogle.

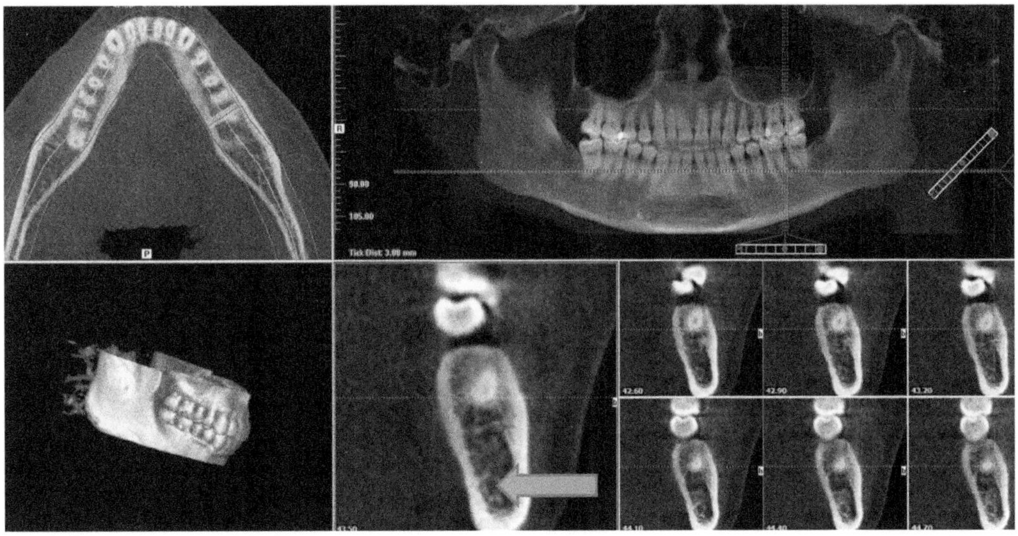

Figure 8.1 CBCT image, with the arrow indicating the position of the inferior alveolar nerve canal.

the utilization of implant planning software, static surgical guides for implant placement can be fabricated by sending the digital files to the dental lab, or can be made by the clinician directly using a 3D printing device. In addition, using computer-aided design and computer-aided manufacturing (CAD/CAM) software and machinery, provisional or permanent restorations can be fabricated chairside and delivered at the same appointment.

Computerized Implant Planning Technology

Using 3D imaging, precise implant placement design pertaining to depth, angulation, location, proximity to vital structures, and relation to opposing dentition can be achieved with the aid of computerized implantology. Virtual treatment planning allows for highly predictable results, and has been known to significantly reduce surgical complications such as inferior alveolar nerve injury, sinus perforation, and dehiscence. In this way, virtual implant planning and computer-generated static drilling guides allow for more efficient and efficacious placement of dental implants.

Virtual implant planning is generally a three-stage process, with the first stage being CBCT imaging following the required protocol of the proprietary software being used. The 3D image allows for evaluation of bone quantity, anatomic structures, and their relation to the proposed 3D restoration. The restoration is then virtually created and overlaid on the CBCT image. Lastly, implants and abutments can then be virtually fabricated by the clinician and adjusted with regard to an optimally placed prosthesis, within the confines of the bony anatomy. Additionally, bone augmentation procedures, such as sinus lift, can be simulated and factored into treatment planning (Figure 8.2).

Once the treatment plan is set, the clinician can then use this diagnostic information to aid in free-hand placement of the implant, or the plan can be digitally transferred to a variety of stereolithographic surgical drilling guide manufacturers or used with a 3D stereolithographic printer chairside, which will both be discussed later in the chapter. Such drilling guides are used with osteotomy twist drills with "drill stops" which allow for precise control of depth, angulation, and location of implant placement based on the virtual design. Simplant, Blue Sky Bio, and NobelProcera® are a few of the major software programs available [1].

Virtual implant planning has been demonstrated to reduce complications and improve placement accuracy, especially in more complex cases, and has established itself as a tool which is heavily relied upon by the modern implantologist.

Intraoral Optical Impressions and Integration with CBCT, CAD/CAM, and Stereolithography

Intraoral scanners are a relatively new tool available to clinicians for obtaining digital impressions of tooth morphology and adjacent oral structures. Intraoral optical impressions can be used to create a 3D, color-accurate surface representation of the dentition and gingiva. These scanners use a light-emitting diode (LED) or laser to

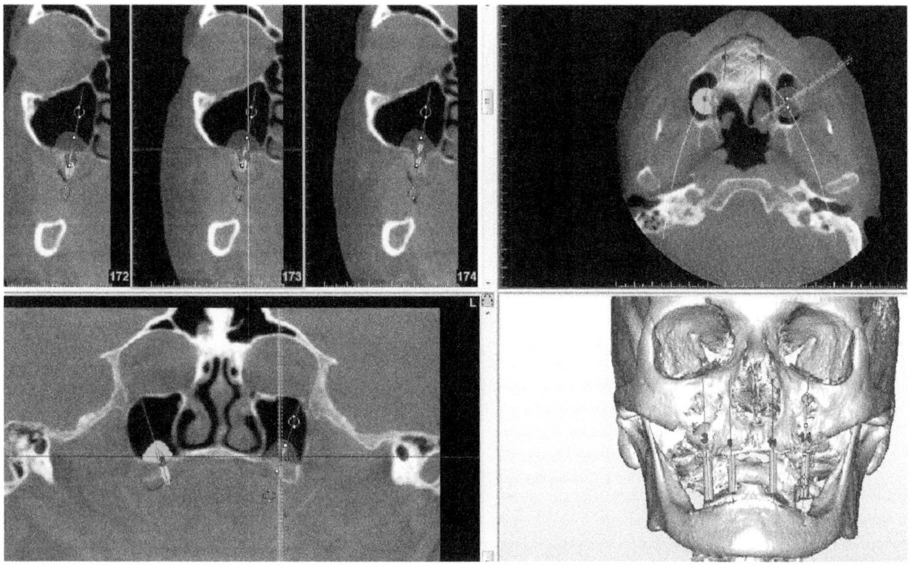

Figure 8.2 Virtual implant treatment work-up with Simplant, allowing for visualization of four maxillary implants in three dimensions, while also simulating sinus augmentation.

convert surface information into a digital stereolithography file, and can obviate the need for taking physical alginate impressions in the dental office [2].

The two main types of optical scanners available are blue LED and laser scanners. LED scanners require a contrasting medium in the form of a powder which is applied to all scanned surfaces, which laser scanners do not require. The iTero™ scanner (Align Technology) was the first standalone optical laser scanner which became widely available to clinicians in 2006. This technology uses still image acquisition via a red laser projected onto the oral tissues with parallel confocal technology, which is similar to creating a panoramic photograph by stitching together multiple images. There are several other manufacturers available today, including Cadent iTero, E4D® by D4D Technologies, Lava™ chairside oral scanner by 3M ESPE , and CEREC® by Sirona. The digital impression allows the user to create a 3D surface-level image of a tooth preparation or abutment, along with opposing dentition, adjacent teeth, and other oral structures [1].

The advantages of digital impressions are numerous. Besides being more time efficient and less invasive than conventional alginate impressions, the digital models can be sent to dental labs directly along with a digital prescription. The lab then uses software to indicate margins, verify occlusion, and provide quality control. The models can be downloaded directly to their milling machines, allowing for CAD/CAM fabrication of restorations (such as the E.max crown) without any need for physical models. Several companies, including Sirona and D4D, also have optional software and milling units available to allow for immediate CAD/CAM fabrication of the final restoration chairside.

Models can be produced from the scanned information in one of two ways. The first utilizes stereolithography by resin photopolymerization in a layer-by-layer fashion to create a 3D object, which can be used for a variety of applications including surgical stents and diagnostic models. Milling is another technique used to fabricate temporary or permanent ceramic restorations from an intraoral scan, and utilizes a precured urethane block which is milled to reduce excess material to a highly precise degree. Several studies have shown digital optical impression accuracy to be equal to or greater than conventional techniques [1]. Chairside STL models and guides have also been demonstrated to have similar accuracy to those fabricated by an outside manufacturer, while increasing convenience and cost-effectiveness [1].

Due to their high degree of precision compared to conventional methods, the use of optical impressions and CAD/CAM restoration fabrication can reduce procedure time, the need for prosthetic adjustments and remakes, and patient and laboratory costs. Additionally, digital impressions can be integrated with CBCT and CAD/CAM milling or 3D printers for a variety of objectives, including production of diagnostic models, implant surgical stent fabrication, and temporary or permanent ceramic restoration fabrication [1].

Surgical Drilling Guide Integration and Fabrication

As previously mentioned, optical surface imaging STL files can be integrated with the CBCT using a variety of software programs, which use corresponding points on the teeth or surrounding structures to overlay the surface data to the CBCT. This process also allows the integration of implant planning software and precise implant placement planning. This information can then be digitally sent to an outside dental stent manufacturer for surgical drilling guide fabrication, which precisely dictates the depth, angulation, and location of the osteotomy. Alternatively, the file can be sent to a chairside 3D printer directly, which allows for the fabrication of custom tooth, mucosa, or bone supported osteotomy guides on the same day, at the cost of only a several dollars per stent (Figure 8.3).

Three-dimensional stereolithographic printers use polymer layering to create the static surgical guide, and although a variety of printing resins can be used, only some are specifically designed and approved for dental implant surgical guide fabrication. Premade metal drilling inserts can then be manually inserted into the drilling guide after the polymer has cured, to allow for guidance of the osteotomy drills.

Static drilling guides have been shown to provide a high level of accuracy relative to standard endosteal implant placement, and can also increase time and cost efficiency, when factoring in reduced postoperative complications due to placement error. However, static guides will occasionally need to be refabricated if they do not seat appropriately on the teeth, bone, or mucosa. Additionally, if changes are required during osteotomy preparation regarding desired implant location or dimensions, the guide must be abandoned and the traditional free-hand approach used, due to the lack of adjustability in the static guide. In the posterior arch, the bulkiness of the guide combined with the length of the osteotomy drill may prohibit use in some situations, especially for patients with limited opening [1].

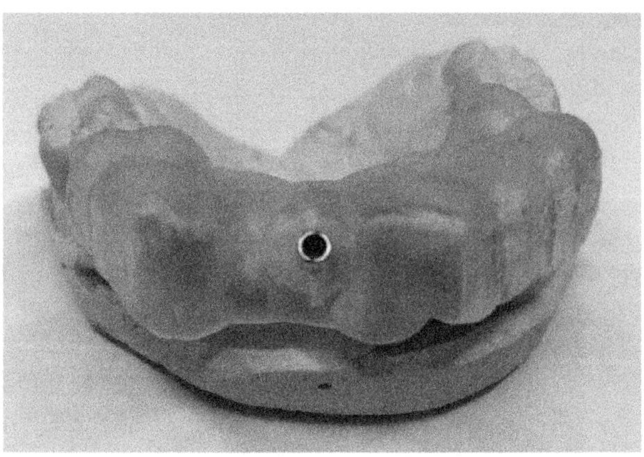

Figure 8.3 A static surgical pilot drilling guide with metal drilling insert for a maxillary anterior implant.

Guided Navigation in Osteotomy Preparation and Implant Placement

Dynamic navigation is a newly developed method for implant placement, and allows for real-time 3D visualization of the preparation with high magnification on a computer monitor. This technology allows for the placement of dental implants using an array on the implant handpiece, an array attached to the patient's arch, and two overheard cameras to track and guide implant placement. Passive array systems reflect light emitted from a light source back to the stereo cameras while active array systems emit light directly, which is then tracked by the stereo cameras.

Passive optical dynamic navigation systems employ the use of fiducial markers, which are securely attached to the patient's arch prior to CBCT scanning. These markers allow for registration of the patient's arch to the stereo cameras, with the aid of the attached light-reflecting array. This array is placed extraorally, and attaches to the fiducial markers via a clip. Using this array and a second array attached to the handpiece, the stereo cameras allow for triangulation and thus "dynamic navigation" of the osteotomy preparation by displaying 3D images on a computer monitor and requiring little to no direct visualization.

Some important considerations are the fact that the drill and patient-mounted arrays must be in sight of two overhead cameras, and a small flap must also be established using traditional methods. Passive optical dynamic navigation systems require the use of an overhead blue light, which is reflected by the arrays and received by the stereo cameras. Generally, minimal computer experience is required by the clinician. Additionally, only a small flap is required, as visualization of the bony contour is not required to establish necessary osteotomy angulation and location, thus allowing the procedure to be more minimally invasive.

The standard workflow starts with CBCT imaging of the arch with the secured fiducial marker, which contains three metallic segments. The DICOM (Digital Imaging and Communications in Medicine) file is then uploaded to the navigation system software, and a virtual implant is placed and modified as necessary. Additionally, a radiopaque tooth can be placed prior to scanning if desired for implant planning. Drill lengths and diameters intended for use are then registered into the navigation system.

The next step is the surgical phase, in which the fiducial marker is again placed on the patient's arch, this time with an attached light-reflecting array, compatible with the navigation system being used, via a plastic clip. A second compatible array is also attached to the handpiece at this time. Traditional local anesthesia is provided and a small full-thickness mucoperiosteal flap can be prepared. The patient is then positioned to allow direct vision of the arrays via the two overhead cameras. The drills are then oriented per the 3D images displayed on the screen, and the osteotomy is carried out using indirect visualization via the computer monitor. After osteotomy preparation, final implant placement can be done indirectly or with direct visualization, depending on clinician preference [3].

One clear advantage of this technology compared to static surgical drilling guides is the ability to make any necessary changes to the planned implant position during the osteotomy preparation. Dynamic navigation has also been shown to have improved accuracy, time efficiency, and cost-effectiveness, compared to static guides [1]. It is also associated with improved operator ergonomics compared to standard and static drill guide implant placement, and also allows for minimally invasive flap reflection. Without the need for direct visualization, dynamic navigation systems may be particularly useful in patients with limited opening, and for posterior regions in which direct visualization can be compromised.

Although a learning curve does exist, these systems do not require extensive computer expertise by the clinician and are intended to be relatively straightforward to use. This being said, several case experiences may be necessary to establish clinical proficiency, and usage requires training of both the clinician and their support staff. Additionally, dynamic navigation cannot be used for edentulous cases, as intrabony fiducial markers are not currently available. In this scenario, a static guide would be preferential. For the same reason, the fiducial marker often cannot be adequately stabilized by periodontally compromised teeth or provisional restorations. In this case, static guides would also be preferential (Figure 8.4).

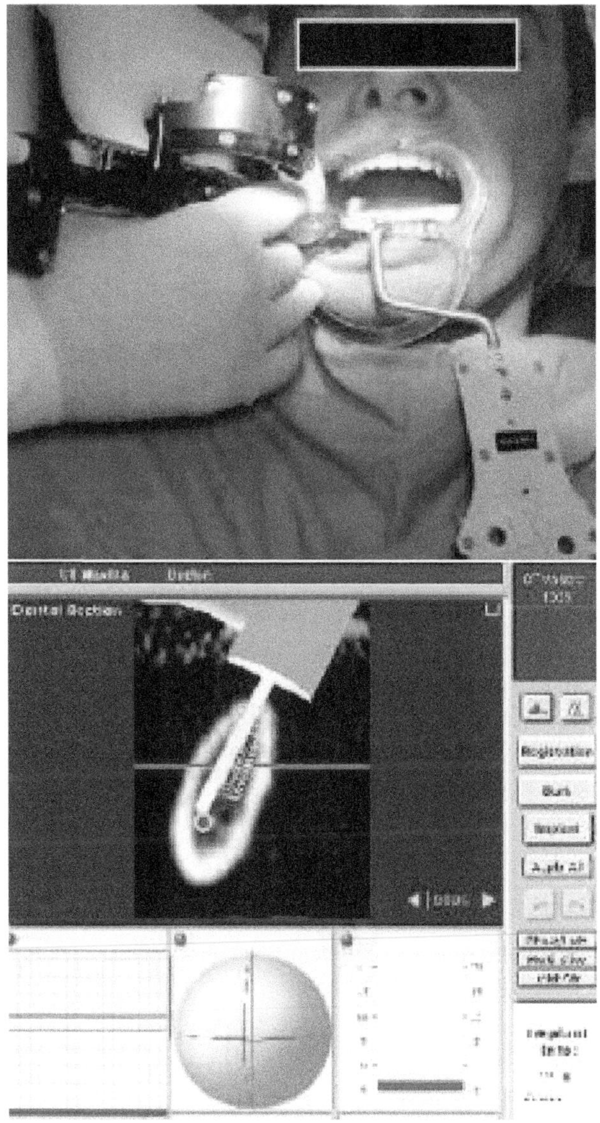

Figure 8.4 Guided navigation dental implant surgery. The array attached to the patient's arch and the array attached to the surgical handpiece can be visualized, while the stereo cameras are outside the frame. The lower image shows the osteotomy preparation in real time. *Source:* This article was published in Contemporary Implant Dentistry, 3rd Edition, Carl Misch, Diagnostic Casts and Surgical Templates, Page 289, Copyright Elsevier 2008, and is used with permission.

In summary, both static guides and dynamic navigation systems are very useful, accurate, and accessible ways to improve implant placement. Indications for use of either of these systems over the free-hand method are numerous, and include situations in which flapless approaches or minimally invasive flaps are required, such as after ridge augmentation, to allow preservation of all crestal bone. They are also very helpful when there is very limited space, and interimplant or implant–tooth distances require superior accuracy. Additionally, they can aid in angulation when screw-retained implants are desired, or if one is working in the esthetic zone and emergence profile is key. Lastly, when you expect the implant to be in close relation to adjacent vital structures such as the sinus membrane or inferior alveolar nerve, the high degree of accuracy provided by these systems is preferred.

Membranes for Bone Grafting

Numerous resorbable and nonresorbable membranes are currently available for use in guided bone regeneration (GBR) prior to planned implant placement, with many having specific advantages and disadvantages. Classically, polytetrafluoroethylene membranes have been used as a nonresorbable option to allow for GBR. Although providing good long-term material stability, exposure can occur, prolonging the healing phase or resulting in graft loss or infection. Collagen resorbable membranes have also classically been used for GBR with success, allowing for improved patient tolerance resulting from a reduced number of required procedures. However, collagen membranes are also associated with cytotoxicity, hastened degradation associated with graft site collapse, and impedance of bone regeneration. Additionally, they can be challenging to adapt and suture clinically.

More recently, silkworm cocoon-derived silk membranes have been shown to be superior to traditional membranes in several aspects. Silk membranes were shown to have greater tensile yield strength in recent studies, and were associated with significantly increased bone volume at 4 and 8 weeks postoperatively, with increased histological bone formation and osteoblasts noted [1].

Amnion-chorion membrane barriers have also recently been proposed for GBR and sinus perforation repair during maxillary sinus augmentation. Hyperdry amniotic membrane, a preservable human amnion, has also been proposed as a sound dressing material for surgical defects of the oral mucosa, with studies suggesting its clinically usefulness. With regard to dental implants, there is reason to believe that it may be a useful mucosal cover for sites of bone augmentation or implant placement, when primary closure cannot be achieved, allowing for reduced infection and tissue contracture risk while eliminating the need for harvest site morbidity associated with donor sites [4].

BMP, PRGF, and PRP

Bone morphogenetic protein (BMP) is a naturally occurring protein within the extracellular matrix of bone, with multiple varieties having been identified and evaluated for their osteoinductive potential with regard to bone augmentation in preparation for dental implant placement. BMP-2 has been particularly associated with stimulation of osteogenesis in multiple studies, and was approved for use in sinus lift and ridge augmentation surgery by the FDA in 2007. A 2011 study by Gonzalez et al. showed excellent long-term dental implant stability in the posterior maxilla after use of BMP-2 in conjunction with sinus augmentation surgery [5] (Figure 8.5).

For sinus augmentation, BMP-2 can be reconstituted with normal saline and placed on a collagen carrier, which is then secured beneath the sinus membrane after lateral window establishment. No additional bone grafting is required, but allogenic or xenograft bone can be combined with the BMP collagen carrier for even greater augmentation [1]. BMP-2 is also particularly useful for the challenge of producing increased vertical bone height. A 2017 study using BMP-2 for ridge augmentation showed an average vertical gain for 3.6 mm in the maxilla and 2.32 mm in the mandible, with results similar to that of alveolar distraction osteogenesis. Benefits of BMP include the reduced need for donor site morbidity in securing autogenous bone, as well as its reliable osteogenic potential in producing quality bone.

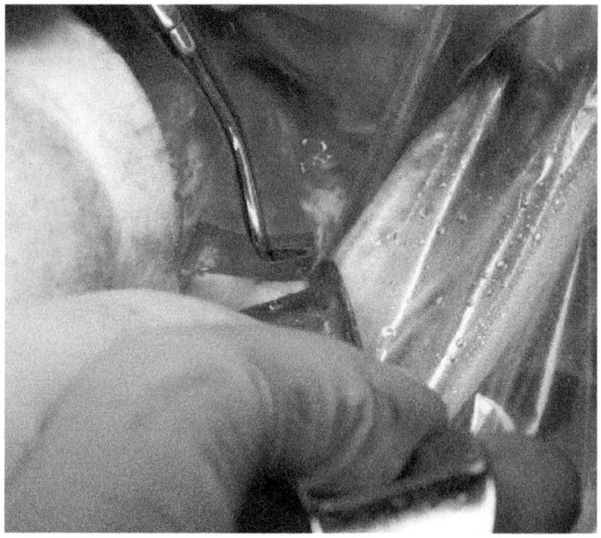

Figure 8.5 Sinus augmentation surgery, with reflection of the sinus membrane in preparation for BMP placement.

Plasma rich in growth factors (PRGF) and platelet-rich plasma (PRP) are also currently being used for bone and soft tissue regeneration for dental implant placement. PRGF and PRP are prepared by centrifuge of autologous blood from the patient, and then activated using a 10% calcium chloride, or similar, solution. This process allows the extraction of concentrated platelets in a small volume of plasma containing several growth factors from the patient's blood, which can be used to promote bone regeneration. PRGF, in contrast to PRP or serum, contains higher levels of transforming growth factor (TGF)-beta and platelet-derived growth factor (PDGF)-BB. PRGF is also leukocyte free while PRP includes leukocytes. A 2011 study focusing on bone formation in rat calvaria suggested PRGF could have significant use as a potential method for bone regeneration [5] (Figure 8.6).

In contrast to PRGF, PRP has demonstrated efficacy in many human studies. PRP includes three isomeres of platelet-derived growth factors (PDGF$\alpha\alpha$, PDGF$\beta\beta$, and PDGF$\alpha\beta$), as well as TGF-beta (TGF-beta 1 and TGF-beta 2), vascular endothelial growth factor, and epithelial growth factor. The plasma in PRP also contains three blood

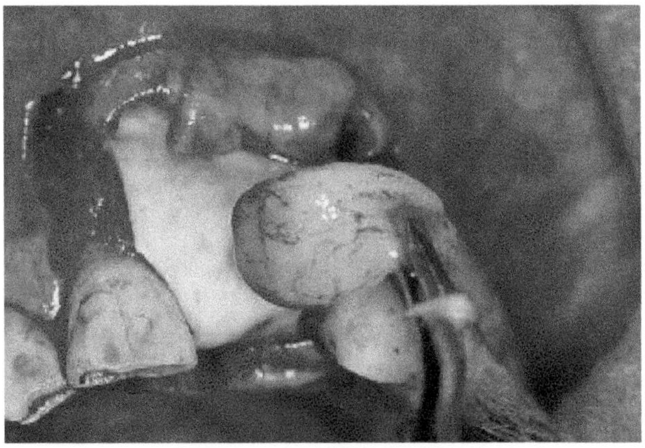

Figure 8.6 Use of PRP in alveolar ridge augmentation. *Source:* This article was published in Contemporary Implant Dentistry, 3rd Edition, Carl Misch, Keys to Bone Grafting and Bone Grafting Materials, Page 844, Copyright Elsevier 2008, and is used with permission.

proteins, fibrin, fibronectin, and vitronectin, which are known to act as cell adhesion molecules for osteoconduction, bone matrix formation, and connective tissue and epithelial cell migration. For this reason, PRP has been used for its potential in both hard and soft tissue regeneration.

Platelet-rich plasma centrifugation has been developed for use in the office setting or operating room, with multiple centrifuge devices being available for this purpose. Although the majority of publications have shown significant healing enhancement with PRP usage, due to variance in the efficacy of different machines, some studies have shown mixed results. Studies have shown wide-ranging use in the clinical setting, with positive results demonstrated in horizontal and vertical alveolar ridge augmentation using autogenous bone or bone substitutes, sinus augmentation surgery, treatment of bony periodontal defects and periimplant defects. PRP has also been shown to allow for earlier implant loading and improved osteointegration in patients with reduced bone quality due to radiotherapy or osteoporosis [4]. With regard to soft tissue regeneration, PRP has shown improved healing of connective tissue grafts, gingival grafts, and palatal grafts. PRP is a valuable asset for use in bone regeneration and skin or mucosa healing, and should be considered as an adjunct in cases where hard or soft tissue augmentation is required.

Implant-Supported, Full-Arch, Fixed Prostheses with Immediate Loading and "All-on-Four"

Implant-supported, full-arch, fixed prostheses with immediate loading have become an increasingly popular treatment option for the fully edentulous mandible and maxilla, with growing evidence to support their use. The most popular technique has been termed "all-on-four" and was introduced by Dr Paulo Malo, in Portugal, in 1998. This technique was developed to maximize the use of available bone and allow for immediate functioning.

The all-on-four technique uses four implants in the edentulous jaw, efficiently utilizing bone by tilting the posterior implants in a posterior direction, to allow for longer implants than could otherwise be accommodated with the available space. Thus, a secure, immediate loading prosthesis can be delivered even with minimal bone support in the maxilla or mandible. More recently, other techniques using similar principles but a different number of implants have been described and studied [4]. In one such study, five or six implants were placed in each arch, yielding an implant success rate of 93% with an immediate, computer-guided restoration success rate of 100% at 16 months [6].

The primary considerations include the ability to achieve primary stability of the implant (35–45 Ncm torque), as well as the absence of parafunctional habits in the patient. In the maxilla, the procedure is indicated with a minimal bone width of 5 mm and height of 10 mm from canine to canine. Regarding the mandible, 5 mm width is minimally required, with 8 mm of bone height between the mental foramina. The posterior implants can then be tilted to a maximum of 45° but if the angulation exceeds 30°, splinting is needed. Ideally, the screw access holes of the tilted posterior implants should be located in the region of the occlusal surface of the planned first molar, second premolar, or first premolar. The posterior implants used are ideally 4–4.3 mm in diameter, and the immediate loaded fixed prosthesis should have a maximum of 12 teeth. As with all multiunit fixed prostheses, the angulation after abutment placement needs to allow for a single path of insertion.

The basic workflow for all-on-four mandibular implants involves making a midcrestal, full-thickness, mucoperiosteal flap. Identification of the mental foramen is important as the final implant should be at least 6 mm anterior to the foramen to avoid the anterior loop. Additionally, proper identification and marking of the midline are critical. A static drilling guide can then be seated, and a twist drill is used to initiate the posterior osteotomy with a maximum angulation of 45°. After angulation is verified, the osteotomy is enlarged as needed and the implant is installed. Next, the anterior implant sites are prepared with as much interimplant space as possible, without interfering with the apex of the posterior implants. Straight or 17° multiunit abutments are then placed to allow for proper emergence of the prosthetic screw. After suturing, an open tray impression can be taken if the immediate restoration has not already been fabricated along with the surgical guide (Figures 8.7 and 8.8).

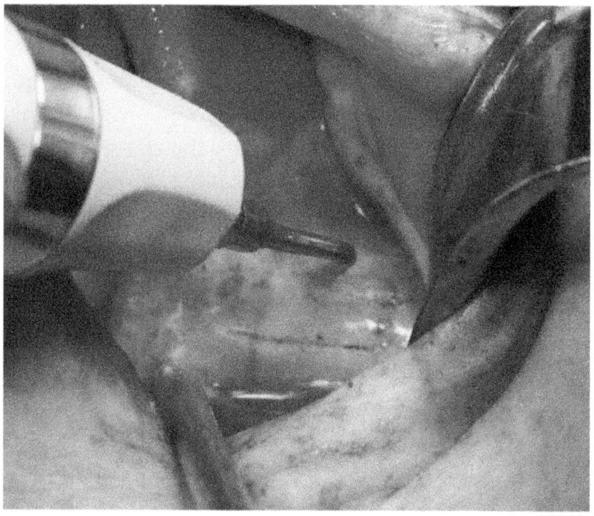

Figures 8.7 Identification and surgical access of the anterior maxillary sinus wall.

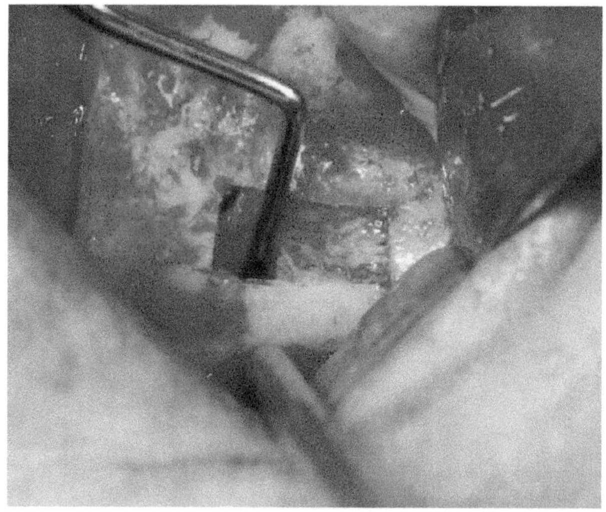

Figures 8.8 Exploration of the anterior maxillary sinus wall. A small perforation can be seen.

With the edentulous maxilla, a few additional steps are necessary. The anterior wall of the maxillary sinus must be identified by making a small osteotomy and verifying its location. Once the anterior wall has been identified and explored with a probe, the posterior osteotomy can be initiated as posteriorly as possible while staying at least 4 mm from the anterior sinus wall. Again, the posterior implants are tilted posteriorly to a maximum of 45°, to minimize the cantilever.

Zygomatic Implants

Zygomatic implants are dental implants that achieve their stability in the zygomatic buttress rather than the maxilla, and can currently provide dental rehabilitation in the setting of severe posterior maxillary atrophy. Generally, zygomatic implants should be considered when sufficient anterior maxillary bone exists or can be established, but the posterior alveolar crest has severe atrophy and is unsuitable for dental implants with or without bone grafting. In such cases, bilateral, posterior zygomatic implants can be placed in combination with two anterior standard implants, to offer adequate support for a fixed prosthesis or overdenture (Figures 8.9–8.12).

The process for zygomatic implants involves exposure of the palatal crest, the creation of a 10 × 5 mm window in the lateral wall of the sinus, and elevation of the sinus membrane from the posterior wall, ideally without perforation. This allows for direct visualization of the path of the drill during osteotomy preparation, which is a critical aspect. The osteotomy is then initiated at a site on the alveolar crest determined by the final restoration, and

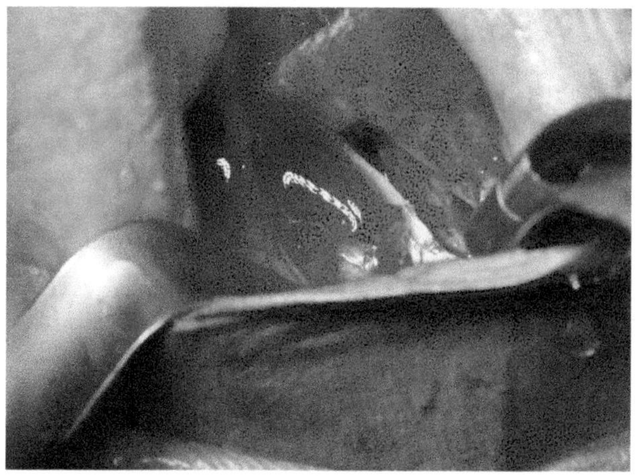

Figure 8.9 Establishment of a lateral maxillary sinus window in preparation for the zygomatic implant osteotomy.

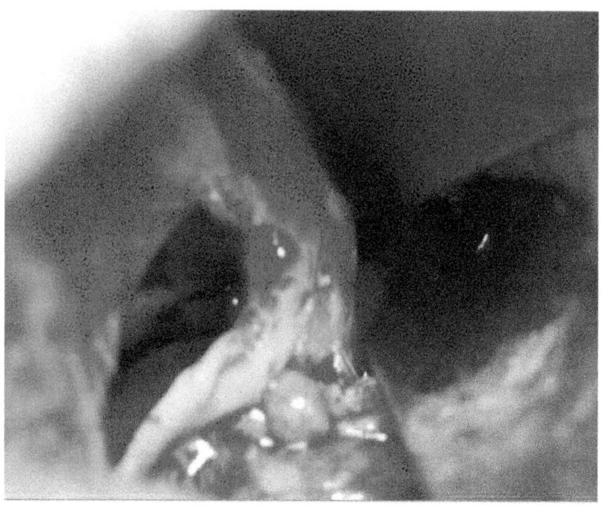

Figure 8.10 Zygomatic implant osteotomy preparation with retraction of the soft tissue.

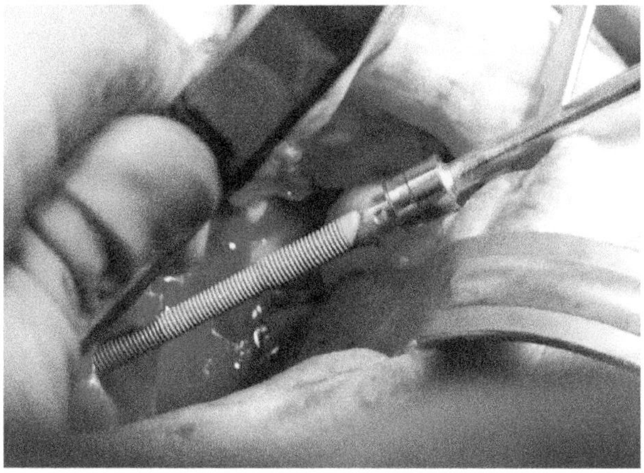

Figure 8.11 Zygomatic implant placement.

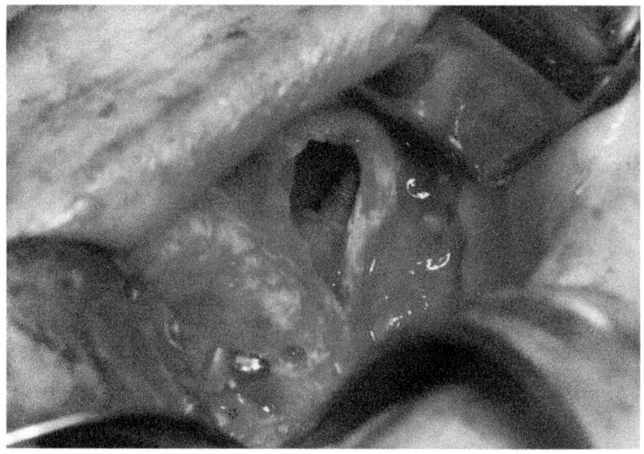

Figure 8.12 The zygomatic implant in its final position, via the lateral maxillary sinus window.

proceeds either through the sinus itself or in the outer cortical bone of the maxilla and zygoma, with careful retraction and protection of the soft tissue. The osteotomy is then widened with twist drills and the depth of the prepared site, based on the radiographically predetermined implant length, is verified with a depth indicator. The implant is then installed using the zygoma handpiece, with visualization through the lateral sinus window, until the apex of the implant engages in the zygomatic bone, torqued to 45 Ncm. The cover screws are then placed and water-tight, tension-free primary closure should be achieved. Healing abutments can be placed either as a one-stage or two-stage protocol, as with standard endosteal implants [7].

Different variations of insertion of the zygomatic implant placement are shown in Figure 8.13.

Lasers

Diode lasers can be a useful adjunctive tool in dental implant therapy. Lasers have a variety of uses in dentistry and can be very useful for uncovering implants or elastically recontouring the gingiva. They provide better safety than electrosurgery, maintain a temperature within the zone of safety for bone, and do not cause tissue shrinkage which can affect esthetic outcome. The diode laser's tip allows simultaneous cutting and coagulation providing excellent hemostasis and improving surgical visualization as well as allowing for immediate impression taking. Thus, lasers can be a useful clinical tool in stage two dental implant surgery, for gingival debridement prior to prosthesis placement, and for flap creation in patients with an increased risk of bleeding.

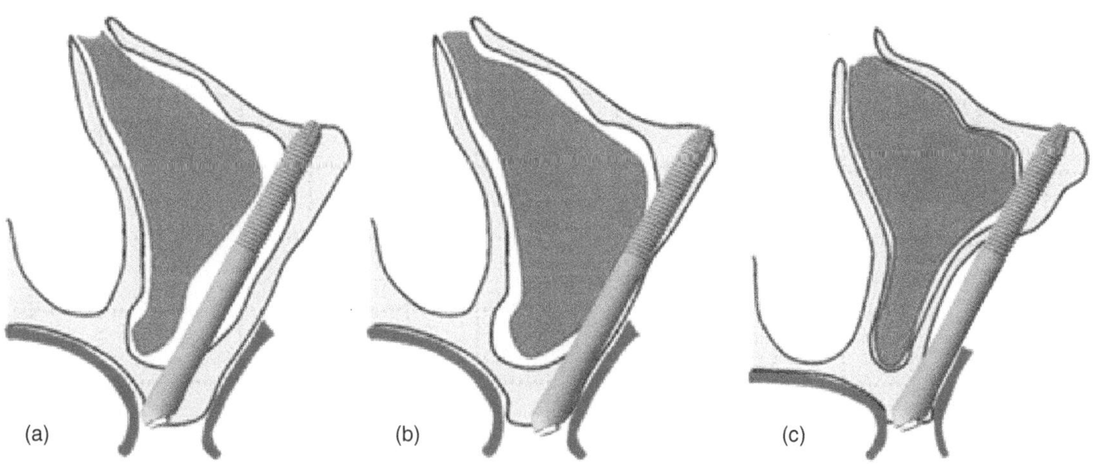

Figure 8.13 Zygomatic implant placement techniques: intrasinus (a), in the wall of the maxilla (b), and extrasinus (c). *Source:* Davó R et al., 2020/MDPI/Licensed under CC BY 4.0.

Conclusion

In summary, the many technologic, material, and procedural innovations in dental implant therapy offer a tremendous benefit to patients and clinicians alike. As dental implant therapy moves forward, these advancements will only become more valuable and relevant to the practice of implant therapy. Being open to such advancements, while integrating one's own clinical experience and expertise, will almost certainly allow for improved treatment outcomes, time and cost efficiency, and ultimately, improved doctor and patient satisfaction.

References

1 Orentlicher, G. and Goldsmith, D. (2007). Computer-guided implantology – a new era. *J. Oral Maxillofac. Surg.* 65: 71.
2 Scherer M.A contemporary approach to intraoral optical scanning and in-office 3-D printing. www.michaelscherermd.com/wp-content/uploads/2015/09/SchererMD-DentistryToday_122015.pdf
3 Block M, E.R. (2016). Static or dynamic navigation for implant placement – choosing the method of guidance. *J. Oral Maxillofac. Surg.* 74: 269–277.
4 Dym H (2015). Implant procedures for the general dentist. *Dent. Clin. North Am.* 59: 271.
5 Gonzalez, M., Fuentes, R., Triplett, R., and Triplett, S. (2011). BMP-2 used for maxillary sinus augmentation and implant placement: 15 years follow-up after final restorations. *J. Oral Maxillofac. Surg.* 69 (9), Supplement: e51.
6 Reuss J, Pi-Anfruns J, and Moy P (2018). Is bone morphogenetic protein-2 as effective as alveolar distraction osteogenesis for vertical bone regeneration? *J. Oral Maxillofac. Surg.* 76: 752–760.
7 Singh, P. and Cranin, A. (2010). *Atlas of Oral Implantology*, 3e, 275–283. St Louis, MO: Mosby Elsevier.

Part IV

Trauma

9

Diagnosis and Management of Dentoalveolar Trauma

Justine S. Moe and Shelly Abramowicz

Introduction

Dentoalveolar injuries make up 5% of all facial fractures in the pediatric population [1] and have a prevalence of approximately 17.5% among children and adolescents [2]. Frequent causes include falls in toddlers [3, 4], sports [5–7], and playground accidents [5, 8, 9] in children and motor vehicle accidents [10–12], assault [10, 13, 14], industrial accidents [15–17], and endotracheal intubation [18–20] in teenagers and adults. Boys are affected twice as often as girls with a peak incidence at 2–4 years and 8–10 years [21].

Evaluation

Dentoalveolar injuries can occur in isolation or in association with multisystem injury. As such, the maxillofacial trauma evaluation should be completed as part of the initial evaluation and management of the trauma patient as per advanced trauma life support (ATLS) guidelines [22]. The comprehensive maxillofacial evaluation is completed once life-threatening injuries are identified and treated. An understanding of the patient's overall status and injuries is important to plan for the appropriate timing of the management of dentoalveolar trauma.

History

When possible, a comprehensive history should be taken from the patient or parental guardian. The nature of the injury (location, timing, mechanism of injury, etc.) should be noted. Dentoalveolar injuries can arise from direct trauma, such as blunt force to the anterior teeth, or from indirect trauma, such as a blow to the chin [23]. The location of injury may give information regarding the degree of bacterial contamination. Events surrounding the accident which may increase suspicion of concomitant injuries or child abuse should be noted [24].

In the event of tooth avulsion, the timing of the injury, use of storage medium, and time to implantation should be recorded. If the location of the tooth is not identified, accidental inhalation or ingestion should be ruled out. The patient should be questioned about change in dental occlusion, tooth mobility, intraoral bleeding, and pain following the injury. In addition, information regarding demographic data, medical and dental history, medication allergies, tetanus vaccination status, last oral intake, and last menstrual cycle in female patients should be obtained.

Physical Examination

A comprehensive maxillofacial examination should be completed. The face, chin, forehead, scalp, and neck should be evaluated. Palpation of the facial skeleton should be completed to assess for tenderness or step deformities to rule out facial fracture. The intraoral soft tissues, including the oral mucosa, gingiva, lips, tongue, floor of mouth, soft palate, and oropharynx, should be evaluated for lacerations, contusions, debris, or foreign bodies. The maxilla and mandible should be evaluated for step-off deformities, gross malocclusion, mobility, or displacement of fractured segments.

Finally, the dentition should be evaluated. In the pediatric patient, the clinician should be mindful of the stage of dentition and the normal eruption sequence in order to distinguish physiologic mobility of erupting permanent teeth and exfoliating primary teeth from pathologic findings. Infraction lines can be identified by transillumination along the long axis of the tooth [25]. Crown fractures

Oral and Maxillofacial Surgery, Medicine, and Pathology for the Clinician, First Edition. Edited by Harry Dym, Leslie R. Halpern, and Orrett E. Ogle.

should be identified with evaluation of the exposed structures. Tooth mobility and tooth displacement, including direction and amount, should be assessed. Percussion sensitivity can be indicative of injury to the periodontal ligament (PDL). Tooth vitality testing is not reliable in the acute setting due to variable patient cooperation and false-negative results [26, 27]. Sensitivity responses can be temporarily decreased, notably after displacement injuries; however, repeated testing has shown that normal reactions can return after a few weeks or months [27].

Radiographic Studies

Radiographic imaging is indicated in dentoalveolar injuries to evaluate root injuries, PDL injuries, alveolar injuries, and jaw fractures. In addition, radiographs provide information on root development, size of the pulp chamber and root canal, and proximity of the succedaneous tooth to the injured tooth.

Ideally, dentoalveolar injuries should be evaluated by different angulations using standardized projection techniques [28] including occlusal, periapical, and panoramic films. Computed tomography has limited utility for dentoalveolar injuries but may be obtained if concomitant maxillofacial factures are suspected. Chest and/or abdominal radiographs should be considered if a high suspicion of inhalation or ingestion of an avulsed tooth or dental appliance exists.

Diagnosis and Management of Dentoalveolar Injuries

Diagnosis of dentoalveolar injuries has been facilitated following the development of multiple classification schema [29–33]. Tooth fractures have been classified by Ellis and Davey [34]. Class I fractures extend through enamel only, class II fractures extend through enamel and dentin, class III fractures extend through the pulp, and class IV fractures are root fractures. Andreasen's classification [21] is a modification of the World Health Organization (WHO) classification [32] and is now the most widely used classification in the literature.

Prompt diagnosis and management of dentoalveolar injuries are crucial as delayed treatment can have a deleterious effect on prognosis. In young patients, the goal is to maintain pulp vitality to ensure continued root growth and development and an intact dentition. Guidelines for the management of dentoalveolar injuries have been established by the International Association of Dental Traumatology [28, 35, 36].

Injuries to the Dental Hard Tissue and Pulp

For injuries involving tooth structure, the goals of treatment are to maintain pulp vitality, minimize thermal stimuli and bacterial contamination to the pulp, and to restore tooth form and function. If indicated, restoration with a prosthetic crown should be delayed until pulp testing is no longer required [37].

Crown Infraction

Crown infraction refers to the incomplete fracture of enamel without loss of tooth substance [28]. Craze lines can be seen in a vertical, horizontal, or oblique orientation depending on the location and direction of trauma [38]. However, these injuries may be easily missed and may require direct transillumination to diagnose [23].

No immediate treatment is indicated for tooth infraction. Outpatient dental follow-up should be established. Dental infractions may require sealant to prevent further discoloration and the status of the pulp should be monitored [28].

Crown Fracture

Crown fractures account for 60–70% of all traumatic injuries seen in the dental office [39] (Figure 9.1). Crown fractures may be complicated or uncomplicated. Uncomplicated crown fracture refers to the loss of tooth substance involving the enamel, or enamel and dentin, without pulp exposure [28]. Dentinal sensitivity to hot, cold, and mastication is often seen. Complicated crown fracture refers to the loss of tooth substance involving the enamel, dentin, and pulp. Patients may complain of pain and sensitivity.

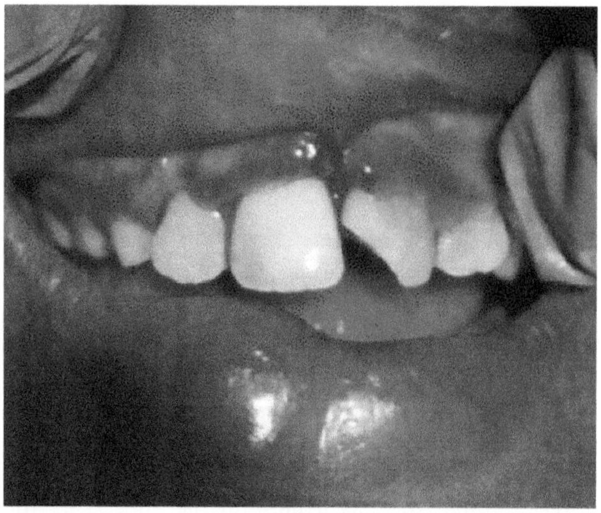

Figure 9.1 Crown fracture of the central incisor.

Enamel fractures may be treated by smoothing sharp edges, with a composite restoration, or the enamel fragment may be bonded to the tooth. Fractures involving enamel and dentin can be treated with glass ionomer cement or other restorative material as a temporizing measure until a permanent composite restoration can be fashioned [28]. If available, the tooth fragment can also be bonded to the tooth. Uncomplicated crown fractures have excellent prognosis with nearly 100% pulp survival [40] and treatment can be delayed for greater than 24 hours with no effect on outcome [37].

For crown fractures involving the pulp, the prognosis is best for fractures treated within the first 2 hours [41] but can be treated up to 24 hours [37]. Direct pulp cap using calcium hydroxide is indicated for pinpoint exposures and for exposures up to 1.5 mm if seen within 24 hours. In teeth with an open apex, exposures greater than 1.5 mm and smaller exposures over 24 hours are treated with pulpotomy, in which the superficial pulp is removed and calcium hydroxide or mineral trioxide aggregate (MTA) is placed [42]. In teeth with a closed apex, exposures larger than 1.5 mm and exposures over 24 hours are treated with root canal therapy. Teeth with a necrotic pulp should be treated with root canal therapy if the apex is mature or apexification if the apex is immature.

Crown-Root Fracture

Crown-root fractures are delineated as uncomplicated or complicated. Uncomplicated crown-root fractures involve enamel, dentin, and root structure in the absence of pulp exposure. Complicated crown-root fractures involve enamel, dentin, and root structure with pulp exposure. Even in the presence of pulp exposure, symptoms may be mild and limited to sensitivity to hot, cold, and mastication [28].

The coronal fragment should be removed to evaluate the fracture level to assess for restorability. Fractures that are longitudinal or that involve greater than one-third of the root are generally indications for extraction. If the fracture involves the coronal root and is horizontally angulated, dental restoration may be possible in conjunction with gingivectomy, ostectomy, and/or orthodontic extrusion [28]. Complicated crown-root fractures that are deemed restorable will also require pulp extirpation in the closed root apex and pulp capping or pulpotomy in the open root apex.

Root Fracture

Root fractures most often occur in teeth with complete root development [39]. Horizontal and oblique root fractures may be missed on initial radiographic exam. Fractures in the coronal third are associated with a mobile or displaced coronal fragment. Root fractures in the middle or apical third may be asymptomatic with no excess mobility.

Apical and middle third root fractures with mobility should be treated with a flexible splint for 4 weeks [28]; no treatment is required in the absence of excessive mobility. Cervical root fractures may require splinting for up to 4 months [28]. If pulpal necrosis develops, endodontic therapy of the coronal segment is indicated [28].

Vertical root fractures generally require extraction. Cervical root fractures may be treated with extraction or with orthodontic extrusion of the root following root canal therapy.

Injuries to the Periodontal Tissues

For injuries involving the PDL, the goals of treatment are to preserve PDL vitality, prevent sequelae of PDL necrosis, including replacement and inflammatory resorption, and to manage pulpal necrosis in the event of neurovascular bundle injury.

Concussion

Dental concussion refers to the injury of the tooth-supporting structure without abnormal mobility or displacement. The tooth may be percussion sensitive and may exhibit symptoms of hyperemia [28]. Treatment involves removing the tooth from occlusion. The tooth should be monitored for later reaction to the trauma [28].

Subluxation

Dental subluxation is injury to the tooth-supporting structure with abnormal loosening without tooth displacement [37]. Patients often exhibit tenderness to palpation and/or percussion. The tooth has increased mobility and bleeding from the gingival sulcus may be present.

Treatment includes occlusal adjustment to ensure the tooth is out of function and monitoring with vitality testing. Normally, a splint is not required but may be placed for 2 weeks for patient comfort [28]. Following concussion, the frequency of pulpal necrosis is approximately 26% and external resorption is 4% [39]; patients should thus be counseled on the possible need for future root canal therapy.

Intrusion

Intrusion, or intrusive luxation, is the displacement of the tooth apically into the alveolar bone. Clinically, the crown appears shortened, there is gingival bleeding and the tooth may be immobile. The displaced root apex may be palpable along the alveolar ridge.

Teeth with incomplete root formation should be monitored for spontaneous eruption. If reeruption does not occur after a few weeks, orthodontic repositioning is recommended [28]. If the tooth is intruded more than 7 mm, it should be positioned surgically or manually. Root canal therapy is only indicated in the event of pulpal necrosis [43].

Teeth with completed root formation that are intruded less than 3 mm should be monitored for eruption, and should undergo orthodontic or surgical repositioning if no movement is seen in 2–4 weeks [28]. Teeth intruded more than 3 mm should be immediately repositioned surgically or orthodontically. Teeth intruded more than 7 mm should be repositioned surgically [28]. Surgically repositioned teeth should be stabilized with a flexible splint for 4–8 weeks [28]. The frequency of pulpal necrosis is approximately 96% [39] and external resorption is 92.8% [44]; endodontic therapy should thus be undertaken 10–14 days following the injury. Pulpectomy and placement of calcium hydroxide in the canal is recommended to prevent inflammatory resorption followed by conventional root canal therapy at a later date [28].

Extrusion

Extrusion, or partial avulsion, is the subtotal displacement of the tooth from the dental socket [28]. The tooth is elongated with excess mobility. There is often gingival sulcular bleeding [28] (Figure 9.2).

Extruded teeth should be manually repositioned in the tooth socket and stabilized for 2 weeks using a flexible splint [28]. The tooth should be monitored with vitality testing; the frequency of pulpal necrosis is approximately 64% and external resorption is 7% following extrusion [39].

Lateral Luxation

Lateral luxation refers to the tooth displaced in the labial, lingual or mesial, or distal directions (Figure 9.3). Luxation is often associated with an alveolar fracture and gingival lacerations [45]. The tooth may be immobile if lodged in position in the socket. Malocclusion may result if the luxated tooth creates an occlusal interference.

Laterally luxated teeth should be manually repositioned into their original location and stabilized for 4 weeks with a flexible splint [28]. Pulp vitality is monitored following the trauma. If pulp necrosis develops, pulpectomy and endodontic treatment with calcium hydroxide are indicated to prevent root resorption. If resorption is arrested or nonexistent, a formal root canal may be performed at a later date [28].

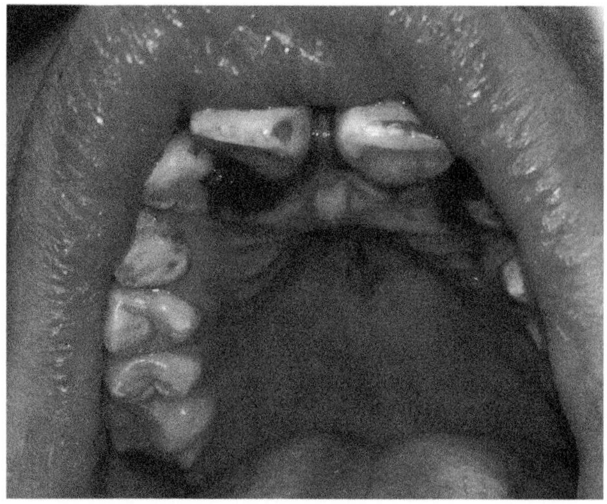

Figure 9.2 Lateral luxation of permanent central incisors.

Avulsion

Tooth avulsion, or exarticulation, is the complete displacement of the tooth from its dental socket and encompasses 0.5–3% of dental injuries [36, 43, 46]. Avulsion most commonly occurs in children between age 7 and 10 due to the immature condition of the PDL during tooth eruption, and most commonly involves the maxillary central incisor [43] (Figure 9.4).

Avulsion of the permanent tooth is a critical injury as prognosis depends on the immediate postinjury management. The probability of survival depends on the vitality of the PDL prior to replantation, more so than the time to replantation [47–49]. Treatment is aimed at maintaining PDL vitality and, in immature teeth, allowing revascularization of the pulp space [36].

When indicated, immediate replantation is ideal. The tooth should be handled without touching the root, washed

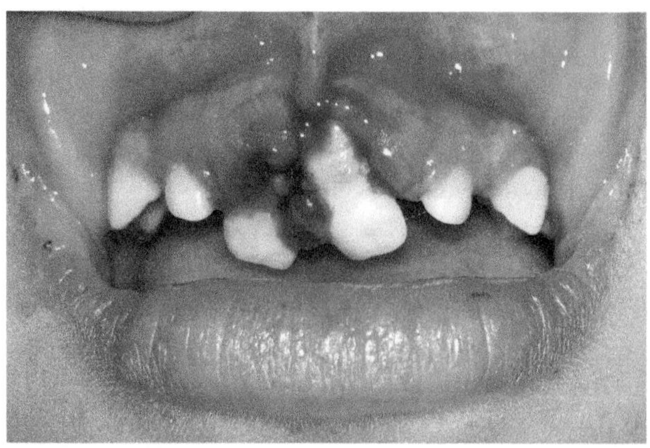

Figure 9.3 Extrusion of primary central incisors with associated gingival contusion and laceration.

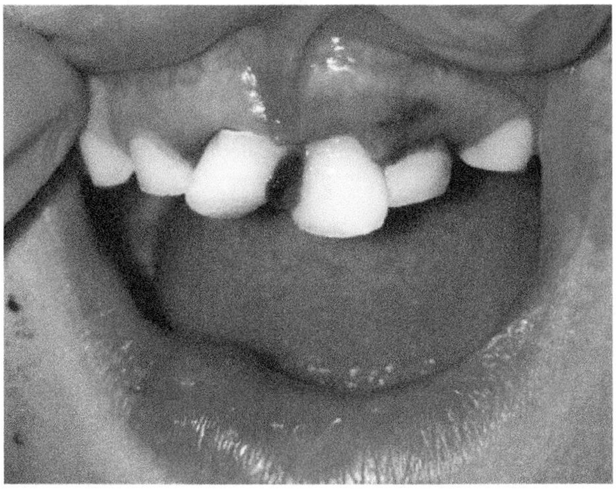

Figure 9.4 Luxation of exfoliating primary central incisors.

briefly with cool water and repositioned in the tooth socket. Possible contraindications to replantation include extensive caries, periodontal disease, alveolar fractures, and immunocompromised state [50].

If replantation is not possible, the tooth should be stored in physiologic medium which can maintain the pH, osmolality, and cell metabolites of the PDL [51]. Hank's balanced salt solution (HBSS) is a commercially available solution that is considered the gold standard due to its ability to maintain PDL vitality for an extended period of time [51, 52]. UW solution is a cold organ transplant storage medium that is effective for avulsed teeth but is not easily accessible [53]. Regular pasteurized whole milk is the most frequently recommended and has the best prognosis among other easily accessible solutions [51, 54, 55]. Milk has shown clinical efficacy equivalent to HBSS [52]. Saliva is no longer considered an effective transport medium due to a nonphysiologic osmolarity and high microbial load [51, 56].

Avulsed teeth which have not been replanted immediately should be replanted as soon as possible. The tooth should be rinsed with saline, the soft tissue on the root surface should not be removed, and the alveolar socket should be debrided only with saline irrigation prior to replantation. A flexible splint is applied for 14 days [36].

If a tooth is avulsed for longer than 2 hours, it has a poor prognosis. In this situation, replantation may still be beneficial up to 24 hours in order to maintain alveolar bone support during maxillary growth and to serve as a space maintainer. In these cases of delayed replantation, however, the PDL is necrotic and the expected outcome is replacement resorption, ankylosis, and eventual loss of the tooth [36]. The frequency of external resorption is approximately 89% [44].

Following replantation and splint application, the area should be cleaned gently with water, saline, or chlorhexidine. The tooth should be taken out of function. Gingival lacerations should be closed. Tetanus coverage should be ensured and the patient should receive systemic antibiotics for 7–10 days. Close dental follow-up should be established.

Teeth with closed apices will require endodontic therapy approximately 7–10 days following replantation. Intracanal calcium hydroxide treatment up to 1 month is recommended to prevent root resorption. Formal root canal therapy may be completed following cessation or absence of root resorption [49]. Extraoral endodontic therapy prior to replantation has also been described [57]. A metaanalysis found no significant difference in radiographic resorption between immediate extraoral endodontics and intraoral endodontic therapy at 1 week in teeth with greater than 60 minutes of dry time [58].

Replanted teeth with open apices may require root canal therapy if revascularization of the pulp space does not occur. Crown discoloration is common and may be treated with internal bleaching, veneers, or crowns at a later date [59, 60].

Various external root treatments have been suggested prior to replantation with the aim of minimizing external root resorption. For avulsed teeth with open apices less than 2 hours, some authors recommend soaking the tooth in HBSS and tetracycline [49, 61]. For avulsed teeth with closed apices less than 2 hours, some authors recommend soaking the tooth in HBSS [49]. For avulsed teeth greater than 2 hours, some authors recommend PDL removal mechanically or with sodium hypochlorite solution, endodontic therapy, and external root treatment with citric acid, stannous fluoride, and doxycycline prior to replantation [49, 61–63]. However, no single treatment has been shown to prevent inflammatory or replacement resorption [64–66].

Dentoalveolar Injuries in the Primary Dentition

Most dentoalveolar injuries in the primary dentition commonly occur while the child is learning to walk around 1.5–2.5 years of age [67]. However, child abuse should be ruled out [67]. Displacement injuries are more common than tooth fractures in the primary dentition [67]. When determining the appropriate treatment, the patient's maturity, time to exfoliation, and dental occlusion should be kept in mind [35]. A conservative approach to treatment is often indicated to minimize emotional trauma to the patient [67]. The main goal of treatment is to preserve the underlying permanent tooth germ.

Class I crown fractures may be smoothed and observed. Large class II fractures may require calcium hydroxide and/or glass ionomer base and acid-etch resin restoration. Class III fractures with a vital pulp may be treated with calcium hydroxide pulpotomy followed by glass ionomer lining and composite restoration [35]. Class III fractures with nonvital pulp or greater than 24 hours are often treated with extraction [35].

Root fractures occur rarely and may require removal of a mobile coronal segment. The apical fragment should not be removed if there is a risk to the developing permanent tooth, and it often undergoes normal resorption or exfoliation [35].

Intruded primary teeth with apices displaced toward the developing permanent tooth should be extracted immediately. Otherwise, intruded primary teeth may be monitored for reeruption for a few weeks. Extraction should be completed if reeruption does not occur or if acute inflammation and gingival swelling occur during reeruption [35].

Subluxated and concussed primary teeth should be observed. Luxated primary teeth should be extracted if there is a risk of injury to the underlying permanent tooth germ (Figure 9.5). If the primary tooth is displaced away from the permanent tooth germ and does not interfere with occlusion, it may be monitored for spontaneous repositioning [35]. Luxated teeth with occlusal interference may be repositioned manually and often do not require splinting. Minimally displaced extruded teeth may be observed for spontaneous alignment. Severely extruded teeth should be extracted.

Avulsed primary teeth should not be replanted due to the risk to the succedaneous permanent tooth [35, 68–70]. Following eruption of the primary canines, anterior maxillary arch space is not affected by premature loss of primary incisors [71]. A fixed or removable partial denture may be fabricated for esthetic concerns [67].

Splinting

A flexible splint is desirable for injuries of the PDL to allow for physiologic tooth movement to reduce the risk of ankylosis and external root resorption. Splints are most commonly made using acid-etched bonding in combination with wire, nylon line, fiberglass or a titanium splint [37] (Figure 9.6).

Injuries to the Gingiva or Oral Mucosa

Gingival injuries include contusions, abrasions, lacerations, and avulsions. Gingival injuries should be addressed after the management of concomitant dental or alveolar injuries. Contusions do not require treatment. Abrasions should be debrided to remove foreign material. Lacerations should be cleaned, repositioned, and repaired with resorbable suture. Gingival avulsions occur infrequently. If associated with underlying dental or alveolar injury, a local soft tissue flap should be advanced to cover the alveolar bone. Isolated gingival avulsions should be observed to allow for granulation.

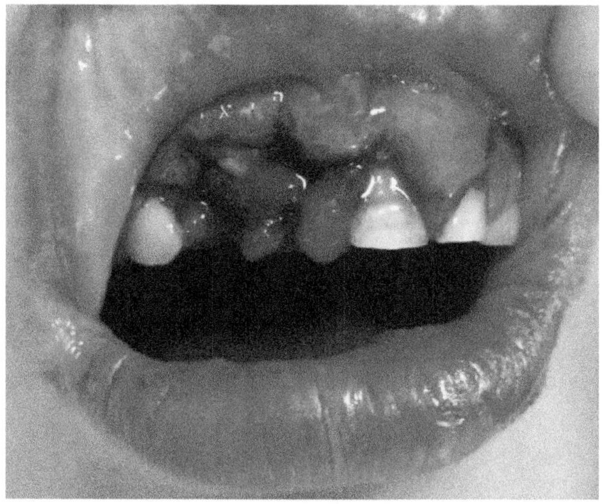

Figure 9.5 Avulsion of primary central and lateral incisors.

Injuries to Supporting Bone

Alveolar socket fractures and comminution are often associated with dental injuries and treatment guidelines follow those for the associated dental injury. Alveolar process fractures may have one or several teeth in the segment and may occur in isolation or with dental, maxillofacial, and/or

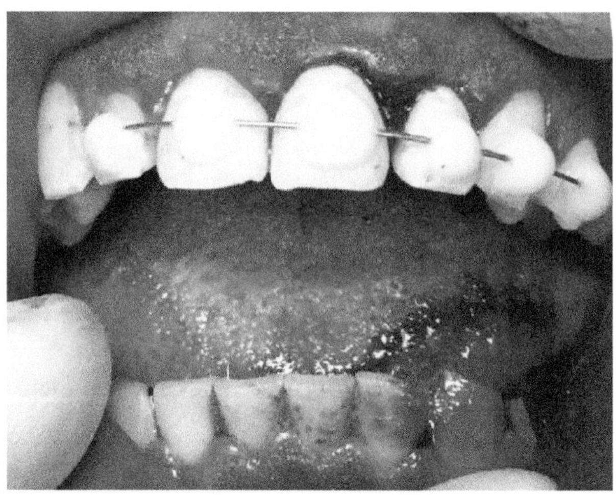

Figure 9.6 Flexible splint fabricated with acid-etched resin and stainless steel wire.

mucosal injuries. Isolated alveolar fractures involving primary or permanent teeth are treated with manual reduction and rigid stabilization with a rigid splint, such as an arch bar, Essig wire or acrylic splint for 4 weeks [28, 35]. Occasionally, open reduction and internal fixation with surgical techniques may be required [37]. Tetanus coverage and systemic antibiotics are recommended. Follow-up should be established to monitor for osseous healing and tooth vitality.

Follow-Up

Patient compliance with follow-up visits and home care is imperative to optimize healing. Guidelines for follow-up schedules are given elsewhere [28]. Patients should be counseled at the time of injury on the need for multiple postinjury appointments [72]. In addition, up to 30% of patients experience multiple dental trauma episodes [72]; preventive strategies should thus be discussed with the patient and may also be effective as public educational initiatives.

Conclusion

Patients with dentoalveolar injuries should be managed with a multidisciplinary approach involving emergency medical staff, restorative dentistry, prosthodontics, orthodontics, and oral and maxillofacial surgery. Prompt diagnosis and treatment are essential to allow for physiologic healing and to minimize the risks of complications.

References

1 James, D. (1985). Maxillofacial injuries in children. In: *Maxillofacial Injuries* (ed. N.L. Rowe and J.L.L. Williams). Edinburgh: Churchill Livingstone.

2 Azami-Aghdash, S., Ebadifard Azar, F., Pournaghi Azar, F. et al. (2015). Prevalence, etiology, and types of dental trauma in children and adolescents: systematic review and meta-analysis. *Med. J. Islam. Repub. Iran* 29 (4): 234.

3 Hasan, A.A., Qudeimat, M.A., and Andersson, L. (2010). Prevalence of traumatic dental injuries in preschool children in Kuwait – a screening study. *Dent. Traumatol.* 26 (4): 346–350.

4 Govindarajan, M., Reddy, V.N., Ramalingam, K. et al. (2012). Prevalence of traumatic dental injuries to the anterior teeth among prevalence of traumatic dental injuries to three to thirteen-year-old school children of Tamilnadu. *Contemp. Clin. Dent.* 3 (2): 164–167.

5 Sgan-Cohen, H.D., Megnagi, G., and Jacobi, Y. (2005). Dental trauma and its association with anatomic, behavioral, and social variables among fifth and sixth grade schoolchildren in Jerusalem. *Community Dent. Oral. Epidemiol.* 33 (3): 174–180.

6 Altun, C., Ozen, B., Esenlik, E. et al. (2009). Traumatic injuries to permanent teeth in Turkish children. *Ank. Dent. Traumatol.* 25 (3): 309–313.

7 Bendo, C.B., Paiva, S.M., Oliveira, A.C. et al. (2010). Prevalence and associated factors of traumatic dental injuries in Brazilian school children. *J. Public Health Dent.* 70 (4): 313–318.

8 Schuch, H.S., Goettems, M.L., Correa, M.B. et al. (2013). Prevalence and treatment demand after traumatic dental injury in South Brazilian school children. *Dent. Traumatol.* 29 (4): 297–302.

9 Noori, A.J. and Al-Obaidi, W.A. (2009). Traumatic dental injuries among primary school children in Sulaimani city, Iraq. *Dent. Traumatol.* 25 (4): 442–446.

10 Thelen, D.S. and Bårdsen, A. (2010). Traumatic dental injuries in an urban adolescent population in Tirana, Albania. *Dent. Traumatol.* 26 (5): 376–382.

11 Huang, B., Marcenes, W., Croucher, R., and Hector, M. (2009). Activities related to the occurrence of traumatic dental injuries in 15- to 18-year-olds. *Dent. Traumatol.* 25 (1): 64–68.

12 Jorge, K.O., Moysés, S.J., Ferreira e Ferreira, E. et al. (2009). Prevalence and factors associated to dental trauma in infants 1–3 years of age. *Dent. Traumatol.* 25 (2): 185–189.

13 Pattussi, M.P., Hardy, R., and Sheiham, A. (2006). Neighborhood social capital and dental injuries in Brazilian adolescents. *Am. J. Public Health* 96 (8): 1462–1468.

14 Fakhruddin, K.S., Lawrence, H.P., Kenny, D.J., and Locker, D. (2008). Impact of treated and untreated dental injuries on the quality of life of Ontario schoolchildren. *Dent. Traumatol.* 24 (3): 309–313.

15 Trullás, J.M., Ballester, M.L., Bolíbar, I. et al. (2013). Frequency and characteristics of occupational dental trauma. *Occup. Med.* 63 (2): 152–155.

16 Ramli, R., Rahman, N.A., Rahman, R.A. et al. (2011). A retrospective study of oral and maxillofacial injuries in Seremban hospital, Malaysia. *Dent Traumatol.* 27 (2): 122–126.

17 Hächl, O., Tuli, T., Schwabegger, A., and Gassner, R. (2002). Maxillofacial trauma due to work-related accidents. *Int. J. Oral Maxillofac. Surg.* 31 (1): 90–93.

18 Vogel, J., Stübinger, S., Kaufmann, M. et al. (2009). Dental injuries resulting from tracheal intubation – a retrospective study. *Dent. Traumatol.* 25 (1): 73–77.

19 Mańka-Malara, K., Gawlak, D., Hovhannisyan, A. et al. (2015). Dental trauma prevention during endotracheal intubation – review of literature. *Anaesthesiol. Intensive Ther.* 47 (4): 425–429.

20 Owen, H. and Waddell-Smith, I. (2000). Dental trauma associated with anaesthesia. *Anaesth. Intensive Care* 28 (2): 133–145.

21 Andreasen, J.O. (ed.) (1981). *Traumatic Injuries of the Teeth*, 2e. Copenhagen: Munksgaard.

22 American College of Surgeons (2013). *ATLS Advanced Trauma Life Support for Doctors – Student Course Manual*, 9e. Chicago, IL: American College of Surgeons.

23 Moule, A.J. and Moule, C.A. (2009). Minor traumatic injuries to the permanent dentition. *Dent. Clin. North Am.* 53 (4): 639–659.

24 Avsar, A., Akbaş, S., and Ataibiş, T. (2009). Traumatic dental injuries in children with attention deficit/hyperactivity disorder. *Dent. Traumatol.* 25 (5): 484–489.

25 Liewehr, F.R. (2001). An inexpensive device for transillumination. *J. Endod.* 27 (2): 130–131.

26 Bastos, J.V., Goulart, E.M., and de Souza Côrtes, M.I. (2014). Pulpal response to sensibility tests after traumatic dental injuries in permanent teeth. *Dent. Traumatol.* 30 (3): 188–192.

27 Andreasen, F.M. and Kahler, B. (2015). Pulpal response after acute dental injury in the permanent dentition: clinical implications – a review. *J. Endod.* 41 (3): 299–308.

28 Diangelis, A.J., Andreasen, J.O., Ebeleseder, K.A. et al.., for the International Association of Dental Traumatology. (2012). International Association of Dental Traumatology guidelines for the management of traumatic dental injuries: 1. Fractures and luxations of permanent teeth. *Dent. Traumatol.* 28 (1): 2–12.

29 Sanders, B., Brady, F.A., and Johnson, R. (1979). *Pediatric Oral and Maxillofacial Surgery*. St Louis, MO: CV Mosby.

30 Sweet, C.A. (1955). A classification and treatment for traumatized anterior teeth. *J. Dent. Child.* 22: 144.

31 Ingle, J.J. and Beveridge, E.E. (ed.) (1976). *Endodontics*, 2e. Philadelphia, PA: Lea & Febiger.

32 World Health Organization (1995). *Application of the International Classification of Diseases and Stomatology, IDC-DA*. Geneva: World Health Organization.

33 Feliciano, K.M.P.C. and de Franca Caldas, A. (2006). A systematic review of the diagnostic classifications of traumatic dental injuries. *Dent. Traumatol.* 22 (2): 71–76.

34 Ellis, R.G. and Davey, K.W. (1970). *The Classification and Treatment of Injuries to the Teeth of Children*. Chicago, IL: Year Book Medical Publishers.

35 Malmgren, B., Andreasen, J.O., Flores, M.T. et al.., for the International Association of Dental Traumatology.(2012). International Association of Dental Traumatology guidelines for the management of traumatic dental injuries: 3. Injuries in the primary dentition. *Dent. Traumatol.* 28 (3): 174–182.

36 Andersson, L., Andreasen, J.O., Day, P. et al.., for the International Association of Dental Traumatology.(2012). International Association of Dental Traumatology guidelines for the management of traumatic dental injuries: 2. Avulsion of permanent teeth. *Dent. Traumatol.* 28 (2): 88–96.

37 Jaramillo, D.E. and Bakland, L.K. (2009). Trauma kits for the dental office. *Dent. Clin. North Am.* 53 (4): 751–760.

38 Lubisich, E.B., Hilton, T.J., Ferracane, J., and Northwest Precedent (2010). Cracked teeth: a review of the literature. *J. Esthet. Restor. Dent.* 22 (3): 158–167.

39 Andreasen, J.O. (1970). Etiology and pathogenesis of traumatic dental injuries: a clinical study of 1,298 cases. *Scand. J. Dent. Res.* 78: 329–342.

40 Robertson, A., Andreasen, F.M., Andreasen, J.O., and Norén, J.G. (2000). Long-term prognosis of crown-fractured permanent incisors. The effect of stage of root development and associated luxation injury. *Int. J. Paediatr. Dent.* 10 (3): 191–199.

41 Miloro, M., Ghali, G.E., Larsen, P., and Waite, P. (ed.) (2012). *Peterson's Principles of Oral and Maxillofacial Surgery*, 3e. Shelton, CT: People's Medical Publishing House.

42 Bakland, L.K. (2009). Revisiting traumatic pulpal exposure: materials, management principles, and techniques. *Dent. Clin. North Am.* 53 (4): 661–673.

43 Andreasen, J.O., Bakland, L.K., and Andreasen, F.M. (2006). Traumatic intrusion of permanent teeth. Part 2. A clinical study of the effect of preinjury and injury factors, such as sex, age, stage of root development, tooth location, and extent of injury including number of intruded teeth on 140 intruded permanent teeth. *Dent. Traumatol.* 22 (2): 90–98.

44 Soares, A.J., Souza, G.A., Pereira, A.C. et al. (2015). Frequency of root resorption following trauma to permanent teeth. *J. Oral Sci.* 57 (2): 73–78.

45 Andreasen, J.O. and Ravn, J.J. (1972). Epidemiology of traumatic dental injuries to primary and permanent teeth in a Danish population sample. *Int. J. Oral Surg.* 1 (5): 235–239.

46 Glendor, U., Halling, A., Andersson, L., and Eilert-Peterson, E. (1996). Incidence of traumatic tooth injuries in children and adolescents in the county of Va ¨stmanland, Sweden. *Swed. Dent. J.* 20 (1,2): 15–28.

47 Raphael, S.L. and Gregory, P.I.J. (1990). Parental awareness of the emergency management of avulsed teeth in children. *Aust. Dent. J.* 35 (2): 130–133.

48 Blomlof, L. (1981). Milk and saliva as possible storage media for traumatically exarticulated teeth prior to replantation. *Swed. Dent. J. Suppl.* 8: 1–26.

49 Krasner, P. and Rankow, H.J. (1995). New philosophy for the treatment of avulsed teeth. *Oral Surg. Oral Med. Oral Pathol. Oral Radiol. Endod.* 79 (5): 616–623.

50 American Academy on Pediatric Dentistry Council on Clinical Affairs (2008-2009). Guideline on management of acute dental trauma. *Pediatr. Dent.* 30 (7 Suppl): 175–183.

51 Malhotra, N. (2011). Current developments in interim transport (storage) media in dentistry: an update. *Br. Dent. J.* 211 (1): 29–33.

52 Blomlöf, L., Otteskog, P., and Hammarström, L. (1981). Effect of storage media with different ion strengths and osmolalities on human periodontal ligament cells. *Scand. J. Dent. Res.* 89 (2): 180–187.

53 Hiltz, J. and Trope, M. (1991). Vitality of human lip fibroblasts in milk, Hanks balanced salt solution and Viaspan storage media. *Endod. Dent. Traumatol.* 7 (2): 69–72.

54 Doyle, D.L., Dumsha, T.C., and Sydiskis, R.J. (1998). Effect of soaking in Hank's balanced salt solution or milk on PDL cell viability of drystored human teeth. *Endod. Dent. Traumatol.* 14 (5): 221–224.

55 Poi, W.R., Sonoda, C.K., Martins, C.M. et al. (2013). Storage media for avulsed teeth: a literature review. *Braz. Dent. J.* 24 (5): 437–445.

56 Layug, M.L., Barrett, E.J., and Kenny, D.J. (1998). Interim storage of avulsed permanent teeth. *J. Can. Dent. Assoc.* 64 (5): 357-363.

57 Giannetti, L. and Murri, A. (2006). Clinical evidence and literature to compare two different therapeutic protocols in tooth avulsion. *Eur. J. Paediatr. Dent.* 7 (3): 122–130.

58 Day, P. and Duggal, M. (2019). Interventions for treating traumatised permanent front teeth: avulsed (knocked out) and replanted. *Cochrane Database Syst. Rev.* 2: CD006542.

59 Ebelseder, K., Friehs, S., Ruda, C. et al. (1998). A study of replanted permanent teeth in different age groups. *Endod. Dent. Traumatol.* 14 (6): 274–278.

60 Pohl, Y., Filippi, A., and Kirschner, H. (2005). Results after replantation of avulsed permanent teeth. I. Endodontic considerations. *Dent. Traumatol.* 21 (2): 80–92.

61 Cvek, M., Cleaton-Jones, P., Austin, J. et al. (1990). Effect of topical application of doxycycline on pulp revascularization and periodontal healing in reimplanted monkey incisors. *Endod. Dent. Traumatol.* 6 (4): 170–176.

62 Selvig, K.A., Bjorvatn, K., Bogle, G.C., and Wikesjo, U.M.E. (1992). Effect of stannous fluoride and tetracycline on periodontal repair after delayed tooth replantation in dogs. *Scand. J. Dent. Res.* 100 (4): 200–203.

63 Selvig, J.A., Bjorvatn, K., and Claffey, N. (1990). Effect of stannous fluoride and tetracycline on repair after delayed replantation of root-planed teeth in dogs. *Acta Odontol. Scand.* 48 (2): 107–112.

64 Barbakow, F.H., Cleaton-Jones, P.E., Austin, J.C., and Vierra, E. (1981). Healing of replanted teeth following topical treatment with fluoride solutions and systemic admission of thyrocalcitonin: a histometric analysis. *J. Endod.* 7 (7): 302–308.

65 Filippi, A., Pohl, Y., and von Arx, T. (2002). Treatment of replacement resorption with Emdogain – a prospective clinical study. *Dent. Traumatol.* 18 (3): 138–143.

66 Schjutt, M. and Andreasen, J.O. (2005). Emdogain does not prevent progressive root resorption after replantation of avulsed teeth: a clinical study. *Dent. Traumatol.* 21 (1): 46–50.

67 McTigue, D.J. (2009). Managing injuries to the primary dentition. *Dent. Clin. North Am.* 53 (4): 627–638.

68 Assuncao, L.R., Ferelle, A., Iwakura, M.L., and Cunha, R.F. (2009). Effects on permanent teeth after luxation injuries to the primary predecessors: a study in children assisted at an emergency service. *Dent. Traumatol.* 25 (2): 165–170.

69 Andreasen, J.O. and Ravn, J.J. (1971). The effect of traumatic injuries to primary teeth on their permanent successors. II. A clinical and radiographic follow-up study of 213 injured teeth. *Scand. J. Dent. Res.* 79: 284–294.

70 Zamon, E.L. and Kenny, D.J. (2001). Replantation of avulsed primary incisors: a risk-benefit assessment. *J. Can. Dent. Assoc.* 67 (7): 386–389.

71 Rock, W.P., British Society of Paediatric Dentistry.(2002). UK National Clinical Guidelines in Paediatric Dentistry. Extraction of primary teeth – balance and compensation. *Int. J. Paediatr. Dent.* 12 (2): 151–153.

72 Al-Jundi, S.H. (2004). Type of treatment, prognosis, and estimation of time spent to manage dental trauma in late presentation cases at a dental teaching hospital: a longitudinal and retrospective study. *Dent. Traumatol.* 20 (1): 1–5.

Part V

Pathology

10

Biopsy Technique: When, Where, and How?

Steven Caldroney and Pushkar Mehra

Introduction

A biopsy is an examination of tissue removed from a living body to discover the presence, cause, or extent of a disease. The aim of biopsy is to define a lesion based on its histopathology. Tissue diagnoses establish a prognosis in malignant or premalignant lesions, facilitate the prescription of specific treatment, contribute to the assessment of the efficacy of the treatment, and act as a document with medical-legal value [1]. Biopsies act as a diagnostic tool allowing a practitioner to garner a diagnosis and formulate an appropriate surgical treatment plan. The differential diagnosis of an oral cavity lesion seen clinically or radiographically is diverse and must be diagnosed accurately. Although the majority of oral cavity lesions are benign, early detection of malignant or potentially precancerous lesions is paramount for a favorable patient outcome.

Worldwide, head and neck and oral cavity cancer accounts for more than 550 000 cases and 380 000 deaths annually [2]. In the United States, head and neck cancer accounts for 3% of malignancies, with approximately 63 000 Americans developing head and neck cancer annually and 13 000 dying from the disease [3]. The early diagnosis of oral cancer is crucial and reducing diagnostic delays may have the highest impact for improving survival and cure rates. A longer time interval from first symptom to referral for diagnosis is a risk factor for advanced stage and mortality of oral cancer [4]. Therefore, knowledge and proficiency in the recognition of a potentially malignant oral lesion, followed by the correct implementation of a biopsy technique, have a profound effect on morbidity and mortality. The aim of this chapter is to provide insight into the management of an oral lesion from presentation to biopsy, with discussion of adjunctive techniques. Common pearls/pitfalls will also be discussed.

Patient Evaluation: Health History, Medications

If a patient presents with an abnormal oral lesion, a clinician should be able to clinically characterize the lesion. It is important to have an orderly checklist that is followed closely, so that important steps are not overlooked (Figure 10.1).

A clinical encounter must first start with a thorough health and social history, including current medications. The effect of systemic health on oral disease is well documented. Some of the more common systemic categories with oral manifestations are autoimmune, endocrine, immunologic, hematologic, gastrointestinal, and hypersensitivity reactions. Because many systemic diseases often present with abnormalities of the mouth and jaws, it is essential that these be appropriately recognized to provide a possible diagnosis and referral for appropriate treatment. Oftentimes, dentists and oral surgeons contribute to or are the first to diagnose a systemic disease through its oral manifestations (Table 10.1).

Therefore, the medical history should be carefully considered and a high index of suspicion maintained when encountering an oral lesion. Additionally, history of smoking, chewing tobacco, alcohol consumption, oral human papilloma virus infection, and trauma should be elucidated. Oral infection with HPV-16 confers an approximately 50-fold increase in risk for HPV-positive oropharyngeal squamous cell carcinoma [5].

An understanding of the relationship between systemic disease, current medications and possible surgically related side-effects is of paramount importance prior to initiating treatment. It may be necessary to organize a physician consultation, especially for clients with uncontrolled medical problems (uncontrolled diabetes, hypertension) requiring medical optimization. The benefit-to-risk ratio of stopping an anticoagulant to minimize bleeding and the risk of a thrombotic event may also need to be discussed prior to a

Oral and Maxillofacial Surgery, Medicine, and Pathology for the Clinician, First Edition. Edited by Harry Dym, Leslie R. Halpern, and Orrett E. Ogle.

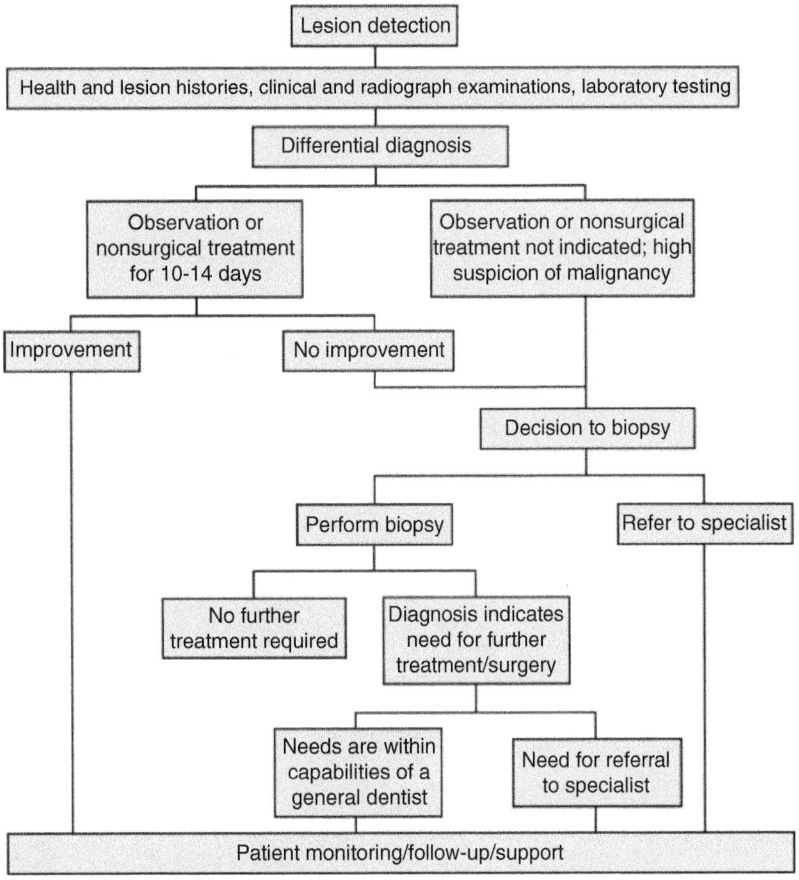

Figure 10.1 Decision tree for treatment of oral lesions. *Source:* Adapted from Ellis E. Principles of differential diagnosis and biopsy. In: Hupp J, Ellis E, Tucker MR (eds). Contemporary Oral and Maxillofacial Surgery, 6th edn. St Louis: Mosby, 2014: 422-447.

surgical procedure. It can be considered as below the standard of care to perform an invasive therapy without garnering a thorough, accurate and up-to-date health history.

Lesion History

The oral cavity is lined with stratified squamous epithelium overlying mesenchymal tissues, such as connective tissue, adipose, nerves, muscles, cartilage, salivary tissue, and bone. Benign and malignant lesions may originate from any of these tissues. The first step, and one of the keys in successful therapeutic management of an oral tissue lesion, is formulating a differential diagnosis. Clinical differential diagnosis is the cognitive process of applying logic and knowledge to create a list of possible diagnoses. Therefore, a thorough history of the lesion is prudent. Frequently, a working diagnosis can be formulated based on the patient's medical, dental, and/or social history.

Once an oral lesion has been identified, the clinician should undertake a standard protocol, beginning with eliciting and documenting the pertinent history, including duration, any antecedent event, symptoms and changes in appearance, as well as prior diagnostic and therapeutic measures [6]. It is important to know when the patient first noticed the lesion and/or how long the lesion has been present. Generally, oral lesions should be evaluated in relation to their association with local irritating or traumatic factors, which should be addressed. If the lesions persist after a period of 2–3 weeks, biopsies and histopathologic evaluations are necessary. If the area is deemed especially suspicious for a premalignant or malignant process, referral to a health are provider with expertise in the field may be warranted.

Lesion evolution, such as changes in size, especially rapid growth, ulceration, or induration should be noted. Slow-growing lesions tend to be benign while malignant processes exhibit more rapid turnover. It is important to know if there are any associated symptoms, either localized or systemic. The presence or absence of symptoms such as pain, paresthesia, dysphagia, swelling or lymph node enlargement can help focus the differential diagnosis.

Table 10.1 Common systemic diseases and their clinical oral manifestations.

Category	Disease	Oral manifestations
Autoimmune	Sjogren syndrome	Xerostomia, candidiasis, parotid enlargement
	Lupus	Oral discoid lesions, erythema, purpura, petechiae, raised keratotic plaques, ulcers, chelitis
	Pemphigoid	Diffuse painful ulceration
	Pemphigus	Diffuse painful ulceration, Nikolsky sign
	Behçet syndrome	Numerous aphthous ulcers (soft palate/oropharynx)
Endocrine	Diabetes mellitus	Periodontitis, candidiasis, atrophy of tongue papilla, delayed wound healing
	Addison disease	Melanin hyperpigmentation, candidiasis
	Parathyroid disease	Loss of lamina dura of teeth, radiolucent jaw lesions
Immune	HIV	Candida, Kaposi sarcoma, linear gingival erythema, necrotizing ulcerative gingivitis, hemorrhage
	Epstein–Barr	Oral hairy leukoplakia
	Cytomegalovirus	Oral ulcerations, sialadenitis of major salivary glands
Hematologic	Anemia	Mucosal pallor, atrophic glossitis, angular cheilitis, gingival hypertrophy
	Leukemia	Bleeding, ulceration, diffuse or localized gingival hypertrophy, boggy gingiva, secondary infections (herpes, candidiasis)
	Non-Hodgkin lymphoma	Erythema, ulcerations, nodular swelling, ulcerated masses, tooth mobility or loss, lymphadenopathy
	Thrombocytopenia	Petechiae, purpura, ecchymosis, hematoma
Gastrointestinal	Inflammatory bowel disease	Pyostomatitis vegetans, mucosal erythema
	Crohn's disease	Diffuse mucosal swelling, cobblestone mucosa, ulcers with erythematous base, fibrous tissue tags
	Gastroesophageal reflux disease	Water brash, xerostomia, palatal erythema
	Celiac disease (gluten insensitivity)	Aphthous or hemorrhagic ulcers
	Bulimia/anorexia	Sialadenitis, bilateral parotid enlargement

Clinical Examination

Once a thorough medical and lesion history has been performed, attention should next be directed to performing a systematic head and neck exam. Oral cancer and premalignant oral lesions may develop at any site, so it is important to develop a consistent examination sequence to ensure that no sites are overlooked. A detailed description on how to perform a head and neck exam is beyond the scope of this chapter but a complete extraoral and intraoral examination, including palpation of the neck, is essential (Figure 10.2). At a minimum, the extraoral clinical exam should include examination of the face, parotid glands, neck musculature and lymph nodes, midline neck

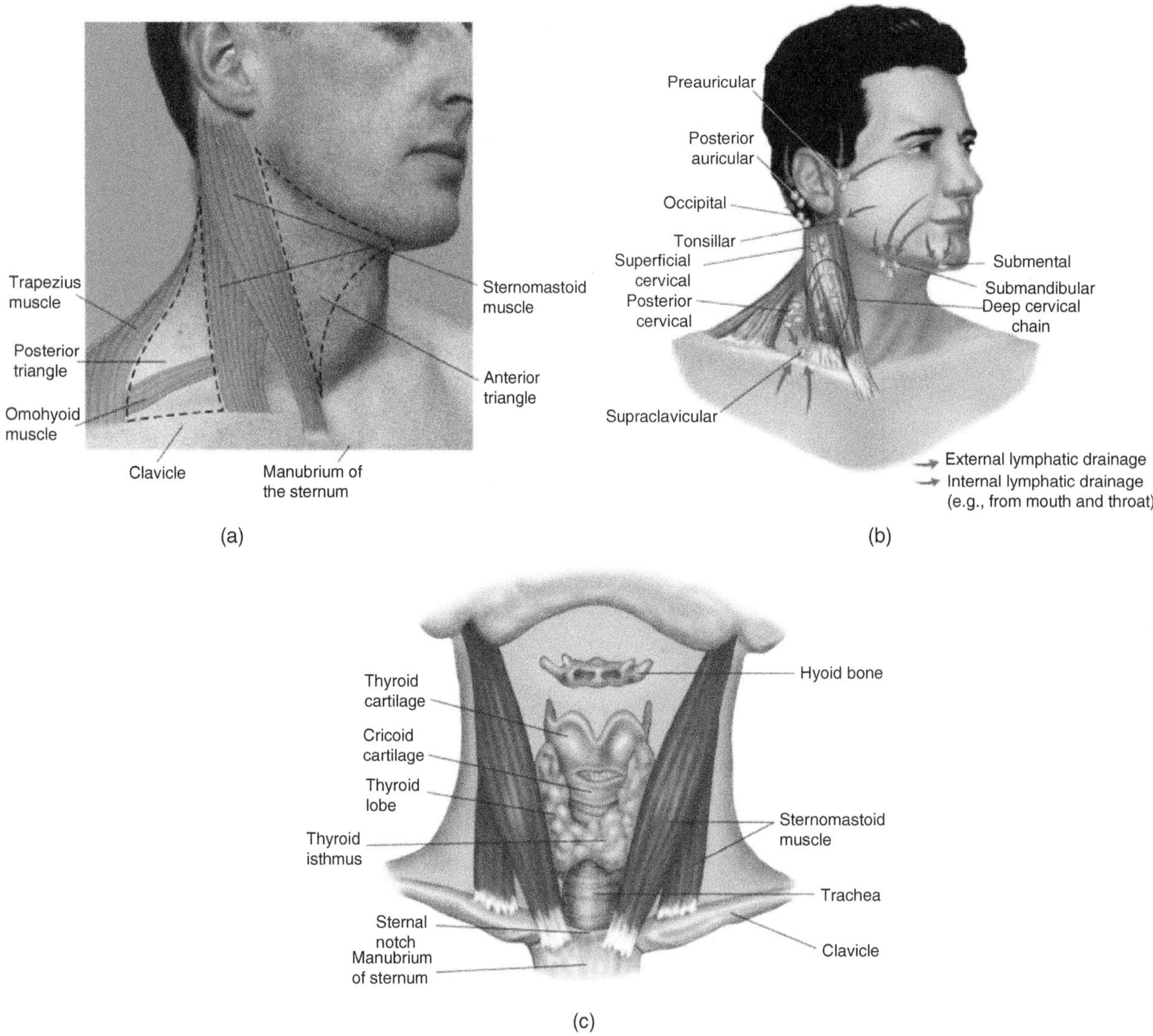

Figure 10.2 (a) Anterior and posterior triangles of the neck. The landmarks of these triangles should be identified and palpated for any abnormalities. (b) Lymph node basins of the face and neck. A thorough and methodical palpation of all lymph node levels should be performed bilaterally in all head and neck exams. Any abnormalities should be documented (size, firmness, pain on palpation, fixed or moveable). (c) Midline structures of the neck including hyoid bone, thyroid, hyoid and cricoid cartilages, thyroid gland and tracheal rings should be inspected for any abnormalities. *Source:* Bickley L, Szilagyi P, Hoffman R (eds). Bates' Guide to Physical Examination, 9th edn. Philadelphia: Lippincott-Raven, 2007; 23, 25, 26.

structures, and lips/commissures of the mouth, with special attention paid to any evidence of asymmetry. Intraorally, the buccal mucosa, floor of mouth, tongue (all surfaces), tonsils and tonsillar pillars, hard and soft palate, posterior pharyngeal wall, retromolar area, gingiva, and teeth should be thoroughly inspected (Table 10.2). The sequence used in performing an extraoral examination and subsequently the intraoral examination is not as important as performing each examination the same way each time. Consistency allows these examinations to be performed quickly and efficiently while still maintaining the ability to identify abnormal versus normal conditions.

Once the head and neck examination is complete, attention should next be addressed to a thorough examination of the lesion in question. Location, size, color, consistency, and texture of the lesion should be documented. As mentioned previously, a lesion can arise from any tissue within the oral environment. The location or type of tissue affected can aid in formulating a focused differential diagnosis. The overall appearance of the lesion should be carefully evaluated, with special emphasis on the size, shape, consistency, and surface appearance of the lesion. For example, a red/white and indurated lesion may be highly suspicious for a carcinoma.

Table 10.2 Head and neck examination sequence.

Extraoral examination	Intraoral examination
1. Overall facial symmetry (eyes, nose, ears), including skin of face	1. Floor of mouth/ sublingual glands
2. Cranial nerve examination (CN I–XII)	2. Tonsils/tonsillar pillars, uvula, posterior pharyngeal wall, base of tongue
3. Parotid glands	3. Hard/soft palate
4. Neck (lymph nodes -anterior/ posterior triangle), musculature, midline structures - hyoid, trachea, thyroid	4. Retromolar area, lingual gutter, tuberosity area
5. Lips/commissures	5. Gingiva, alveolar bone
	6. Teeth
	7. Tongue (dorsal, ventral, lateral surfaces)

A variety of benign and malignant lesions may also occur within the hard tissues of the maxilla and mandible. Careful consideration of the patient history and the location of the lesion within the mandible, its borders, its internal architecture, and its effects on adjacent structures generally makes it possible to narrow the differential diagnosis.

Although the radiologic findings in some bony lesions may be nonspecific, there are often clues for histologic diagnosis within the anatomy surrounding each lesion. In many cases, the clinical history alone is crucial in reaching a correct diagnosis. Precise radiologic evaluation of a lesion can have a significant impact on diagnosis and subsequent patient treatment and at a minimum, a panoramic radiograph should be an integral part of the clinical examination. A cone beam CT or medical-grade CT offers the ability to more accurately diagnose a lesion, especially three-dimensionally, and may be warranted. Imaging is not always expected to provide a specific diagnosis but should help narrow the differential diagnosis, thereby helping to guide patient treatment. For example, a benign lesion may appear as a well-circumscribed radiolucency, while a malignancy may appear with irregular borders, moth-eaten, and not well defined. A mixed radiolucent/radiopaque lesion may signify a fibroosseous lesion. Furthermore, radiographic findings may help focus the differential based on growth pattern, as is the case with an odontogenic keratocyst, which has a propensity for anterior posterior growth rather than jaw expansion (Figure 10.3).

Knowledge of the history and clinical nature of a lesion is only one step in the pathway toward a correct diagnosis and proper management of the patient. Other steps include selection of the type of biopsy, correct implementation of the biopsy technique, and transfer of adequate and complete clinical information to the pathologist, which are all necessary to achieve the best results [7–9].

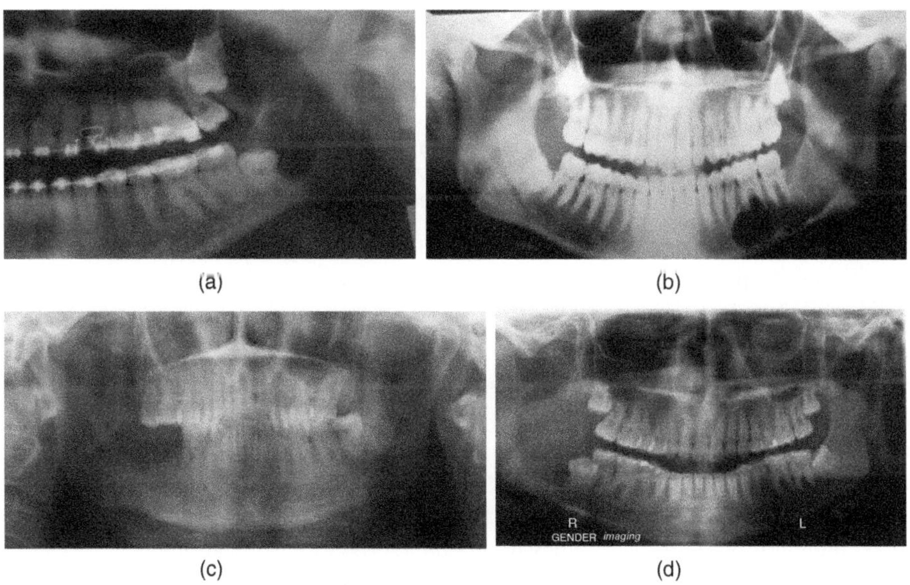

Figure 10.3 (a) Well-circumscribed radiolucency; dentigerous cyst. (b) Cystic appearing lesion exhibiting anterior/posterior growth; odontogenic keratocyst. (c) Ill-defined radiolucency of alveolar ridge; squamous cell carcinoma. (d) Ill-defined moth-eaten radiolucency with extensive bone destruction; ameloblastic carcinoma.

Indications for Biopsies

It is an accepted fact that microscopic analysis is the gold standard to establish confirmative diagnosis of most oral lesions. A biopsy is indicated when a diagnosis cannot be made based on medical history, clinical history, and examination alone. Indications for performing a biopsy are given in Boxes 10.1 and 10.2. Contraindications to biopsy are usually relative, and some examples are listed in Box 10.3.

Precancerous Lesion: "Potentially Malignant Disorders"

Precancerous lesions of the oral mucosa consist of a group of oral diseases that should be given special emphasis and have clear indications for biopsy and diagnosis at an early stage. In a World Health Organization workshop held in 2005, the terminology, definitions, and classifications of oral lesions with a predisposition to malignant transformation were discussed and the term "potentially malignant disorders" was recommended to eliminate confusion [10]. The most common premalignant conditions of the oral cavity are leukoplakia, erythroplakia, lichen planus, and oral epithelial dysplasia. The clinical significance of oral squamous epithelial dysplasia (OED) lies in its association with malignant transformation into oral squamous cell carcinoma (OSCC) [11]. OED can present clinically as leukoplakia: homogeneous (flat, thin, uniform white) and nonhomogeneous (white and red/erythroleukoplakia, speckled, nodular, or verrucous leukoplakia) [10] or erythroplakia [12].

Box 10.1 Biopsy indications (soft tissue lesions)

1. Confirmation of a clinical diagnostic suspicion
2. Any lesion that persists for more than 2 weeks with no apparent etiologic basis, including local irritative factors
3. Any inflammatory lesion that does not respond to treatment or proves refractory after 2 weeks
4. Any "potentially malignant disorder": leukoplakia, erythroleukoplakia, erythroplakia, lichen planus, or hyperkeratotic lesion
5. Any lesion suspected as a malignancy or neoplasm
6. The detection of certain systemic illnesses requiring histologic confirmation in order to establish the definitive diagnosis, e.g. lupus, amyloidosis, scleroderma, Sjögren syndrome
7. Confirmation of the diagnosis of vesiculobullous diseases affecting the oral mucosa, such as pemphigus or pemphigoid
8. New or enlarging pigmented lesions, especially those with an irregular border and nonhomogenous coloration
9. Any abnormal tissue removed from the oral cavity should be sent for histopathological analysis, however confident the clinician may be with the diagnosis

Box 10.2 Biopsy indications (hard tissue lesions)

1. Bony lesions accompanied by pain, swelling, paresthesia, or other symptoms
2. To confirm a radiographic diagnosis
3. Bone lesions showing rapid expansion as evidenced by consecutive radiographic or clinical examinations
4. Lesions with rapid bone loss, periodontal widening, root resorption, or tooth mobility in the absence of trauma
5. Radiolucent lesions showing displacement of teeth

Box 10.3 Biopsy contraindications: may require referral to specialist

1. Severe underlying medically compromised patients or those with poorly controlled systemic disease, where a biopsy procedure may result in complications
2. Patients with significant risk of bleeding. Patients with an underlying bleeding diathesis related to anticoagulants. Those with an inherited coagulopathy, including, but not limited to, hemophilia or von Willebrand disease
3. Patients undergoing bisphosphonate therapy or radiotherapy due to risk of exposing underlying bone
4. Biopsies are not necessary in lesions with a known etiology or anatomic/physiologic variations
5. Any "potentially malignant disorder." A lesion with a high suspicion for carcinoma, or any lesion that has the potential to transform into carcinoma requires referral to a specialist for management.

Leukoplakia is defined as “a white plaque of questionable risk having excluded known diseases or disorders that carry no increased risk for cancer” (Figure 10.4). Clinically, leukoplakia may affect any part of the oral and oropharyngeal cavity and can be divided into two subtypes: homogeneous and nonhomogeneous [12]. Homogeneous lesions are uniformly flat, thin, uniformly white in color, and exhibit shallow cracks of the surface keratin [10, 13]. Nonhomogeneous lesions have been defined as a white and red lesion (known as erythroleukoplakia or speckled leukoplakia) that may be either irregularly flat (speckled) or nodular (Figure 10.5).

Speckled leukoplakia was first described in 1963 by Pindborg [14]. In a retrospective analysis of 248 mouth cancers, Pindborg noted that 64% arose in an area of speckled leukoplakia [15]. Histopathologically, two distinct appearances may be seen as dysplastic or nondysplastic leukoplakia. Oral dysplastic leukoplakia has a fivefold greater risk of malignant change than nondysplastic oral leukoplakia. Overall, 6% of oral leukoplakia can be expected to become malignant [16].

Verrucous leukoplakia is another type of nonhomogeneous leukoplakia. First described by Hansen in 1985, proliferative verrucous leukoplakia (PVL) is a unique form of oral leukoplakia that has a high risk for becoming dysplastic and transforming into squamous cell carcinoma (Figure 10.6). Hansen followed 30 patients with PVL – nine transformed to verrucous carcinoma, 12 transformed to papillary carcinoma, and five changed to squamous carcinoma [17]. Silverman prospectively followed 54 patients with PVL for a mean time of 7.7 years and showed a 70.3% transformation rate into squamous cell carcinoma [18]. Because the clinical appearance alone cannot differentiate between leukoplakia with or without oral epithelial dysplasia, versus squamous cell carcinoma, a biopsy is prudent (Figure 10.7).

A study by Liu et al. showed that high-grade dysplasia had a higher incidence of malignant change than low-grade dysplasia (5-year oral cancer-free survival 59% vs 90.5%) [19]. Ho et al. reported a relatively high overall malignant transformation rate of 22% at 5 years among patients diagnosed with OED undergoing long-term

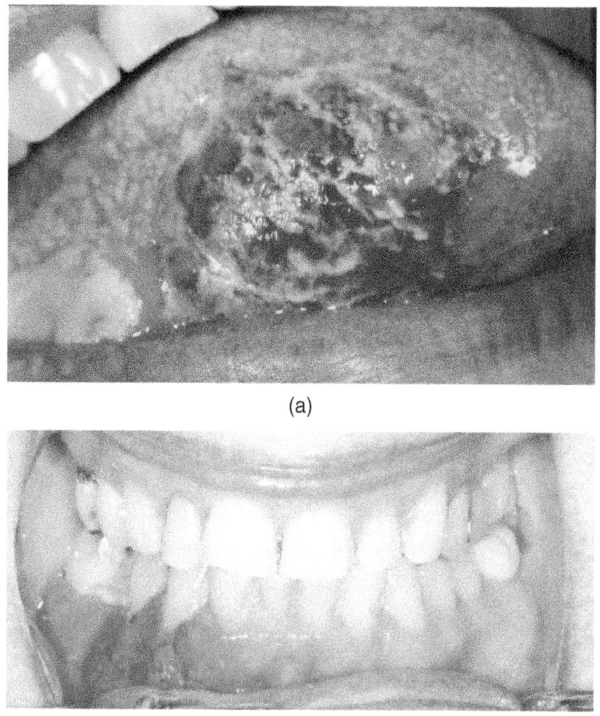

(a)

(b)

Figure 10.5 (a) Speckled leukoplakia. (b) Erythroleukoplakia.

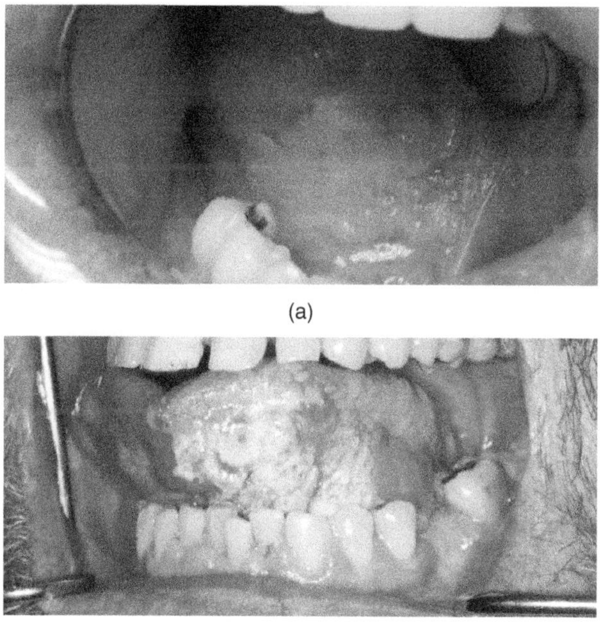

(a)

(b)

Figure 10.4 (a) Homogenous leukoplakia. (b) Nonhomogenous leukoplakia.

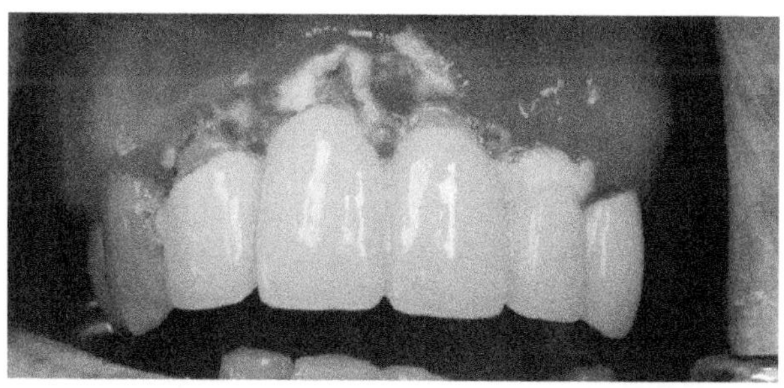

Figure 10.6 Proliferative verrucous leukoplakia. Biopsy of red lesion on the interdental papilla between central incisors exhibited squamous cell carcinoma.

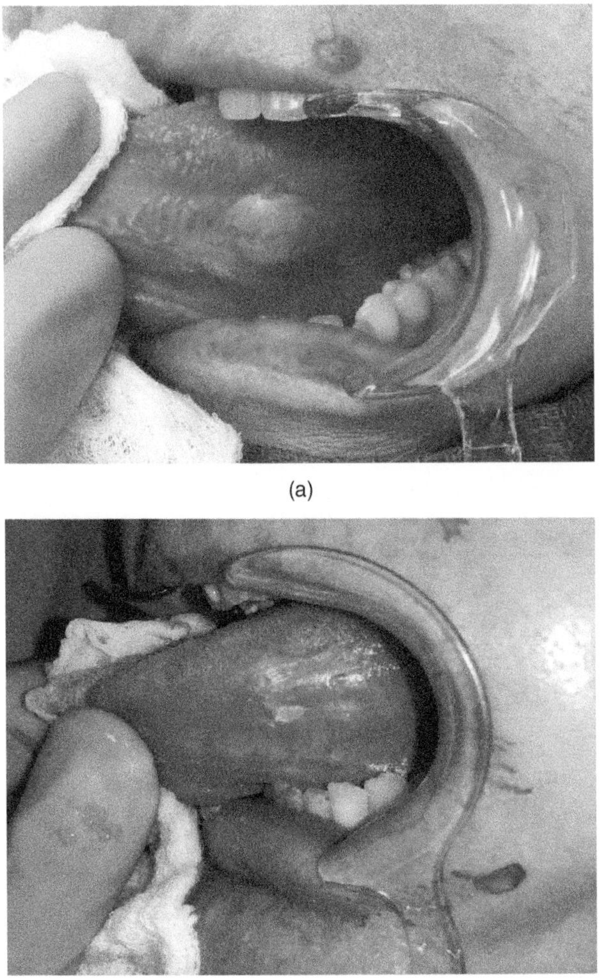

(a)

(b)

Figure 10.7 (a) Severe dysplasia. (b) Squamous cell carcinoma. These photos portray why it is prudent to biopsy a potentially malignant lesion. Although the lesion in (a) seems more suspicious, the lesion in (b) turned out to be squamous cell carcinoma.

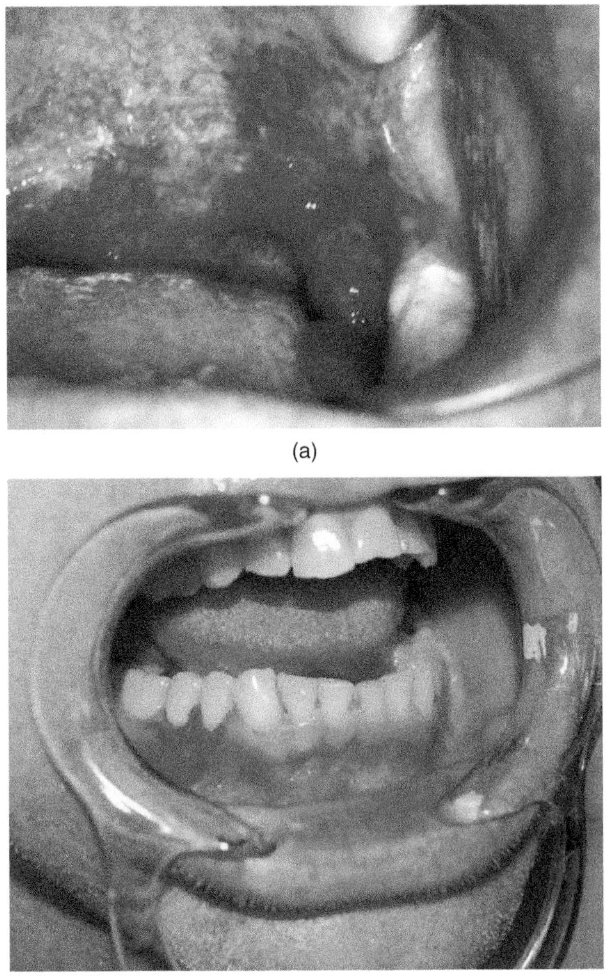

(a)

(b)

Figure 10.8 (a, b) Clinical examples of erythroplakia.

follow-up. Factors such as nonsmoking, size greater than 200 mm^2, lateral tongue site, severe dysplasia, and nonhomogeneous appearance were all associated with a 5-year malignant transformation rate of around 40% or greater. Nonsmokers were 7.1 times more likely to undergo malignant transformation compared to heavy smokers. Malignant transformation occurred after a median of 48 months following diagnosis of dysplasia [20].

Erythroplakia (Figure 10.8) is defined as any lesion of the oral mucosa that presents as bright red velvety plaques, which cannot be characterized clinically or pathologically as any other recognizable condition [21]. It has been reported that up to 91% of lesions demonstrate severe dysplasia, carcinoma *in situ* (CIS), or invasive carcinoma [22].

Oral lichen planus (OLP), described by Erasmus Wilson in 1869, is a chronic, autoimmune, inflammatory disease that affects the skin, oral mucosa, genital mucosa, scalp, and nails [23, 24]. The prevalence of OLP has been reported in the literature as ranging between 0.5% and 3%. Clinically, OLP may be seen as six types: papular, reticular, plaque-like, atrophic, erosive, and bullous. What makes OLP interesting is its ability to transform into malignancy. Transformation rate has been reported up to 10%, with the risk being greater in erosive and atrophic forms [23]. A prospective study with a mean follow-up of 31.9 months by Van der Meij showed an overall transformation rate of 1.7% with an annual transformation rate of 0.65% [25].

The importance of awareness of these "potentially malignant disorders" cannot be overstated. Practitioners must have a high index of suspicion, knowledge, and ability to recognize such lesions. Biopsy or prompt referral is mandatory.

Biopsy Techniques

After deciding that biopsy of an oral cavity lesion is warranted, a practitioner must decide if they have the necessary expertise and proper instrumentation to perform the biopsy (Figure 10.9). It is recommended that if a lesion is highly suspicious for a potential malignancy, referral be made to a facility or practitioner with the proper resources if in fact the lesion turns out to be positive for carcinoma.

Biopsies are typically classified based on lesion characteristics, the technique employed, and the materials used. The most common types of biopsy techniques are incisional biopsy, excisional biopsy, and punch biopsy.

Incisional Biopsy

Incisional biopsy, usually performed with a scalpel, is the most common biopsy procedure. The main indication for an incisional biopsy is to provide the pathologist with a representative sample of the lesion for diagnostic purposes. Incisional biopsy is used for lesions suspected of malignancy or in precancerous lesions. It is also used for chronic ulcers, squamous cell carcinoma, leukoplakia, erythroplakia, lichen planus, and when lesion size does not allow for removal of the whole lesion. If the lesion is extensive, multiple biopsies can be taken. It is important to label and send the biopsies separately. Whenever possible, multiple biopsy sites can be marked on a drawing or photograph and sent with the specimen to the pathologist.

Classic teaching includes selecting a site at the periphery of the lesion to ensure inclusion of healthy tissue in the sample. However, the main principle guiding site selection should be acquisition of the most representative sample; an attempt to include tissue from the periphery may inadvertently lead to underdiagnosis [26, 27]. In terms of the precancerous lesions of leukoplakia and erythroplakia, the adequate and correct sampling of lesions may prove difficult. Sampling errors are common, especially in larger lesions. As discussed previously, lesions showing a nonhomogeneous or speckled appearance and lesions of erythroplakia are potentially more serious with a generally higher incidence of dysplasia and malignant transformation. These areas, if present, should be the sites of choice for biopsy. If the lesion is extensive or there are numerous erythematous regions it may be prudent to biopsy more than one area [28]. Care should also be taken to avoid necrotic areas. If a clinician is uncertain of the most appropriate site from which to obtain a biopsy sample, referral to a specialist is necessary [27].

It is important to note that if a lesion is highly suspicious for carcinoma, a biopsy should be taken with an adequate depth, including the basement membrane and underlying connective tissue and muscle. A prospective randomized controlled study by D'Cruz et al. showed the benefit of elective neck dissection at the time of primary surgery, as compared with watchful waiting followed by therapeutic neck dissection for nodal relapse, in patients with early-stage, clinically node-negative oral squamous

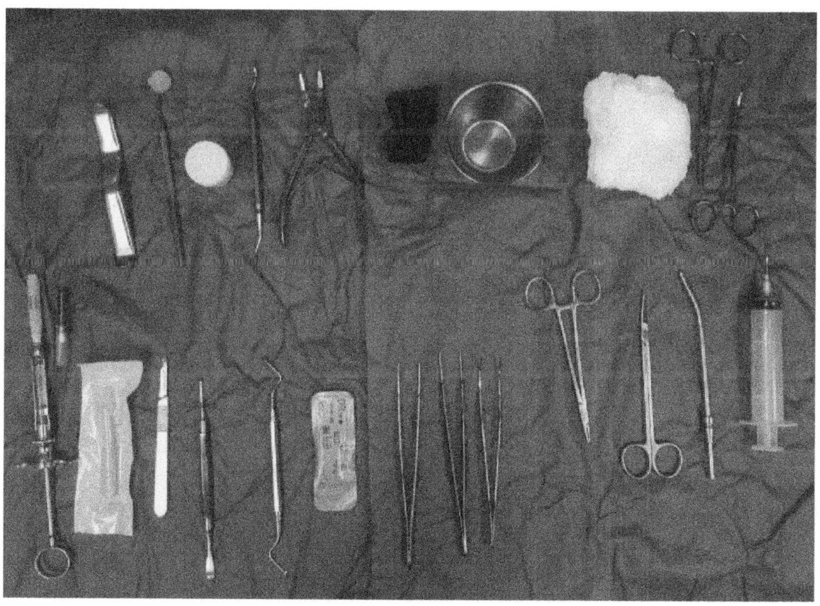

Figure 10.9 Hard/soft tissue biopsy armamentarium.

cell carcinoma. The results show an absolute overall survival benefit of 12.5% and a disease-free survival benefit of 23.6% [29]. The indication to perform a neck dissection in a clinically node-negative patient is based on tumor depth. In a metaanalysis by Huang et al. [30], 4 mm was the suggested optimal depth. It was also the depth suggested in the randomized prospective study by Kligerman et al. [31]. More recently, a study by Zhang et al. recommended that a 3 mm cut-off showed a better balance between sensitivity (92.9%) and specificity (43.1%) [32].

Excisional Biopsy

An excisional biopsy is the complete removal of a lesion. This type of biopsy serves both a diagnostic and therapeutic role. It is recommended to take a small peripheral safety margin on normal tissue. Excisional biopsies are usually elliptical shaped in a 3:1 length to width ratio. The blade is angled toward the center, removing a wedge-shaped piece of tissue and facilitating a simple straight-line closure. Small pedunculated lesions that are easily accessible, such as fibromas, papillomas, pyogenic granulomas, or mucoceles, are amenable to excisional biopsy. An excisional biopsy is only indicated if the lesion is almost certainly benign [33]. Not infrequently, the correct clinical diagnosis of a carcinoma will not be made, and an excisional biopsy will be performed on a presumed benign lesion.

In a paper by Bailey et al., it was noted that with excision biopsies of a malignant lesion, microscopic tumor may remain, and the usual landmarks that enable the surgeon to plan a safe margin are destroyed. Suturing of the inadequate incision may further distort the anatomy and implant the foci more deeply. The loss of these original dimensions of the primary tumor prevents clinical TMN staging. The only guidelines the surgeon has for conceptualizing the shape and size of the original tumor are preoperative clinical description and the gross pathologic specimen. This creates a situation where one must assume residual carcinoma is present, but with a paucity of information on which to base a sound surgical approach. Also, because the lesion was initially thought to be benign, it is likely the tumor depth is not accurate, thus complicating the clinical decision of whether or not to treat the neck. In these situations, it is best to avoid an excisional biopsy on a potentially malignant lesion. The authors recommend that if malignancy is suspected, the lesion should be referred to an oncologic surgeon, so that the original primary lesion, the clinical Tstage, and clinical depth of invasion can be evaluated effectively [34].

Punch Biopsy

A punch biopsy is a rapid and simple technique used to obtain a representative sample of an oral lesion. A biopsy punch is a sterile, disposable instrument with a cylindrical cutting blade connected to a handle. There are both short and long versions. These punches come in various sizes – 2, 3, 4, 5, 6, or 8 mm – allowing a cylinder of tissue 2–8 mm in diameter to be taken.

The punch is placed over the lesional tissue, and a downward twisting motion is applied. The cylindrical tissue core is amputated at its base with a blade or scissor. Presumed advantages of the punch biopsy are its ease of use, less patient anxiety, and the ability to leave the wound open to heal with secondary intention. However, it is recommended to close the wound with sutures to aid in hemostasis. The indication for its use lies mainly in its ability to obtain several samples from different locations within the oral cavity.

Disadvantages of the punch biopsy include its inability to remove larger lesions. It is also not recommended to use the punch biopsy for vesiculobullous diseases as the twisting action can detach the epithelium, preventing proper assessment of the epithelium–connective tissue interface that is necessary for the classification of such lesions [35]. Finally, the punch biopsy is not applicable to deep lesions, so it is not recommended for use in lesions where an accurate measurement of depth is required (Box 10.4).

Adjunctive Techniques

The term "adjunctive technique" may be applied to any technology or device that can help detect oral cancer or precancerous lesions, aid in the characterization of lesions detected during a routine examination, and/or facilitate the selection of appropriate sites for further diagnostic evaluation (i.e., biopsy). Its application should accelerate the pathway to a definitive diagnosis, improve diagnostic accuracy, and reduce false-negative rates due to sampling error. A "screening adjunctive technique" would be applied to a general population and be part of a routine examination, whereas a "diagnostic adjunctive technique" would only be used following the detection of an oral abnormality to facilitate the diagnostic process [38].

Accurate clinical identification of high-risk premalignant lesions either at initial evaluation or during follow-up is key in patient management. For that reason, clinical assessment methods or adjunctive clinical techniques that may help predict the presence of severe dysplasia or

Box 10.4 Special considerations/pitfalls of the biopsy procedure

1. Written and verbal consent should be obtained prior to any surgical procedure, including a biopsy. The proposed treatment, why it is necessary, as well as risks, benefits, and potential complications should be discussed in detail. The need for future surgery or referral should also be discussed
2. *Local anesthesia*: if a clinician is going to mark the site of proposed biopsy, it should be done prior to the administration of local anesthetic. The anesthesia should be administered deep into the surgical field of the proposed biopsy site so as to not cause tissue edema or distortion of the specimen. Care should be taken to avoid injection directly into the biopsy site
3. If the biopsy site involves the gingiva or hard palate, healing by secondary intention may be necessary. Patients must be advised that there may be prolonged discomfort as the area heals secondarily. The risk of gingival recession must be discussed preoperatively
4. When a palatal swelling is encountered, such as in the case of a suspected minor salivary gland tumor, an incisional biopsy down to bone should be performed. The palatal mucosa may be thick and a shallow biopsy may not include a representative sample of the lesion. A palatal biopsy must also account for the underlying vascular anatomy. Care must be taken to avoid the palatine artery and nerves
5. Use a surgical blade/scalpel whenever possible. Use of an electrocautery or laser may cause a thermal artifact. Fulguration artifact is an important problem induced during electrosurgical or laser cutting of tissue. The resulting effect of a layer of carbonized tissue, a zone of thermal necrosis, and a zone of tissue exhibiting thermal damage makes histopathologic interpretation more difficult [35]
6. When performing a biopsy on the lip, brisk bleeding may be encountered. One way to mitigate this is by having the assistant grasp the lip between thumb and index finger on either side of the lesion. A chalazion clamp may also be used (Figure 10.10). If the lesion involves the vermilion border, a thorough discussion about possible esthetic compromise must be initiated
7. When performing labial gland biopsies in the diagnosis of Sjögren syndrome, a minimum of five minor salivary glands is necessary. When removing a mucocele, inclusion of the associated minor salivary gland is essential to prevent recurrence

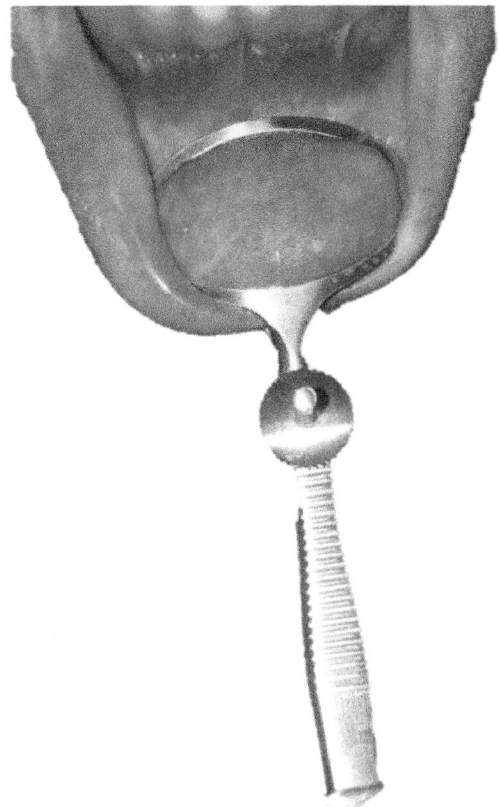

Figure 10.10 Chalazion clamp. A chalazion clamp is an excellent tool for lip biopsies. The ring is centered over the lesion and tightened. It provides excellent hemostasis and traction.

8. Tongue wounds are prone to dehiscence. Deep muscular sutures and placing mucosal sutures very close together may help mitigate this. If dehiscence occurs, the clinician should recommend that the patient keep the area clean and monitor for healing by secondary intention. It is not advisable to resuture the wound
9. Mucosal biopsies that are superficial and that typically do not include underlying muscle tissue tend to curl and distort. This creates some difficulty in proper measurement and orientation of the specimen for tissue processing. This may be overcome by immediately following the biopsy with spreading the specimen onto a piece of stiff card, paper or plastic prior to dropping it (mounted on the stiff paper or plastic) into the formalin fixative [36]

(Continued)

Box 10.4 (Continued)

10. When performing a bone biopsy, it is recommended that an aspiration be performed first to rule out a possible vascular lesion
11. After removal, the biopsy specimen should be immediately placed in a fixative solution due to tissue autolysis. The most commonly used fixative is 10% neutral buffered formalin. If more than one biopsy is taken, they should be placed in separate fixative containers. Most pathology laboratories will provide specimen containers and biopsy processing forms at no charge
12. The fixative container should be labeled. Patient's name, date of birth, other identifying information such as chart number, location and type of biopsy, practitioner's name, and date of biopsy should be provided as a minimum
13. Special care should be taken with biopsies of a suspected autoimmune disease such as pemphigus/pemphigoid. Two specimens should be sent – one in 10% neutral buffered formalin and one in Michel's solution for direct immunofluorescence [37]
14. *Biopsy processing form*. The importance of the biopsy processing form cannot be overstated. In addition to both the patient's and practitioner's information, a detailed description of the biopsy procedure must be included. It is important to include a lesion history, including associated signs or symptoms. A detailed clinical description, including size, shape, color, location, type of biopsy, and clinical impression, is required. The sending of clinical photographs and/or radiographs for bone pathology can be extremely helpful. Accurate clinical and radiographic information is paramount
15. If the diagnosis does not corroborate the clinical picture, a practitioner must rely on clinical judgment. The patient may require an additional biopsy from an adjacent area of the lesion, or a referral to a specialist may be warranted

carcinoma within a lesion have clinical utility, in accelerating biopsy and avoiding sampling errors [39]. It is imperative for clinicians to understand that adjunctive techniques do not replace the need for a careful visual and tactile examination, and that the gold standard for the definitive diagnosis of oral cancer and precancerous lesions remains a tissue biopsy followed by submission for histopathologic evaluation [38].

Lugol's Iodine

The French physician Lugol first made Lugol's iodine in 1829. It is a solution of elemental iodine and potassium iodide in water [40]. The technique of vital tissue staining with Lugol's iodine is also called Schiller's test, as Schiller first used it as a diagnostic aid in gynecological lesions in 1933 [41].

In the head and neck region, Lugol's iodine was first used in the detection of esophageal diseases. Shiozaki first described the potential role of Lugol's iodine in OSCC detection [42]. The study by Kurita et al. is the first that points out the importance of Lugol's iodine in the delineation of the margins of dysplastic oral lesions. In their study, iodine color lining identified the boundary of dysplastic or malignant epithelium [43]. The structure of the mucosal surfaces of the mouth and oropharynx are very similar to the proximal esophagus and the risk factors for neoplastic transformation at these sites are similar.

The mechanism of action of vital staining with Lugol's iodine is based on the fact that the majority of the oral cavity and oropharynx is covered by nonkeratinized, glycogen-containing squamous epithelium. Iodine is glycophilic and normal nonkeratinized mucosa readily takes up the stain and turns a mahogany brown color. In contrast, dysplastic and invasive cancer cells contain little or no glycogen so they do not take up the stain and appear as pale areas [44]. Lugol's iodine is not beneficial in keratinized areas of the oral cavity such as the gingiva.

The technique is simple and consists of applying Lugol's iodine to the suspicious oral lesion with a cotton-tip applicator. Iodine may need to be applied for 1–2 minutes (Figure 10.11). McMahon et al., in their comparative study, evaluated the efficacy of Lugol's solution in the determination of extension of suspicious lesions. These authors demonstrated a significantly lower incidence of dysplasia or carcinoma among the margins of resection of lesion stained with Lugol's solution [45]. Lugol's iodine is cheap, easy to use, and effective in delineating dysplastic and malignant superficial lesions of the oral epithelium. It is a helpful adjunct leading to early diagnosis and better patient management.

Toluidine Blue

Toluidine blue (TB), also known as tolunium chloride, is a cationic metachromatic dye that may selectively bind to free anionic groups such as sulfate, phosphate, and carboxylate

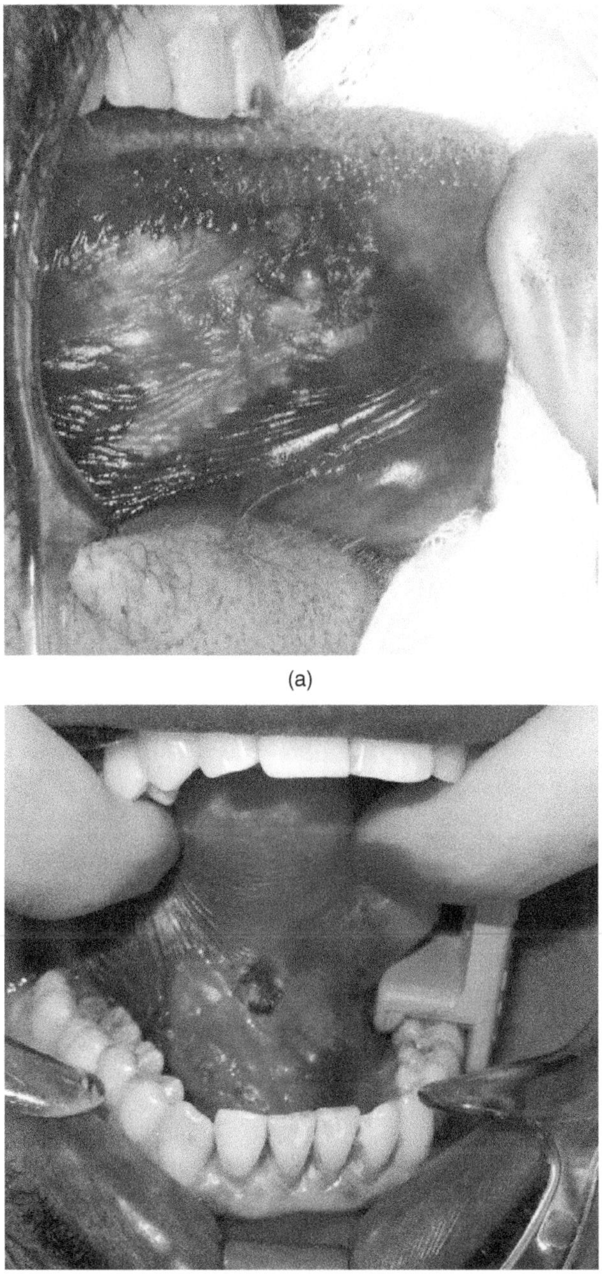

Figure 10.11 Lugol's iodine is applied to a suspicious lesion of the nonkeratinized oral mucosa. Normal tissue stains mahogany brown while dysplastic tissue remain pale. (a) Lateral surface of the tongue. (b) Floor of mouth.

radicals of large molecules [46]. It is used as an *in vivo* stain based on the fact that dysplastic and anaplastic cells may contain quantitatively more nucleic acids than normal tissues. Also, malignant epithelium may contain intracellular canals that are wider than normal epithelium, which may facilitate penetration of the dye. TB staining is a highly reliable, cost-effective, noninvasive, and easy method for the detection of *in situ* and invasive carcinomas. Staining should be routinely used to assist in the choice of biopsy site and in the follow-up of premalignant lesions. In experienced hands, marginal demarcation of malignant lesions enables an intervention method to be adopted earlier for these diseases which carry a high rate of morbidity and mortality.

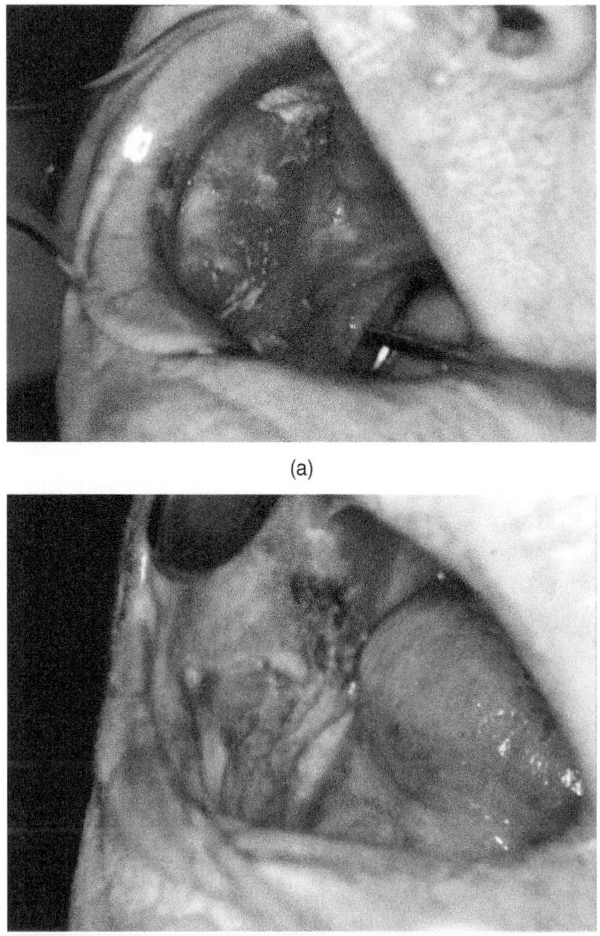

Figure 10.12 (a) Lesion of the right buccal mucosa prior to application of toluidine blue. (b) After application of toluidine blue (dark blue areas should undergo biopsy).

The technique is relatively simple and user-friendly kits may be purchased commercially. The lesion is first swabbed with 1% acetic acid to remove any salivary debris. The acetic acid is washed off with saline and TB is swabbed on for at least 20 seconds. Finally, the area is swabbed again with acetic acid to remove excess TB. The lesion is evaluated for retention of blue stain. A dark blue color is considered positive (Figure 10.12).

The true efficacy of TB lies in guiding biopsy site selection and reducing sampling error, especially with larger, nonhomogeneous, mixed or multifocal lesions where variable histopathology can exist within a lesion or between lesions. Toluidine blue also has utility in monitoring high-risk patients with a past history of squamous cell carcinoma or dysplasia [38].

Brush Biopsy/Cytology

Oral brush biopsies provide a sample for histopathologic examination in a less painful way than traditional scalpel or punch biopsy. The accuracy of brush tests has been the subject of many published studies. In every study in which oral lesions have been simultaneously assessed by both a brush biopsy and surgical biopsy, this test has been shown to have both sensitivity and specificity well over 90%. In a study by Mehrotra, minimally suspicious lesions were brushed and the results compared to matched histopathology. The sensitivity and specificity were 96% and 100%, respectively. The authors go on to say that as an adjunct to oral cancer examination, brush biopsy has the potential to reduce the poor mortality rate associated with oral malignancies [47]. The importance of oral brush biopsy was emphasized in a multicenter study in which nearly 5% of clinically benign-appearing oral mucosal lesions were sampled using this technique and later confirmed using scalpel biopsy to represent dysplastic epithelial changes or invasive cancer [48].

Currently, the only cytopathologic test commercially available in the United States is the Oral CDx BrushTest® (CDx Laboratories, Suffern, NY). The OralCDx brush biopsy is a minimally invasive screening method for surveillance of leukoplakia, erythroleukoplakia, and early detection of innocuous-appearing OSCC [49]. OralCDx consists of two components: (i) the OralCDx brush obtains a complete transepithelial biopsy specimen, collecting cells from all three layers of the epithelium: superficial, intermediate and basal; (ii) the analysis of the OralCDx sample is computer generated. Each kit comes with detailed instructions. A final test report with color microscopic images is then sent to the submitting clinician within 2 weeks. There are four possible results: negative, positive, atypical, and inadequate. Any positive or atypical result warrants further evaluation, and may require the patient to undergo scalpel biopsy and histopathologic evaluation [38].

A brush biopsy is a noninvasive, painless, outpatient procedure. It is an excellent addition to a clinician's armamentarium, especially when confronted with a suspicious lesion. However, confirmation of a cytologically generated diagnosis must be followed by a formal tissue biopsy. The oral brush biopsy overcomes obstacles that have affected early oral cancer detection by eliminating guesswork about which lesion requires surgical biopsy, reducing the tendency to delay referral of patients for scalpel biopsy, and reducing the hesitation of patients to comply with follow-up surgical biopsy [50].

References

1. Saini, R., Santosh, S., and Suganda, S. (2010). Oral biopsy: a dental gawk. *J. Surg. Tech. Case Rep.* 2 (2): 93.
2. Fitzmaurice, C., Allen, C., Barber, R.M. et al. (2017). Global, regional, and national cancer incidence, mortality, years of life lost, years lived with disability, and disability-adjusted life-years for 32 cancer groups, 1990 to 2015: a systematic analysis for the global burden of disease study. *JAMA Oncol.* 3 (4): 524.
3. Siegel, R.L., Miller, K.D., and Jemal, A. (2017, 2017). Cancer statistics. *CA Cancer J. Clin.* 67 (1): 7.
4. Seoane, J., Alvarez-Novoa, P., Gomez, I. et al. (2016). Early cancer diagnosis: the Aarhus statement. A systematic review and meta analysis. *Head Neck* 38: E2182–E2189.
5. Gillison, M.L., Broutian, T., Pickard, R.K. et al. (2012). Prevalence of oral HPV infection in the United States, 2009–2010. *JAMA.* 307 (7): 693.
6. Sylvie-Louis, A. and Hagen, K. (2012). Oral soft tissue biopsy: an overview. *J. Can. Dent. Assoc.* 78: c75.
7. Kahn, M.A., Lynch, D.P., Turner, J.E. et al. (1998). The do's and don't's of an oral mucosal biopsy performed by the general dentist. *J. Tenn. Dent. Assoc.* 78: 28–31.
8. Zargaran, M., Baghaei, F., Moghimbeigi, A. et al. (2012). Evaluation of pre-analytical biopsy specimen errors in the pathology laboratory of Hamadan school of dentistry (2009–2010). *J. Dent.* 13: 103–139.
9. Pippi, R. (2006). Technical notes about soft tissue biopsies of the oral cavity. *Minerva Stomatol.* 55: 51–56.
10. Van der Waal, I. (2009). Potentially malignant disorders of the oral and oropharyngeal mucosa: terminology, classification and present concepts of management. *Oral Oncol.* 45: 317–323.
11. Brennan, M., Migliorati, C.A., Lockhart, P.B. et al. (2007). Management of oral epithelial dysplasia: a review. *Oral Surg. Oral Med. Oral Pathol. Oral Radiol. Endod.* 103 (Suppl): S19.e1–e12.
12. Jaber, M.A., Porter, S.R., Speight, P. et al. (2003). Oral epithelial dysplasia: clinical characteristics of western European residents. *Oral Oncol.* 39 (6): 589–596.
13. Warnakulasuriya, S., Johnson, N.W., and van der Waal, I. (2007). Nomenclature and classification of potentially malignant disorders of the oral mucosa. *J. Oral Pathol. Med.* 36: 575–580.

14 Pindborg, J., Renstrup, G., Poulsen, H. et al. (1963). Studies in oral leukoplakias: clinical and histologic signs of malignancy. *Acta Odontol. Scand.* 21: 407–414.

15 Pindborg, J., Daftary, D., and Mehta, F. (1968). Studies in oral leukoplakia: a preliminary report on the period prevalence of malignant transformation in leukoplakia based on a follow-up study of 248 patients. *Am. Dent. Assoc.* 76 (4): 767–771.

16 Van der Waal, I. (2010). Potentially malignant disorders of the oral and oropharyngeal mucosa: present concepts of management. *Oral Oncol.* 46: 423–425.

17 Hansen, L., Olsen, J., and Silverman, S. (1985). Proliferative verrucous leukoplakia: a long term study of thirty patients. *Oral Surg. Oral Med. Oral Pathol.* 60 (3): 285–298.

18 Silverman, S. and Gorsky, M. (1997). Proliferative verrucous leukoplakia: a follow-up study of 54 cases. *Oral Surg. Oral Med. Oral Pathol. Oral Radiol. Endod.* 84: 154–157.

19 Liu, W., Shi, L., Wu, L. et al. (2012). Oral cancer development in patients with leukoplakia – clinicopathological factors affecting outcome. *PLoS One* 7 (4): e34773.

20 Ho, M., Risk, J., Woolgar, J. et al. (2012). The clinical determinants of malignant transformation in oral epithelial dysplasia. *Oral Oncol.* 48: 969–976.

21 World Health Organization Collaborative Reference Centre for Oral Precancerous Lesions (1978). *Application of the International Classification of Diseases to Dentistry and Stomatology*. Geneva: WHO.

22 Shafer, W.G. and Waldron, C.A. (1975). Erythroplakia of the oral cavity. *Cancer* 36: 1021–1028.

23 Farhi, D. and Dupin, N. (2010). Pathophysiology, etiologic factors, and clinical management of oral lichen planus, part I: facts and controversies. *Clin. Dermatol.* 28: 100–108.

24 Ismail, S.B., Kumar, S.K., and Zain, R.B. (2007). Oral lichen planus and lichenoid reactions: etiopathogenesis, diagnosis, management and malignant transformation. *J. Oral Sci.* 49: 89–106.

25 Van der Meij, E.H., Schepman, K.P., and Van der Waal, I. (2003). The possible premalignant character of oral lichen planus and oral lichenid lesions: a prospective study. *Oral Surg. Oral Med. Oral Pathol. Oral Radiol. Endod.* 96 (2): 164–171.

26 Melrose, R.J., Handlers, J.P., Kerpel, S. et al., for the American Academy of Oral and Maxillifacial Pathology. (2007). The use of biopsy in dental practice. The position of the American Academy of Oral and Maxillofacial Pathology. *Gen. Dent.* 55 (5): 457–461.

27 Poh, C.F., N, S., Berean, K.W. et al. (2008). Biopsy and histopathologic diagnosis of oral premalignant and malignant lesions. *J. Can. Dent. Assoc.* 74 (3): 283–288.

28 Speight, P.M. and Morgan, P.R. (1993). The natural history and pathology of oral cancer and precancer. *Comm. Dent. Health* 10 (1): 31–41.

29 D'Cruz, A., Vaish, R., Kapri, N. et al. (2015). Elective versus therapeutic neck dissection in node-negative oral cancer. *N. Engl. J. Med.* 373: 521–529.

30 Huang, S.H., Hwang, D., Lockwood, G. et al. (2009). Predictive value of tumor thickness for cervical lymph-node involvement in squamous cell carcinoma of the oral cavity: a meta-analysis of reported studies. *Cancer* 115: 1489.

31 Kligerman, J., Lima, R.A., Soares, J.R. et al. (1994). Supraomohyoid neck dissection in the treatment of T1/T2 squamous cell carcinoma of oral cavity. *Am. J. Surg.* 168: 391.

32 Zhang, T., Lubek, J., Salama, A. et al. (2014). Treatment of cT1N0M0 tongue cancer: outcome and prognostic parameters. *J. Oral Maxillofac. Surg.* 72: 406–414.

33 Oliver, R.J., Sloan, P., and Pemberton, M.N. (2004). Oral biopsies: methods and applications. *Br. Dent. J.* 196 (6): 329–333.

34 Bailey, J., Blanchaert, R., and Ord, R. (2001). Management of oral squamous cell carcinoma treated with inadequate incision. *J. Oral Maxillofac. Surg.* 59: 1007–1010.

35 Avon, S.L. and Hagen, B.E. (2012). Oral soft-tissue biopsy: an overview. *J. Can. Dent. Assoc.* 78 (c75): 1–9.

36 Rosebush, M., Anderson, M., and Rawal, S. (2010). The oral biopsy: indications, techniques and special considerations. *J. Tenn. Dent. Assoc.* 90: 17–20.

37 Milner, Y. and David, K. (1973). Preservation of tissue-fixed immunoglobulins in skin biopsies of patients with lupus erythematosus and bullous diseases – preliminary report. *J. Invest. Dermatol.* 59: 449–452.

38 Kerr, R. and Shah, S. (2013). Standard examination and adjunctive technique for detection of oral premalignant and malignant lesions. *J. Calif. Dent. Assoc.* 41: 329–341.

39 Patton, L.L., Epstein, J.B., and Kerr, A.R. (2008). Adjunctive techniques for oral cancer examination and lesion diagnosis: a systematic review of the literature. *J. Am. Dent. Assoc.* 139: 896–905.

40 Petruzzi, M., Lucchese, A., Baldoni, E. et al. (2010). Use of Lugol's iodine in oral cancer diagnosis: an overview. *Oral Oncol.* 46: 811–813.

41 Schiller, W. (1933). Early diagnosis of carcinoma of the cervix. *Surg. Gynecol. Obstet.* 56: 210–222.

42 Shiozaki, H., Tahara, H., Kobayashi, K. et al. (1990). Endoscopic screening of early esophageal cancer with the Lugol dye method in patients with head and neck cancers. *Cancer* 66: 2068–2071.

43 Kurita, H. and Kurashina, K. (1996). Vital staining with iodine solution in delineating the border of oral

dysplastic lesions. *Oral Surg. Oral Med. Oral Pathol. Oral Radiol. Endod.* 81: 275–280.

44 McCaul, J., Cymerman, J., Hislop, S. et al. (2013). LIHNCS – Lugol's iodine in head and neck cancer surgery: a multicentre, randomised controlled trial assessing the effectiveness of Lugol's iodine to assist excision of moderate dysplasia, severe dysplasia and carcinoma in situ at mucosal resection margins of oral and oropharyngeal squamous cell carcinoma: study protocol for a randomised controlled trial. *Trials* 14: 310.

45 McMahon, J., Devine, J., McCaul, J. et al. (2010). Use of Lugol's iodine in the resection of oral and oropharyngeal squamous cell carcinoma. *Br. J. Oral Maxillofac. Surg.* 48: 84–87.

46 Giovanacci, I., Vescovi, P., Manfredi, M. et al. (2016). Non-invasive tools for diagnosis of oral cancer and dysplasia: a systematic review. *Med. Oral Patol. Oral Cir. Bucal* 21: e305–e315.

47 Mehrotra, R., Mishra, S., Singh, M. et al. (2011). The efficacy of oral brush biopsy with computer assisted analysis in identifying precancerous and cancerous lesions. *Head Neck Oncol.* 3: 1–7.

48 Sciubba, J.J. (1999). Improving detection of precancerous and cancerous oral lesions. Computer-assisted analysis of the oral brush biopsy. *J. Am. Dent. Assoc.* 130: 1445–1457.

49. Kosicki, D., Riva, C., Pajarola, G. et al. (2007). OralCDx brush biopsy – a tool for early diagnosis of oral squamous cell carcinoma. *Schweiz. Monatsschr. Zahnmed.* 117: 222–227.

50. Zunt, S.L. (2001). Transepithelial brush biopsy: an adjunctive diagnostic procedure. *J. Indiana Dent. Assoc.* 80: 6–8.

11

Diagnosis and Management of Recurrent Lesions of the Oral Mucosa

Mihai Radulescu

Introduction

Recurrent lesions of the oral mucosa indicate that the balance between destructive and reparatory events is periodically lost. It can be difficult to determine the etiology, and sometimes there may be a combination of several factors: traumatic, infective, immunologic, and nutritional deficiencies. To complicate the situation even more, different types of lesions can have the same clinical appearance at different stages. Vesicular lesions are generally short-lived in the mouth and are most often "caught" in the ulcerative phase. A chronic lesion that is generally silent may manifest periodic symptomatic exacerbations and remissions, thus mimicking the pattern of recurrent lesions.

This chapter will review the clinical features, diagnosis, and management of the classic conditions that should be considered in the differential diagnoses of recurrent mucosities of the oral cavity: aphthous stomatitis, herpetic lesions, candidiasis, lichen planus, pemphigus vulgaris, erythema multiforme (EM), and fixed drug reactions.

Aphthous Lesions and Recurrent Aphthous Stomatitis

Aphthous lesions, also known colloquially as "canker sores," are the most common form of oral ulcerations. As the etymology of the term suggests (*aphtai* = burn in ancient Greek), aphthae are usually associated with pain.

Presentation

The clinical presentation is a white-grayish pseudomembranous membrane over an area of necrosis and surrounded by an erythematous halo. It typically involves the nonkeratinized mucosa. It is classified by size: minor (<10 mm), major (>10 mm), and herpetiform (many small aphthae at the same time).

The overall prevalence of aphthae in the US population is approximately 20% [1] and it is most frequently found in children. Minor aphthae usually heal without treatment within 1–2 weeks while major aphthae may take more than 6 weeks and may heal with scarring. Most of these lesions are sporadic, but some patients develop recurrent aphthous stomatitis (RAS). Among the RAS forms, approximatively 70% are minor, 10% major, and 10% herpetiform [2]. It seems to be more frequent in women, patients under 40 years, white, nonsmokers and of high socioeconomic status [3]. In the Caucasian population, the prevalence of RAS is 2–5% [4].

Etiology

Recurrent aphthosis can be caused by a multitude of factors. Genetic influence has long been suspected: children of RAS+ parents have a 90% chance of developing RAS during their lifetime [5]. Possible theories suggest that genes associated with the human leukocyte antigen (HLA) complex, heat-shock proteins, tumor necrosis factor (TNF)-alpha, or vascular endothelial growth factor (VEGF) could induce the deregulation in the local immune response [6].

Oral and Maxillofacial Surgery, Medicine, and Pathology for the Clinician, First Edition. Edited by Harry Dym, Leslie R. Halpern, and Orrett E. Ogle.

However, the genetic predisposition is not the unique determining factor: the identical twins of a RAS+ individual may never develop RAS symptoms.

Diagnosis

The clinician needs to investigate and possibly eliminate the factors that could trigger recurrent oral aphthosis. This is not an easy task. First, a traumatic etiology has to be ruled out: mechanical irritation from dental prosthetics, tooth brushing, oral habits. Fixed drug reactions and possible hypersensitivity to foods need to be ruled out also. The most commonly associated drugs are naproxen, cotrimoxazole, tetracyclins, barbiturates, and carbamazepine [3]. The toothpaste surfactant sodium lauryl sulfate [7] and cinnamon flavor [8] have also been associated with RAS.

Primary RAS is a diagnosis of exclusion. A complete medical history and review of systems is warranted in order to identify possible extraoral pathology with secondary manifestations of RAS. In particular, the clinician should investigate the presence of extraoral lesions of the skin or mucosae, cyclic fever, gastrointestinal symptoms, articular symptoms, lymphadenopathy, weight loss, and fatigue.

Several diseases of immune dysregulation are known to cause RAS: Behçet disease, Crohn's disease, gluten enteropathy, cyclic neutropenia, PFAPA syndrome (Periodic Fever, Aphthous stomatitis, Pharyngitis, cervical Adenitis), Reiter syndrome, Sweet syndrome, MAGIC syndrome (Mouth And Genital ulcers with Inflamed Cartilage), lupus erythematosus, and HIV [9]. Some of these are summarized in Table 11.1. Vitamin B12 deficiency, atopical reaction to drugs or diet, stress, and smoking cessation have also been associated with increased risk of aphthae [10]. It is important to consider that vesicular lesions of the mouth are often short-lived and can present as ulcerations by the time the patient comes for clinical exam. Thus, viral or desquamative etiologies such as pemphigus and pemphigoid should also be considered in the differential diagnosis of RAS.

Table 11.1 Systemic conditions that would commonly present with oral recurrent aphthous lesions.

Behçet disease	Vasculitis of small and medium sized vessels causing recurrent aphthous ulcers, as well as recurrent genital ulceration, ocular disease and a range of neurologic, renal, and hematologic abnormalities
Cyclic neutropenia	Cyclic reduction in the circulating levels of neutrophils, causing recurrent oral ulcerations, fever, upper respiratory tract infections, and lymphadenopathy approximatively every 21 d
PFAPA syndrome	Periodic fever, aphthous ulceration, pharyngitis, and cervical adenitis; it occurs mostly in children and the condition usually improves with tonsillectomy
Reiter syndrome	Immune condition causing arthritis, urethritis, conjunctivitis, and oral ulcers
Sweet syndrome	Patients have aphthous lesions accompanied by fever, leukocytosis and well-demarcated, plum-colored skin papules or plaques. There is an associated malignancy (such as acute myeloid leukemia) in half of patients

Treatment

The treatment for aphthous ulcers is palliative, the goal being to reduce the duration, size, and recurrence of lesions. Local interventions are also an important adjuvant in controlling a secondary RAS that is not well covered by systemic treatment, thus avoiding increase of immunosuppressive drug dosage and the many associated side-effects.

First-line treatment options include antiseptics (chlorhexidine), topical antiinflammatory drugs (Amlexanox®), muccoprotective agents (sucralfate), and analgesics (lidocaine) for as long as the lesions persist [11] (Table 11.2). Laser therapy with low pulse Nd:YAG or chemical cauterization with silver nitrate can also provide pain relief, likely via disruption of local nerve impulses [11].

Topical steroids can decrease symptoms and improve healing time, but do not affect recurrence rate. If multiple lesions are present, an aqueous solution is preferred. A dexamethasone rinse can be considered [4]. In the case of isolated lesions, a high-potency topical steroid (Kenalog®, clobetasol, or fluocinomide [12]) in an adherent carrier such as Orabase® or denture adhesive paste can be applied in small amounts to the specific area [13]. Steroids should not be used for more than 2 weeks and the patient should be monitored for yeast superinfection. Also, topical steroids should not be placed on viral lesions, as they could aggravate the lesion.

Minocycline, an antibiotic with immunomodulatory effect suppressing neutrophils, T lymphocytes, and collagenase activity, can also be used. A blind cross-over study demonstrated a significant reduction in duration and severity of pain compared to placebo [14]. Daily administration of vitamin B12 sublingually can reduce the frequency and severity of the lesions; it has also shown benefit in non-B12-deficient patients, and has no side-effects. A small study showed lower RAS recurrence in subjects using chewable nicotine tablets [11].

Intralesional treatment with triamcinolone (0.1–0.5 mL per lesion) can be considered for a painful single aphtha [15]. For severe lesions resistant to topical or local treatment, a systemic steroid such as prednisone can be recommended. It can be started at 1 mg/kg/d as a single dose in patients with severe lesions and tapered after

Table 11.2 Topical medications for recurrent aphthous ulcers.

Medication	Class	Form	Dispense	Instructions	Side-effects
Chlorhexidine	Antibiotic	0.12%	480 mL bottle	15 mL rinse and spit tid	Safe
Lidocaine	Analgesic	3%	28 mg tube	Prn to affected areas q4–6 h	Safe
Amlexanox	Antiinflammatory	5% paste	5 g tube	Apply to affected areas bid	Safe
Sucralfate	Mucoprotective	Suspension	415 mL bottle	5 mL qid with applicator to affected area	Safe
Dexamethasone	Steroid	Elixir 0.05/5 mL	100 mL bottle	5 mL rinse and spit tid	Mucosal atrophy Systemic absorption with prolonged use
Minocycline	Antibiotic	0.2% aqueous solution	200 mL bottle	5 mL rinse and spit qid for 10 d	safe
Kenalog (triamcinolone)	High-potency steroid	0.1% or 0.5% ointment in Orabase	15 g tube	Apply to affected areas tid	Mucosal atrophy Systemic absorption with prolonged use
Clobetasol	High-potency steroid	0.05% ointment in Orabase	15 g tube	Apply to affected areas tid	Mucosal atrophy Systemic absorption with prolonged use
Fluocinomide	High-potency steroid	0.05% ointment in Orabase	15 g tube	Apply to affected areas tid	Mucosal atrophy Systemic absorption with prolonged use

1–2 weeks [16]. The recommendation is to use less than 50 mg per day, preferably in the morning, for 5 days [4].

Severe cases of RAS are usually treated with colchicine, pentoxifylline, dapsone, or infliximab but these modalities should be reserved to oral medicine specialists due to the multiple side-effects.

Herpetic Lesions

In oral herpes, the principal symptom is the appearance of vesicles and ulcers that heal spontaneously within 5–10 days: the "cold sores." The cause is most often herpes simplex virus type 1 (HSV-1) but epidemiology has been changing and HSV-2, which is commonly associated with herpes genitalis, can also be found in herpes labialis [17].

Course of the Disease

The primary HSV oral infection can be anything from asymptomatic to severe gingivostomatitis with fever and lymphadenopathy. Following this, the virus ascends along the sensory axons of the trigeminal nerve, establishing latency in the gasserian ganglion. From there, it can become reactivated by various stimuli: stress, fever, ultraviolet light, trauma, menstruation [18]. As the virus travels distally along the afferent fibers, the patient experiences prodromal symptoms: itching, burning, or paresthesia [19]. The first mucosal lesions develop as vesicles that eventually erupt, forming ulcerations and ultimately scabbing. The recurrent herpes labialis occurs typically at the junction of the vermilion and the cutaneous lip. Intraorally, it usually occurs on the keratinized mucosa, which distinguishes it from recurrent aphthous lesions that tend to occur mostly on the free gingiva [20].

Diagnosis

The diagnosis is based on clinical presentation and history. In cases of recurrent intraoral lesions with unobserved vesicular stages, a viral culture can be useful in order to rule out recurrent aphthosis.

Treatment

The aim of antiviral therapy is to block viral replication. All the antiviral medications in Table 11.3 work by mimicking guanosine and blocking the viral DNA polymerase. Thus, for the treatment to be effective, aciclovir, famciclovir, or valaciclovir should be started at the first signs, ideally

Table 11.3 Medications for recurrent herpes labialis.

Medication	Form	Dispense	Instructions	Notes
Aciclovir	5% ointment	15 g	Every 3–4 h for 4 d	Must be started at first prodromal signs
Penciclovir	1% ointment	5 g	Every 2 h, for 4 d	Must be started at first prodromal signs
Aciclovir	200 mg	25 tabs	1 tab 5 times daily for 5 d	Must be started at first prodromal signs Can cause headache, gastrointestinal (GI) disturbance, rash
Famciclovir	750 mg	2 tabs	2 tabs as a single dose	Must be started at first prodromal signs Can cause headache, GI disturbance, nausea
Valaciclovir	500 mg	8 tabs	2 g bid for 1 d	Must be started at first prodromal signs Can cause headache, GI disturbance, rash

during the prodromal stage. Peak viral titers are reached in the first 24 hours after lesion onset, when most lesions reach the vesicular stage, and by that time it is already too late to start treatment [19]. Topical antivirals such as aciclovir and penciclovir are also available, but tend to be less effective. For pain management, a topical anesthetic such as viscous lidocaine or benzocaine can be administrated [21]. Zilactin®, a topical medication containing hydroxypronyl cellulose that adheres to the mucosa, may be used to protect the lesions from irritants [22].

For prophylaxis treatment, such as before dental procedures, valaciclovir (1 g or 2 g bid) or acyclovir (400 mg bid or tid) can be prescribed [21]. Patients with severe recurrent lesions who do not experience prodromal symptoms may be candidates for long-term antiviral therapy.

Candidiasis

Candidiasis is the most common mycosis of the oral cavity. *Candida albicans* is a normal inhabitant of the oral flora and its growth is controlled by the immune system and competitive microbiota. A decrease in the host defense mechanism, broad-spectrum antibiotics, topical or inhaled corticosteroids can alter the balance and promote candidiasis. Other risk factors include smoking, xerostomia, diabetes mellitus, endocrinopathies, pregnancy, immunosuppressive conditions, malignancies, and nutritional deficiencies.

Clinical Presentation

The pseudomembranous form, often referred as "thrush," is the classic presentation. The white plaques represent cellular debris and fungal proliferation and wipe off with gauze, revealing an erythematous mucosal bed with *Candida* invasion. Sometimes, the erytemateous form predominates, especially under dentures. On the tongue, it can cause atrophy of the papillae. When it develops in the middle of the dorsum of the tongue, in a diamond-shaped pattern, it is called median rhomboid glossitis. The hyperplastic form is usually more severe or chronic; it elicits hyperplastic tissue response with acantholysis and hyperkeratosis and it is less likely to scrape off. Angular cheilitis is a mixed infection of *C. albicans* and salivary species of streptococci at the level of the oral commissure.

Diagnosis

The diagnosis is most often based on the clinical presentation and associated symptoms. For microscopic confirmation, a lesion scraping can be smeared on a glass slide and fixed with alcohol or allowed to air dry. For a chairside diagnosis, a drop of 10% potassium hydroxide can be placed on the slide to dissolve the keratinocytes, and the sample can be inspected for the presence of hyphae. Alternatively, it can be sent to the lab for periodic acid–Schiff (PAS) stain, which preferentially stains the fungal glycogen. Another diagnostic modality is via culture on Sabouraud medium. Mucosal biopsy is also an alternative [23].

Treatment

Oral candidiasis is most often treated with topical antifungal agents, such as nystatin ointment and clotrimazole troches (Table 11.4). For patients experiencing xerostomia and having difficulty dissolving the troches, nystatin or amphotericin suspensions can be prescribed. Angular cheilitis responds well to a combination of antifungal and a topical steroid, such as nystatin-triamcinolone acetonide ointment [24].

For patients with refractory candidiasis, muccocutaneous candidosis, women with concurrent candida vaginitis or patients in whom compliance is a problem, a systemic antifungal therapy with ketoconazole or fluconazole is recommended. Patients should be informed that the systemic use of these drugs can cause hepatotoxicity. Liver function

Table 11.4 Topical medications for oral candidiasis.

Medication	Form	Dispense	Instructions	Notes
Nystatin	Ointment	30 g tube	Apply to affected area or to denture base and insert denture tid	Safe Inexpensive
Clotrimazole	10 mg troches	70 troches	Dissolve in mouth 5 times daily for 14 d	Safe High sugar content Expensive
Nystatin	100 000 IU/mL oral suspension	60 mL bottle	Swish with 5 mL qid allowing suspension to be retained in the mouth as long as possible. Continue treatment for 24 h after symptoms disappear	Safe Inexpensive Poor penetration
Amphotericin	Oral suspension 100 mg/mL	48 mL	Swish with 1 mL for 3 min qid, and swallow	Topical and systemic effects Expensive
Nystatin-triamcinolone acetonide	Ointment	15 g tube	Apply to corners of mouth after meals and at bedtime, for 2 wk	Safe Inexpensive

tests should be performed if the medication is used for more than 2 weeks [25].

Lichen Planus

Oral lichen planus is a chronic inflammatory lesion that presents with relapse and remissions. It has a prevalence of 0.5–2%, with a 2:1 female-to-male ratio and a general age at onset of 30–60 years. The underlying etiology is unclear. It involves a T-cell-mediated reaction with complex interplay between CD4, CD8, and local mast cells, macrophages, eosinophils, and basophils [26].

Clinical Presentation

The most common presentation of oral lichen planus is the reticular form, often bilateral and asymptomatic, and recognized by the presence of white, interlacing Wickham striae. There are several other variations of lichen planus (plaque-like, atrophic, ulcerative, papullar, and bullous). The patient may also present with cutaneous lichen planus, which manifests as purple, itchy, polygonal plaques or papules that may also display Wickham striae. The exacerbation of the oral lesions often coincides with periods of physiologic stress [27].

Diagnosis

Clinical diagnosis of oral lichen planus is usually sufficient for lesions with classic bilateral presentation. Several forms can be present at the same time and a biopsy is indicated whenever in doubt. The clinician needs to bear in mind that the ulcerative form has a lifetime risk of malignant transformation estimated at 0.5–2% [28].

The differential diagnoses include candida, pemphigus, pemphigoid, chronic ulcerative stomatitis, erythema multiforme, lupus erythematosus, and leukoplakia. Oral lichenoid reactions resemble lichen planus and can be caused by contact hypersensitivity to dental materials, graft-versus-host disease, and lichenoid reaction caused by drugs: NSAIDs, antihypertensives (beta-blockers, angiotensin-converting enzyme inhibitors [ACEI], diuretics), dapsone, oral hypoglycemics (sulfonylurea), phenothiazines, antimalarial drugs, and phenothiazines.

Treatment

The literature agrees that only the erosive, ulcerative or symptomatic lesions need to be treated. The first line of treatment consists of high-potency topical steroids, often coadministered with a topical antifungal to prevent oral candidiasis [29] (Table 11.5a). For patients who do not improve or who cannot tolerate topical corticoids for reasons such as allergic contact mucositis or recurrent oropharyngeal candidiasis, the second line of treatment consists of topical calcineurin blockers and intralesional steroids (Table 11.5b). Intralesional injections with betamethasone have the advantage of delivering a high local concentration yet repeated injections raise concerns regarding systemic absorption, the potential suppression of the hypothalamic-pituitary-adrenal axis and resulting side-effects [29]. Finally, patients with severe and refractory disease that cannot be managed with topical therapy may be considered for systemic glucocorticoids such as prednisone or systemic immunomodulatory agents such as azathioprine, ciclosporin, methotrexate, thalidomide, mycophenolate, or rituximab.

Table 11.5a Medications used for lichen planus – first line of treatment.

Medication	Class	Form	Dispense	Instructions	Notes
Dexamethasone	Steroid	Elixir 0.5 mg/5 mL	237 mL	5 mL rinse and split 6 times per day	Risk of candidiasis
Clobetasol	High-potency steroid	Ointment 0.05%	15 g	Dry area with gauze and apply tid	Opportunistic candidiasis
Fluocinonide	High-potency steroid	Ointment 0.05%	15 g	Dry area with gauze and apply tid	Eating and drinking should be avoided for 30 min
Betamethasone	High-potency steroid	Ointment 0.05%	15 g	Dry area with gauze and apply tid	Can be administered in gingival trays or dental base carrier Systemic absorption has been documented yet the risk of adrenal suppression appears to be low

Table 11.5b Medications used for lichen planus – second line of treatment.

Medication	Class	Form	Administered	Notes
Pimecrolimus	Topical calcineurin inhibitor	1% cream	Dry area with gauze and apply tid	Concerns of increased risk of cancer
Tacrolimus	Topical calcinerium inhibitor	0.1% ointment	Dry area with gauze and apply tid	Concerns of increased risk of cancer
Triamcinolone	High-potency corticosteroid	10–40 mg/mL	Intralesional injections in submucosa q2–4 wk	Hypopigmentation Systemic absorption Risk of increased glucose level in diabetics Risk of increased blood pressure

Additional therapies that have been reported to be effective include topical retinoids, oral retinoids, hydroxychloroquinone, topical rapamycin, oral dapsone, oral metronidazole, cryotherapy, and laser therapy [30].

Pemphigus Vulgaris

Pemphigus is a relatively rare (1–5 cases/million/year) but potentially fatal blistering disease causing lesions of the skin, mucosa, or both. Six forms of pemphigus have been identified (pemphigus vulgaris, paraneoplastic pemphigus, pemphigus foliaceus, pemphigus erythematosus, pemphigus vegetans, and IgA pemphigus). Out of these, pemphigus vulgaris and paraneoplastic pemphigus are the most likely to be found in the mouth, and pemphigus vulgaris is the most common [31].

Clinical Presentation

Pemphigus vulgaris itself has two clinical forms: muccocutaneous and mucous. In mucous pemphigus, the patient does not develop skin lesions and oral lesions are consistently found. In 50–79% of pemphigus vulgaris patients, the first lesions occur in the oral cavity [32].

The intraoral vesiculobullous lesions in pemphigus vulgaris are usually short-lived due to masticatory trauma and rupture, leaving painful ulceration. As these heal, new lesions develop. The clinical presentation can be sometimes confusing: the lesions can appear to heal spontaneously and can be misdiagnosed as recurrent aphthous stomatitis [33]. This can be complicated by the fact that pemphigus vulgaris may undergo an unpredictable course with apparent curing, followed by remission [34].

Etiology

The underlying pathology is B-cell dysfunction with production of autoantibodies against the cadherin-type cell adhesion glycoproteins desmoglein-1 (expressed in the superficial epidermis and mucosa) and desmoglein-3 (in the suprabasal mucosa only). Circulating antidesmoglein-1 is involved in mucocutaneous pemphigus and causes loss of intercellular adhesion. In mucosal pemphigus, antidesmoglein-3 produces epithelial detachment from the basal layer. In both cases, blisters are produced.

Direct immunofluorescent tagging of antidesmoglein-3 IgG is used for diagnosis [35].

Diagnosis

Early detection based on oral presentation plays an important role. The lesions can be induced clinically on manual pressure or with a cotton swab (positive Nikolsky sign), but this is not specific enough. The diagnosis is made by biopsy, which should be within 1 cm and taken from intact perilesional mucosa. A sample from the ulcerated center would miss the epithelium and cannot be used to detect the loss of hemidesmosomal attachments. The tissue must be handled carefully to prevent inadvertent detachment of the epithelial layer.

Two samples need to be submitted to pathology: one in 10% formalin solution for histologic study and one fresh sample in Michel solution for immunohistochemical study. Formalin preserves the tissue by forming intermolecular bridges between proteins. This inhibits tissue autolysis but interferes with immunofluorescent antibody staining. It is important to call the lab in advance and confirm it provides services for direct immunofluorescent evaluation and to submit the specimen in Michel solution quickly in order to preserve antibody detection [35].

Treatment

If left untreated, pemphigus vulgaris is potentially fatal from dehydration or systemic infections due to loss of epithelial protection. Mild forms of oral pemphigus may be controlled with topical corticosteroids such as 0.1% triamcinolone acetonide, 0.05% fluocinolone acetonide, or 0.005% clobetasol proprionate in Orabase, applied 3–4 times a day for 9–24 weeks [36]. For patients who find direct application of topical applications difficult, gingival trays can be fabricated and left in place for 10–20 minutes per treatment. Alternatively, dexamethasone 0.1 mg/mL as a 5 mL bid or tid "swish and spit" can be prescribed. When using topical steroids, patients should be monitored for oropharyngeal candidiasis.

For lesions that do not respond sufficiently to local measures, intralesional corticosteroid could be used, such as triamcinolone acetonide (10 mg/mL) in 0.1–0.5 mL per injection side. The recommendation is to use no more than 20 mL per treatment session [37].

For multifocal pemphigus, systemic glucocorticoids (prednisone, prednisolone, methylprednisone) and immunomodulatory agents (azathioprine, mycophenolate mofetil, ciclosporin) can be used. The treatment goals are to stop disease progression and improve symptoms. A typical regimen can start with 60 mg prednisolone per day and be augmented gradually up to 240 mg per day, until the disease is controlled. Then, the dose is gradually tapered weekly, and then monthly, till the minimal dose that can control the disease is reached. On long-term therapy, patients are at risk of developing Cushing symptoms [38].

Erythema Multiforme

The first description of erythema multiforme was published in 1866 by von Hebra who described it as a benign condition affecting the skin, with characteristic erythematous lesions in target form, and a tendency for recurrence. Since then, the understanding of this disease has evolved. It is classified as a reactive mucocutaneous condition, likely precipitated by a viral infection and having a minor and a major form. Stevens–Johnson syndrome (SJT) and toxic epidermal necrolysis (TEN) are more extensive conditions that were previously considered part of the EM spectrum, but now are understood as different entities and attributed to drug reactions [39, 40].

Clinical Presentation

Erythema multiforme is a relatively rare disease, with an incidence of less than 1/100 000 cases per year. It is most commonly seen in individuals between 20 and 40 years old. Children and adolescents are affected in 20% of cases, but are more likely to have a recurrent form [41]. EM minor typically affects only one mucosa and may be associated with bilateral skin lesions on the extremities, while EM major typically involves two or more mucosae and has variable skin involvement that is usually more extensive than in EM minor but less than 10% of the body surface [42, 43].

Erythema multiforme presents with mucosal lesions 25–60% of the time. It is usually accompanied by skin lesions, but it can also precede them by several days. The oral mucosa is involved 70% of the time; other sites include pharyngeal, upper respiratory, ocular or genital [44]. Due to the fact that the oral mucosa is so often involved, some authors even consider oral EM as a distinct category in itself that presents with bilateral cutaneous targetoid lesions 25% of the time. The oral lesions of EM are usually painful and can have variable presentation: bullae, erosions, ulcerations with or without a pseudomembrane, or nonspecific hyperkeratotic plaques with interspersed erythematous changes [45].

Recurrent EM shows an average of six episodes per year and the literature reports a clear association with HIV infection in 23–100% of cases. A study using the polymerase chain reaction (PCR) has identified HSV DNA in 50%

of biopsies of patients diagnosed with idiopathic recurrent EM, raising the probability that a subclinical HSV could also be involved. Other conditions that have been associated with recurrent EM include *M. pneumoniae* infections, hepatitis C, vulvovaginal candidiasis, menstruation, complex aphthosis, and the food preservative benzoic acid [45].

Regarding the involvement of oral lesions in recurrent EM, the 1993 study by Schofield et al. identified that in a series of 65 patients, 69% had oral mucous membrane lesions. The most common precipitating factor was a preceding HSV infection [46]. These findings are consistent with those of Farthing et al., who examined a series of 82 patients with recurrent EM and found that 70% had oral lesions. The most commonly affected intraoral sites were the buccal mucosa and tongue [47]. Celentano et al. investigated 60 patients with oral mucous lesions from EM, and found that 52% had previous recurrences. The most common causative factors were drugs (47%) and HSV (30%) [48].

Prodromal symptoms of malaise, fever, and pain are common in mucosal EM. They appear a week or more before the onset of EM but it is not clear if they are part of the disease or a precipitating infection that may have triggered EM [45]. The lesions appear over 3–5 days, are painful and resolve over 1–3 weeks [48].

Diagnosis

The diagnosis of EM is one of exclusion. Biopsy in this case is useful only to rule out other pathologies. The differential diagnostic of recurrent EM affecting the oral cavity should include RAS, Behçet disease, recurrent HSV, lichen planus, cyclic neutropenia, drug reactions, and pemphigus.

Treatment

The most effective treatment for patients with HSV-associated EM is continuous antiviral prophylaxis for more than 6 months. The options include aciclovir 400 mg bid, valaciclovir 500 mg qd, and famciclovir 250 mg qd. If nonresponsive, the dose can be increased or another antiviral may be tried. If the treatment is effective, it should be continued for 1–2 years before it is discontinued. If lesions relapse, the lowest effective dose should be reinstalled and cessation reattempted after 6–12 months [45].

For patients not responding to antiviral therapy, the treatment can be azathioprine, dapsone, mycophenolate mofetil, immunoglobulin, hydroxychloroquine, thalidomide, and ciclosporin [45].

Fixed Drug Eruptions

Fixed drug eruptions (FDE) are recurrent and site-specific lesions of the skin, moccosa, or both that occur each time a specific drug is taken.

Clinical Presentation

The lesions usually appear 30 minutes to 8 hours after drug intake, within a mean length of time of 2 hours. The lesion resolves after the causative drug is stopped, and leaves areas of hyperpigmentation. If reexposed to the drug, local reeruption occurs at the same spot, though it sometimes may involve additional areas [49, 50]. Most often, the skin is involved but oral lesions may occur at the same time. Sometimes, oral mucosa may be the only involved site, or in conjunction with genital or other mucosal areas [51].

Most of the oral cases of FDE are case reports. The most extensive study to date, Özkaya (2013), identified that among 176 patients with FDE, 61 (35%) presented oral mucosal lesions [51]. Among those, 69% had orogenital lesions, 16% had oral and skin lesions, and 15% had only oral lesions. The most commonly involved intraoral sites were the dorsum of the tongue and hard palate. Less often, the inner lip mucosa and ventrolateral tongue were involved. The study reports the lip lesions as a different group, and involved more often than the intraoral lesions, namely in 19% of the FDA cases [52].

An older study by Browne (1964) investigated 145 patients with FDE from dapsone and found that 14% had oral mucosal lesions, with the most common site being the hard palate, followed by the tongue and the gingiva. He also reported that lip lesions were involved more often than intraoral lesions, namely in 42% of the FDE cases [52].

Özkaya identifies the type of intraoral FDE lesions as vesicular (77%), aphthous (20%), and erythematous (3%). He describes that 44% of the patients were initially misdiagnosed with herpes simplex, Behçet disease, pemphigus vulgaris, EM, erosive lichen planus, oral candida, or vitamin deficiency. The drugs responsible for the intraoral lesions included naproxen, trimethroprim-sulfamethoxazole, piroxicam, dipyrone, etodolac, phenobarbital, and ornidazole [51? >].

Etiology

The current understanding is that FDE are mediated by resident CD8+ T cells residing in the epidermis at the specific sites where the lesions would develop. These T cells appear to be effector-memory cells that have migrated from the circulation second to repeated infections in those areas [51]. There, they can become reactivated by drug-stimulated keratinocytes via ICAM-1 (intracellular adhesion molecule-1), and release interferon-γ, causing the inflammatory flare-up at the site [53].

Diagnosis

The gold standard diagnostic procedure is the drug rechallenge test, where the patient is administered the drug starting at 1/10th of the therapeutic dose and observed to see if the lesions recur. A second alternative is topical provocation by patch testing over the previous area of eruption. Topical testing may be preferred in patients at risk of extensive lesions, yet it is less sensitive [54].

Treatment

The treatment of mild lesions is with topical corticosteroids. If there is severe involvement, oral corticosteroids can be administered. One regimen is methylprednisolone 0.5 mg/kg/d for 3–5 days. The causative agent and cross-reacting substances should be avoided. Extensive cases can be difficult to differentiate from EM major, Stevens–Johnson syndrome, and TEN. Successful desensitization with allopurinol has been reported [54, 55].

References

1 Messadi, D.V. and Younai, F. (2010). Aphthous ulcers. *Dermatol. Ther.* 23: 281–290.
2 Edgar, N., Saleh, D., and Miller, R. (2017). Recurrent aphthous stomatitis: a review. *J. Clin. Aesthet. Dermatol.* 10 (3): 26–36.
3 Scully, C. and Porter (2006). Clinical practice. Aphthous ulceration. *N. Engl. J. Med.* 13 (355): 165–172.
4 Altenburg, A., El-Haj, N., Micheli, C. et al. (2014). The treatment of chronic recurrent oral aphthous ulcers. *Dtsch. Arztebl. Int.* 111: 665–673.
5 Ship, I.I. (1972). Epidemiologic aspects of recurrent aphthous ulcerations. *Oral Surg. Oral Med. Oral Pathol.* 33: 400–406.
6 Dan, S., Jinwei, Z., Qiang, Z. et al. (2017). Exploring the molecular mechanism and biomarker of recurrent aphthous stomatitis based on gene expression microarray. *Clin. Lab* 63 (2): 249–253.
7 Fakhry-Smith, S., Din, C., Nathoo, S.A., and Gaffar, A. (1997). Clearance of sodium lauryl sulphate from the oral cavity. *J. Clin. Periodontol.* 24: 313–317.
8 Renton, M.I., Li, M.K., and Parsons, L.M. (2015). Cinnamon spice and everything not nice: many features of intraoral allergy to cinnamic aldehyde. *Dermatitis* 26 (3): 116–121.
9 Riera Matute, G. and Riera Alonso, E. (2011). Recurrent aphthous stomatitis in rheumatology. *Rheumatol. Clin.* 7 (5): 323–328.
10 Baccaglini, L., Lalla, R.V., Bruce, A.J. et al. (2011). Urban legends: recurrent aphthous stomatitis. *Oral Dis.* 17: 755–770.
11 Belenguer-Guallar, I., Jiminez-Soriano, Y., and Claramunt-Lozano, A. (2014). Treatment of recurrent aphthous stomatitis. A literature review. *J. Clin. Exp. Dent.* 6 (2): 168–174.
12 Ship, J. (1996). Recurrent aphthous stomatitis: an update. *Oral Surg. Oral Med. Oral Pathol.* 80 (2): 141–147.
13 Munoz-Corcuera, M., Esparza-Gomez, G., Gonzalez-Moles, M., and Bascones-Martinez, A. (2009). Oral ulcers: clinical aspects. A tool for dermatologists. Part I. Acute ulcers. *Clin. Exp. Dermatol.* 34: 289–294.
14 Gorsky, M., Epstein, J., Raviv, A. et al. (2008). Topical minocycline for managing symptoms of recurrent aphthous stomatitis. *Spec. Care Dent.* 28: 27–31.
15 Altenburg, A. and Zouboulis, C.C. (2008). Current concepts in the treatment of recurrent aphthous stomatitis. *Skin Ther. Lett.* 13: 1–4.
16 Healy, C.M. and Thornhill, M.H. (1995). An association between recurrent oro-genital ulceration and non-steroidal anti-inflammatory drugs. *J. Oral Pathol. Med.* 24: 46–48.
17 Arduino, P.G. and Porter, S.R. (2008). Herpes simplex virus type 1 infection: overview on relevant clinico-pathological features. *J. Oral Pathol. Med.* 37: 107–121.
18 Cunningham, A., Griffiths, P., Leone, P. et al. (2012). Current management and recommendations for access to antiviral therapy of herpes labialis. *J. Clin. Virol.* 53: 6–11.
19 Fatahzadeh, M. and Schwartz, R.A. (2007). Human herpes simplex virus infections: epidemiology, pathogenesis, symptomatology, diagnosis, and management. *J. Am. Acad. Dermatol.* 57: 737–763.
20 Woo, S.-B. and Challacombe, S. (2007). Management of recurrent oral herpes simplex infections. *Oral Surg. Oral Med. Oral Pathol.* 103: 12–18.
21 Vestey, J.P. and Norval, M. (1992). Muccocutaneous infections with herpes simplex and their management. *Clin. Exp. Dermatol.* 17 (4): 221.

22 Rodu, B. and Mattingly, G. (1992). Oral mucosal ulcers: diagnosis and management. *J. Am. Dent. Assoc.* 123 (10): 83.

23 Giannini, P.J. and Shetty, K.V. (2011). Diagnosis and management of oral candidiasis. *Otolaryngol. Clin. North Am.* 44: 231–240.

24 Sheikh, S., Gupta, D., Pallagatti, S. et al. (2013). Role of topical drugs in the treatment of oral mucosal disease. *N. York State Dent. J.* 11: 58–64.

25 Muzyka., B.C. (2013). Update on fungal infections. *Dent. Clin. North Am.* 57: 561–581.

26 Alrashdan, M., Cirillo, N., and McCullough, M. (2016). Oral lichen planus: a literature review and update. *Arch. Dermatol. Res.* 308: 539–551.

27 Ivanovski, K., Nakova, M., Warburton, G. et al. (2005). Psychological profile in oral lichen planus. *J. Clin. Periodontol.* 32: 1034–1040.

28 Stoopler, E. and Sollecito, T. (2014). Recurrent gingival and oral mucosal lesions. *JAMA* 312 (17): 1794–1795.

29 Liu, C., Xie, B., Yang, Y. et al. (2013). Efficacy of intralesional betamethasone for erosive oral lichen planus and evaluation of recurrence: a randomized, controlled trial. *Oral Surg. Oral Med. Oral Pathol. Oral Radiol.* 116: 584–590.

30 Yang, H., Wu, Y., Ma, H. et al. (2016). Possible alternative therapies for oral lichen planus cases refractory to steroid therapies. *Oral Surg. Oral Med. Oral Pathol. Oral Radiol.* 121: 496–509.

31 Scully, C. and Mignogna, M. (2008). Oral mucosal disease: pemphigus. *Br. J. Oral Maxillofac. Surg.* 46: 272–277.

32 Robinson, J.C., Lozada-Nur, F., and Frieden, I. (1997). Oral pemphigus vulgaris: a review of the literature and a report on the management of 12 cases. *Oral Surg. Oral Med. Oral Pathol. Oral Radiol. Endod.* 84 (4): 349–355.

33 Femiano, F., Gombos, F., Nunziata, M. et al. (2005). Pemphigus mimicking aphthous stomatitis. *J. Oral Pathol. Med.* 34: 508–510.

34 Darling, M. and Daley, T. (2006). Blistering mucocutaneous diseases of the oral mucosa – a review: part 2. Pemphigus vulgaris. *J. Can. Dent. Assoc.* 72 (1): 63–66.

35 Oliver, R.J., Sloan, P., and Pemberton, M.N. (2004). Oral biopsies: methods and applications. *Br. Dent. J.* 196: 329–333.

36 Ata-Ali, F. and Ata-Ali, J. (2011). Pemphigus vulgaris and mucous membrane pemphigoid: update on etiopathogenesis, oral manifestations and management. *J. Clin. Exp. Dent.* 3 (3): 246–250.

37 Knudson, R.M., A, N., and Kalaaji, Bruce A. (2010). The management of mucous membrane pemphigoid and pemphigus. *Dermatol. Ther.* 23: 268–280.

38 Scully, C. and Challacombe, S.J. (2002). Pemphigus vulgaris: update on etiopathogenesis, oral manifestations, and management. *Crit. Rev. Oral Biol. Med.* 13 (5): 397–408.

39 Bastuji-Garin, S., Rzany, B., Stern, R. et al. (1993). Clinical classification of cases of toxic epidermal necrolysis, Stevens–Johnson syndrome, and erythema multiforme. *Arch. Dermatol.* 129 (1): 92–96.

40 Auquier-Dunant, A., Mockenhaupt, M., Naldi, L. et al. (2002). Correlations between clinical patterns and causes of erythema multiforme majus, Stevens–Johnson syndrome, and toxic epidermal necrolysis. *Arch. Dermatol.* 138 (8): 1019–1024.

41 Jawetz, R., Elkin, A., Michael, L. et al. (2007). Erythema multiforme limited to the oral mucosa in a teenager on oral contraceptive therapy. *J. Pediatr. Adolesc. Gynecol.* 20 (5): 309–313.

42 Chan, H.L., Stern, R.S., Arndt, K.A. et al. (1990). The incidence of erythema multiforme, Stevens–Johnson syndrome, and toxic epidermal necrolysis. A population-based study with particular reference to reactions caused by drugs among outpatients. *Arch. Dermatol. Res.* 126: 43–47.

43 Scully, C. and Bagan, J. (2008). Oral mucosal diseases: erythema multiforme. *Br. J.Oral Maxillofac. Surg.* 46 (2): 90–95.

44 Sokumbi, O. and Wetter, D. (2012). Clinical features, diagnosis, and treatment of erythema multiforme: a review for the practicing dermatologist. *Int. J. Dermatol.* 51: 889–902.

45 Ayangco, L. and Rogers, R.S. (2003). Oral manifestations of erythema multiforme. *Dermatol. Clin.* 21: 195–205.

46 Schofield, J.K., Tatnall, F.M., and Leigh, I.M. (1993). Recurrent erythema multiforme: clinical features and treatment in a large series of patients. *Br. J. Dermatol.* 128 (5): 542–545.

47 Farthing, P.M., Maragou, P., Coates, M. et al. (1995). Characteristics of the oral lesions in patients with cutaneous recurrent erythema multiforme. *J. Oral Pathol. Med.* 24 (1): 9–13.

48 Celentano, A., Tovaru, S., Yap, T. et al. (2015). Oral erythema multiforme: trends and clinical findings of a large retrospective European case series. *Oral Surg. Oral Med. Oral Pathol. Oral Radiol.* 120 (6): 707–716.

49 Korkij, W. and Soltani, K. (1984). Fixed drug eruption. A brief review. *Arch. Dermatol.* 120 (4): 520–524.

50 Shiohara, T. (2009). Fixed drug eruption: pathogenesis and diagnostic tests. *Curr. Opin. Allergy Clin. Immunol.* 9: 316–321.

51 Özkaya, E. (2013). Oral mucosal fixed drug eruption: characteristics and differential diagnosis. *J. Am. Acad. Dermatol.* 69 (2): e51–e58.

52 Browne, S.G. (1964). Fixed eruption in deeply pigmented subjects: clinical observations on 350 patients. *Br. Med. J.* 2 (5416): 1041–1044.

53 Özkaya, E. (2008). Fixed drug eruption: state of the art. *J. Dtsch. Dermatol. Ges.* 6 (3): 181–188.

54 Andrade, P., Brinca, A., and Goncalo, M. (2011). Patch testing in fixed drug eruptions a 20-year review. *Contact Derm.* 65: 195–201.

55 Teraki, Y. and Shiohara, T. (2004). Successful desensitization to fixed drug eruption: the presence of CD25+CD4+ T cells in the epidermis of fixed drug eruption lesions may be involved in the induction of desensitization. *Dermatology* 209: 29–32.

12

Benign Pediatric Pathology: Diagnosis and Management

Dina Amin and Shelly Abramowicz

Introduction

Pediatric head and neck tumors are rare. Nevertheless, it is essential for healthcare providers to be familiar with their clinical presentation, behavior, and management. Pediatric head and neck tumors can be categorized into: (i) odontogenic cysts and tumors, (ii) nonodontogenic cysts and tumors, (iii) soft tissue lesions, and (iv) salivary gland lesions. This chapter will discuss presentation and management of some of the more common benign head and neck cysts and tumors.

Odontogenic Cysts

A cyst is an epithelium-lined cavity that is filled with fluid. Cysts are broadly classified according to their cell of origin: odontogenic and nonodontogenic. They are further subclassified into inflammatory and developmental categories. Inflammatory odontogenic cysts result from local inflammation. Developmental odontogenic cysts have an unknown etiology but known cells of origin [1].

Periapical Cyst

A periapical cyst results from an infection causing accumulation of purulent material at the apex of a tooth. The source of infection is decay or injured pulp. The associated tooth can be tender to percussion and palpation, and there may be gingival swelling and/or fistula. If the inflammation is contained within the associated bone, a periapical abscess or cyst may form.

Radiographically, a periapical cyst and abscess have the same appearance. It is a well-defined, round, unilocular radiolucency at the tooth apex (Figure 12.1). Treatment depends on the restorability of the tooth: if restorable, endodontic treatment and cyst enucleation or, if not restorable, extraction of involved tooth and enucleation of associated cyst. Recurrence is rare [1, 2].

Buccal Bifurcation Cyst

Buccal bifurcation cyst (BBC) develops along the buccal surface of the roots of the mandibular first or second molars. The typical age of onset is 6–12 years when these teeth erupt into the oral cavity. The true cause behind the inflammatory response leading to cyst formation is unclear. The proposed etiology is extension of enamel onto the roots which results in loss of periodontal attachment along the buccal root surface and extending to the root bifurcation.

Clinically, BBC presents with a vital tooth, buccal soft tissue swelling, delayed eruption or altered eruption of the involved tooth, and an increase in periodontal pocket depth in the affected area. Radiographically, this cyst presents as a well-defined, unilocular radiolucency at the furcation or buccal aspect of the involved tooth that tilts the involved molar with the root apices pointing toward the mandibular lingual cortex. In some cases, a periosteal reaction on the buccal surface of the mandible can be seen. Treatment is enucleation of the cyst with periodontal scaling and root planing; tooth extraction is not recommended [3, 4].

Dentigerous Cyst

A dentigerous cyst is the second most common odontogenic cyst with an incidence of 1.44 per 100 impacted teeth. It develops from the proliferation of a remnant of the enamel organ. This cyst has a wide age range from 10 years to 30 years with a slight male predilection [4]. Mandibular

Oral and Maxillofacial Surgery, Medicine, and Pathology for the Clinician, First Edition. Edited by Harry Dym, Leslie R. Halpern, and Orrett E. Ogle.

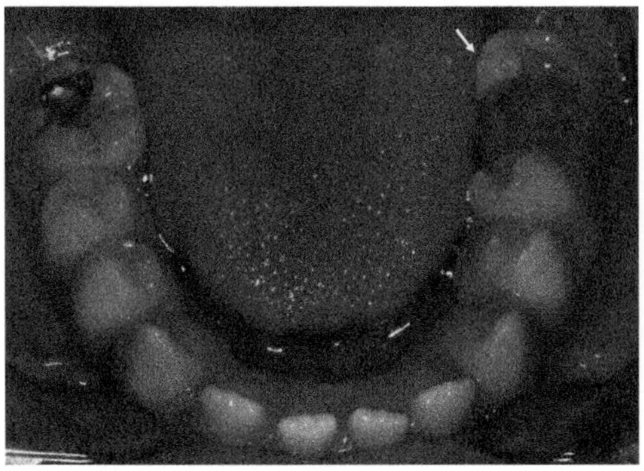

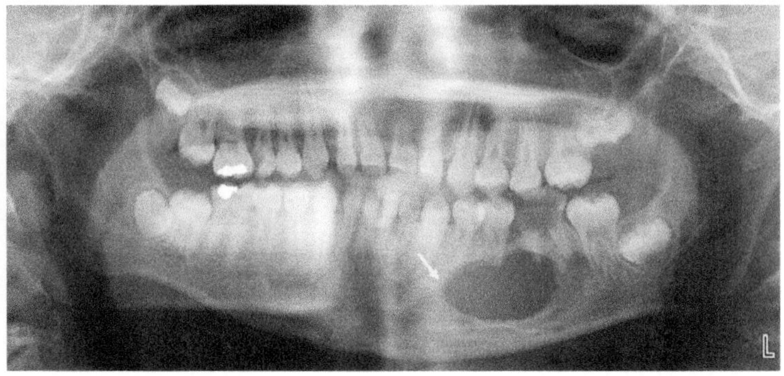

(a) (b)

Figure 12.1 Periapical cyst. Panoramic radiograph demonstrating a 3.5 cm unilocular radiolucent lesion in the left side of the mandibular body causing root resorption of mandibular first molar and second premolar.

third molars, maxillary third molars, maxillary canine, and mandibular second premolar are the most common locations.

Dentigerous cyst can be asymptomatic and incidentally discovered or, when it is large, it can cause a significant expansion of the buccal cortex. Radiographically, this cyst appears as a well-defined, unilocular radiolucency that is associated with the crown of an unerupted tooth and is attached to the cementoenamel junction [1, 4].

There are two treatment options: (i) marsupialization or (ii) enucleation and curettage with extraction of the impacted tooth. Marsupialization is indicated to allow decompression of a large lesion and allow tooth eruption, or when enucleation and curettage may result in a pathologic fracture or neurosensory nerve dysfunction. Recurrence is rare [5].

Eruption Cyst

Eruption cyst is the soft tissue variant of the dentigerous cyst. Eruption cyst forms during tooth eruption through the soft tissue, specifically when the dental follicle separates from the crown. The exact cause is unknown, but trauma and infection are risk factors. Eruption cyst is most commonly found in children aged 6–9 years. Central incisors and the permanent first molar are the most common locations. Clinically, eruption cyst is associated with an unerupted tooth and presents as a bluish purple fluctuant lesion over the alveolar mucosa. No treatment is indicated unless the cyst causes a delay in tooth eruption or infection; in these scenarios, unroofing of the tooth is the only necessary treatment [4, 6].

Odontogenic Keratocyst

In 2005, the World Health Organization (WHO) reclassified odontogenic keratocyst (OKC) from a cyst to keratocystic odontogenic tumor (KCOT). This decision was based on its aggressive growth, specific histologic features suggestive of neoplastic tendencies, high recurrence rate, the evidence of a "solid" variant, and the association with the PATCH tumor suppressor gene [7, 8]. However, in 2017, the WHO moved odontogenic keratocystic tumor back to the cyst category, citing insufficient evidence to justify reclassification as a neoplasm [8].

OKC has two variants: sporadic and syndromic. In both situations, the cyst is derived from remnants of the dental lamina. Although it has a wide range of age occurrence, 60% are found in patients aged 10–40 years. OKC has a slight male predilection. Approximately 60–80% of cases involve the posterior mandible and ramus. Clinically, OKC presents with normal mucosa and slight buccal and lingual plate expansion. Radiographically, OKC is a well-defined, unilocular or multilocular radiolucency that is usually associated with an impacted tooth [9].

Histologic presentation consists of a uniform layer of stratified squamous epithelium that is 6–8 cells in thickness and has a corrugated parakeratinized surface with a thin friable wall. Daughter cysts and epithelial budding may be present. The latter two features indicate an aggressive behavior and high recurrence rate. The presence of daughter cysts is more commonly noted in syndromic cases. Syndromic OKC is associated with nevoid basal cell carcinoma syndrome, also known as Gorlin syndrome, and basal cell nevus syndrome. This is an autosomal dominant syndrome caused by the mutation of the PATCH tumor suppressor gene mapped on chromosome 9q22.3-q31. The syndrome is characterized by the tendency to develop multiple basal cell carcinomas that may affect both sun-exposed and nonsun-exposed areas of the skin, multiple OKCs, palmar plantar pits, frontal bossing, hypertelorism, mandibular prognathism and calcified falx cerebri, among other clinical features. An OKC could be the first sign of the syndrome. Therefore, any patients with multiple OKCs should be assessed for this condition. Syndromic OKC is characterized by a high recurrence rate or the presence of new cystic lesions. Sporadic and syndromic cysts cannot be distinguished histologically [9, 10].

Many surgeons believe that OKC's histologic features play a significant role in recurrence. Therefore, many treatment strategies have been proposed for OKC with the ultimate goal of decreasing recurrence: enucleation and curettage [11], enucleation and curettage with peripheral ostectomy [1, 12], enucleation and curettage with cryotherapy [13], enucleation and curettage with Carnoy's solution [14], excision of the overlying mucosa with cyst enucleation and bone cavity treatment with Carnoy's solution [15], marsupialization [16], decompression and marsupialization followed by enucleation of the remaining cyst [17], and marginal resection [18]. In some studies, marsupialization has been shown to result in complete resolution with no histologic or radiographic signs of cystic remnants [16].

The recurrence rate varies according to the treatment and ranges from no recurrence to 50%, depending on the study [18]. A high recurrence rate is associated with nevoid basal cell carcinoma syndrome [10].

There are multiple suggested mechanisms for recurrence. There may be a remnant of the dental lamina within the jaw not associated with the first KCOT. The original OKC may not have been completely removed secondary to a thin friable lining and cortical perforation with adherence to the adjacent soft tissue. Rests of the dental lamina and satellite cysts may remain after enucleation [1].

Odontogenic Tumors

Odontoma

Odontoma is considered a hamartomatous developmental malformation of dental tissues and is the most frequent type of odontogenic tumor in the pediatric population. It arises from the odontogenic epithelium and mesenchyme that produce enamel and dentine. These tumors are subdivided into compound and complex odontoma [1]. Clinically, they are asymptomatic and discovered incidentally during routine radiographic examination. Odontoma may cause delayed teeth eruption [19]. Radiographic presentation is a dense radiopaque tooth-like structure surrounded by a radiolucent rim associated with an unerupted tooth (compound odontoma) or a dense radiopaque irregular amorphous structure (complex odontoma) [20] (Figure 12.2). Treatment consists of enucleation and curettage. Recurrence is rare [21] (Table 12.1).

Ameloblastoma

Ameloblastoma is the second most common benign odontogenic tumor after odontoma [1] and accounts for 1% of all tumors of the jaws. It is locally aggressive with a propensity to recur. It arises from the odontogenic epithelium. In 2005, the WHO classified ameloblastoma into solid/multicystic, extraosseous/peripheral, desmoplastic, and unicystic types [8]. In the 2017 update, ameloblastoma classification was narrowed to ameloblastoma, unicystic ameloblastoma, and extraosseous/peripheral types. The adjective "solid/multicystic" for the conventional ameloblastoma was dropped because it has no biologic significance and leads to confusion [8]. In general, in adults, histologic features dictate treatment for an ameloblastoma which consists of resection with 1–1.5 cm margin and one barrier in soft tissue [22, 23]. Further discussion of ameloblastoma in adults is beyond the scope of this chapter and can be found elsewhere in this book.

Unicystic ameloblastoma (UA) was recognized as a distinct subtype based on distinct clinical, radiographic, and

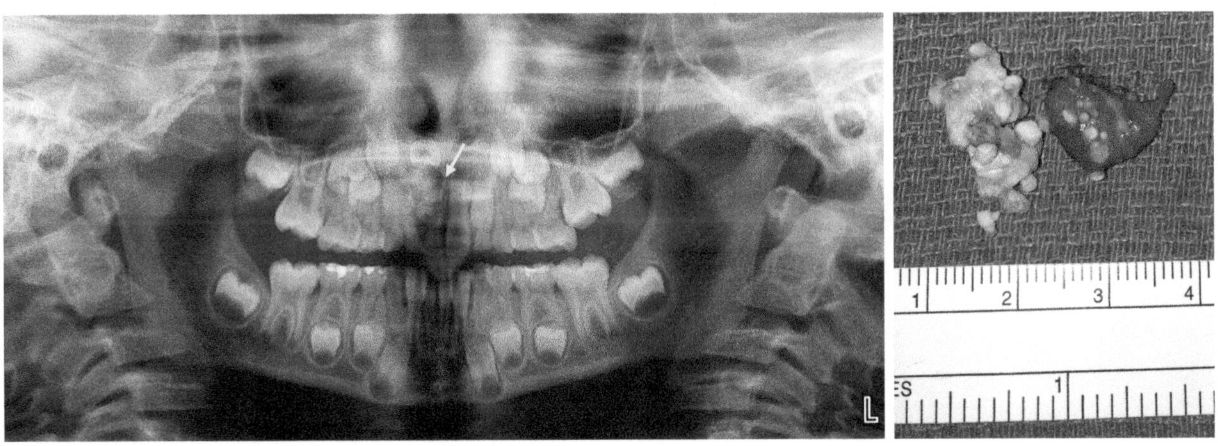

(a) (b)

Figure 12.2 Compound odontoma. (a) Seven-year-old boy with a lesion on the right maxilla adjacent to maxillary primary lateral and central incisors. (b) Intraoperative view demonstrating multiple small tooth-like structures.

Table 12.1 Odontoma.

	Compound odontoma	Complex odontoma
Location	Anterior maxilla	Posterior maxilla
Clinical features	Radiopaque, multiple small tooth-like structures	Radiopaque, irregular mass that does not resemble tooth morphology
Radiographic appearance	Multiple small tooth-like structures	Confused with other calcified lesions such as osteoma
Treatment	Enucleation and curettage	Enucleation and curettage

Source: Based on [1, 21].

histopathologic features [8, 23]. UA accounts for 10–46% of all intraosseous ameloblastomas and occurs most commonly in a younger population [24]. UA is typically found in the posterior mandible.

Clinically, ameloblastoma causes asymptomatic expansion. Radiographically, it is a well-defined unilocular radiolucency associated with the crown of an impacted tooth. Its radiographic features resemble a dentigerous cyst. An ameloblastoma may displace or resorb adjacent roots and has the capacity to expand and perforate the jaw [10] (Figure 12.3). Histologically, it is divided into three subtypes according to the pattern of proliferation of the ameloblastomatous epithelium: luminal, intraluminal, and mural [25, 26].

Treatment of UA is dictated by histologic subtype. Luminal and intraluminal UA are treated via enucleation and curettage with peripheral ostectomy [8, 26]. Treatment of mural UA involves resection with 1–1.5 cm in bone and one barrier in soft tissue [25]. The recurrence rate of UA is correlated with the histologic subtype and the applied treatment. Mural UA has high recurrence rates following simple enucleation (60–80%). However, surgical resection with a 1–1.5 cm bony margin and a margin of one plane in soft tissue is associated with a recurrence rate close to zero [22, 24]. The reported recurrence rate after treatment for luminal and intraluminal UA ranges from 10% to 25% [27]; a higher recurrence rate is observed with enucleation (30.5%) [27, 28]. However, a lower rate is observed with enucleation and peripheral ostectomy (16%) [27] as well as with resection (0%) [28].

Ameloblastic Fibroma

Ameloblastic fibroma (AF) is a true mixed odontogenic tumor in which the odontogenic epithelium and mesenchymal origins are neoplastic. AF represents 2% of odontogenic tumors [20]. The age range is 6–12 years [29]. Approximately 80% occur in the posterior mandible. Its clinical presentation is a slow-growing, asymptomatic expansile lesion. AF is frequently discovered during routine dental radiographs. Radiographically, AF presents with a well-defined unilocular or multilocular radiolucency associated with an unerupted tooth that may displace adjacent teeth [29]. Treatment depends on the size of the lesion [30]. AF smaller than 3 cm is treated with enucleation and curettage [30]. Larger and destructive AF are treated with *en bloc* resection [30]. The AF recurrence rate ranges from 18.3% to 43.5% and it is associated with malignant transformation [31].

Ameloblastic fibrosarcoma is the malignant counterpart of AF [32]. An ameloblastic fibrosarcoma can arise from a recurrent AF or *de novo* [32, 33]. It is composed of benign epithelium and malignant mesenchymal components. Clinical signs are rapid increase in size, indistinct radiographic borders, pain, or paresthesia [32]. Treatment is resection with 1.5–2 cm. Because it is a low-grade sarcoma, chemotherapy and radiation therapy are not required [30].

Non-dontogenic Cysts

Idiopathic Bone Cavity

Idiopathic bone cavity (IBC) is an empty bone cavity. The etiology is unknown, but the most accepted theory is bony trauma that leads to formation of an intraosseous hematoma. Local clots break down and cause an osteolytic bone reaction which resembles a lesion on panoramic radiograph. Other etiologic theories include cystic degeneration of a primary tumor of bone, such as a giant cell lesion (GCL), ischemic necrosis of bone/fatty marrow, and possibly a defect in calcium metabolism [34]. IBC has a wide age range but most commonly occurs in young adults aged 10–20 years with no gender predilection [35]. IBC occurs exclusively in the mandible and favors the anterior region. Clinically, IBC presents with asymptomatic expansion that is associated with vital teeth. It is discovered with routine dental X-ray. The radiographic appearance is a well-defined radiolucency with sclerotic and distinguished scalloped borders. Treatment is exploratory surgery to confirm the diagnosis and curettage. There is no recurrence [34].

Aneurysmal Bone Cyst

Aneurysmal bone cyst (ABC) is an uncommon lesion of the jaws with an unknown etiology. Like IBC, ABC does not have an epithelial lining but is filled with blood. The WHO describes ABC as an expansile, multilocular,

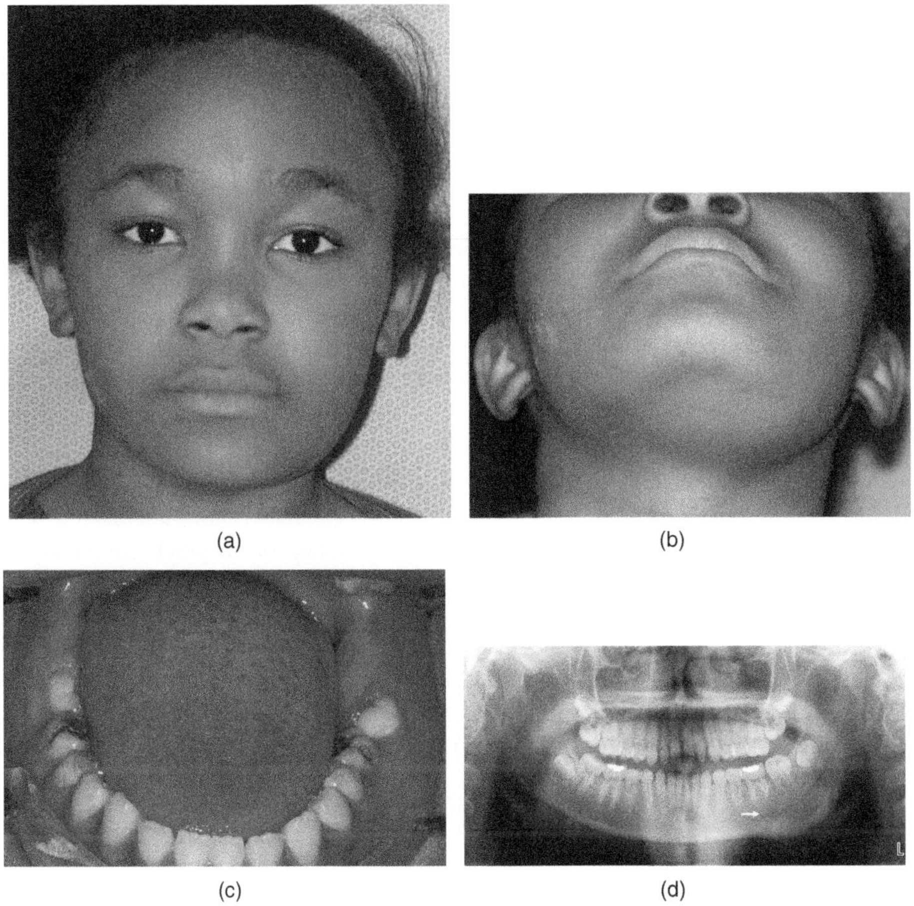

(a) (b) (c) (d)

Figure 12.3 Unicystic ameloblastoma. (a) Frontal photograph of a 13-year-old girl with swelling of left mandible. (b) Submental photograph showing mandibular asymmetry. (c) Intraoral picture showing partially erupted mandibular left second molar with slight buccal expansion. (d) Panoramic radiograph demonstrating a 4 cm unilocular radiolucent lesion in the left side of the mandibular body causing expansion of the inferior border of the mandible and root resorption of mandibular first molar.

osteolytic lesion with blood-filled spaces separated by fibrous septa-containing osteoclast-type giant cells and reactive bone [36]. Multiple theories have been proposed, ranging from vascular malformation, reactive factors and genetic predisposition [35, 37]. ABC can occur at any age but is more common in patients younger than 30 [35]. ABC has no gender predilection.

Clinically, it presents as painless swelling without thrill or bruit on auscultation. There may be displacement, loosening, and/or resorption of adjacent teeth. Radiographically, this is a well-defined unilocular or multilocular radiolucency with occasional root resorption and/or cortical plate perforation. When present as a multilocular lesion, it is often described as having a "soap bubble" appearance. Treatment is enucleation and curettage. However, due to the high recurrence rate, *en bloc* resection is sometimes advocated [35, 38]. Other treatments that have been suggested as adjuncts to surgery include cryotherapy, steroids, calcitonin, and embolization [35].

Nonodontogenic Tumors

Congenital Epulis

Congenital epulis is also known as gingival cyst of the newborn or granular cell tumor. Congenital epulis is a benign tumor of mesenchymal origin that occurs almost exclusively in the anterior maxillary alveolar ridge of newborns [12]. Although it has an unclear etiology, endocrine [39] and reactive theories have been suggested [40]. Congenital epulis has a striking female predilection with a 10:1 female-to-male ratio. Clinically, it is a sessile, firm, nonpainful tumor that is similar in color and consistency to normal mucosa. Congenital epulis may lead to mechanical obstruction resulting in respiratory distress and difficulty in feeding. Treatment is surgical excision, and recurrence is rare even with incomplete excision [12, 41].

Melanotic Neuroectodermal Tumor of Infancy

Melanotic neuroectodermal tumor of infancy is a benign tumor that is neural crest in origin; 82% occur in infants younger than 6 months. This tumor occurs in the maxilla (68–80%) more frequently than the mandible (5.8%) [42]. Clinically, it appears as a rapidly growing, nonulcerated, sessile mass with a blue color. Diagnostic work-up should include urine test to look for high levels of vanillylmandelic acid. Radiographically, it is an ill-defined radiolucency with tooth buds floating in space. Treatment is wide local excision with 5 mm margins. Recurrence is 10–20% with wide local excision [1, 12, 42].

Juvenile Ossifying Fibroma

In contrast to other fibroosseous lesions, juvenile ossifying fibroma (JOF) represents a true neoplasm [43]. It is distinguished from other fibroosseous lesions primarily by its age of onset, clinical and radiographic presentation, and high recurrence tendency [44]. JOF has two clinical variants based on its histopathologic features: trabecular (TJOF) and psammomatoid (PsJOF) [45, 46]. The site of involvement aids in differentiating between the trabecular subtype and the psammomatoid subtype, with PsJOF primarily occurring in the paranasal sinuses and TJOF with a gnathic predilection that primarily occurs in the maxilla [45]. Psammomatoid ossifying fibroma (PsOF) occurs most commonly between 16 and 33 years of age. In contrast, trabecular ossifying fibroma occurs at a younger age between 8 and 12 years old. Both variants have the same clinical appearance.

Clinically, JOF may exhibit slow or rapid and aggressive growth patterns. Small lesions are discovered incidentally during routine X-ray. In contrast, large lesions show painless swelling and facial asymmetry, nasal obstruction, sinusitis, headaches, proptosis, diplopia, and blindness. Radiographically, PsJOF is a ground-glass radiopaque lesion with a well-defined, discrete border and associated bony expansion demonstrating a spherical configuration. In contrast, TJOF presents with a well-defined border that is primarily radiolucent with irregular and scattered calcifications and is distinct from the normal surrounding bone; associated bony expansion is similar to PsJOF with a spherical configuration [47].

There are two treatment options for JOF. Small lesions should be enucleated with peripheral ostectomy to level of normal bone and with preservation of adjacent vital structures to the extent possible. Resection with 5 mm margins should be considered when it shows aggressive behavior such as invading adjacent bony cavities, or where preservation of the inferior border is not possible [44, 48, 49]. The recurrence rate is 38% after enucleation and curettage [46, 50].

Fibrous Dysplasia

Fibrous dysplasia (FD) is caused by sporadic mutation in the GNAS gene during early embryogenesis. Instead of normal bone deposition, there is deposition of immature woven bone within a stroma of abnormal fibrous connective tissue forms. FD is classified as a dysplastic process because of its self-limited growth and apparent responsiveness to the hormonal changes of puberty [10].

Fibrous dysplasia has three types depending on when the GNAS mutation occurs: monostotic, polyostotic, and syndromic. The monostotic type occurs in 70% of cases and is limited to one bone. Polyostotic FD is caused by mutation during postnatal life and affects several bones. In approximately 3% of patients, polyostotic FD occurs as a part of a syndrome: McCune–Albright syndrome (cafe-au-lait spots and endocrine abnormalities) or Jaffe–Lichtenstein syndrome (skin pigmentation). Other clinical manifestations include mandibular buccal expansion, bowing of the inferior border, superior displacement of the inferior alveolar canal, displacement of the sinus floor, and obliteration of the maxillary sinuses. Radiographically, FD exhibits an ill-defined margin that blends into surrounding bone and appears as a diffuse radiopaque lesion with a characteristic "ground-glass" appearance, narrowing of the periodontal ligament space and ill-defined lamina dura that blends with abnormal bone [43, 51].

Fibrous dysplasia frequently stabilizes during or shortly after puberty; therefore, surgical intervention should be deferred until the disease is quiescent. Surgical contouring or debulking procedures may be performed when there is facial deformity or obliteration of vital structures. Regrowth of surgically recontoured FD is observed in approximately 25% of cases. Radiation therapy is contraindicated because of the risk for postirradiation osteosarcoma [1] (Figure 12.4).

Giant Cell Lesion

Gian cell lesion is a benign proliferative vascular lesion dependent on angiogenesis [52]. The lesion occurs at all ages but is predominantly observed in children and young adults [43]. The mandible is affected more than the maxilla. GCL is classified and treated based on the related biological behavior [52–54] (Table 12.2). Clinically, the symptoms of GCL range from incidental discovery during a routine X-ray to discomfort and/or pain and paresthesia [43]. Radiographically, GCL presents as a multilocular, mixed radiolucent/radiopaque lesion. Occasionally, there is loss of lamina dura, cortical bone thinning or perforation, root resorption, and displacement of teeth [43, 55]. If multifocal or bilateral tumors are present, hyperparathyroidism, cherubism, and Noonan syndrome should be ruled out [55].

Treatment of GCL is dictated by the type; nonaggressive GCL of the jaws predictably responds to enucleation/curettage [53, 56]. The use of adjuvant or alternative

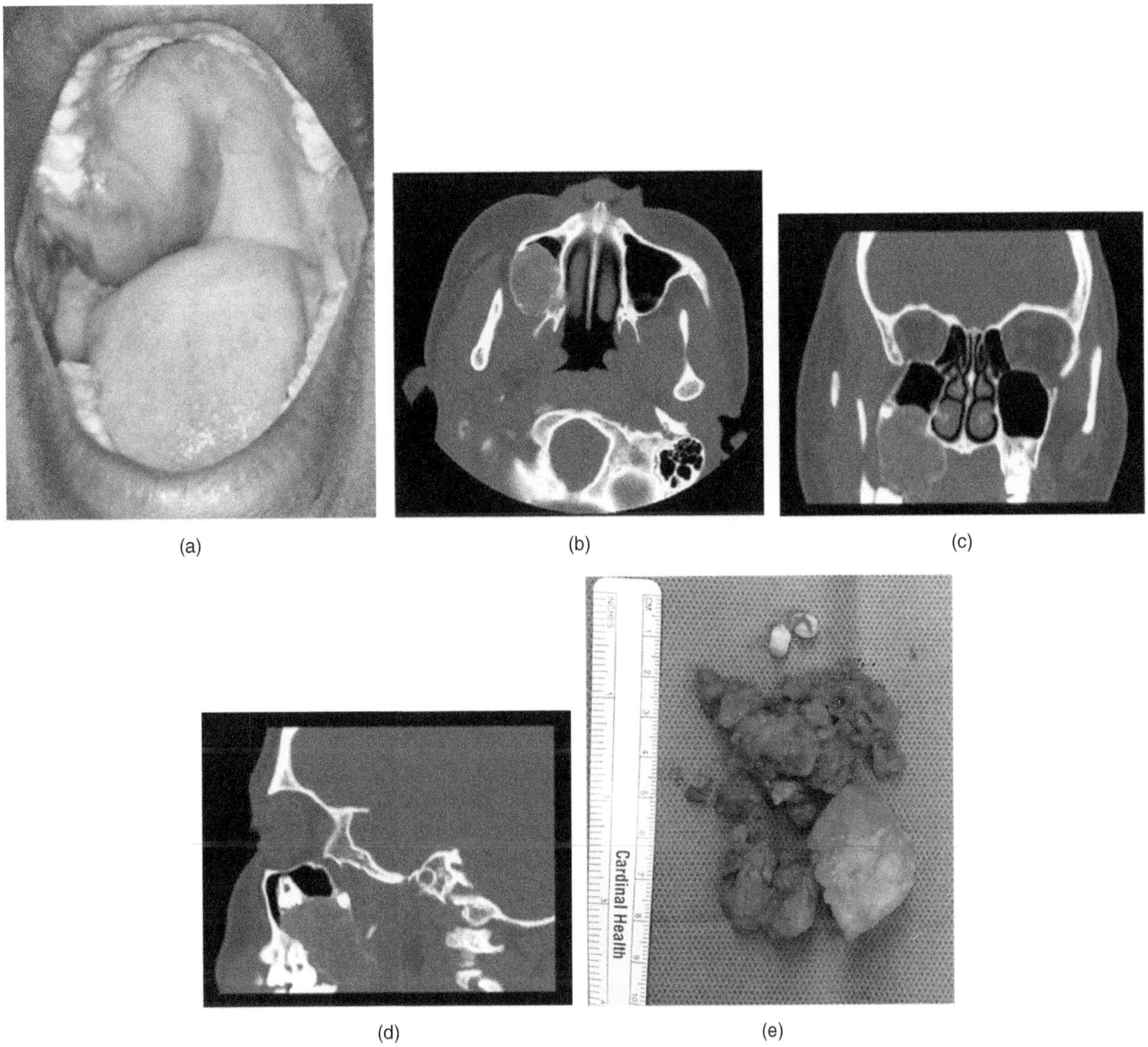

Figure 12.4 Fibrous dysplasia. (a) A 16-year-old female with a slow-growing lesion of the right maxilla. This caused nasal obstruction and difficulty swallowing. (b) Axial CT image demonstrates increased density of the right maxilla and obliteration of the maxillary sinus. (c) Coronal CT image demonstrates diffuse radiopaque lesion with a characteristic "ground-glass appearance." (d) Resected specimen

therapies such as intralesional steroids [52, 57] and systemic [58, 59] or nasal [60, 61] calcitonin is unnecessary because patients with nonaggressive lesions can be predictably cured with curettage/enucleation alone [55]. Aggressive GCLs can be treated with tumor debulking and postoperative antiangiogenic agents such as interferon (IFN)-alpha or bisphosphonates. IFN appears to inhibit osteoclasts and stimulate osteoblasts [62, 63]. Bisphosphonates inhibit the formation, activation, and survival of osteoclasts [64]. Aggressive GCLs treated by enucleation alone have a recurrence rate approaching 70% [52].

Cherubism

Cherubism is an autosomal dominant disease caused by a mutation in the SH3BP2 gene on chromosome 4p16 [65]. The disease has variable penetrance, with 100% in males and 50–70% in females [66]. Sporadic cases have been reported [67]. Clinically, there are symmetric bilateral intraosseous lesions in mandibular angles, ascending rami

Table 12.2 Classification of giant cell lesions.

	Nonaggressive	Aggressive
Clinical behavior	Asymptomatic Incidental discovery Does not meet criteria for an aggressive tumor	Size greater than 5 cm Rapid growth Recurrence after treatment
Radiographic appearance	1 No cortical thinning/perforation 2 No tooth displacement 3 No root resorption	Cortical bone thinning/perforation Tooth displacement Root resorption

Lesions with at least three characteristics are considered aggressive. *Source:* [54]/with permission of Elsevier.

and coronoids, but condyles are spared. Maxillary involvement shows thickening of the alveolar ridge and a V-shaped palate. Maxillary with orbital involvement gives cherubism its name: the lateral and inferior orbital walls may tilt the eyeballs upward and retract the lower lid, thereby exposing the sclera "eyes toward heaven" with cheek fullness to give the patient a cherubic appearance [1, 65]. Teeth displacement, mobility, and/or failure of eruption are frequently observed. Radiographically, there is bilateral multilocular radiolucencies. Extensive involvement may cause an unaesthetic appearance and functional impairment (i.e., speech or visual disturbances) [1, 68].

When a child reaches puberty, cherubism stabilizes and slowly regresses. If possible, surgical recontouring should be deferred until then (Table 12.3).

Soft Tissue Lesions

Fibroma

Fibroma is the most common soft tissue lesion in the oral cavity. It is reactive in nature and is caused by repeated local trauma. It most commonly presents in the cheek at the level of the occlusal plane. Clinically, the fibroma is an asymptomatic, well-circumscribed lesion with a color similar to the oral mucosa. It is sessile or pedunculated. Treatment consists of surgical excision and removal of the traumatic stimulus. Recurrence is rare [2, 12].

Pyogenic Granuloma

Pyogenic granuloma is a common lesion in the pediatric population. The name is a misnomer because it does not exhibit granulomatous features [12]. Pyogenic granuloma is a hyperplastic tissue response to local irritation or trauma in which the microorganisms enter the abraded surface and stimulate the proliferation of connective tissue. It bleeds easily and can resemble a malignant lesion (such as leukemia). The most common locations are the lips, interdental papilla or buccal mucosa along the occlusal level. Clinically, pyogenic granuloma presents as an asymptomatic slow-growing mass that is red to purple in color, depending on how long the lesion has been present, with a smooth surface or lobulated appearance. Pyogenic granuloma is extremely friable and bleeds easily [12]. Treatment is surgical excision [2] (Figure 12.5).

Branchial Cleft Cyst

Branchial cleft cyst is a developmental cyst. It comprises 20% of pediatric congenital head and neck lesions [2]. Although it is present at birth, it is typically only discovered during adolescence after an upper respiratory infection. The most common type is the second branchial cleft cyst, which is found anterior to the sternocleidomastoid muscle. If the cyst arises from the first branchial arch, it may be found in the preauricular area or along the mandible. Clinically, it is soft, mobile, and nontender and may be associated with a small skin pit that drains. Treatment is surgical excision [69].

Hemangioma

Hemangioma is a benign tumor of infancy. One-third of hemangiomas are found in the head and neck, and 14% are found within the oral cavity [2, 70]. Hemangioma has a female predilection with an increase in frequency in whites

Table 12.3 Cherubism classification.

Grade	Location
Grade I	Involves bilateral mandibular ascending rami
Grade II	Involves bilateral maxillary tuberosities and mandibular ascending rami
Grade III	Involves maxilla and mandible and may include coronoids and condyles

Source: Based on [68].

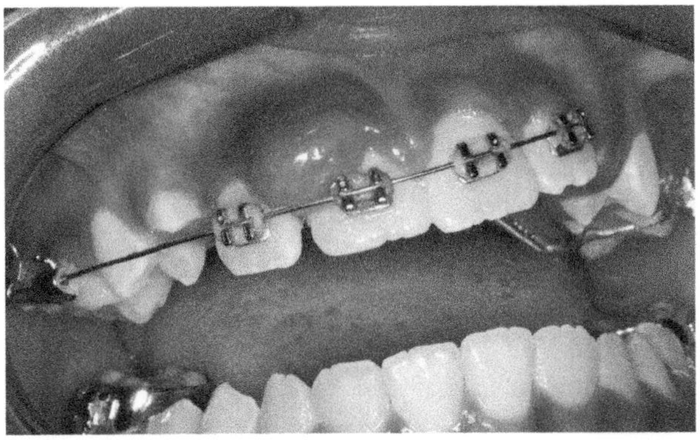

Figure 12.5 Pyogenic granuloma. Intraoral view of 2.5 × 1 cm, erythematous, smooth surface lesion in the interdental papilla between maxillary right lateral and central incisors. It was diagnosed as a pyogenic granuloma. Note that the orthodontic appliance may have contributed to local irritation in the area.

and premature infants. Clinically, it is firm to palpation and does not blanch with pressure (Figure 12.6). Hemangioma occurs in single (80%) or multiple lesions (20%) and exhibits a characteristic life cycle [70] (Table 12.4).

Treatment is not indicated unless the tumor causes destruction, distortion, or obstruction (e.g., subglottic narrowing or blockage of visual axis) [71]. Intralesional corticosteroid injection is recommended for small, well-localized hemangiomas that are less than 2 cm in diameter. This injection has antiangiogenic properties that accelerate involution [72]. Daily oral prednisolone is recommended for hemangiomas that are large, rapidly growing, and causing distortion of facial features, ulceration, and/or impinging on anatomic structures [70]. Propranolol (oral or intravenous) has also been successfully used by some centers to reduce volume, color, and elevation [73].

If the patient fails intralesional steroids and propranolol and if there are contraindications to prolonged corticosteroid treatment, the next line of therapy is vincristine (IFN-alpha) [74]. Resection is considered if there is obstruction of a vital structure, recurrent bleeding, and/or ulceration [70]. After involution, there may be residual fibrofatty tissue or redundant or damaged skin. If there are esthetic concerns, residual fibrofatty tissues can be excised after the lesion involutes [75].

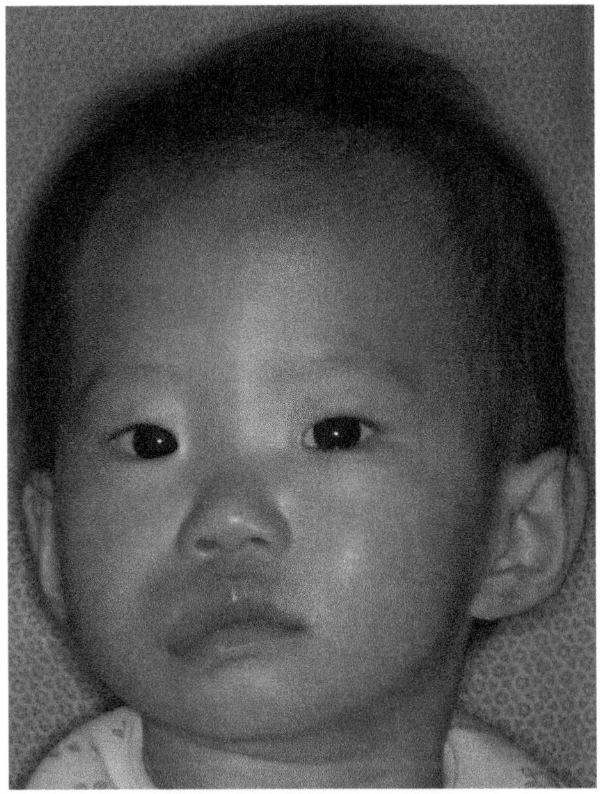

(a)

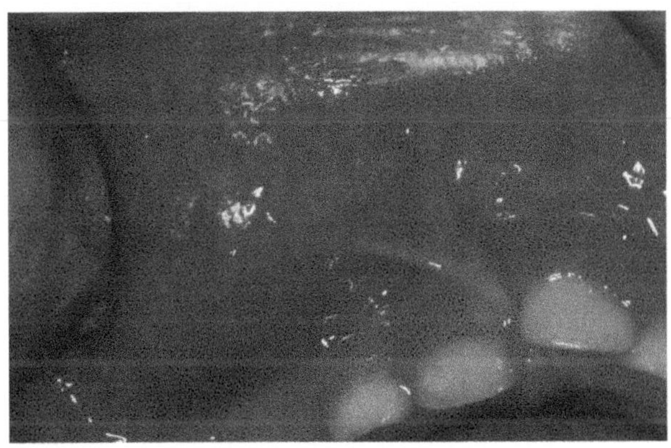

(b)

Figure 12.6 Hemangioma. (a) Frontal photograph of an 8-month-old boy with hemangioma of the upper lip causing downward displacement of the right lip commissure. (b) Intraoral view of above.

Vascular Malformation

Vascular malformation is a structural anomaly of blood vessels. Although it may be present at birth, this malformation does not become clinically obvious until late in infancy or childhood [2]. Vascular malformation (VM) is categorized according to the type of vessel involved: low-flow vascular malformations (capillary, venous, and lymphatic malformations [LM]) or fast-flow vascular malformations (arterial or arteriovenous malformations [AVM]) [70]. Ultrasound helps in distinguishing between AVM, VM, and LM [76]. MRI is the gold standard to determine the type and extent of the lesion. Depending on the type, vascular malformations can cause skeletal abnormalities (i.e., skeletal hypertrophy) in 35% of cases [2] or local

Table 12.4 Hemangioma life cycle.

Phase	Age (years)	
Proliferating phase	0–1	Growth factors stimulate proliferation of endothelial cells
Involuting phase	1–5	Minimal changes/progression
Involuted phase	5–7 and beyond	Lesion is replaced with fibro-fatty tissue

Source: Based on [70].

complications (i.e., destruction of anatomic structures, infection, obstruction, pain, thrombosis, or ulceration). High-flow vascular malformation can also lead to disseminated intravascular coagulation, pulmonary embolism, thrombocytopenia, and congestive heart failure [70].

Treatment of vascular malformations is challenging because complete resection of this lesion is usually clinically devastating. Before surgical intervention, embolization or sclerotherapy is usually necessary to provide temporary occlusion of the nidus. Embolization alone results in transient improvement due to the recruitment of new vessels by the nidus [2].

Verrucous Vulgaris and Condyloma Acuminatum

Human papilloma virus (HPV) is a DNA virus that can infect injured skin and/or mucosa. The virus subtype dictates the clinical manifestations. Verrucous vulgaris (also known as the common wart) is caused by HPV subtypes 2 and 4. It has contact transmission with injured skin and is incorporated in the host DNA. The most common locations are the lips, oral mucosa, and fingers. Clinically, it is a white lesion with an exophytic, granular or cauliflower-like surface. Condyloma acuminatum is caused by HPV subtypes 6 and 11 and is most commonly found on the genitalia. Clinically, condyloma acuminatum appears as asymptomatic, multiple pink or white nodules that can grow and coalesce to form a broad-based, exophytic mass. Transmission to the oral cavity can occur.

Treatment for both lesions is the same. Lesions should be excised and the bed cauterized to kill any remaining virus. Recurrence is common because the virus remains latent within the cells or is reinoculated from an infected or untreated person. If condyloma acuminatum is found in a child, sexual activity and possible abuse should be suspected [2].

Salivary Gland Lesions

Mucocele

Mucocele is a mucus retention cyst that occurs exclusively in the minor salivary gland. It is the second most common benign lesion in the oral cavity after fibroma. Trauma is the typical etiology. A mucocele results from the rupture of a salivary gland duct and leakage of mucin into the surrounding tissues. The lower lip is the most common location. Treatment is surgical excision and removal of associated inflamed minor salivary glands [1].

Ranula

Ranula is a mucus-filled lesion that arises from the sublingual gland and is most frequently found in children and young adults. Most common etiologies are congenital, trauma, and sublingual salivary gland anomalies [77]. The plunging ranula is a variant which presents as an intraoral swelling with an extension into submental space by perforating the mylohyoid muscle [54, 78]. Clinically, ranula appears as a blue, dome-shaped, fluctuant swelling in the floor of the mouth that is lateral to the midline. Treatment includes excision of the ranula and associated sublingual gland [77–79] (Figure 12.7).

Pleomorphic Adenoma

Pleomorphic adenoma (PA) is the most common salivary gland tumor. It has epithelial and mesenchymal components. It arises from the parotid gland (85%), submandibular gland (8%), sublingual gland (0.1%) or minor salivary

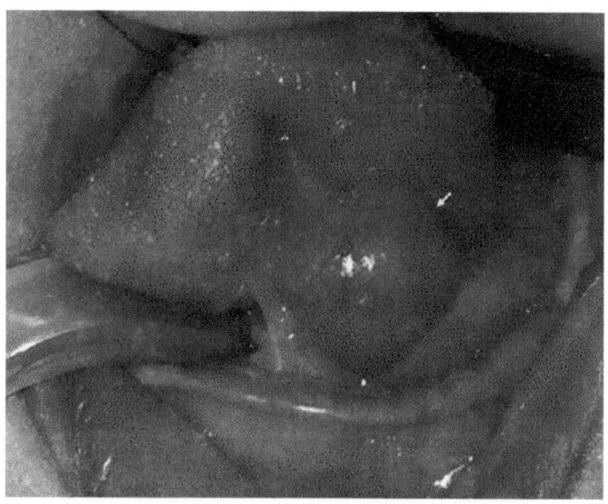

Figure 12.7 Intraoral view of a ranula in the left floor of the mouth.

gland (7%) [80, 81]. In the minor salivary glands, it most commonly occurs in the palate (60%), followed by the upper lip [1, 82]. Clinically, it is a painless, slow-growing lesion with normal overlying skin and/or mucosa. In the parotid gland, 90% of PA originate superficial to the facial nerve. MRI and CT with contrast or ultrasound are used to identify PA and its relationship with adjacent structures [83].

Treatment depends on site involved. Parotid PA is treated with parotidectomy with preservation of the facial nerve. Submandibular PA is treated with surgical excision of the gland and the associated tumor. Minor salivary gland PA is treated with excision with 5 mm margin including one anatomical barrier (periosteum), sparing the bone [80, 82]. The recurrence rate is 1% [83].

References

1 Neville, B., Damm, D., Allen, C., and Chi, A. (2015). *Oral and Maxillofacial Pathology*, 4e. Philadelphia, PA: Saunders.
2 Abramowicz, S. (2011). Pediatric head and neck tumors: benign lesions. In: *Current Therapy in Oral and Maxillofacial Surgery* (ed. S. Bagheri, R. Bell and H.A. Khan), 1136. Saunders.
3 Corona-Rodriguez, J., Torres-Labardini, R., Velasco-Tizcareno, M., and Mora-Rincones, O. (2011). Bilateral buccal bifurcation cyst: case report and literature review. *J. Oral Maxillofac. Surg.* 69 (6): 1694–1696.
4 Arce, K., Streff, C.S., and Ettinger, K.S. (2016). Pediatric odontogenic cysts of the jaws. *Oral Maxillofac. Surg. Clin. North. Am.* 28 (1): 21–30.
5 Allon, D.M., Allon, I., Anavi, Y. et al. (2015). Decompression as a treatment of odontogenic cystic lesions in children. *J. Oral Maxillofac. Surg.* 73 (4): 649–654.
6 Anderson, R.A. (1990). Eruption cysts: a retrograde study. *ASDC J. Dent. Child.* 57 (2): 124–127.
7 Wright, J.M., Odell, E.W., Speight, P.M., and Takata, T. (2014). Odontogenic tumors, WHO 2005: where do we go from here? *Head Neck Pathol.* 8 (4): 373–382.
8 Wright, J.M. and Vered, M. (2017). Update from the 4th edition of the World Health Organization classification of head and neck tumours: odontogenic and maxillofacial bone tumors. *Head Neck Pathol.* 11 (1): 68–77.
9 Pogrel, M.A. (2013). The keratocystic odontogenic tumor. *Oral Maxillofac. Surg. Clin. North. Am.* 25 (1): 21–30.
10 Regezi, J.A. (2002). Odontogenic cysts, odontogenic tumors, fibroosseous, and giant cell lesions of the jaws. *Mod. Pathol.* 15 (3): 331–341.
11 Al-Moraissi, E.A., Pogrel, M.A., and Ellis, E. 3rd. (2016). Enucleation with or without adjuvant therapy versus marsupialization with or without secondary enucleation in the treatment of keratocystic odontogenic tumors: a systematic review and meta-analysis. *J. Craniomaxillofac. Surg.* 44 (9): 1395–1403.
12 Glickman, A. and Karlis, V. (2016). Pediatric benign soft tissue oral and maxillofacial pathology. *Oral Maxillofac. Surg. Clin. North. Am.* 28 (1): 1–10.
13 Schmidt, B.L. and Pogrel, M.A. (2001). The use of enucleation and liquid nitrogen cryotherapy in the management of odontogenic keratocysts. *J. Oral Maxillofac. Surg.* 59 (7): 720–725.
14 Tagesen, J., Jensen, J., and Sindet-Pedersen, S. (1990). Comparative study of treatment of keratocysts by enucleation, enucleation combined with cryotherapy or fixation of the cyst membrane with Carnoy's solution followed by enucleation: a preliminary report. *Tandlaegebladet* 94 (16): 674–679.
15 Stoelinga, P.J.W. (2001). Long-term follow-up on keratocysts treated according to a defined protocol. *Int. J. Oral Maxillofac. Surg* 30 (1): 14–25.
16 Pogrel, M.A. and Jordan, R.C. (2004). Marsupialization as a definitive treatment for the odontogenic keratocyst. *J. Oral Maxillofac. Surg.* 62 (6): 651–655.
17 Marker, P., Brøndum, N., Clausen, P.P., and Bastian, H.L. (1996). Treatment of large odontogenic keratocysts by decompression and later cystectomy. *Oral Surg. Oral Med. Oral Pathol. Oral Radiol. Endod* 82 (2): 122–131.
18 Kaczmarzyk, T., Mojsa, I., and Stypulkowska, J. (2012). A systematic review of the recurrence rate for keratocystic odontogenic tumour in relation to treatment modalities. *Int. J. Oral Maxillofac. Surg.* 41 (6): 756–767.
19 Tomizawa, M., Otsuka, Y., and Noda, T. (2005). Clinical observations of odontomas in Japanese children: 39 cases including one recurrent case. *Int. J. Paediatr. Dent.* 15 (1): 37–43.
20 Abrahams, J.M. and McClure, S.A. (2016). Pediatric odontogenic tumors. *Oral Maxillofac. Surg. Clin. North. Am.* 28 (1): 45–58.
21 An, S.Y., An, C.H., and Choi, K.S. (2012). Odontoma: a retrospective study of 73 cases. *Imaging Sci. Dent.* 42 (2): 77–81.
22 Pogrel, M.A. and Montes, D.M. (2009). Is there a role for enucleation in the management of ameloblastoma? *Int. J. Oral Maxillofac. Surg.* 38 (8): 807–812.
23 Carlson, E.R. and Marx, R.E. (2006). The ameloblastoma: primary, curative surgical management. *J. Oral Maxillofac. Surg.* 64 (3): 484–494.

24 Zhang, J., Gu, Z., Jiang, L. et al. (2010). Ameloblastoma in children and adolescents. *Br. J. Oral Maxillofac. Surg.* 48 (7): 549–554.

25 Dammer, R., Niederdellmann, H., Dammer, P., and Nuebler-Moritz, M. (1997). Conservative or radical treatment of keratocysts: a retrospective review. *Br. J. Oral Maxillofac. Surg.* 35 (1): 46–48.

26 Ackermann, G.L., Altini, M., and Shear, M. (1988). The unicystic ameloblastoma: a clinicopathological study of 57 cases. *J. Oral Pathol.* 17 (9–10): 541–546.

27 Seintou, A., Martinelli-Kläy, C.P., and Lombardi, T. (2014). Unicystic ameloblastoma in children: systematic review of clinicopathological features and treatment outcomes. *Int. J. Oral Maxillofac. Surg.* 43 (4): 405–412.

28 Lau, S.L. and Samman, N. (2006). Recurrence related to treatment modalities of unicystic ameloblastoma: a systematic review. *Int. J. Oral Maxillofac. Surg.* 35 (8): 681–690.

29 Marx, R.S.D. (2012). *Oral and Maxillofacial Pathology: A Rationale for Diagnosis and Treatment*, 2e. Chicago, IL: Quintessence.

30 Marx, R.E. (2011). *Jaw Cysts, Benign Odontogenic Tumors of the Jaws, and Fibro-osseous Diseases*. Philadelphia, PA: Saunders.

31 Pereira, K.D., Bennett, K.M., Elkins, T.P., and Qu, Z. (2004). Ameloblastic fibroma of the maxillary sinus. *Int. J. Pediatr. Otorhinolaryngol.* 68 (11): 1473–1477.

32 Reichart, P.A. and Zobl, H. (1978). Transformation of ameloblastic fibroma to fibrosarcoma. *Int. J. Oral Surg.* 7 (5): 503–507.

33 Kobayashi, K., Murakami, R., Fujii, T., and Hirano, A. (2005). Malignant transformation of ameloblastic fibroma to ameloblastic fibrosarcoma: case report and review of the literature. *J. Cranio-Maxillofac. Surg.* 33 (5): 352–355.

34 Hatakeyama, D., Tamaoki, N., Iida, K. et al. (2012). Simple bone cyst of the mandibular condyle in a child: report of a case. *J. Oral Maxillofac. Surg.* 70 (9): 2118–2123.

35 Jones, R.S. and Dillon, J. (2016). Nonodontogenic cysts of the jaws and treatment in the pediatric population. *Oral Maxillofac. Surg. Clin. North. Am.* 28 (1): 31–44.

36 Barnes, L. (2005). *World Health Organization Classification of Tumors: Pathology and Genetics of Head and Neck Tumors*, 326. Lyon: IARC Press.

37 Panoutsakopoulos, G., Pandis, N., Kyriazoglou, I. et al. (1999). Recurrent t(16;17)(q22;p13) in aneurysmal bone cysts. *Genes Chromosomes Cancer* 26 (3): 265–266.

38 Kumar, V.V., Malik, N.A., and Kumar, D.B. (2009). Treatment of large recurrent aneurysmal bone cysts of mandible: transosseous intralesional embolization as an adjunct to resection. *Int. J. Oral Maxillofac. Surg.* 38 (6): 671–676.

39 Bilen, B.T., Alaybeyoglu, N., Arslan, A. et al. (2004). Obstructive congenital gingival granular cell tumour. *Int. J. Pediatr. Otorhinolaryngol.* 68 (12): 1567–1571.

40 Williams, R.W., Grave, B., Stewart, M., and Heggie, A.A. (2009). Prenatal and postnatal management of congenital granular cell tumours: a case report. *Br. J. Oral Maxillofac. Surg.* 47 (1): 56–58.

41 Kumar, R.M., Bavle, R.M., Umashankar, D.N., and Sharma, R. (2015). Congenital epulis of the newborn. *J. Oral Maxillofac. Pathol.* 19 (3): 407.

42 Gupta, R., Gupta, R., Kumar, S., and Saxena, S. (2015). Melanotic neuroectodermal tumor of infancy: review of literature, report of a case and follow up at 7 years. *J. Plast. Reconstr. Aesthet. Surg.* 68 (3): e53–e54.

43 Dyalram, D., Aslam-Pervez, N., and Lubek, J.E. (2016). Nonodontogenic tumors of the jaws. *Oral Maxillofac. Surg. Clin. North Am.* 28 (1): 59–65.

44 Tolentino, E.S., Centurion, B.S., Tjioe, K.C. et al. (2012). Psammomatoid juvenile ossifying fibroma: an analysis of 2 cases affecting the mandible with review of the literature. *Oral Surg. Oral Med. Oral Pathol. Oral Radiol.* 113 (6): e40–e45.

45 El-Mofty, S. (2002). Psammomatoid and trabecular juvenile ossifying fibroma of the craniofacial skeleton: two distinct clinicopathologic entities. *Oral Surg. Oral Med. Oral Pathol. Oral Radio.l Endod.* 93 (3): 296–304.

46 Slootweg, P.J., Panders, A.K., Koopmans, R., and Nikkels, P.G. (1994). Juvenile ossifying fibroma. An analysis of 33 cases with emphasis on histopathological aspects. *J. Oral Pathol. Med.* 23 (9): 385–388.

47 Owosho, A.A., Hughes, M.A., Prasad, J.L. et al. (2014). Psammomatoid and trabecular juvenile ossifying fibroma: two distinct radiologic entities. *Oral Surg. Oral Med. Oral Pathol. Oral Radiol.* 118 (6): 732–738.

48 Yang, H.Y., Zheng, L.W., Luo, J. et al. (2009). Psammomatoid juvenile cemento-ossifying fibroma of the maxilla. *J. Craniofac. Surg.* 20 (4): 1190–1192.

49 Zama, M., Gallo, S., Santecchia, L. et al. (2004). Juvenile active ossifying fibroma with massive involvement of the mandible. *Plast. Reconstr. Surg.* 113 (3): 970–974.

50 Sarode, S.C., Sarode, G.S., Waknis, P. et al. (2011). Juvenile psammomatoid ossifying fibroma: a review. *Oral Oncol.* 47 (12): 1110–1116.

51 Barker, B.F., Carpenter, W.M., Daniels, T.E. et al. (1997). Oral mucosal melanomas: the WESTOP Banff workshop proceedings. Western Society of Teachers of Oral Pathology. *Oral Surg. Oral Med. Oral Pathol. Oral Radiol. Endod.* 83 (6): 672–679.

52 Kaban, L.B., Troulis, M.J., Wilkinson, M.S. et al. (2007). Adjuvant antiangiogenic therapy for giant cell tumors of the jaws. *J. Oral Maxillofac. Surg.* 65 (10): 2018–2024. discussion 2024.

53 Chuong, R., Kaban, L.B., Kozakewich, H., and Perez-Atayde, A. (1986). Central giant cell lesions of the jaws: a clinicopathologic study. *J. Oral Maxillofac. Surg.* 44 (9): 708–712.

54 Kaban, L. (2004). *Pediatric Oral and Maxillofacial Surgery*. Philadelphia, PA: Saunders.

55 Abramowicz, S., Goldwaser, B.R., Troulis, M.J. et al. (2013). Primary jaw tumors in children. *J. Oral Maxillofac. Surg.* 71 (1): 47–52.

56 Kruse-Losler, B., Diallo, R., Gaertner, C. et al. (2006). Central giant cell granuloma of the jaws: a clinical, radiologic, and histopathologic study of 26 cases. *Oral Surg. Oral Med. Oral Pathol. Oral Radiol. Endod.* 101 (3): 346–354.

57 Comert, E., Turanli, M., and Ulu, S. (2006). Oral and intralesional steroid therapy in giant cell granuloma. *Acta Otolaryngol.* 126 (6): 664–666.

58 Harris, M. (1993). Central giant cell granulomas of the jaws regress with calcitonin therapy. *Br. J. Oral Maxillofac. Surg.* 31 (2): 89–94.

59 Pogrel, M.A. (2003). Calcitonin therapy for central giant cell granuloma. *J. Oral Maxillofac. Surg.* 61 (6): 649–653. discussion 653–6544.

60 de Lange, J., van den Akker, H.P., van den Berg, H. et al. (2006). Limited regression of central giant cell granuloma by interferon alpha after failed calcitonin therapy: a report of 2 cases. *Int. J. Oral Maxillofac. Surg.* 35 (9): 865–869.

61 de Lange, J., van den Akker, H.P., Veldhuijzen van Zanten, G.O. et al. (2006). Calcitonin therapy in central giant cell granuloma of the jaw: a randomized double-blind placebo-controlled study. *Int. J. Oral Maxillofac. Surg.* 35 (9): 791–795.

62 Kaban, L.B., Troulis, M.J., Ebb, D. et al. (2002). Antiangiogenic therapy with interferon alpha for giant cell lesions of the jaws. *J. Oral Maxillofac. Surg.* 60 (10): 1103–1111. discussion 1111–1112.

63 Kaban, L.B., Mulliken, J.B., Ezekowitz, R.A. et al. (1999). Antiangiogenic therapy of a recurrent giant cell tumor of the mandible with interferon alfa-2a. *Pediatrics* 103 (6 Pt 1): 1145–1149.

64 Landesberg, R., Eisig, S., Fennoy, I., and Siris, E. (2009). Alternative indications for bisphosphonate therapy. *J. Oral Maxillofac. Surg.* 67 (5 Suppl): 27–34.

65 Peters, W.J. (1979). Cherubism: a study of twenty cases from one family. *Oral Surg. Oral Med. Oral Pathol.* 47 (4): 307–311.

66 Faircloth, W.J. Jr., Edwards, R.C., and Farhood, V.W. (1991). Cherubism involving a mother and daughter: case reports and review of the literature. *J. Oral Maxillofac. Surg.* 49 (5): 535–542.

67 Grunebaum, M. and Tiqva, P. (1973). Non familial cherubism: report of two cases. *J. Oral Surg.* 31 (8): 632–635.

68 Kalantar Motamedi, M.H. (1998). Treatment of cherubism with locally aggressive behavior presenting in adulthood: report of four cases and a proposed new grading system. *J. Oral Maxillofac. Surg.* 56 (11): 1336–1142.

69 Gonzalez-Perez, L.M., Prats-Golczer, V.E., Montes Carmona, J.F., and Heurtebise Saavedra, J.M. (2014). Bilateral first branchial cleft anomaly with evidence of a genetic aetiology. *Int. J. Oral Maxillofac. Surg.* 43 (3): 296–300.

70 Abramowicz, S. and Padwa, B.L. (2012). Vascular anomalies in children. *Oral Maxillofac. Surg. Clin* 24 (3): 443–455.

71 Greene, A.K. (2011). Management of hemangiomas and other vascular tumors. *Clin. Plast. Surg.* 38 (1): 45–63.

72 Crum, R., Szabo, S., and Folkman, J. (1985). A new class of steroids inhibits angiogenesis in the presence of heparin or a heparin fragment. *Science* 230 (4732): 1375–1378.

73 Hogeling, M., Adams, S., and Wargon, O. (2011). A randomized controlled trial of propranolol for infantile hemangiomas. *Pediatrics* 128 (2): e259–e266.

74 Perez, J., Pardo, J., and Gomez, C. (2002). Vincristine – an effective treatment of corticoid-resistant life-threatening infantile hemangiomas. *Acta Oncol.* 41 (2): 197–199.

75 Mulliken, J.B., Fishman, S.J., and Burrows, P.E. (2000). Vascular anomalies. *Curr. Probl. Surg.* 37 (8): 517–584.

76 Paltiel, H.J., Burrows, P.E., Kozakewich, H.P. et al. (2000). Soft-tissue vascular anomalies: utility of US for diagnosis. *Radiology* 214 (3): 747–754.

77 Kokong, D., Iduh, A., Chukwu, I. et al. (2017). Ranula: current concept of pathophysiologic basis and surgical management options. *World J. Surg.* 41: 1476–1481.

78 de Visscher, J.G., van der Wal, K.G., and de Vogel, P.L. (1989). The plunging ranula. Pathogenesis, diagnosis and management. *J. Craniomaxillofac. Surg.* 17 (4): 182–185.

79 Mahadevan, M. and Vasan, N. (2006). Management of pediatric plunging ranula. *Int. J. Pediatr. Otorhinolaryngol.* 70 (6): 1049–1054.

80 Ord, R.A. (2004). Salivary gland tumors in children. In: *Pediatric Oral and Maxillofacial Surgery* (ed. L.B. Kaban and M.J. Troulis), 202–211. Philadelphia, PA: Saunders.

81 Mehta, D. and Willging, J.P. (2006). Pediatric salivary gland lesions. *Semin. Pediatr. Surg.* 15 (2): 76–84.

82 Carlson, E.R. and Ord, R.A. (2016). Benign pediatric salivary gland lesions. *Oral Maxillofac. Surg. Clin. North Am.* 28 (1): 67–81.

83 Kakimoto, N., Gamoh, S., Tamaki, J. et al. (2009). CT and MR images of pleomorphic adenoma in major and minor salivary glands. *Eur. J. Radiol.* 69 (3): 464–472.

13

Diagnosis and Management of Salivary Gland Pathology

Prince Dhillon and Michael Turner

Introduction

Salivary gland diseases occurs in approximately 1% of the population [1]. The different types of salivary gland diseases can be categorized as follows: obstructive (including secondary bacterial infections), viral infections, autoimmune disease, and benign and malignant tumors. This chapter will review the diagnosis, pathophysiology, and management of these disease processes.

A common presenting sign of a salivary gland disorder is inflammation, referred to as sialadenitis, and when it occurs in the parotid gland, it is termed parotitis.

A decrease in salivary flow is termed hyposalivation and is an objective finding. Xerostomia is the feeling of dry mouth and is a subjective finding. Salivary glands can have a decrease in function, but the total salivary output can be maintained by the remaining salivary glands. Alternatively, a patient can have hyposalivation if there is a systemic etiology affecting all the major salivary glands. For example, a local obstruction like a sialolith, malignancy, stricture or adhesion can be responsible for hyposalivation from a single gland and most likely will not cause symptoms of xerostomia. That being said, hyposalivation is a critical risk factor for developing infectious sialadenitits. Severe hyposalivation can also put one at risk for caries, candida infections, and mucositis.

The main etiologies of hyposalivation are dehydration, medications, radiation, Sjögren syndrome, and uncontrolled diabetes mellitus [2]. Medications that have anticholinergic properties are common in today's pharmacologic landscape, and include antihistamines, antiemetics, antidepressants, benzodiazepines, chemotherapeutics, and diuretics [3]. Patients with multiple medications have a higher incidence of polypharmacy-induced hyposalivation [4]. A practitioner can diagnose a systemic etiology of inadequate salivary flow by inquiring about symptoms of inadequate salivary flow like xerostomia, the subjective feeling of a dry mouth, the constant need to drink water with meals, waking up in the night to take a sip of water, and difficulty swallowing food.

Evaluation and diagnosis of salivary gland infections begins with a comprehensive history and physical exam. A history of symptomatology is important, starting with open-ended questions. The salivary glands are examined carefully, comparing each side and paying attention to swelling, erythema, tenderness, and warmth. An acute infectious process will have these cardinal signs of infection like any other organ, but chronically infected glands may not follow in the same pattern. Hence, imaging can be important to obtain a diagnosis.

Obstructive Salivary Gland Disorders

Obstructive salivary gland disorders occur when the duct system of one of the major salivary glands becomes either occluded or partially occluded, resulting in cessation of salivary flow. This results in the gland becoming swollen and sometimes painful. Typically, this resolves over 2–3 hours. Obstructions can be divided into sialoliths, foreign bodies, strictures, and mucous plugs.

Sialolithiasis (Salivary Gland Stones)

Etiology

Sialolithiasis is the formation of calculi in the duct system of the salivary glands. Intermittent salivary stasis and turbulence result in alteration of the mucoid elements of saliva, leading to the formation of an organic scaffold. Subsequently, a variety of salivary minerals precipitate on

Oral and Maxillofacial Surgery, Medicine, and Pathology for the Clinician, First Edition. Edited by Harry Dym, Leslie R. Halpern, and Orrett E. Ogle.

this scaffold and a calculus is formed. Because the submandibular gland secretes both mucinous and serous components, approximately 80–90% of sialoliths occur in this organ. The remaining sialoliths occur in the parotid gland, typically 10–20%, with 1% or less in the sublingual glands [5]. Minor salivary gland calculi are rare, occurring most often in the upper lip and buccal mucosa. About 25% of patients with sialolithiasis have multiple, unilateral stones, but bilateral salivary stones occur only in 2.2% of cases [6].

In the submandibular gland, salivary calculi are located most commonly in three specific regions: the ductal opening, the area where the lingual nerve and the submandibular gland cross, and at the hilum of the gland. These areas are more susceptible to turbulence and salivary stasis. As stated above, the submandibular saliva has a higher mucin and calcium content so in areas of turbulence, sialolithiasis tend to form.

The risk factors associated with salivary gland stones include dehydration, diuretics, anticholinergic medications, trauma to the region, and gout [7]. Hypercalcemia, however, is not related to stone formation [8].

Patients with salivary obstruction caused by a sialolithiasis typically present with pain and swelling of the gland, particularly following gustatory stimulation. Submandibular stones present with painless swelling approximately 30% of the time [9]. Not all salivary gland stones are symptomatic. Asymptomatic sialoliths are typically noted incidentally on physical exam or on radiographs.

When patients report intermittent symptoms, this is most likely secondary to the presence of a partial obstruction. Patients can function with a partial obstruction without symptoms until the remaining lumen of the duct becomes obstructed by a mucous plug. Once the mucous plug is disrupted, salivary flow then resumes.

During the physical examination of the patient with suspected salivary stone, attention should be focused on the flow of saliva from the respective duct, recognizing whether there is a complete or partial obstruction. In the submandibular region, bimanual palpation of the floor of the mouth and the neck should be performed. Parotid glands should be palpated from behind the gland, moving in a forward direction.

Sialolithiasis Imaging

Imaging studies should be obtained in most instances. There are a multitude of options for this.

Computed tomography (CT) scanning is one of the two modalities of choice for the evaluation of salivary stones. Most stones are calcified enough to be visible with noncontrast imaging. CT scans have a 10-fold greater sensitivity in detecting stones compared with plain films. Sensitivity for the identification of parotid tumors with CT approaches 100% [6, 10].

Ultrasound is the second most common imaging modality and is now being used more frequently. More than 90% of stones 2 mm in diameter or larger can be detected by ultrasound [11]. It is able to detect radiolucent or radiopaque stones and is not susceptible to artifact from adjacent dental restorations. Finally, and importantly, there is no radiation associated with ultrasound, limiting patient exposure [12].

Plain films can be effective in detecting radiopaque stones. This is very useful in detecting submandibular calculi, which are radiopaque in 80–95% of cases, although with the onset of CT and ultrasound, they are no longer typically used.

Plain film sialography is rarely utilized now because of increased access to in-office cone beam CT scans (CBCT). CBCT sialography allows for a 3D rendered image of the salivary gland and duct system. In this technique, the salivary duct is cannulated and a radiopaque dye is infiltrated into the gland prior to imaging. It is useful in diagnosing stricture, sialectasis, and cystic degeneration of the duct and gland, as in patients with Sjögren syndrome [13].

Magnetic resonance imaging (MRI) is not widely used for initial obstructive gland imaging. An MRI with contrast or sialography can have superior sensitivity compared with ultrasound and a lower procedural failure rate than standard sialography for evaluation of a stricture or stenosis [14]. Visualization of sialoliths can sometimes be challenging because of their low water content [15]. Cost should also be considered when imaging the salivary glands. Ultrasound is relatively inexpensive compared to a contrast MRI.

Management of Sialolithiasis

Initial care of patients with sialolithiasis is management of their obstruction and, if indicated, treatment of their concurrent infection. The majority of patients with acute obstruction can be resolved with hydration to increase the serous component of their saliva. This creates a conducive environment which can result in displacement of the obstructing mucous plug and conversion back to a partial obstruction. Sialolithiasis can lead to concurrent infections as a result of ductal obstruction, stasis, and retrograde contamination. If there is purulence, cutaneous erythema, and systemic signs of infection, patients should be treated with either amoxicillin/clavulanate potassium combination or azithromycin for 7–10 days. Chronic obstruction may result in atrophy and dysfunction of the affected salivary gland. If the obstruction is removed, a gland can regain function up to 75% of the time, as long as the duct remains patent [16].

To restore patency to the gland, sialolithectomy and possibly a sialodochoplasty should be performed. This can be achieved utilizing multiple techniques dependent upon the location, size, and shape of the sialolith.

Smaller anterior located stones in the submandibular gland (Figure 13.1) can be removed by either dilating the duct to allow the stone to pass or making an incision overlying the stone and removing it. A surgical stent should be placed to prevent stricture of the duct. Note that the parotid duct is highly susceptible to the formation of strictures and incisions into this duct should be avoided at all costs. If an incision is made into Stenson's duct, a stent should be sutured into the lumen for at least 4 weeks. Postoperative dilation may be indicated following this for an extended period of time until stable patency is achieved.

Sialendoscopy is a minimally invasive procedure for visualization and instrumentation of various salivary gland diseases. A sialendoscopy is performed using semi-rigid endoscopes that have diameters of approximately 1–1.5 mm. The sialendoscope is placed into the duct of the gland and the stone is visualized and, if possible, removed with a retrieval basket.

Submandibular stones can also be removed via a transoral approach, particularly if they are palpable [9]. Parotid stones, on the other hand, are less likely to be removed transorally. When approaching the submandibular gland via the transoral approach, care must be taken to avoid trauma to the duct and associated lingual glands, as this can lead to ranula formation. Proximal stones are more challenging to remove transorally, as the increased dissection required through a limited exposure increases the risk of trauma to surrounding nerves [5]. Combining endoscopic and open intraoral techniques has led to improved success rates in removing proximal stones [5].

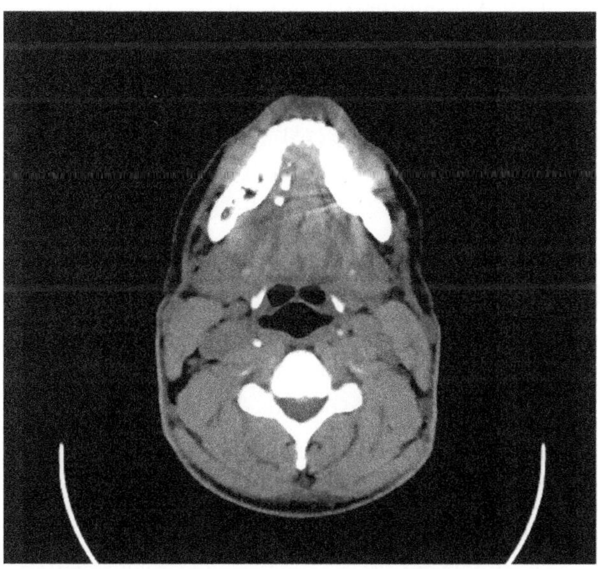

Figure 13.1 Axial CT of distal salivary gland stones.

For parotid stones, a combined transfacial and sialendoscopic approach can be used to remove stones that are not near the distal aspect of the orifice of Stensen's duct. A small percentage of patients with persistent symptoms due to salivary stones will require gland removal [5]. For parotid stones, parotidectomy is a last resort, reserved for patients who have failed less invasive approaches and whose unrelenting symptoms warrant the additional risk to the auriculotemporal nerve and facial nerve during dissection of the gland [17]. For the submandibular gland, a transcervical excision has a risk of injury to the lingual, facial, and hypoglossal nerves, so it is reserved for cases where transoral or minimally invasive approaches have not been successful [18].

Extracorporeal lithotripsy uses shock waves to fragment sialoliths so they can pass through the duct. This is considered when stones are in the proximal ducts or in the salivary glands themselves and thus a simple transoral approach is not possible. In one prospective study, 76 patients with parotid stones were treated with extracorporeal shock wave therapy after failure of conservative therapy. Fifty percent were free of stones after a follow-up period of 48 months. Twenty-six percent had residual stone fragments detected but were asymptomatic. Extracorporeal lithotripsy can be used for stones that are intraductal and are smaller than 7 mm [19]. Unfortunately, in the United States, there is not an FDA-approved device for this procedure.

Bacterial Salivary Gland Infections

Bacterial infections are the most common type of salivary gland infections. Acute bacterial salivary gland infections can present as a painful swelling, sometimes coupled with systemic signs of infection such as fevers, chills, and malaise. Systemic signs of an infection such as leukocytosis, fevers, and chills should prompt the provider to consider an inpatient admission. Hyposalivation or absence of salivary flow from the glands allows for oral bacteria to ascend in a retrograde fashion into the duct and then into the parenchyma. Acute bacterial salivary gland infections are typically concurrent with an obstructive salivary gland disorder but can also occur independently.

Acute parotid infections can occur in hospitalized patients as well. Patients requiring inpatient hospital stays can be dehydrated perioperatively, and sometimes malnourished, leading to lack of salivary gland stimulation and ductal stasis. These factors put these patients at increased risk for an ascending bacterial infection. Generally, these infections are seen on postoperative days 5–7 [19]. The organisms responsible for these infections are gram-negative bacteria but as for most oral infections, they also have other components: *Eikenella*, *Escherichia coli*, *Fusobacterium*, *Haemophilus influenzae*, *Klebsiella*, *Prevotella*, *Proteus*, and *Pseudomonas* species as well as methicillin-resistant *Staphylococcus aureus* (MRSA) [20].

For salivary glands with minimal or no purulence and no systemic signs of infection, conservative management is indicated. This would include digital massage, oral antibiotics, warm compresses, hydration, and sialagogs. As the clinical severity of the infection increases, IV antibiotics and possible drainage may be indicated if an abscess is seen on imaging.

A chronic salivary gland infection is one that lasts more than 1 month, due to either delayed evaluation or recurrent episodes. It can present as a painless swelling, unilateral or bilateral in nature, and can be easily confused for a salivary gland neoplasm. This inflammation that occurs secondarily can last for days, weeks or months with periods of quiescence that can result in ductal wall irregularities and strictures.

Treatment of salivary gland infections is difficult. Antibiotics, steroids, sialagogs, and warm compresses have been used with mixed results. Sialendoscopy is an effective treatment to clear precipitated serum proteins within the intraductal system, by dilating the ducts, overcoming strictures, and flushing out the ductal systems. Severe infections can result in significant impairment of quality of life and may warrant a sialadenectomy, but the benefits of this surgery must be weighed against the risks of injury to the various nerves.

Chronic sclerosing submandibular sialadenitis presents in elderly patients with a unilateral, painful, and swollen gland and is usually secondary to a sialolith or chronic infection. It is clinically difficult to distinguish from a neoplasm, and is aptly referred to as a Kuttner tumor.

Actinomycosis is a gram-positive bacterial disease, often exhibiting a clinical picture similar to a fungal infection, as it is often an opportunistic infection, seldom diagnosed outside immunocompromised patients, and difficult to isolate *in vitro*. Like other salivary gland infections, actinomycosis is thought to ascend in a retrograde fashion into the salivary ducts, followed by a painless, indurated enlargement of the gland, sometimes with multiple draining cutaneous fistulae [21]. It also can present as a typical pyogenic abscess. Definitive diagnosis is made by positive cultures and histopathologic analysis is warranted. Treatment involves an extended period of high-dose penicillin with the possible need for surgical drainage.

Viral Diseases

Viral Sialadenitis

Viral infections occur when a hematogenous virus infiltrates a salivary gland. Many viruses can cause sialadenitis, and can present similarly, but the most common entity is the mumps.

Mumps is an acute, bilateral, nonsuppurative viral parotitis which is usually caused by the paramyxovirus, but can also be caused by coxsackie A, coxsackie B, Epstein–Barr virus, influenza, parainfluenza, and HIV. Parotitis is preceded by prodromal symptoms of low-grade fever, preauricular pain, headache, myalgia, anorexia, arthralgia or malaise. It is then followed by either unilateral or bilateral parotid swelling roughly 30 days later. It then typically progresses to a bilateral involvement in almost all cases for up to 10 days [22]. Since the widespread administration of the MMR vaccine in USA, the incidence of mumps has significantly subsided, but incidences of resurgence are starting to occur on a more frequent basis.

Generally, mumps is self-limiting but complications like mumps orchitis, which is present in 15–30% of cases, can occur about 10 days after parotitis and is bilateral in 25% of all cases [23]. To prevent the onset of orchitis in young males, male patients are treated prophylactically with interferon to prevent the occurrence of sterility. Other complications like oophoritis, meningitis, encephalitis deafness, and, less commonly, arthritis, pancreatitis, and myocarditis can occur. Treatment hinges on supportive care with adequate hydration and minimizing stimulation of the parotid glands.

HIV has numerous effects on oral health, including decreasing salivary flow, but without a significant increase in sialolithiasis rates [24]. HIV-associated salivary gland disease (HIV-SGD) refers to the high prevalence of salivary gland swelling in patients with HIV with a parotid gland enlargement. This occurs in up to 10% of patients with HIV. Usually the swelling occurs in a slow fashion, is asymptomatic, and when it is persistent, it is usually due to benign lymphoepithelial cysts within the gland which have numerous names in the literature: benign lymphoepithelial cysts or lesions, MAIDS-related lymphadenopathy, diffuse infiltrative lymphocytosis syndrome, cystic lymphoid hyperplasia, and HIV-SGD [25]. These cysts are caused by lymphocytosis, diffuse lymphocytic infiltration, and cervical lymphadenopathy, and can be diagnosed on ultrasound, CT or MRI [26].

While aspiration can temporarily ameliorate the cystic swellings, treatment involving sclerotherapy, radiation therapy, and antiretroviral therapies may sometimes be definitive, but ultimately surgical removal of the gland may be warranted to treat the cosmetic deformity.

Granulomatous Disease of the Salivary Gland

Granulomatous diseases of the salivary gland are rare and often diagnosed by their extraglandular manifestations. *Mycobacterium tuberculosis* is ever prevalent in developing nations, and commonly affects the lungs with progression leading to miliary tuberculosis; however, it can sometimes affect the salivary glands through localized infiltration from adjacent lymph nodes. Even in developing nations, where tuberculosis is largely unchecked, it is still a rare form of extrapulmonary tuberculosis [27]. An infiltration of the salivary gland is similar in appearance to a parotid tumor and is diagnosed during histologic evaluation of the specimen. Otherwise, diagnosis is by fine-needle aspiration biopsy and the treatment is antituberculous chemotherapy.

Nontuberculous mycobacterial (NTM) infections involving the salivary glands are rare, but when they do occur, they generally affect parotid glands of children or immunocompromised adults [28]. The organisms responsible are predominantly of the *Mycobacterium avium intracellulare* family, and *Mycobacterium abscessus*, although there are many other NTM species [29]. NTM do not exhibit human-to-human transmission but are instead acquired from the environment or animals. Lymph node involvement is a hallmark of this disease, and the clinical course is generally indolent and can form cutaneous fistulae. Prolonged antibiotics are generally necessary, but the most definitive treatment is surgical excision of the salivary gland and affected nodes [30].

Sarcoidosis is a systemic granulomatous disease most commonly affecting the pulmonary and lymphatic organs with an increased predilection in younger females and people of African descent, and in 5–10% of cases can involve the salivary glands. The glands will show a chronic, painless, diffuse parotid swelling, with symptoms of xerostomia. Extraglandular symptoms include persistent cough, fatigue, weight loss, fever, night sweats, skin changes, and hypercalcemia from the production of calcitriol by activated macrophages. Other signs include facial nerve palsy, uveoparotitis (Heerfordt syndrome) and Melkersson–Rosenthal syndrome, which is marked by recurrent facial swelling, fissured tongue, and spontaneously resolving facial paralysis. Biopsies show noncaseating granulomas, which typically resolve spontaneously. If no resolution occurs, systemic treatment with steroids and immunosuppressive drugs is warranted [31].

Autoimmune Diseases

Sjögren Syndrome

The most common autoimmune disease of the salivary glands is Sjögren syndrome (SS) with a 9:1 female-to-male ratio, which generally affects 40–50-year-old females. Primary SS is not associated with other autoimmune diseases, and secondary SS presents with concurrent autoimmune disease: systemic lupus erythematosus, rheumatoid arthritis, and scleroderma. SS affects the salivary and lacrimal glands which leads to xerostomia and keratoconjunctivitis sicca. Dry mouth symptoms and dry eye symptoms become persistent, and on clinical exam symmetric parotid swelling is seen. With this disease, there can be extraglandular involvement such as rashes, musculoskeletal symptoms, fatigue, pulmonary, renal and hepatic involvement. Most concerning is the 5–10% prevalence of non-Hodgkin B-cell lymphoma in these patients [32].

The most commonly used classification system is the 2002 US–European Classification system. The two absolute criteria for the diagnosis are a lower lip biopsy including 10 minor salivary glands showing a collection of 50 lymphocytes within 4 cm^2 and positive serum antibodies SS-A (anti-Ro) and SS-B (anti-La) [33].

Management of SS necessitates a multidisciplinary approach, involving a rheumatologist, oral and ocular care specialists, but generally only requires supportive care by prescribing salivary substitutes, lubricating eye drops, and sialagogs. Pilocarpine or cevimeline can be used three times a day prior to meals to promote salivary function. Chewing gum, preferably sugar free and containing xylitol, can increase salivary production through gustatory and masticatory stimulation. Salivary substitutes and lubricants, containing water, electrolytes, glycoproteins, carboxymethylcellulose, mucins, and fluoride, can be bought over the counter as gums, tablets, solutions or sprays. Initial attempts at treating the etiology of SS with B-cell depletion therapy using rituximab have been disappointing [34].

Most concerning in SS is the high risk of developing lymphomas, although mucosal-associated lymphoid tissue (MALT) lymphomas are the most common type of lymphoma seen in SS patients and carry a favorable prognosis [35].

Salivary Gland Tumors

The World Health Organization (WHO) classification of salivary gland tumors lists 23 malignant epithelial salivary gland tumors (SGTs), 10 benign epithelial and four nonepithelial neoplasms. Despite the heterogeneity of histologic subtypes, over half of all SGTs are composed of more than one cell type and are labeled pleiomorphic adenomas. The heterogeneity of SGTs is highly variable, making classification challenging. Prognosis for SGTs is generally best correlated with histologic type, but grading of tumors also has a role in determining prognosis in mucoepidermoid carcinomas, adenocarcinomas, salivary duct carcinomas, and acinic cell carcinomas [36].

Overall, SGTs are rare, comprising only 5% of all head and neck cancers. The parotid is the most common site of SGTs (80%), with 75% of these being benign. Minor salivary glands are responsible for only 9–23% of all SGTs but have a high risk of malignancy, roughly 40–90%. This is the highest when compared to all other salivary glands [36, 37].

The most frequently diagnosed benign SGT is the pleomorphic adenoma. Other benign tumors are Warthin tumor, basal cell adenoma, and canalicular adenoma. The most common malignant neoplasms are mucoepidermoid and adenoid cystic carcinomas (ACC), which account for roughly half of all malignancies in the salivary glands [38]. Mucoepidermoid carcinomas are the most common neoplasm in pediatric patients, who are also at increased risk for mesenchymal tumors and malignant epithelial tumors compared to adult patients. The average age of a patient with a SGT is 45 years old.

When evaluating a patient with a suspected SGT, the basic history of the present illness and physical exam should be performed, with particular attention paid to any facial nerve involvement, trismus, and cervical lymphadenopathy. CT and MRI imaging are equally effective in diagnostic accuracy of salivary gland cancers [39]. Contrast enhancement can help delineate the extent of the lesion, irregular margins, bony resorption, perineural invasion, and involvement of lymph nodes [40].

Ultrasound is a safe and inexpensive imaging modality with a sensitivity close to 100%, but is limited as it cannot identify lesions of the deep parotid lobe. Ultimately, tissue diagnosis by fine needle aspiration or ultrasound-guided core needle biopsy for surgical planning is best. Intraoperative frozen sections have variable accuracy and are highly dependent on the expertise of the pathologist [41]. If metastatic disease or lymph node involvement needs to be ruled out, 18F-fluorodeoxyglucose positron emission tomography (PET) has been shown to have good diagnostic accuracy [42].

Treatment of SGTs is surgical excision. A superficial parotidectomy is indicated if the lesion is superficial to the facial nerve, although if the deep lobe is involved, a total parotidectomy should be performed. Involvement of the facial nerve is a major risk of a total parotidectomy, although sacrificing a branch of the facial nerve is predictable if there is a preoperative weakness or signs of involvement on imaging [43]. When there is evidence of extracapsular disease, mandibulectomy, partial maxillectomy or removal of skin may be necessary. Low-grade submandibular neoplasms confined within the parenchyma of the gland only necessitate removal of the gland. Sublingual gland malignancies can often be accessed intraorally but since this gland is not encapsulated by cervical fascia, surgery may necessitate removal of the submandibular gland, the floor of the mouth mucosa and its associated vital structures. Malignancies of the minor salivary glands require excision with wide, adequate margins.

In those 15% of salivary gland malignancies where there is lymph node involvement, a radical neck dissection needs to be performed [44]. For high-grade malignancies with clinically negative neck lymph nodes, a prophylactic neck dissection is also recommended [45]. Adjuvant therapy for malignant SGTs involves postoperative radiation therapy. In the case of local recurrence, repeat surgery, irradiation, and/or palliative chemotherapy are also options. For metastatic disease, chemotherapy has not been shown to increase survival but does have significant palliative benefits [46]. Hematogenous spread is the main source for salivary malignancies, with metastasis most often being located in the lungs (80%), bone (15%), and other sites [46].

Pleomorphic Adenoma

Pleomorphic adenoma is the most common SGT, making up one-half to two-thirds of all benign SGTs [47]. It occurs in the fourth to fifth decades of life and has a slight female predilection. Risk factors include prior radiation exposure and tobacco use. It is described as a benign mixed epithelial tumor characterized by its microscopic diversity, in that it is composed of both epithelial and myoepithelial cells in varying proportions. Classic pleomorphic adenomas are described as having an even mixture of cells and stroma, whereas atypical types are described as cellular or myxoid [48]. Grossly, they either resemble cartilage or a firmer type tumor that is tan-white in color. The mass is surrounded by a pseudocapsule, which projects outgrowths of the tumor into the surrounding normal glandular tissue.

Recurrence of pleomorphic adenoma is most likely due to inadequate margins, rather than the characteristics of the neoplasm itself. Malignant transformation is rare, but possible and is rediagnosed as a carcinoma ex pleomorphic adenoma.

Warthin Tumor

Warthin tumor (also known as adenolymphoma or papillary lymphomatous cystadenoma) is the second most common benign SGT. There is a strong male predilection (4:1) and the peak incidence is in the sixth and seventh decades of life [49]. Ninety percent of cases are found in the superficial lobe of the parotid gland. The classic presentation of Warthin tumor is an elderly male with a smoking history, where a mass is found incidentally on examination. Smoking has been shown to confer an eightfold increased risk for this tumor. While generally asymptomatic, occasionally the tumor can cause pain and pressure because of its rapid growth. Occasionally it can even rupture [50].

On MRI, the tumor demonstrates well-defined margins and multifocal lesions. Interestingly, diagnosis of a Warthin tumor necessitates a thorough clinical and radiographic examination of the contralateral parotid gland as this tumor presents bilaterally in 7–10% of cases [51].

Postsurgical recurrence is rare and malignant transformation occurs in only 0.3% of cases. The rates of metastatic transformation and recurrence, however, may be overestimated owing to the fact that this tumor is known to present multifocally, and second primaries can be confused with metastatic disease or recurrence.

Mucoepidermoid Carcinoma

Mucoepidermoid carcinoma is the most frequently occurring malignancy of the salivary glands, accounting for about 35% of all SGT malignancies [52]. The most common site of occurrence is the parotid for the major salivary glands and the palate for the minor salivary glands. A lesion of the palate will appear as a fluctuant submucosal lump, possibly with a bluish tinge. There is a known female predilection, and this tumor can occur in almost any decade of life. It contains both mucus-producing and epidermoid cells, and their common progenitor, all in varying proportions. The heterogeneity explains the clinical and phenotypic variability of mucoepidermoid carcinoma [53]. The 5-year survival is around 70%, but high-grade and low-grade 5-year survivals vary greatly [54].

Diagnosis at an advanced stage, perineural invasion, positive surgical margins, and the primary located in the submandibular gland also predict an unfavorable prognosis [54].

Adenoid Cystic Carcinoma

Adenoid cystic carcinoma is a highly infiltrative and aggressive basaloid tumor displaying both luminal and abluminal myoepithelial cells. ACC displays an indolent but relentless disease course with poor long-term survival. It is more common at minor salivary gland sites, but still more of these lesions appear in the parotid than anywhere else. Like the pleomorphic adenoma, there is a slight female predilection, but incidence peaks in the fifth to sixth decades.

Adenoid cystic carcinoma, along with undifferentiated carcinoma, ductal carcinoma and carcinoma ex pleomorphic adenoma, shows the highest distant metastasis rate of all salivary gland malignancies [46]. ACC is known to commonly metastasize to the lungs, and can appear decades after the initial primary. ACC can undergo high-grade transformation, which is generally an overgrowth of the ductal component into a pleiomorphic undifferentiated carcinoma or poorly differentiated adenocarcinoma, carrying a 12–36-month median survival time [55].

Polymorphic Low-Grade Adenocarcinoma

Polymorphic low-grade adenocarcinoma (PLGA) resembles an indolent ACC that occurs in a minor salivary gland site. It is an infiltrative tumor consisting of ductal phenotype cells. The palate is the most common site for PLGA, along with lip mucosa and buccal mucosa; less commonly, it will be found in the major salivary glands, with fewer than 50 reported cases worldwide originating in the parotid [56]. Since the palate is a common site for minor SGTs, bony involvement is also common in PLGA. Variable incidence rates have been reported in the literature, possibly owing to variable geographical and ethnic differences [57]. PLGAs generally show limited metastatic behavior and limited local spread but recurrences after 5 years are fairly common and thus warrant long-term follow-up. Despite the name suggesting it is a low-grade variant, higher mitotic rates and nuclear size variation can exist. Generally, treatment includes surgical excision with wide margins, and adjuvant therapy remains controversial [57].

Conclusion

Salivary gland diseases present in various forms, from dry mouth from polypharmacy to aggressive malignant tumors. The ability to recognize, evaluate, diagnose, and manage these disease processes is necessary for the practice of oral and maxillofacial surgery.

References

1 Rauch, S. (1970). Diseases of the salivary glands. In: *Thoma's Oral Pathology*. (ed. K. Thoma, R. Gorlin and H. Goldman), 997–1003. St Louis, MO: Mosby.

2 Sreebny, L.M., Yu, A., Green, A., and Valdini, A. (1992). Xerostomia in diabetes mellitus. *Diabetes Care* 15: 900–904.

3 Wolff, A. (2017). A guide to medications inducing salivary gland dysfunction, xerostomia, and subjective sialorrhea: a systematic review sponsored by the World Workshop on Oral Medicine VI. *Drugs R&D* 17: 1–28.

4 Wu, A.J. and Ship, J.A. (1993). A characterization of major salivary gland flow rates in the presence of medications and systemic diseases. *Oral Surg. Oral Med. Oral Pathol.* 76: 301–306.

5 Zenk, J., Koch, M., Klintworth, N. et al. (2012). Sialendoscopy in the diagnosis and treatment of sialolithiasis: a study on more than 1000 patients. *Otolaryngol. Head Neck Surg.* 147: 858–863.

6 Bryan, R.N., Miller, R.H., Ferreyro, R.I., and Sessions, R.B. (1982). Computed tomography of the major salivary glands. *Am. J. Roentgenol.* 139: 547–554.

7 Huoh, K.C. and Eisele, D.W. (2011). Etiologic factors in sialolithiasis. *Otolaryngol. Head Neck Surg.* 145: 935–939.

8 Paterson, J.R. and Murphy, M.J. (2001). Bones, groans, moans... and salivary stones? *J. Clin. Pathol.* 54: 412.

9 Ellies, M., Laskawi, R., Arglebe, C., and Schott, A. (1996). Surgical management of nonneoplastic diseases of the submandibular gland. A follow-up study. *Int. J. Oral Maxillofac. Surg.* 25: 285–289.

10 Abdullah, A. (2013). Imaging of the salivary glands. *Semin. Roentgenol.* 48: 65–74.

11 Alyas, F., Lewis, K., Williams, M. et al. (2005). Diseases of the submandibular gland as demonstrated using high resolution ultrasound. *Br. J. Radiol.* 78: 362–369.

12 Joshi, A.S. and Sood, A.J. (2014). Ultrasound-guided needle localization during open parotid sialolithotomy. *Otolaryngol. Head Neck Surg.* 151: 59–64.

13 Hasson, O. (2010). Modern sialography for screening of salivary gland obstruction. *J. Oral Maxillofac. Surg.* 68: 276–280.

14 Choi, J.-S. (2015). Usefulness of magnetic resonance sialography for the evaluation of radioactive iodine-induced sialadenitis. *Ann. Surg. Oncol.* 22 (Suppl 3): S1007–S1013.

15 Burke, C.J. (2011). Imaging the major salivary glands. *Br. J. Oral Maxillofac. Surg.* 49: 261–269.

16 Kagami, H. (2000). Salivary growth factors in health and disease. *Adv. Dent. Res.* 14: 99–102.

17 Eisele, D.W., Wang, S.J., and Orloff, L.A. (2010). Electrophysiologic facial nerve monitoring during parotidectomy. *Head Neck* 32: 399–405.

18 Hald, J. and Andreassen, U.K. (1994). Submandibular gland excision: short- and long-term complications. *ORL J. Otorhinolaryngol. Relat. Spec.* 56: 87–91.

19 McQuone, S.J. (1999). Acute viral and bacterial infections of the salivary glands. *Otolaryngol. Clin. North Am.* 32: 793–811.

20 Carlson, E.R. (2009). Diagnosis and management of salivary gland infections. *Oral Maxillofac. Surg. Clin. North Am.* 21: 293–312.

21 Lee, M.W., Bae, J.Y., Choi, J.H. et al. (2004). Cutaneous eosinophilic vasculitis in a patient with Kimura's disease. *J. Dermatol.* 31: 139–141.

22 Hviid, A., Rubin, S., and Muhlemann, K. (2008). Mumps. *Lancet* 371: 932–944.

23 Manson, A.L. (1990). Mumps orchitis. *Urology* 36: 355–358.

24 Ottaviani, F., Galli, A., Lucia, M.B., and Ventura, G. (1997). Bilateral parotid sialolithiasis in a patient with acquired immunodeficiency syndrome and immunoglobulin G multiple myeloma. *Oral Surg. Oral Med. Oral Pathol. Oral Radiol. Endod.* 83: 552–554.

25 Mandel, L., Kim, D., and Uy, C. (1998). Parotid gland swelling in HIV diffuse infiltrative CD8 lymphocytosis syndrome. *Oral Surg. Oral Med. Oral Pathol. Oral Radiol. Endod.* 85: 565–568.

26 Garg, R., Verma, S.K., Mehra, S., and Srivastawa, A.N. (2010). Parotid tuberculosis. *Lung India* 27: 253–255.

27 Kim, Y.H., Jeong, W.J., Jung, K.Y. et al. (2005). Diagnosis of major salivary gland tuberculosis: experience of eight cases and review of the literature. *Acta Otolaryngol.* 125: 1318–1322.

28 Roveda, S.I. (1973). Cervicofacial actinomycosis. Report of two cases involving major salivary glands. *Aust. Dent. J.* 18: 7–9.

29 Sharkawy, A.A. (2007). Cervicofacial actinomycosis and mandibular osteomyelitis. *Infect. Dis. Clin. North Am.* 21: 543–556, viii.

30 Li, T.J., Chen, X.M., Wang, S.Z. et al. (1996). Kimura's disease: a clinicopathologic study of 54 Chinese patients. *Oral Surg. Oral Med. Oral Pathol. Oral Radiol. Endod.* 82: 549–555.

31 Poate, T.W., Sharma, R., Moutasim, K.A. et al. (2008). Orofacial presentations of sarcoidosis – a case series and review of the literature. *Br. Dent. J.* 205: 437–442.

32 Turner, M.D. (2014). Salivary gland disease in Sjogren's syndrome: sialoadenitis to lymphoma. *Oral Maxillofac. Surg. Clin. North Am.* 26: 75–81.

33 Vitali, C., Bombardieri, S., Jonsson, R. et al. (2002). Classification criteria for Sjogren's syndrome: a revised version of the European criteria proposed by the American-European consensus group. *Ann. Rheum. Dis.* 61: 554–558.

34 Verstappen, G.M. (2017). The value of rituximab treatment in primary Sjögren's syndrome. *Clin. Immunol.* 182: 62–71.

35 Ferro, F. (2016). One year in review 2016: Sjögren's syndrome. *Clin. Exp. Rheumatol.* 34: 161–171.

36 Guzzo, M., Locati, L.D., Prott, F.J. et al. (2010). Major and minor salivary gland tumors. *Crit. Rev. Oncol. Hematol.* 74: 134–148.

37 Spiro, R.H. (1986). Salivary neoplasms: overview of a 35-year experience with 2,807 patients. *Head Neck Surg.* 8: 177–184.

38 Xiao, C.C., Zhan, K.Y., White-Gilbertson, S.J., and Day, T.A. (2016). Predictors of nodal metastasis in parotid malignancies: a National Cancer Data base study of 22,653 patients. *Otolaryngol. Head Neck Surg.* 154: 121–130.

39 Liu, Y., Li, J., Tan, Y.R. et al. (2015). Accuracy of diagnosis of salivary gland tumors with the use of ultrasonography, computed tomography, and magnetic resonance imaging: a meta-analysis. *Oral Surg. Oral Med. Oral Pathol. Oral Radiol.* 119 (238–245): e232.

40 Green, B., Rahimi, S., and Brennan, P.A. (2016). Salivary gland malignancies – an update on current management for oral healthcare practitioners. *Oral Dis.* 22: 735–739.

41 Howlett, D.C., Skelton, E., and Moody, A.B. (2015). Establishing an accurate diagnosis of a parotid lump: evaluation of the current biopsy methods – fine needle aspiration cytology, ultrasound-guided core biopsy, and intraoperative frozen section. *Br. J. Oral Maxillofac. Surg.* 53: 580–583.

42 Kim, M.J., Kim, J.S., Roh, J.L. et al. (2013). Utility of 18F-FDG PET/CT for detecting neck metastasis in patients with salivary gland carcinomas: preoperative planning for necessity and extent of neck dissection. *Ann. Surg. Oncol.* 20: 899–905.

43 Bell, R.B., Dierks, E.J., Homer, L., and Potter, B.E. (2005). Management and outcome of patients with malignant salivary gland tumors. *J. Oral Maxillofac. Surg.* 63: 917–928.

44 Armstrong, J.G., Harrison, L.B., Thaler, H.T. et al. (1992). The indications for elective treatment of the neck in cancer of the major salivary glands. *Cancer* 69: 615–619.

45 Han, M.W., Cho, K.J., Roh, J.L. et al. (2012). Patterns of lymph node metastasis and their influence on outcomes in patients with submandibular gland carcinoma. *J. Surg. Oncol.* 106: 475–480.

46 Licitra, L., Grandi, C., Prott, F.J. et al. (2003). Major and minor salivary glands tumours. *Crit. Rev. Oncol. Hematol.* 45: 215–225.

47 Bradley, P.J. and McGurk, M. (2013). Incidence of salivary gland neoplasms in a defined UK population. *Br. J. Oral Maxillofac. Surg.* 51: 399–403.

48 Seethala, R.R. (2017). Salivary gland tumors: current concepts and controversies. *Surg. Pathol. Clin.* 10: 155–176.

49 Yoo, G.H., Eisele, D.W., Askin, F.B. et al. (1994). Warthin's tumor: a 40-year experience at the Johns Hopkins Hospital. *Laryngoscope* 104: 799–803.

50 Batsakis, J.G. and El-Naggar, A.K. (1990). Warthin's tumor. *Ann. Otol. Rhinol. Laryngol.* 99: 588–591.

51 Chung, Y.F., Khoo, M.L., Heng, M.K. et al. (1999). Epidemiology of Warthin's tumour of the parotid gland in an Asian population. *Br. J. Surg.* 86: 661–664.

52 McHugh, J.B., Visscher, D.W., and Barnes, E.L. (2009). Update on selected salivary gland neoplasms. *Arch. Pathol. Lab. Med.* 133: 1763–1774.

53 Boahene, D.K., Olsen, K.D., Lewis, J.E. et al. (2004). Mucoepidermoid carcinoma of the parotid gland: the Mayo Clinic experience. *Arch. Otolaryngol. Head Neck Surg.* 130: 849–856.

54 McHugh, C.H., Roberts, D.B., El-Naggar, A.K. et al. (2012). Prognostic factors in mucoepidermoid carcinoma of the salivary glands. *Cancer* 118: 3928–3936.

55 Seethala, R.R., Hunt, J.L., Baloch, Z.W. et al. (2007). Adenoid cystic carcinoma with high-grade transformation: a report of 11 cases and a review of the literature. *Am. J. Surg. Pathol.* 31: 1683–1694.

56 Uemaetomari, I., Tabuchi, K., Tobita, T. et al. (2007). The importance of postoperative radiotherapy against polymorphous low-grade adenocarcinoma of the parotid gland: case report and review of the literature. *Tohoku J. Exp. Med.* 211: 297–302.

57 Paleri, V., Robinson, M., and Bradley, P. (2008). Polymorphous low-grade adenocarcinoma of the head and neck. *Curr. Opin. Otolaryngol. Head Neck Surg.* 16: 163–169.

14

Odontogenic Cysts and Odontogenic Tumors

Michael A. Gladwell, Nathan Adams, Bryan Trump and Leslie R. Halpern

Introduction

The World Health Organization (WHO) series on histologic and genetic typing of human tumors are updated approximately every 10 years for nearly every organ system. These reference books provide updated tumor classification schemes based on currently available data and diagnostic criteria, as well as an international standard for professionals. The WHO 4th edition of Head and Neck Tumors was published in January 2017 and it is the ninth volume in the 4th edition of the WHO series. The last effective WHO odontogenic cyst scheme was published in 1992. Therefore, the odontogenic cyst classification has been significantly updated since 1992 [1].

This chapter reviews a diverse array of common and uncommon odontogenic cysts and tumors. The clinical presentations, microscopic features, differential diagnosis, prognosis, and treatment are also described.

Basic Embryology

The embryologic cascades associated with tooth development involve a series of steps that follow a timeline with each based upon the previous one, forming a network that will allow for maturation of the enamel, dentin, and pulpal tissues. As tooth development proceeds, other mesenchymal elements will contribute to the layers and create what will be the mature dental structure. Figure 14.1 depicts a bell stage in tooth development that can give rise to a wide variety of odontogenic cysts and tumors due to the diversity of embryonic cells present. Specifically, odontogenic lesions can be a result of changes in ameloblasts, odontoblasts, and other mesenchymal elements that are programmed for normal dental structures.

Odontogenic Cysts

Odontogenic cysts constitute an important aspect of oral and maxillofacial pathology. Odontogenic cysts are encountered commonly in dental practice. They are identified during routine exams and can present with or without signs and symptoms. With rare exceptions, epithelium-lined cysts in bone are seen only in the jaws. Other than a few cysts that may result from the inclusion of epithelium along embryonic lines of fusion, most jaw cysts are lined by epithelium that is derived from odontogenic cysts [2]. Odontogenic cysts are subclassified as developmental or

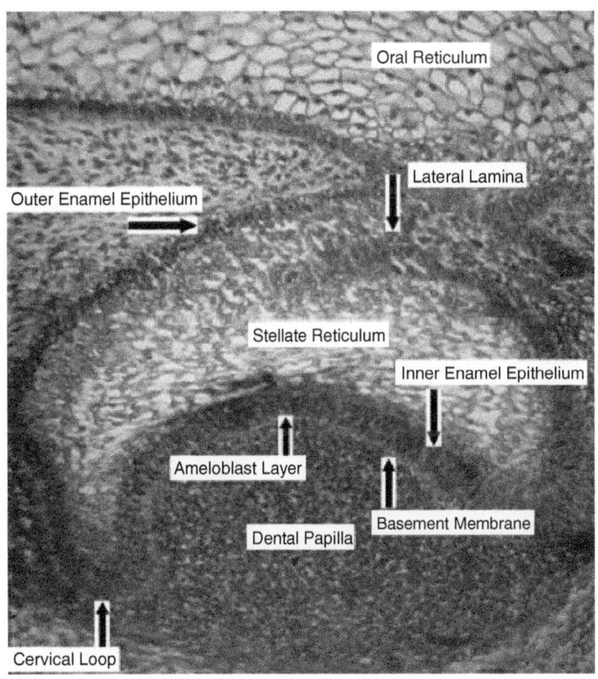

Figure 14.1 Bell stage in tooth development.

Oral and Maxillofacial Surgery, Medicine, and Pathology for the Clinician, First Edition. Edited by Harry Dym, Leslie R. Halpern, and Orrett E. Ogle.

Box 14.1 Classification of Odontogenic Cysts

Developmental origin

1. Dentigerous cyst
2. Odontogenic keratocyst (keratocystic odontogenic tumor)
3. Lateral periodontal and botryoid odontogenic cyst
4. Gingival cyst
5. Glandular odontogenic cyst
6. Calcifying odontogenic cyst
7. Orthokeratinized odontogenic cyst

Inflammatory origin

1. Periapical (radicular) cyst and residual cysts
2. Collateral inflammatory cyst

inflammatory in origin as depicted in Box 14.1. Developmental cysts are of varied embryonic origin but do not appear to be the result of inflammatory reactions. Inflammatory cysts are the result of inflammation [2].

Odontogenic Cysts of Inflammatory Origin

This group of lesions result from the proliferation of epithelium due to inflammation. The periapical (radicular) cyst is formed from inflammation due to a necrotic pulp.

Radicular Cysts

Radicular cysts are inflammatory odontogenic cysts, and overall account for greater than 50% of all the common cysts of the jaws [3]. They are most often associated with the apex of a nonvital tooth (Figure 14.2). A necrotic tooth associated with the cyst is a diagnostic criterion. Often, the tooth is carious or may have a history of trauma. Chronic inflammation in the periradicular tissues results in the periapical granuloma and stimulates the proliferation of the epithelial rests of Malassez. This results in a cavity in the osseous region apical to the necrotic tooth which becomes lined with epithelium. The cyst expansion occurs due to hydrostatic pressure as debris accumulates centrally. Radiographically, these are well-demarcated radiolucent lesions at the apex of a necrotic tooth.

Most of these cysts can be removed *in toto* or curetted out in multiple fragments. Occasional cholesterol deposits can

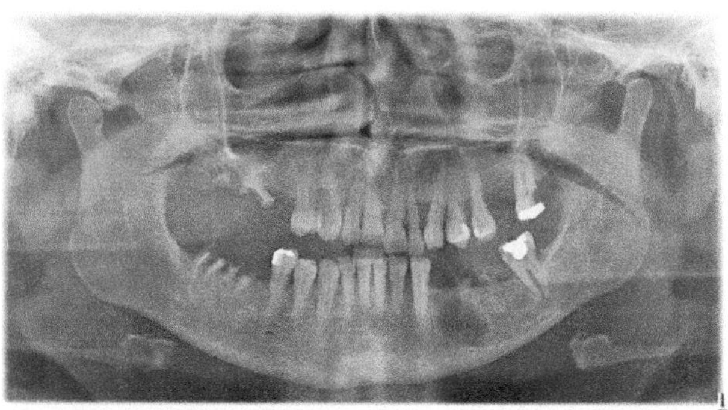

Figure 14.2 Radicular cyst.

be seen. These cysts can also be treated by conventional root canal therapy. Some will resolve while others can persist in the bone when the tooth is extracted. This is referred to as a residual cyst and is discussed in the next section.

Residual Cysts

Residual cysts are radicular cysts that remain in the maxillofacial region after the extraction of a tooth with a periapical cyst. The histopathologic features are the same as a residual cyst. Once the source of the inflammation has been removed, the cell wall will often become noninflamed and the cyst wall will thin (Figure 14.3). These mature noninflamed cysts can be mistaken for developmental odontogenic cysts. The radiographic and clinical history is important in these cases to determine that they are located at a site of a previous tooth extraction or previous tooth treated with root canal therapy. It should be treated by surgical enucleation or curettage.

Collateral Cysts

Collateral cysts occur on the lateral or buccal aspect of a partially erupted vital tooth. The pathogenesis of these cysts is not certain and there is controversy concerning their classification. The most common location is in the posterior mandible associated with partially erupted mandibular third molars. Inflammatory collateral cysts are divided into two main types. Paradental cysts are typically associated with partially erupted lower third molars. The other type occurs in children. The mandibular buccal bifurcation cyst is associated with the buccal aspect of erupting first molars [4].

Developmental Odontogenic Cysts

Developmental odontogenic cysts occur with no known clinical cause. These developmental cysts show some overlap in histopathologic features. This is particularly true with the presence of secondary inflammation. Therefore, histopathologic diagnosis may only be obtained after careful consideration of the clinical and radiographic evidence.

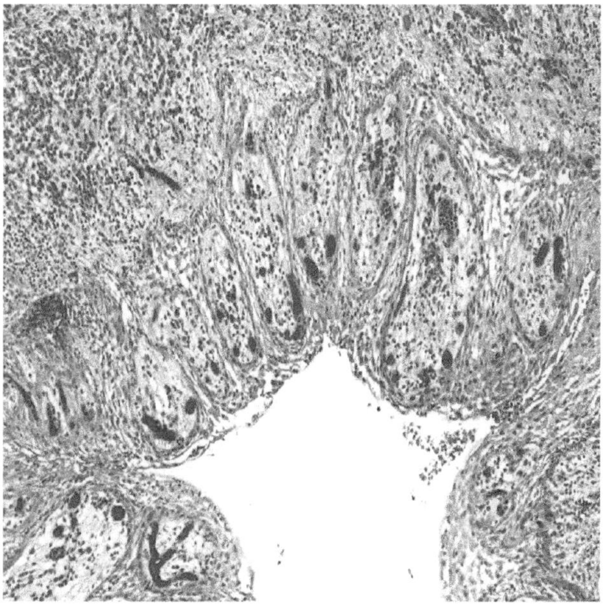

Figure 14.3 Histopathologic features of a residual cyst and a radicular cyst.

Dentigerous Cysts

Dentigerous cyst is the most common developmental cyst of the jaw. A typical dentigerous cyst presents clinically as an asymptomatic unilocular radiolucency enclosing the crown of an unerupted or impacted tooth; the radiolucency usually arises in the cementoenamel junction of the tooth (Figure 14.4). Although it can be associated with any unerupted tooth, the most common tooth is an unerupted mandibular third molar. In most cases, the diagnosis is straightforward, but even a radiographically typical dentigerous cyst can be found to be something else, such as a dental follicle, hyperplastic dental follicle, odontogenic keratocyst (keratocystic odontogenic tumor) or unicystic ameloblastoma [5, 6]. *De novo* dentigerous cysts can also transform into more serious lesions, such as an aggressive ameloblastoma, or present with mucus-containing cells indicative of a mucoepidermoid carcinoma [7].

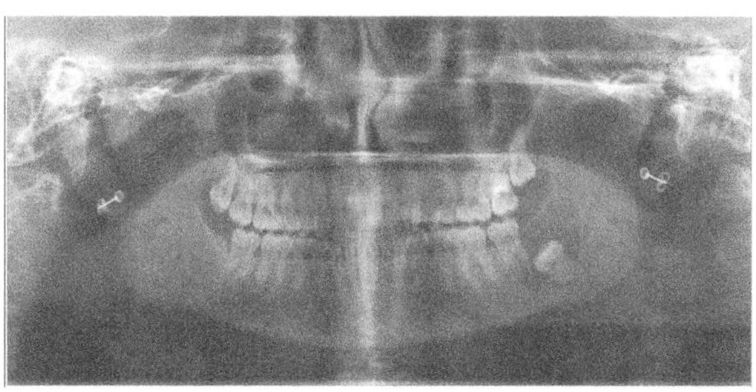

Figure 14.4 Dentigerous cyst.

Dentigerous cysts can mimic other lesions radiographically so histopathologic diagnosis of these lesions is critical [8]. Eruption cysts are dentigerous cysts associated with an unerupted tooth in a normal orientation and has the potential to erupt. This is found primarily in children and occurs twice as often in males as females. The cyst lining of a dentigerous cyst and its soft tissue counterpart (eruption cyst) consists of nonkeratinizing squamous epithelium (Figure 14.5). Often some oral epithelium is noted on the superior aspect of an eruption cyst as the roof of these cysts is usually excised. Treatment is not always required as the cyst may rupture spontaneously. If this does not occur, then simple excision of the roof of the cyst generally results in the eruption of the tooth.

Occasionally, there are cellular elements referred to as Rushton bodies (RBs) in the epithelial lining of odontogenic cysts, mainly radicular, dentigerous, and odontogenic keratocysts. It has two different histomorphological appearances: granular and homogeneous. Although widely speculated upon, the exact pathogenesis and histogenesis of RBs are still under debate [5–7].

The treatment of a dentigerous cyst consists of total enucleation. The pathologist must make sure that the entire cyst is examined since other pathology may be evident. An example is the unicystic ameloblastoma that is often associated with an impacted tooth and can be within the cystic lining of the dentigerous cyst. The most important consideration is to rule out other more aggressive odontogenic lesions such as an aggressive ameloblastoma or odontogenic keratocyst [8]. Cyst removal also includes the tooth and recurrence is rare.

Odontogenic Keratocyst (Keratocystic Odontogenic Tumor)

The odontogenic keratocyst (OKC) is classified as a developmental odontogenic cyst and is believed to arise from the

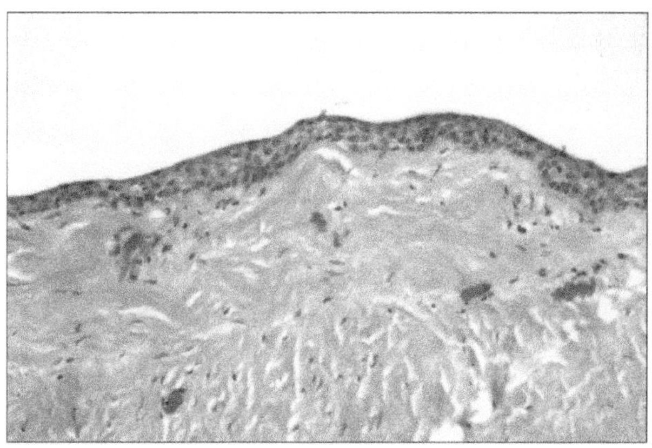

Figure 14.5 The cyst lining of a dentigerous cyst showing nonkeratinizing squamous epithelium.

rests of the dental lamina. Such cysts may be located anywhere in the tooth-bearing portions of the jaws. Most occur in the posterior mandible and ascending ramus; 25–40% are associated with impacted teeth and can resemble a dentigerous cyst on radiographic findings. Odontogenic keratocysts frequently mimic other pathologic entities, such as the dentigerous cyst, lateral periodontal cyst (LPC), and ameloblastoma. Smaller odontogenic keratocysts usually appear as asymptomatic unilocular radiolucencies with corticated borders; larger cysts may be multilocular, cause bony expansion, and be accompanied by pain (Figure 14.6). These lesions are more common in males than females, occur in a wide age range, and are typically diagnosed during the second, third or fourth decade of life [2].

In 2005, the WHO renamed the lesion previously known as an odontogenic keratocyst as the keratocystic odontogenic tumor (KOT or KCOT) [9]. The term "odontogenic keratocyst" was first used by Philipson in 1956 and its clinical and histologic features were confirmed by Browne in 1970 and 1971 [10, 11]. At that time, it was believed to be a benign but potentially aggressive and recurrent odontogenic cyst, and probably represented the lesion previously termed a primordial cyst. Although most of these cysts were lined by parakeratinized epithelium, a few were orthokeratinized. Over the years, it has generally been agreed that the orthokeratinized versions have a lower incidence of recurrence than the parakeratinized version. As initially described, it was believed that the primitive nature of the epithelium may have a premalignant potential, but this is now believed not to be true, and the incidence of malignant transformation is probably extremely low, if it exists at all.

This combination of features led to the 2005 reclassification of this lesion. Even the term KCOT refers only to the parakeratinized version of the odontogenic keratocyst, and this leaves the orthokeratinized version of the cyst without a new designation. Until further reclassification, these orthokeratinized cysts are grouped with other benign odontogenic cysts [12].

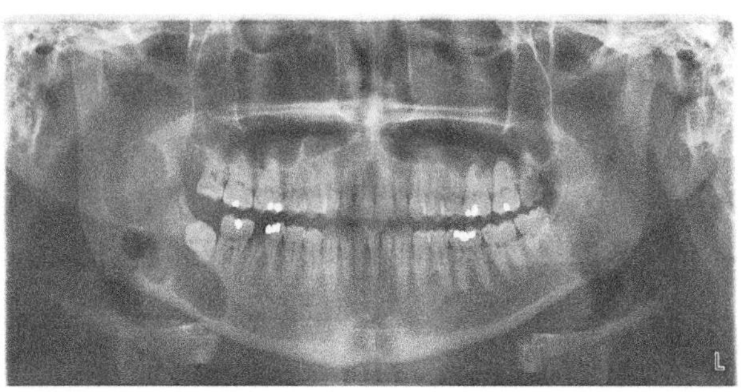

Figure 14.6 Odontogenic keratocyst showing multilocular pattern.

Although the presence of an odontogenic keratocyst may be suspected on clinical or radiographic features, histopathologic diagnosis is required. Grossly, the OKC has a thin friable wall that makes it challenging to enucleate completely. Figure 14.7 depicts the histologic criteria consisting of a uniform layer of stratified squamous epithelium of 5–8 layers in thickness. Below the epithelial lining is a connective tissue wall that is thin and can often separate from friable wall that makes it challenging to enucleate completely. It is often aspirated and the fluid has a creamy or cheesy consistency due to the keratin debris (Figure 14.8). A layer of parakeratin may be seen which indicates aggressive behavior versus orthokeratinized epithelium.

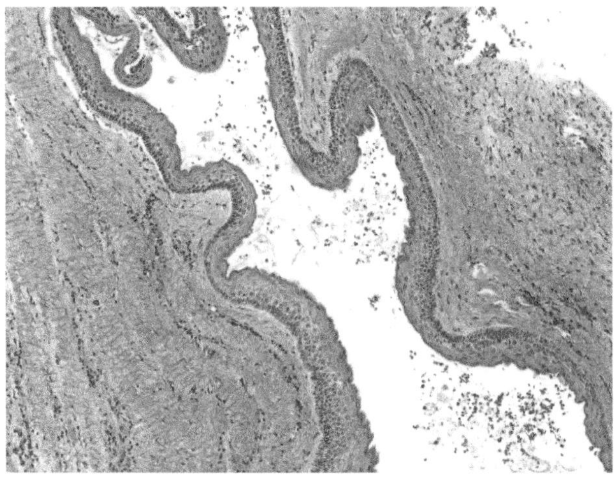

Figure 14.7 The histologic criteria of the odontogenic keratocyst consisting of a uniform layer of stratified squamous epithelium of 5–8 layers in thickness.

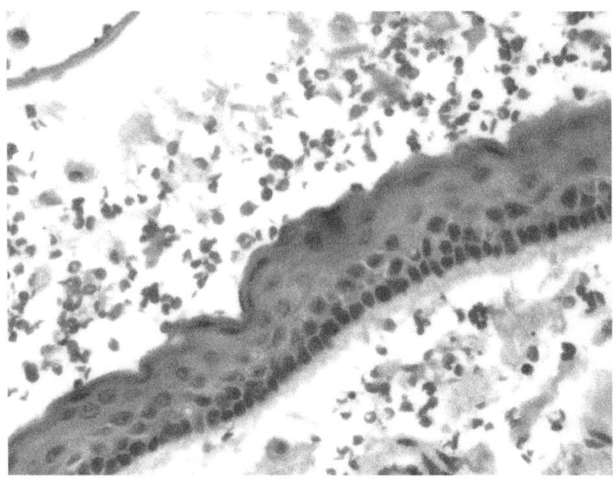

Figure 14.8 Odontogenic keratocyst. Below the epithelial lining is a connective tissue wall that is thin and can often separate from the epithelium. A layer of parakeratin may be seen which indicates aggressive behavior versus orthokeratinized epithelium.

Odontogenic keratocysts are treated similar to other odontogenic cysts which usually involves enucleation and curettage. Complete removal is difficult due to the thin, friable nature of the cyst lining. This also results in a higher recurrence rate of 25–55% [10–12]. Several reports that include a large number of cases indicate a recurrence rate of approximately 30% [2]. Many surgeons recommend peripheral ostectomy of the bony cavity with a bone bur to reduce the frequency of recurrence [2]. Overall prognosis is good.

Most larger OKC lesions require a decompression procedure with unroofing of the lesion and placement of a plastic tube that allows for daily irrigation to cause a metaplastic transformation of the histology into one that provides easier removal. The latter results in a thicker cyst lining and ability to remove more completely [12]. Although most OKCs occur in isolation, some are associated with a hereditary conditon referred to as Gorlin syndrome which is an autosomal dominant trait characterized by the PTCH gene mapped to chromosome 9q22,3-q31 [9]. Associated findings include frontal bossing, basal cell carcinomas of the skin, bifid ribs, calcification of the falx cerebri, and pitting palmar surfaces.

Treatment of cysts in the jaw is based upon acute presentation of pain or inability to chew (the reader is referred to the references for further interest).

Lateral Periodontal Cyst and Botryoid Odontogenic Cyst

The LPCs are developmental cysts thought to arise from rests of the dental lamina. Clinically, these are often incidental findings, usually presenting as well-demarcated unilocular radiolucencies seen between the roots of vital teeth in the mandibular canine to premolar region in 70% of cases (Figure 14.9) [13]. In the maxilla, they most frequently occur in the area of the canine and lateral incisor. Botryoid odontogenic cyst (BOC) is a multilocular variant of the LPCs, first described by Weathers and Waldron in 1973 [14].

The pathogenesis of the LPC and BOC is uncertain, although a number of possible sources of odontogenic epithelium, including the rests of Malassez and reduced enamel epithelium, have been ruled out as candidates [15]. BOCs preferentially involve the mandibular premolar and canine region, followed by the anterior region of the maxilla. They are characterized by multiple cystic spaces and variations in the thickness of the epithelial lining, unlike the LPC which is just a single cystic space. Histopathologic features consist of a thin fibrous wall, with an epithelial lining that is only a few cell layers thick. Some cysts show focal nodular thickenings of the lining epithelium (Figure 14.10). Treatment is usually conservative enucleation [16].

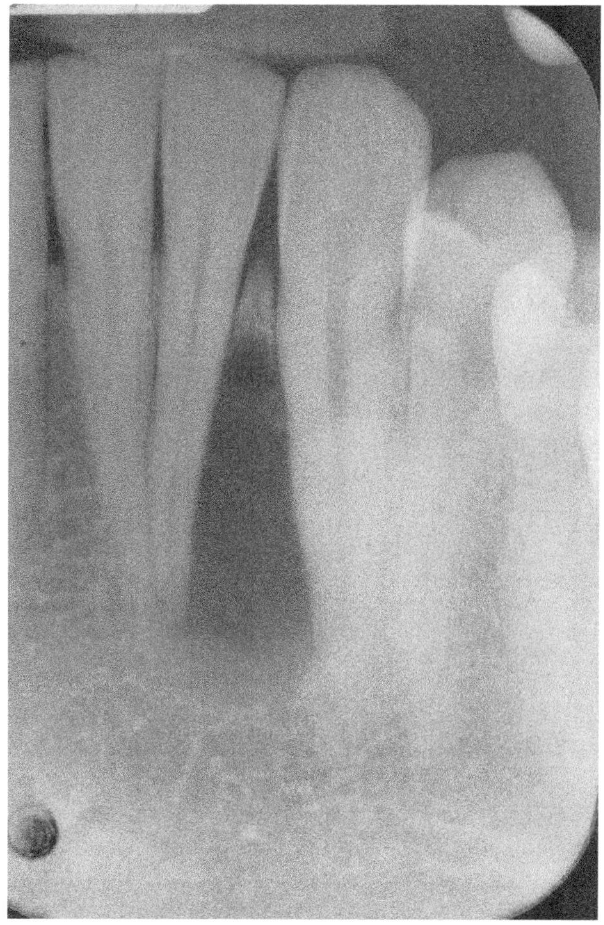

Figure 14.9 Lateral periodontal cysts.

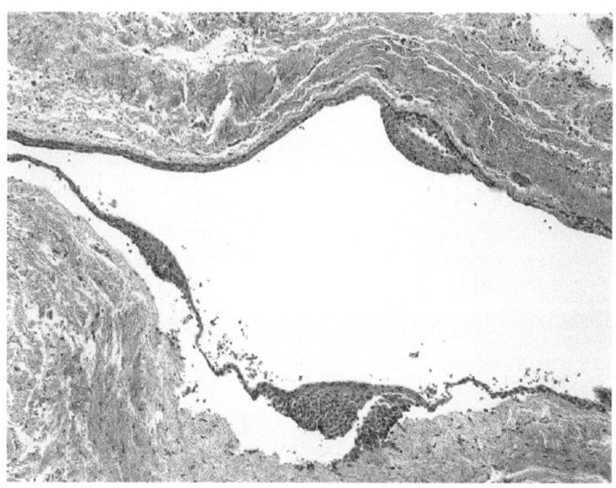

Figure 14.10 Histopathologic features consist of the lateral periodontal cyst showing a thin fibrous wall, with an epithelial lining that is only a few cell layers thick. Some cysts show focal nodular thickenings of the lining epithelium.

Gingival Cyst

Gingival cysts typically occur in two different age groups: gingival cyst of newborns and gingival cyst of adults.

Gingival Cyst of Newborns Gingival cyst of newborns, also known as dental lamina cyst, is a true cyst. It is lined by thin epithelium and shows a lumen usually filled with desquamated keratin, occasionally containing inflammatory cells [17]. These structures originate from remnants of the dental lamina and are located in the corium below the surface epithelium. The nodes are the result of cystic degeneration of epithelial rests of the dental lamina (rests of Serres). After the dental lamina invaginates to form the dental organ, the epithelial pedicle that connects the dental organ to the surface epithelium is broken down, giving rise to the rests of Serres. Occasionally, they may become large enough to be clinically noticeable as discrete white swellings on the ridges. The majority of these cysts degenerate and involute or rupture into the oral cavity within 2 weeks to 5 months of postnatal life [18, 19].

The diagnosis of gingival cyst must be differentiated from three other conditions, which are typically seen during the same time and possibly also have a location similarity. These are natal teeth, Epstein's pearls, and Bohn's nodules. Bohn's nodules, so called after his description of the same in 1866, are scattered over the junction of the hard and soft palate and are derived from minor salivary glands. Bohn also classified cysts in the alveolar ridges as mucous gland cysts. The mechanisms behind the disappearance of the cysts in postnatal life have been attributed to a discharge of cystic keratin at the time of fusion of the cyst walls with the oral epithelium. However, it has been suggested that part of the cystic epithelium may remain inactive even in the adult gingiva.

Gingival Cyst of Adults Gingival cyst of adults is an uncommon lesion. It is considered to represent the soft tissue counterpart of the LPC, being derived from the rests of the dental lamina (rests of Serres). The diagnosis of gingival cyst of the adult should be restricted to lesions with the same histopathologic features as the LPC. On rare occasions, a cyst may develop in the gingiva at the site of a gingival graft; however, such lesions probably represent epithelial inclusion cysts that are a result of the surgical procedure [2].

Glandular Odontogenic Cyst

The glandular odontogenic cyst (GOC), a relatively rare cyst occurring in the tooth-bearing areas, may be of salivary gland origin and has microscopic resemblance to the salivary gland tissue; hence the alternative term "sialoodontogenic cyst." The term GOC was first coined by Gardner [20]. It was later in 1992 that the WHO accepted the GOC as a distinct pathologic entity and included it in the classification as a developmental odontogenic cyst [21]. Histologically, it bears a resemblance to LPC, BOCs, radicular and residual cysts with mucous metaplasia, and low-grade mucoepidermoid carcinoma, thus posing a challenge in making the diagnosis.

Although rare, it has been noted that the GOC has aggressive potential, a high incidence of cortical perforation, and a relatively high rate of recurrence, especially in cases treated conservatively. The lesion is often characterized by squamous epithelium, mucin production, and glandular architecture that is similar to a low-grade mucoepidermoid carcinoma. Therefore, the correct diagnosis is a major challenge and is of extreme clinical importance [22].

The GOC has the potential for rapid growth and bony destruction and treatment consists of aggressive curretage and/or *en bloc* resection.

Calcifying Odontogenic Cyst

The calcifying cystic odontogenic tumor (CCOT), also known as calcifying odontogenic cyst (COC) or Gorlin cyst, is a rare developmental lesion which arises from odontogenic epithelium [23]. Although the lesion has been commonly recognized as a benign odontogenic cyst since Gorlin et al. first described it in 1962 [2], this pathologic entity encompasses a spectrum of clinical behavior and histopathologic features including cystic, solid (neoplastic), and aggressive (malignant) variants [2]. The *World Health Organization Classification of Head and Neck Tumors* classifies the lesion as an odontogenic tumor and names it CCOT [24].

The CCOT can occur in any location of the oral cavity and approximately 65–67.5% of cases occur in the anterior jaws (Figure 14.11) [2]. CCOTs occur with equal frequency in the maxilla and mandible [2] and demonstrate no gender predilection. The lesion occurs in a broad age group with a peak incidence in the second decade of life. The CCOT is believed to arise from odontogenic epithelial remnants trapped within the bones of the maxilla and mandible or gingival tissues, so they can develop either centrally (intraosseous) or peripherally (extraosseous) [25]. The majority of cases (86–98%) demonstrate a cystic architecture while the solid (neoplastic) form comprises 2–16% of cases [2]. Most CCOTs are asymptomatic, often discovered incidentally on radiographic exams. Because the lesion arises in tooth-bearing areas of the jaws or gingiva, they are often located in a periapical or lateral periodontal relationship to adjacent teeth.

Radiographically, CCOTs are well demarcated and appear as a unilocular or multilocular radiolucency [26] with calcifications of variable density noted in one-third to one-half of cases [2]. CCOTs can occur alone or in

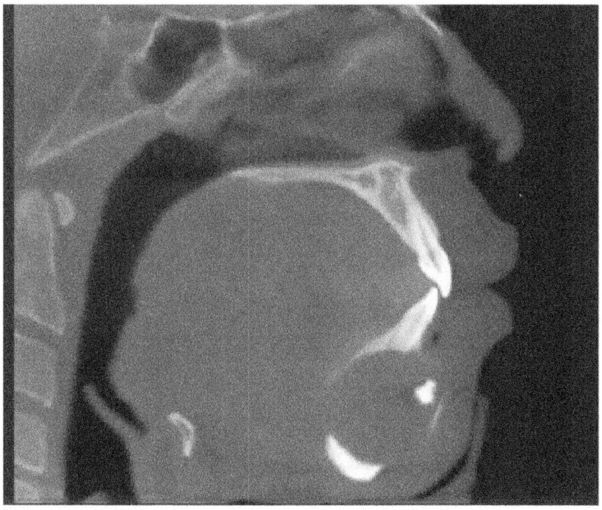

Figure 14.11 CT showing a calcifying odontogenic cyst in the anterior mandible.

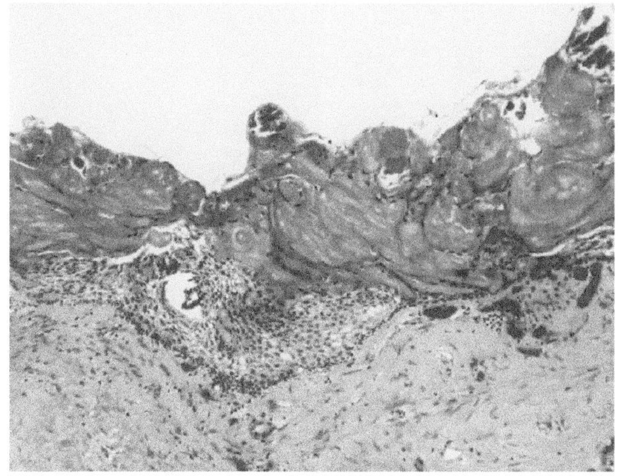

Figure 14.12 Histologic features of the calcifying odontogenic cyst showing a cyst lining composed of an outer layer of basaloid odontogenic epithelium and an inner layer resembling stellate reticulum of the enamel organ. Characteristic features also include the presence of ghost cells and/or calcifications within the cyst lining or fibrous capsule.

association with other odontogenic tumors such as odontomas (20%), adenomatoid odontogenic tumors, and ameloblastomas [2]. Root resorption and divergence are common radiographic findings [2] and an association with an impacted tooth occurs in approximately one-third of cases [2]. Asymptomatic swelling is a common presenting sign in both extraosseous and intraosseous locations, with expansion of the buccal and/or lingual cortical plates often occurring with the latter [24].

Histologic features include a cyst lining composed of an outer layer of columnar basaloid odontogenic epithelium and an inner layer resembling stellate reticulum of the enamel organ. Characteristic features for CCOT include the presence of ghost cells and/or calcifications within the cyst lining or fibrous capsule (Figure 14.12).

Enucleation is the treatment of choice for most intraosseous CCOTs with few recurrences reported in the literature [24]. The extraosseous form is treated with surgical excision and recurrences for this type have not been reported [2]. The prognosis for both intraosseous and extraosseous CCOTs is good.

Orthokeratinized Odontongenic Cyst

Orthokeratinized odontogenic cyst (OOC) occurs predominantly in young adults and shows a 2:1 male-to-female ratio [2]. The mandible is more commonly involved than the maxilla, the most common location being the mandibular molar and the ramus region (Figure 14.13) [27]. The size can vary from <1 cm to >7 cm in diameter [2]. OOCc appear clinically and radiographically representing a dentigerous cyst as they most often involve an unerupted mandibular third molar. Swelling is the most frequent symptom and is accompanied with pain although in most cases, the lesion is asymptomatic. Large lesions can cause cortical expansion [2].

Radiographically, the cyst appears as a well-circumscribed, unilocular, or multilocular radiolucency that occasionally is associated with an unerupted tooth or with the root, without causing resorption. Both the OOC and KCOT show similar findings clinically regarding age, sex, and site of occurrence but OOCs are generally solitary asymptomatic lesions whereas KCOT associated with nevoid basal cell carcinoma syndrome exhibits multiple lesions.

Histologically, OOCs have a thin lining with a flat orthokeratinized stratified squamous epithelium, a prominent granular cell layer, and a flat epithelium connective tissue interface (Figure 14.14) [28]. Basal cells are flat or low cubiodal and not palisaded compared with the KCOT which has a parakeratinized squamous-lined cyst with a palisaded basal layer and a corrugated surface [29]. Satellite or daughter cysts which are common in KCOT are not seen in OOCs [28].

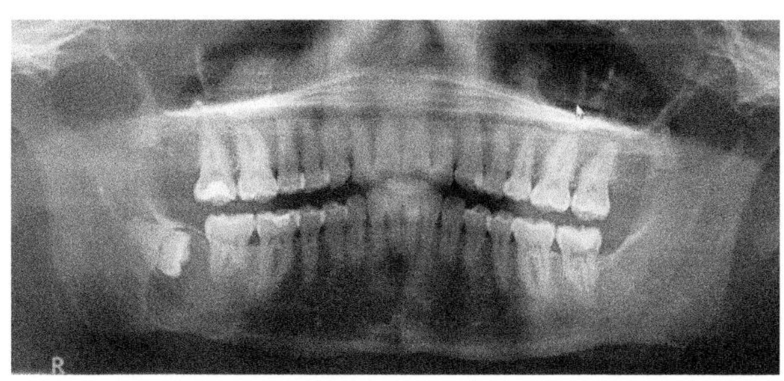

Figure 14.13 Orthokeratinized odontogenic cyst in the mandibular molar region.

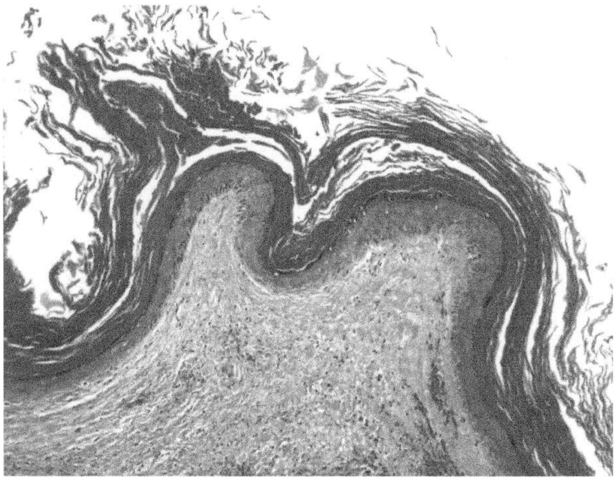

Figure 14.14 Orthokeratinized odontogenic cyst showing a thin epithelial lining of flat orthokeratinized stratified squamous epithelium, a prominent granular cell layer, and a flat epithelium–connective tissue interface.

Keratocystic odontogenic tumor is also called parakeratinized OKC [29]. OOC was more often associated with an impacted tooth (75.7%), when compared with 47.8% for the parakeratinized OKC. Recurrence is seen in 42.6% of parakeratinized OKC cases, compared with only 2.2% for OOC. Due to the less aggressive clinical behavior and recurrence pattern of the orthokeratinized variant, the designation of the orthokeratinized variant warranted a separate entity, "OOC" [30]. Recent immunohistochemical studies comparing OOCs with KCOTs have shown distinct differences in the expression of Ki-67 proliferative index, p53, p63, and bcl-2. Reduced expression of all these markers in OOCs suggests that they have a different cell differentiation and exhibit lower cellular activity than the KCOT tumor [27].

Surgical enucleation with curettage is the treatment of choice for the OOC. Peripheral ostectomy of bony cavity and chemical cauterization with Carnoy's solution is advocated for KCOT due to high recurrence rate [2].

Odontogenic Tumors

The topic of odontogenic tumors covers a broad and extensive group of pathologic lesions, including hamartomas and neoplasms. Great detail is possible regarding the variants of each specific entity, but the goal of this section is to provide the clinician with succinct relevant information for the most common odontogenic tumors by focusing on clinical presentation, histologic features, and treatment (Box 14.2).

Ameloblastoma

Ameloblastic lesions typically present in an asymptomatic fashion. It is unusual to present with any pain or paresthesia associated with this lesion. Therefore, discovery of this tumor is typically a result of expansile extraoral or intraoral swelling or as an incidental finding on routine dental radiographs. Patients are often in their 30s and the condition is suggested to occur with increased frequency in African-Americans [31]. Patients will often present with a painless hard swelling These lesions often exhibit locally aggressive behavior and can spread from the hard tissue to soft tissue surroundings [32, 33]. In dentate areas, ameloblastomas have been noted to cause root resorption (Figure 14.15). This is an important factor to note as unicystic variants of this tumor are more commonly thought to be either dentigerous cysts or odontogenic keratocysts, both of which rarely result in root resorption. Age predilection does not exist with this lesion and it can occur at any age. The lesion can also occur in both the mandible and maxilla although it occurs more frequently in the mandible.

Box 14.2 Odontogenic Tumors

Tumors of odontogenic epithelium

1. Ameloblastoma: malignant ameloblastoma, ameloblastic carcinoma
2. Clear cell odontogenic carcinoma
3. Adenomatoid odontogenic tumor
4. Calcifying epthelial odontogenic tumor
5. Squamous odontogenic tumor

Mixed odontogenic tumors

1. Ameloblastic fibroma
2. Ameloblastic fibrosarcoma
3. Ameloblastic fibroodontoma
4. Odontoameloblastoma
5. Compound odontoma
6. Complex odontoma
7. Calcifying cystic odontogenic tumor/dentinogenic ghost cell tumor; ghost cell odontogenic carcinoma

Tumors of odontogenic ectomesenchyme

1. Odontogenic fibroma
2. Central granular cell odontogenic tumor
3. Odontogenic myxoma

Source: Chi AC, Neville BW 2011/Elsevier.

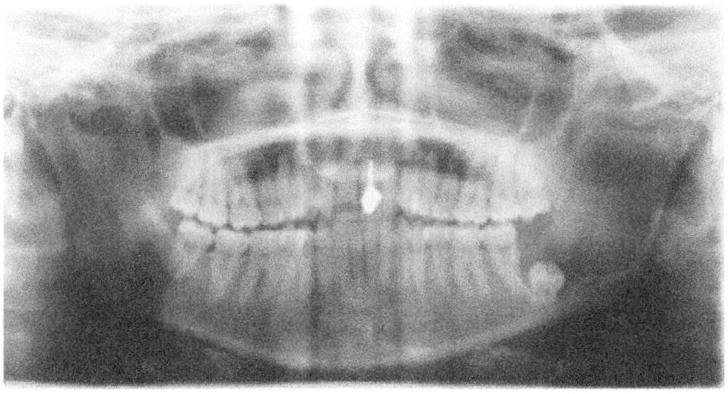

Figure 14.15 Ameloblastoma of posterior mandible with root resorption.

Histologic Features

The major clinicopathologic subtypes of ameloblastoma are solid, multicystic, unicystic, and peripheral, with over 90% representing the multicystic or solid type [31]. There are two main histologic variants, the plexiform and follicular types. Both variants contain mature fibrous stroma, with the plexiform variant presenting with strands of epithelium dispersed throughout the stroma while the follicular type forms epithelial islands (Figure 14.16). The common feature of ameloblastoma is the palisading columnar and cuboidal epithelium with the nuclei polarized away from the basement membrane [32]. Other histologic subtypes of ameloblastoma include the desmoplastic variant, granular cell variant, basal cell variant, and acanthomatous variant. The microscopic cellular type has no bearing on treatment and prognosis (see below). The reader is referred to reference #34 for further interest.

Treatment Considerations

Ameloblastoma is notorious for its aggressive nature despite being a benign tumor. This lesion has a low-grade malignant potential which has created great controversy as well as confusion regarding treatment. Carlson and Marx presented an excellent review of management strategies [33]. This malignant potential coupled with the lesion's predilection for microcystic satellite formation beyond the bone–tumor interface creates a need for more aggressive and definitive treatment. While more conservative methods of treatment such as enucleation, curettage, and peripheral ostectomy have been utilized, reported success rates are naturally lower than for definitive resection of the tumor.

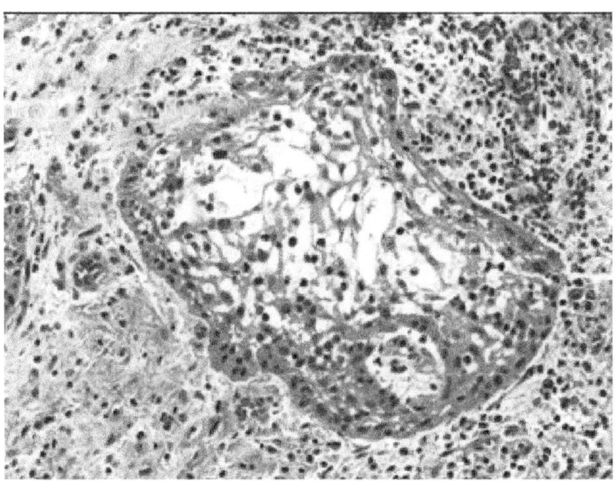

Figure 14.16 Follicular variant of ameloblastoma with epithelial islands.

It is the opinion of the authors that a diagnosis of ameloblastoma should not immediately lead to large resection and subsequent reconstruction. Each case should be evaluated individually to provide the patient with the best potential outcome. The morbidity of resection and reconstruction, despite the highest cure rate, with vascularized and nonvascularized tissues should not be underestimated and should be taken into consideration of the patient's long-term outlook. Therefore, age of patient, location, size, medical comorbidities, and options for reconstruction must be considered when planning treatment of these cases

Calcifying Epithelial Odontogenic Tumor

Clinical Presentation

Calcifying epithelial odontogenic tumor (CEOT), also referred to as a Pinborg tumor, is an uncommon tumor and there is a paucity of published cases [31, 34]. CEOT is a benign neoplasm typically occurring in adults during the second to fifth decades of life. The mandible is affected 70% of the time. It presents as a slow-growing mass, remaining undiagnosed until the swelling becomes visible or until appearance on radiographs is noted. Radiographic appearance is variable but typically presents with scattered radiopacities and radiolucencies throughout a well-circumscribed lesion, expansile in nature, causing thinning of the surrounding bone, and can be associated with impacted teeth (Figure 14.17) [3].

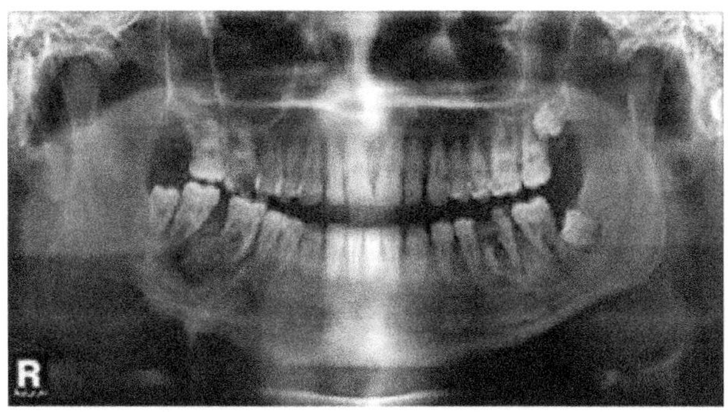

Figure 14.17 Calcifying epithelial odontogenic tumor with scattered radiopacities and radiolucencies throughout a well-circumscribed lesion.

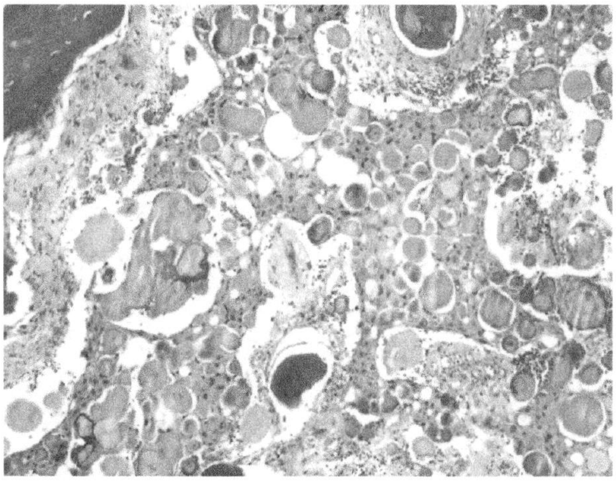

Figure 14.18 CEOT with polyhedral epithelial cells and a well-defined border and intracellular bridges.

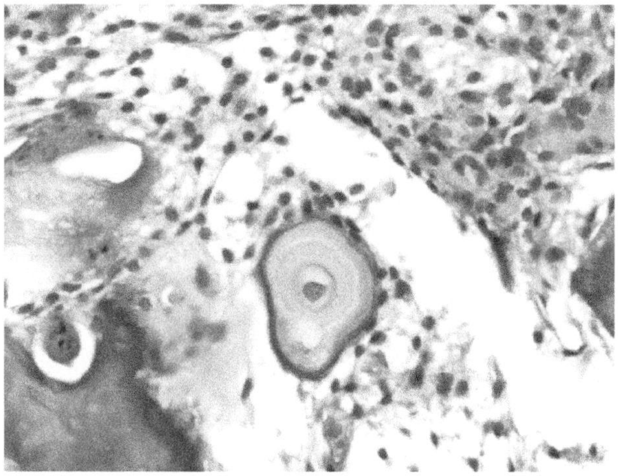

Figure 14.19 CEOT containing cells with calcified material, referred to as Liesegang rings.

Histologic Features

Histologic features of a CEOT include polyhedral epithelial cells with well-defined borders and the presence of intracellular bridges (Figure 14.18). There is often a homogeneous amyloid substance throughout the lesion. Cells containing a calcified material, referred to as Liesegang rings, are pathognomonic of this tumor (Figure 14.19) [4].

Treatment Considerations

An important feature to consider during treatment planning is that although the CEOT appears well circumscribed radiographically, it is not well encapsulated but clinically infiltrative. For this reason, enucleation and curettage alone is associated with the highest recurrence rate. Thus peripheral or marginal ostectomy is required at the time of definitive treatment. As in the case of ameloblastomas, treatment should be influenced by the specific nature and location of the tumor. It can be mistaken for a carcinoma and as such, routine annual follow-up is essential with radiographic surveying as recurrence can occur up to several years following treatment [5, 34].

Adenomatoid Odontogenic Tumor

Clinical Presentation

An adenomatoid odontogenic tumor (AOT) is a lesion that can present in almost any decade of life with a slight maxillary over mandible predilection. AOT typically presents as a slow-growing asymptomatic mass, commonly found incidentally on radiographs of the region (Figure 14.20). Radiographic appearance typically presents with a well-circumscribed radiolucency in a pear shape. It can lie between divergent roots, as a unilocular lesion or associated with an impacted tooth. Small calcifications, radiopacities, are commonly encountered radiographically with this lesion. Root resorption is possible but considered rare.

Histologic Features

Histologically, the lesion is well encapsulated by a fibrous capsule with enlarging odontogenic epithelium protruding from the capsule and filling the lumen of the cavity. This intralesional tissue consists of aggregates of spindle-shaped cells (Figure 14.21).

Treatment Considerations

Due to the well-encapsulated nature of an AOT with it fibrous capsule, treatment typically consists of conservative management with enucleation. Ample visibility by adequate flap reflection is required to ensure full enucleation and prevent tearing of the capsule. Gentle curettage and copious irrigation are also recommended. Recurrence rates following enucleation are extremely low [35].

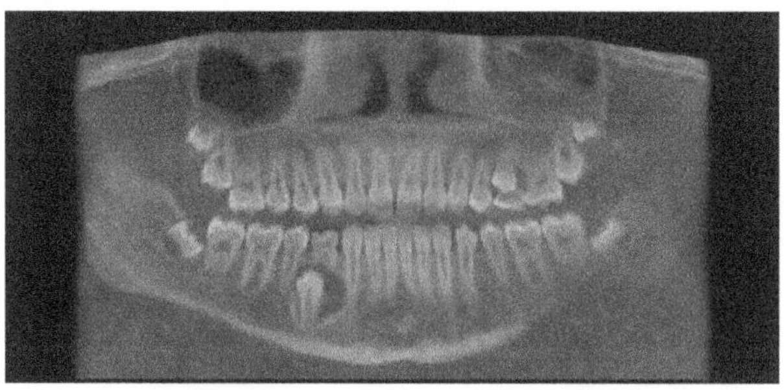

Figure 14.20 Radiograph of adenomatoid odontogenic tumor with a well-circumscribed unilocular radiolucency in a pear-shaped lesion or associated with an impacted tooth.

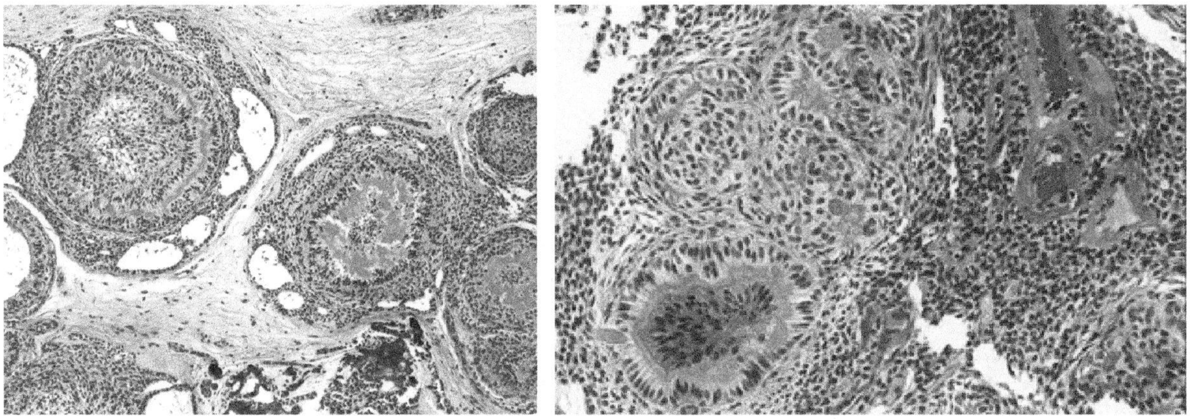

(a) (b)

Figure 14.21 (a, b) Histologically, the adenomatoid odontogenic tumor is well encapsulated by a fibrous capsule with enlarging odontogenic epithelium protruding from the capsule to fill the lumen of the cavity. This intralesional tissue consists of aggregates of spindle-shaped cells.

Squamous Odontogenic Tumor

Clinical Presentation

Squamous odontogenic tumor (SOT) is a relatively uncommon tumor that arises from a proliferation of squamous epithelium originating from both remnants of dental lamina and the rests of Malassez. It is a benign entity most often localized intraosseously (see below) but can be locally infiltrative along the lateral surfaces of adjacent roots (see below) [31]. There is no significant age predilection and the lesion can occur in both the maxilla and mandible. A common complaint is a painless swelling in the alveolar process surrounding the teeth. SOT can be found as a single lesion or in multiple locations of both jaws. Radiographically, it presents as a unilocular radiolucency, appearing as an osseous defect between the roots of adjacent teeth, that can result in root divergence.

Histologic Features

Histologically, SOT consists of a bland squamous epithelium in a cellular fibrous stroma. The epithelium is arranged in islands that can vary in shape and size. These epithelial islands can reveal penetration of the connective tissue wall at the bone interface (Figure 14.22) [7]. This feature, if present histopathologically, becomes clinically significant and would understandably lead the practitioner to consider additional peripheral ostectomy.

Treatment Considerations

Squamous odontogenic tumors are typically amenable to curettage, enucleation or local excision. However, if a preoperative biopsy or fresh frozen pathology reveals a diagnosis of SOT, consideration should be given to performing a thorough curettage of the area as well. If the SOT penetrates the osseous structure, it is recommended to include the overlying tissue in the excision due to the infiltrative nature of the lesion. Recurrence is rare.

Odontogenic Fibroma

Clinical Presentation

Odontogenic fibroma is a rare mesenchymal tumor made up of ectomesenchyme and occasional odontogenic epithelium. It most often occurs during the second or third decade of life with a female prevalence. It can arise in the anterior region of either the maxilla or mandible [31, 36]. The tumor is typically noted on routine radiography as a well-circumscribed radiolucency. It can occur within the bone or on the gingiva. Root resorption is common with this lesion.

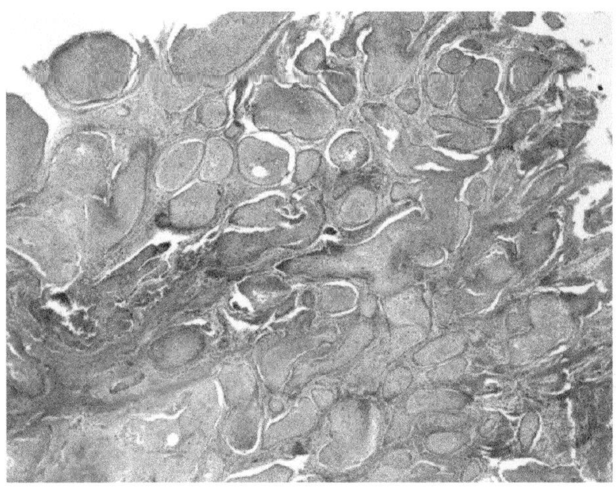

Figure 14.22 Squamous odontogenic tumor.

Histologic Features

The WHO characterizes two histologic variants. Microscopically, odontogenic fibromas consist of fibrous connective tissue with long strands of odontogenic epithelium with varying degrees of cellularity ranging from low to moderate (Figure 14.23) [31, 36].

Treatment Considerations

Surgical removal of odontogenic fibromas is typically straightforward with little attachment to the surrounding bone lending itself to easily enucleation. Enucleation is the treatment of choice for these tumors. Recurrence is rare and the long-term prognosis is excellent [31, 36, 37].

Cementoblastoma

Clinical Presentation

Cementoblastoma is a rare benign neoplasm that is formed by tissue of cementum origin. The defining clinical and radiographic characteristic is a budding nodular mass directly attached to the root of the tooth. Radiographically, the periodontal ligament space goes around the mass attached to the root [12].

Histologic Features

Microscopically, cementoblastoma appears as a calcified mass with sheets of cementum attached to the root structure. The cementoblasts are present throughout a loose connective tissue fibrous stroma with columns of unmineralized tissue oriented in a perpendicular fashion around the periphery (Figure 14.24) [13].

Treatment Considerations

The treatment of choice is excision of the mass with extraction of the affected tooth. Curettage can also be performed to decrease the overall recurrence, but the literature does not definitively support this practice. Increased recurrence has been reported if the affected tooth is left in place following excision [14].

Odontogenic Myxoma

Clinical Presentation

Odontogenic myxoma is a benign, locally aggressive tumor occuring in the maxilla and mandible. Typically, this tumor presents with localized pain and swelling in the orofacial complex. Radiographically, odontogenic myxoma can present with a unilocular or multilocular radiolucency with a honeycomb, ground-glass appearance throughout the lesion with ill-defined borders [15].

Histologic Features

Microscopically, odontogenic myxomas typically consist of stellate to spindle-shaped cells in a loose connective tissue stroma (Figure 14.25). A few cells spread throughout a homogeneous stroma is common [16].

Treatment Considerations

Odontogenic myxomas are locally expansile and aggressive tumors despite being benign. Much debate exists among surgeons as to the ideal treatment method for these tumors to remove the pathology and mitigate risk of recurrence. Some surgeons advocate a more conservative method of treatment consisting of enucleation and peripheral ostectomy. However, due to the microscopic nature of this tumor and its invasion into the marrow spaces of the bone, higher recurrence rates have been reported. Definitive treatment consisting of resection of the mass with 1 cm margins has been shown to have the lowest recurrence rate, but often results in significant morbidity.

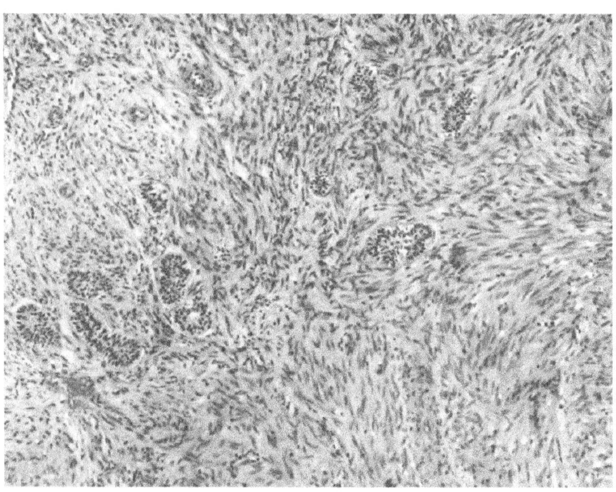

Figure 14.23 Odontogenic fibroma.

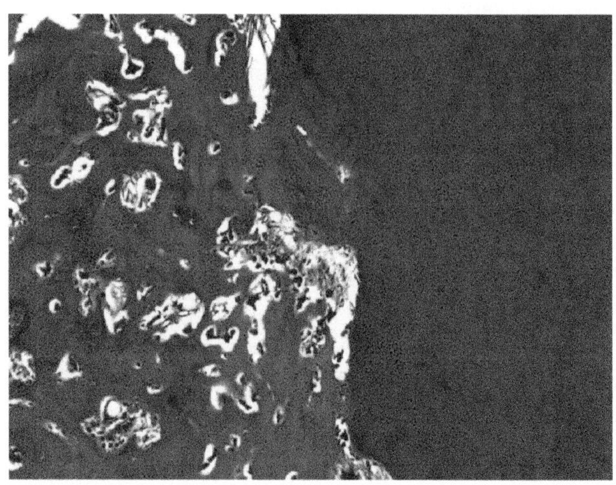

Figure 14.24 Cementoblastoma.

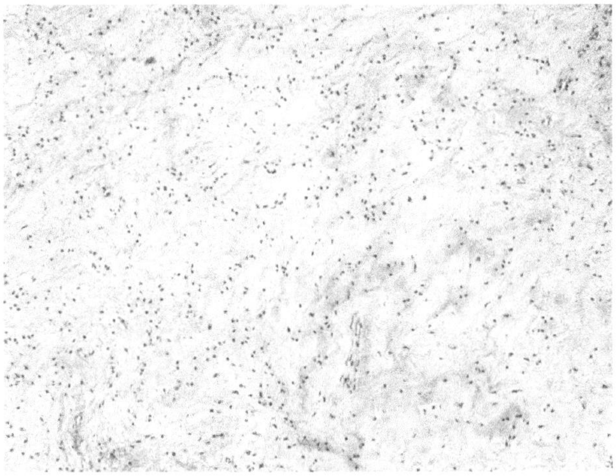

Figure 14.25 Odontogenic myxomas consisting of stellate to spindle-shaped cells in a loose connective tissue stroma.

This morbidity of resection and reconstruction, despite a lower recurrence rate, should not be underestimated and careful consideration should be given in each situation.

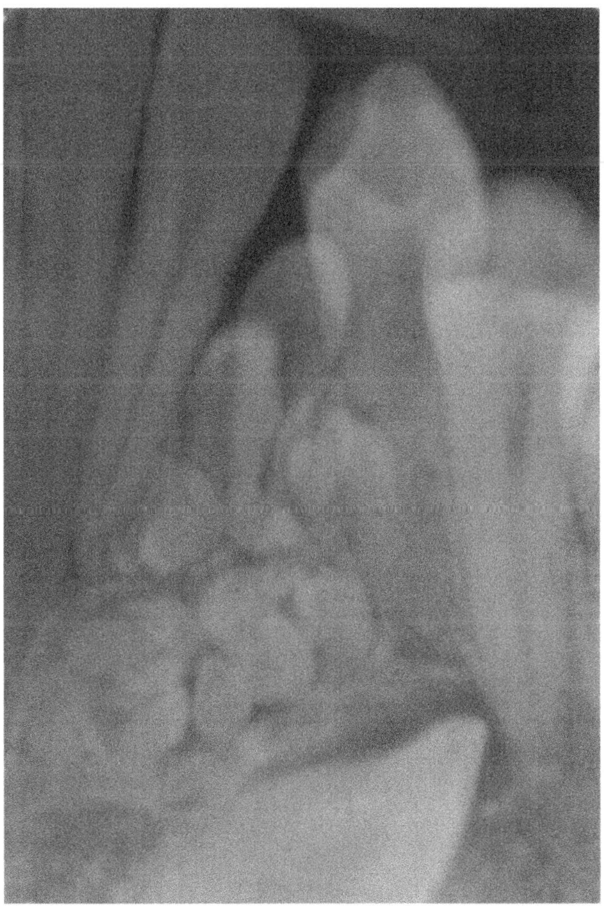

Figure 14.26 Compound odontoma.

Age, location, and size are all contributing factors when treatment method is being determined.

Odontoma

Clinical Presentation

Odontomas are odontogenic tumors that arise from abnormal dental developmental tissues. There are two clinical variants: compound and complex. Compound odontomas give rise to small tooth-like structures whereas complex odontomas form an irregular calcified mass. Clinically, these tumors are slow growing and typically asymptomatic and typically diagnosed on routine radiographs in the dental office. Radiographic presentation is a well-circumscribed radiolucency with multiple radiopacities in the compound variant and an irregular, disorganized radiopacity [17].

Histologic Features

Microscopically, compound odontomas present with aspects of demineralized dental tissues including enamel, dentin, and cementum (Figure 14.26). Complex odontomas present in a very disorganized fashion with variation of dental tissues present (Figure 14.27) [18].

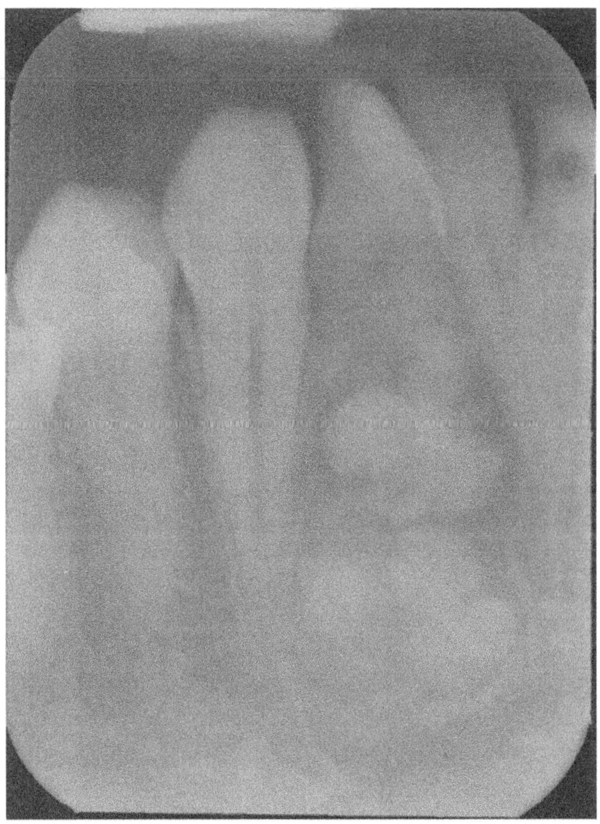

Figure 14.27 Complex odontoma.

Treatment Considerations

Due to the benign and nonaggressive nature of these tumors, conservative management of enucleation and curettage is typically recommended with extremely low rates of recurrence [19]. Care should be taken not to compromise adjacent teeth or injure vital structures.

References

1 Soluk-Tekkesin, M. and Wright, J.M. (2018). The World Health Organization classification of odontogenic lesions: a summary of the changes of the 2017 (4th) edition. *Turk. J. Pathol.* 34 (1): https://doi.org/10.5146/tjpath.2017.01410.

2 Neville, B.W., Damm, D.D., Allen, C.M., and Chi, A.C. (2016). *Oral and Maxillofacial Pathology*. St Louis, MO: Elsevier.

3 Jones, A., Craig, G., and Franklin, C. (2006). Range and demographics of odontogenic cysts diagnosed in a UK population over a 30-year period. *J. Oral Pathol. Med.* 35: 500–507.

4 El-Naggar, A.K., Chan, J.K.C., Grandis, J.R. et al. (ed.) (2017). *World Health Organization Classification of Head and Neck Tumours*, 4e, 232–242. Lyon: IARC.

5 Dunsche, A., Babendererde, O., Lüttges, J., and Springer, I.N. (2003). Dentigerous cyst versus unicystic ameloblastoma – differential diagnosis in routine histology. *J. Oral Pathol. Med.* 32: 486–489.

6 Farah, C.S. and Savage, N.W. (2002). Pericoronal radiolucencies and the significance of early detection. *Aust. Dent. J.* 47: 262–265.

7 Nimonkar, P., Nimonkar, S., Mandlekar, G. et al. (2014). Ameloblastoma arising in a dentigerous cyst: report of three cases. *J. Oral Maxillofac. Surg. Med. Pathol.* 26 (2): 233–237.

8 Zhang, L.L., Yang, R., Zhang, L. et al. (2010). Dentigerous cyst: a retrospective clinicopathological analysis of 2082 dentigerous cysts in British Columbia, Canada. *Int. J. Oral Maxillofac. Surg.* 39: 878–882.

9 Philipsen, H.P., Barnes, L., Eveson, J.W. et al. (2005). *World Health Organization Classification of Tumours. Pathology and Genetics of Head and Neck Tumours*, 306–307. Lyon: IARC.

10 Browne, R.M. (1970). The odontogenic keratocyst. Clinical aspects. *Br. Dent. J.* 128: 225.

11 Browne, R.M. (1971). The odontogenic keratocyst. Histological features and their correlation with clinical behaviour. *Br. Dent. J.* 131: 249.

12 Pogrel, M. (2012). Keratocystic odontogenic tumor. In: *Current Therapy in Oral and Maxillofacial Surgery* (ed. S. Bagheri, R. Bell and H.A. Khan), 380–383. St Louis, MO: Elsevier.

13 Cohen, D.A., Neville, B.W., Damm, D.D. et al. (1984). The lateral periodontal cyst. A report of 37 cases. *J. Periodontol.* 55 (4): 230–234.

14 Weathers, D.R. and Waldron, C.A. (1973). Unusual multilocular cysts of the jaws (botryoid odontogenic cyst). *Oral Surg. Oral Med. Oral Pathol.* 36 (2): 235–241.

15 Carter, L.C., Carney, Y.L., and Perez-Pudlewski, D. (1996). Lateral peridontal cyst: multifactorial analysis of a previously unreported series. *Oral Surg. Oral Med. Oral Pathol.* 81: 210–216.

16 Padayache, A. and Van Wyk, C.W. (1987). Two cystic lesions with features of both the botryoid odontogenic cyst and the central mucoepidermoid tumor: sialo-odontogenic cyst? *J. Oral Pathol.* 16: 499–504.

17 Morelli, J.G. (2007). Disorders of the mucous membranes. In: *Nelson Textbook of Pediatrics*, 18e (ed. R.M. Kliegman, R.E. Behrman, H.B. Jenson and B.F. Staton), 663. Philadelphia, PA: Saunders Elsevier.

18 Flinck, A., Paludan, A., Matsson, L. et al. (1994). Oral findings in group of newborn Swedish children. *Int. J. Pediatr. Dent.* 4 (2): 67–73.

19 Regezi, J.A. (1999). Cyst of jaws and neck. In: *Oral Pathology: Clinical Pathological Correlation*, 4e (ed. J.A. Regezi, J.J. Sciubba and R.C. Jorden), 246. Philadelphia, PA: WB Saunders.

20 Gardner, D.G., Kessler, H.P., Morency, R., and Schaffner, D.L. (1988). The glandular odontogenic cyst: an apparent entity. *J. Oral Pathol.* 17: 359–366.

21 Shear, M. (1992). *Paul Speight Cyst of the Oral and Maxillofacial Region*, 3e. London: Butterworth Heinemann.

22 Kaplan, I., Anavi, Y., and Hirshberg, A. (2008). Glandular odontogenic cyst: a challenge in diagnosis and treatment. *Oral Dis.* 14: 575–581.

23 Gorlin, R.L., Pindborg, J.J., Clausen, F., and Vickers, R.A. (1962). The calcifying odontogenic cyst – a possible analogue of the cutaneous calcifying epithelioma of Malherbe. *Oral Surg. Oral Med. Oral Pathol.* 15: 1235–1243.

24 Barnes, L., Everson, J.W., Reichart, P. et al. (2005). *World Health Organization Classification of Tumours: Pathology and Genetics of Head and Neck Tumours*, 313. Lyon, France: IARC Press.

25 Buchner, A. (1991). The central (intraosseous) calcifying odontogenic cyst: an analysis of 215 cases. *J. Oral Maxillofac. Surg.* 49: 330–339.

26 Iida, S., Fukuda, Y., Ueda, T. et al. (2006). Calcifying odontogenic cyst: radiologic findings in 11 cases. *Oral Surg. Oral Med. Oral Pathol. Oral Radiol. Endod.* 101 (3): 356–362.

27 Swain, N., Shilpa, P., Poonja, L.S. et al. (2012). Orthokeratinized odontogenic cyst. *J. Contemp. Dent.* 2: 31–33.

28 Marx, R.E. and Stern, D. (2012). Odontogenic and nonodontogenic cysts. In: *Oral and Maxillofacial Pathology a Rationale for Diagnosis and Treatment*, 2e, vol. II (ed. R.E. Marx), 616–631. China: Quintessence.

29 Robinson, R.A. (2010). Odontogenic lesions. In: *Head and Neck Pathology Atlas for Histologic and Cytologic Diagnosis*, 1e, 30–36. China: Lippincott Williams and Wilkins.

30 Hemavathy, S., Sahana, N.S., Kumar, V.D. et al. (2013). Orthokeratinized odontogenic cyst: a case report. *Arch. Oral Sci. Res.* 3: 144–150.

31 Chi, A.C. and Neville, B.W. (2011). Odontogenic cysts and tumors. *Surg. Pathol.* 4: 1027–1091.

32 Celur, S. and Babu, K. (2012). Plexiform ameloblastoma. *Int. J. Clin. Pediatr. Dent.* 5 (1): 78–83.

33 Carlson, E.R. and Marx, R.E. (2006). The ameloblastoma: primary, curative surgical management. *J. Oral Maxillofac. Surg.* 64 (3): 484–494.

34 Woods, M. and Reichart, P.A. Surgical management of nonmalignant lesions of the mouth. In: *Maxillofacial Surgery*, 3e, vol. 2 (ed. P. Brennan, H. Schliephake, G. Ghali and L. Cascarini), 1319–1334. Oxford: Churchill Livingstone.

35 Rick, G.M. (2004). Adenomatoid odontogenic tumor. *Oral Maxillofac. Clin. North Am.* 16: 333–354.

36 Dunlap, C.L. (1999). Odontogenic fibroma. *Semin. Diagn. Pathol.* 16: 293–296.

37 Eversole, L.R. (2011). Odontogenic fibroma including amyloid and ossifying variants. *Head Neck Pathol.* 5: 335–343.

15

Osteomyelitis of the Jaw

Junaid Mundiya and Harry Dym

Osteomyelitis is defined as an inflammatory process of the medullary portion of the affected bone but may also affect the periosteum and cortical plates. In the maxillofacial region, the mandible is the bone most frequently affected [1]. The maxilla has a high level of vascularity and thin cortical bone and is therefore less frequently involved [1].

Classification

Osteomyelitis can be classified as acute or chronic. The acute form is differentiated from the chronic form based on the time from initial diagnosis to treatment [2]. If the time between diagnosis and start of treatment is less than 1 month, it is acute osteomyelitis and if it is greater than a month it is classified as chronic osteomyelitis. The acute phase is a suppurative condition. Chronic osteomyelitis can be divided into chronic suppurative and chronic non-suppurative osteomyelitis [2].

Demographic Findings

Some studies have reported a higher male predilection. Others, however, have not found a male predilection to be conclusive due to limited number of patients in the studies [1, 3, 4]. The highest incidence of the disease is commonly reported in the fifth and sixth decades of life which can be associated with higher comorbidities and higher dental pathologies and complications [4, 5].

Clinical Presentation

Osteomyelitis is classically associated with deep, dull pain. The classic clinical presentation consists of pain, swelling, erythema, adenopathy, fever, paresthesia, trismus, and fistulae. Paresthesia can indicate pressure on the inferior alveolar nerve from the inflammatory process. Trismus can indicate inflammation of the muscles of mastication. Acute osteomyelitis is more commonly associated with swelling and erythema and can progress over days to weeks to manifest systemic symptoms such as fever, leukocytosis, lymphadenopathy, and swelling of the affected area [1]. Chronic osteomyelitis is a persistent infection which evolves over months to years [1]. It is characterized by low-grade inflammation, presence of dead bone (Figures 15.1 and 15.2), new bone apposition, and intraoral or extraoral fistulous tracts [1].

Chronic systemic diseases such as hypertension and diabetes can be contributing factors to chronic osteomyelitis and will complicate its treatment. Predisposing factors,

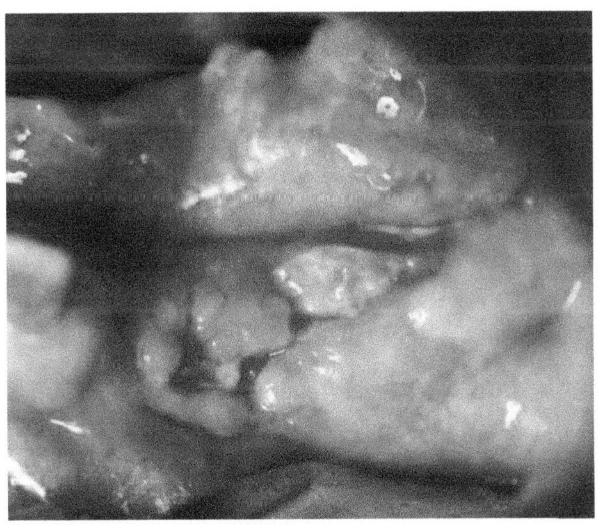

Figure 15.1 Exposed necrotic nonhealing bone of the left mandible. *Source:* Courtesy of H. Dym, DDS, Brooklyn, NY.

Oral and Maxillofacial Surgery, Medicine, and Pathology for the Clinician, First Edition. Edited by Harry Dym, Leslie R. Halpern, and Orrett E. Ogle.

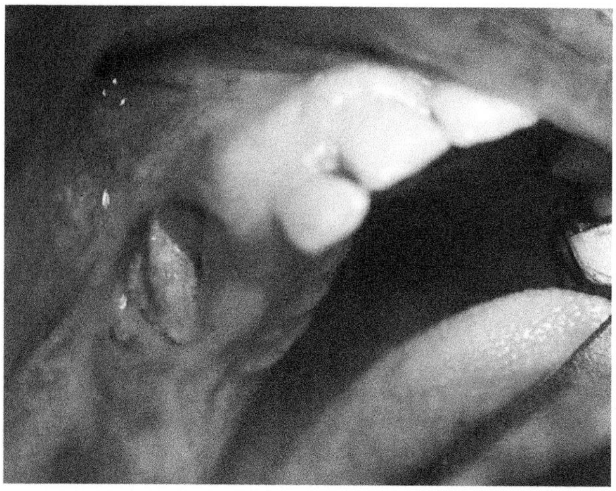

Figure 15.2 Necrotic bone. *Source:* Courtesy of H. Dym, DDS, Brooklyn, NY.

therefore, should be adequately addressed and treated [6]. Patients with hypertension and diabetes are known to show hypertrophic remodeling of the vasculature over time and as a result will have arterial stiffness and microvascular rarefaction to the organisms [1].

Laboratory Analysis

Leukocytosis with left shift is a common presentation with acute osteomyelitis, whereas with chronic osteomyelitis leukocytosis is uncommon. Classic lab values for patients with suspected osteomyelitis are elevated erythrocyte sedimentation rate (ESR) and C-reactive protein (CRP) [7]. The ESR and CRP levels are commonly used to monitor and detect inflammatory disorders [7]. These markers are not specific for any particular illness but correlate with inflammation [7]. CRP is a direct protein measurement whereas ESR is an indirect marker of serum acute-phase protein concentration [7]. ESR measurements can be elevated with conditions other than inflammation, but this is rare with CRP [7]. Since ESR and CRP are nonspecific, they are used as clinical markers for the progression of osteomyelitis. [7].

Radiologic Evaluation

Radiologic evaluation is an important adjunct to the clinical examination to diagnose and determine the extent of the disease. It can also aid in monitoring disease progression and guide treatment. Periapical, panoramic radiograph and cone beam computed tomography (CBCT) scans in a dental office are readily available and should be used in the initial evaluation (Figure 15.3). However, there are limitations to the radiographic modalities available in dental offices. Medical-grade CT scan, magnetic resonance imaging (MRI), and radionuclide imaging (scintigraphy) are advanced imaging studies that can aid in superior evaluation and determining the extend of osteomyelitis.

Radiographic findings can vary when diagnosing osteomyelitis. The initial phase can show radiopacity or osteosclerosis in the region of the jawbone or persistent unremodeled bone in an extraction socket. As the destruction progresses radiographically, lytic, poorly to well-defined radiolucent regions of jawbone spreading from the epicenter can be visualized as mixed or mottled areas [8] (see Figure 15.3). There is evidence of cortical expansion, thinning, erosion, and perforation. Adjacent structures such as nerves, sinus, and teeth can be involved. As the area of the disease progresses, pathologic fracture may be observed.

Magnetic resonance imaging is a useful diagnostic tool due to its nonradiation imaging. However, MRI requires special facilities and will increase the cost for the patient. MRI can well demonstrate the bone marrow changes caused by edema or inflammatory tissue due to increase of water content, which often replaces the normal fatty marrow in the acute stage [8]. When evaluating an MRI, it is useful to evaluate the extent of disease to soft tissue. The T1-weighted images show a decreased signal of bone marrow and in T2-weighted images there is an increased signal [8] (Figure 15.4). Marrow signal changes may take up to 6 months to return to normal after successful therapy [9]. Therefore, MRI is not useful in monitoring treatment during the first 6 months [9].

A radionuclide study uses three-phase imaging and technetium Tc99m-labeled bisphosphonates to demonstrate abnormal radionuclide accumulation in mandibular osteomyelitis due to inflammation and pathologic bone turnover [8, 9]. Radionuclide imaging studies show pathologically increased tracer uptake in affected regions of the jawbone, and the contralateral jawbone, if normal, may be used as an internal control or reference standard [8]. Due to poor spatial resolution, routine radionuclide bone scans have a low specificity [9] (Figure 15.5).

Computed tomography scans are the most common imaging system used in diagnosing osteomyelitis and treatment progression. CT scans can demonstrate early features of impeding cortical perforation and full extent of intramedullary disease [9]. Common CT scan findings are a mixture of radiolucency, sclerosis, cortical erosion, sequestrum, abscess formation, and periosteal new bone enveloping a sequestum [9] (Figure 15.6).

Imaging studies by themselves are not sufficient to diagnose osteomyelitis due to other conditions with similar

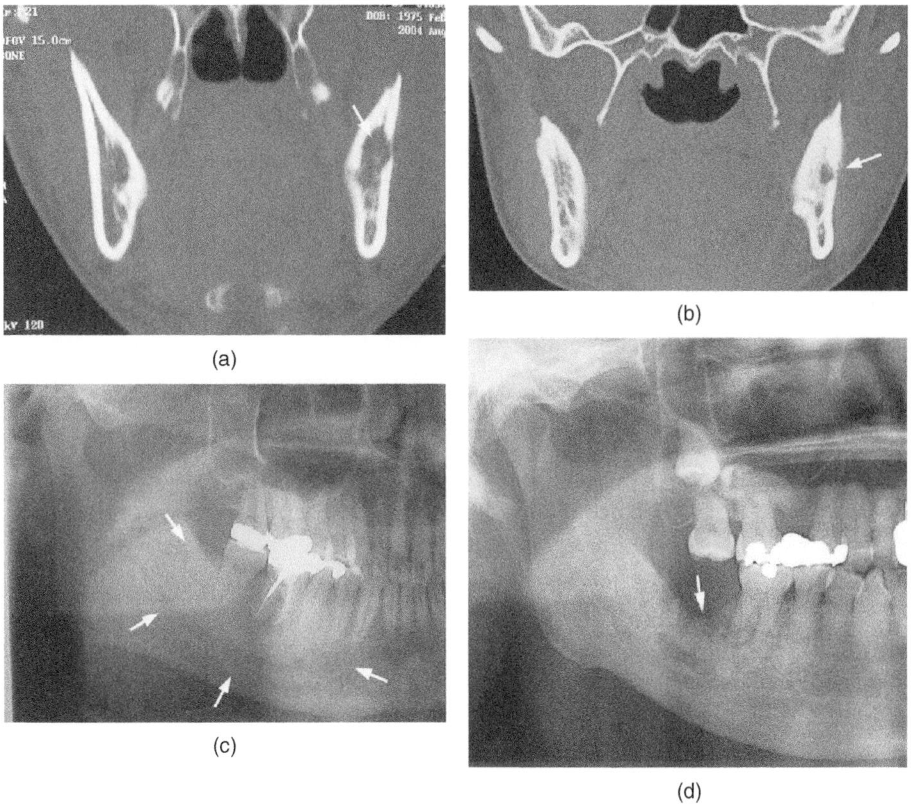

Figure 15.3 Patterns of conventional imaging features. (a) Lytic. (b) Mixed. (c) Sclerotic. (d) Sequestrum. Ranges with changes in bone marrow are indicated with arrows. *Source:* Ariji et al. [8] with permission from Elsevier.

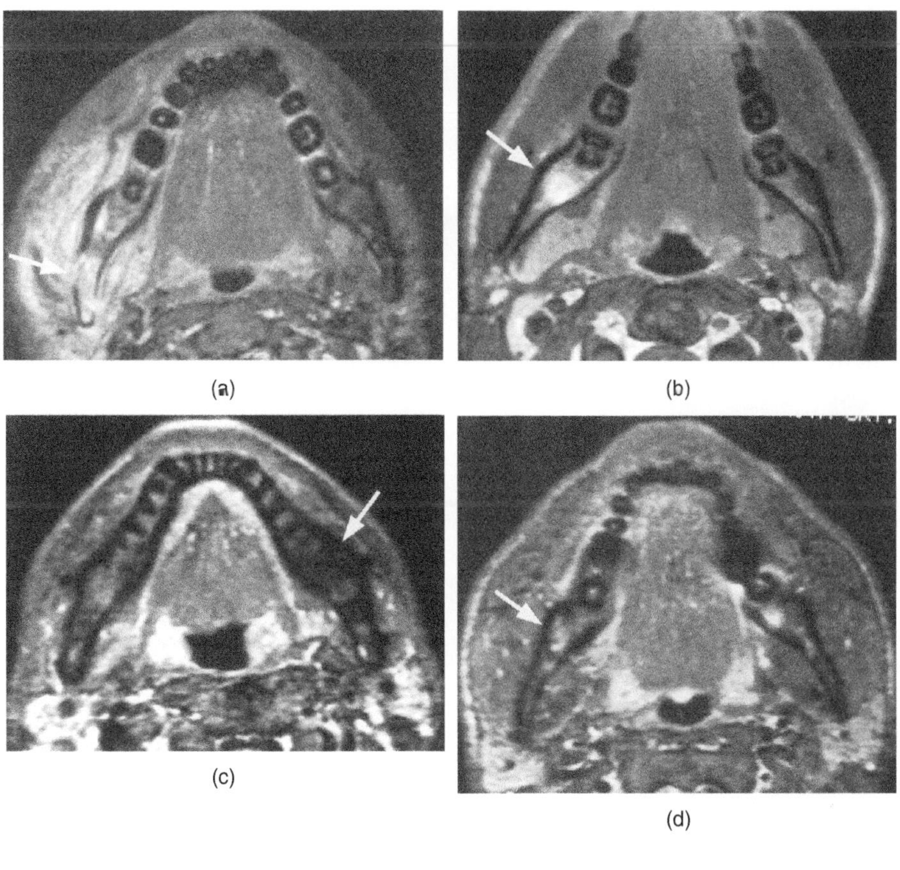

Figure 15.4 Patterns based on the change of signal intensity of the bone marrow on short T1 inversion recovery images. (a) Extensive high. Shows erosion of the cortical bone (arrow) and the adjacent soft tissue swelling with high SI. (b) Focal high (arrow). (c) Low (arrow). (d) No change (arrow). *Source:* Ariji et al. [8] with permission from Elsevier.

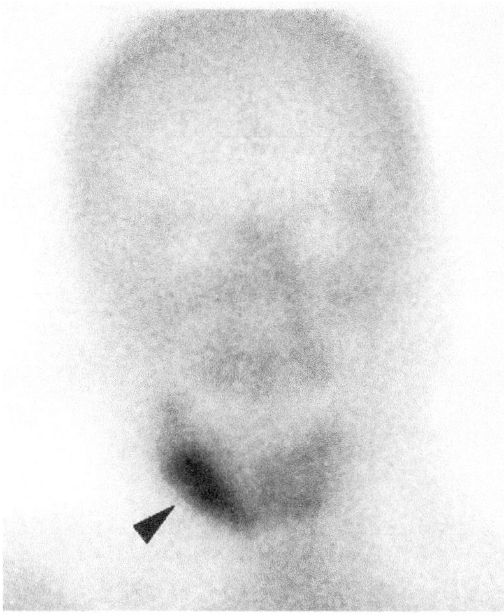

Figure 15.5 Right mandibular osteomyelitis on 99mTc radionuclide bone scan (bone phase image, anteroposterior projection). Arrowhead indicates intense uptake in the right mandibular body.

imaging patterns. A clinical exam, history, and histopathology are also necessary for definitive diagnosis.

Microbiology

Osteomyelitis can be caused by injury, malignant tumors, malnutrition, diabetes, chronic systemic disease, and infectious disease causing hypovascularized bone. However, odontogenic infection is the most common cause of osteomyelitis of the jaw [10]. Gingivitis, chronic periodontitis, endodontic treatment, or previous dental extractions can disturb the dental biofilm harboring anaerobic bacteria which can be the source of osteomyelitis [10].

The most common bacteria associated with osteomyelitis are streptococci, and anaerobic bacteria such as *Bacteroides* and *Peptostreptococcus* [10]. However, many microorganisms have been reported as a source of acute or chronic osteomyelitis such as *Actinomyces*, *Bacteroides*, *Bacillus*, *Candida*, *Eikenella*, Firmicutes, *Fusobacterium*, *Klebsiella*, *Lactobacillus*, *Prevotella*, and many more (Box 15.1) [10].

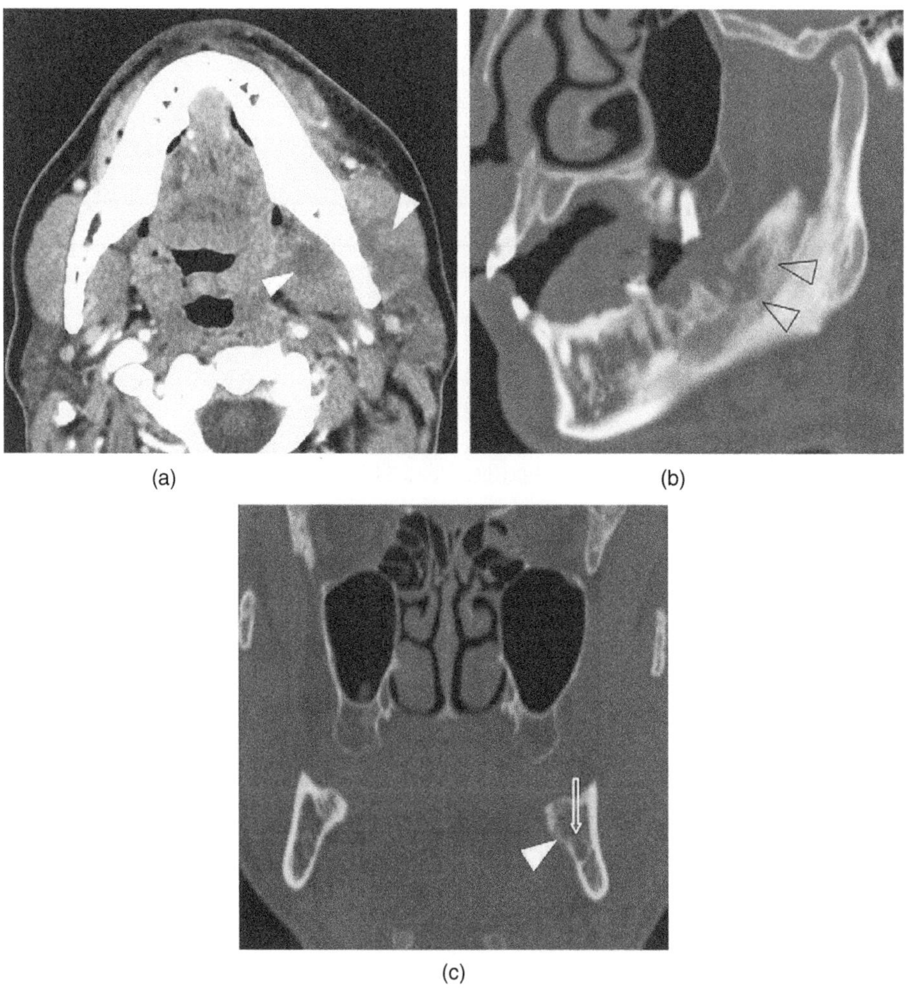

Figure 15.6 (a) Axial contrast-enhanced CT image demonstrates marked left masticator muscle swelling with masticator space abscesses (arrowheads). (b) Sagittal oblique image demonstrates mottled lucency distal to the left third molar extraction socket (arrowheads). (c) True coronal CT image (perpendicular to long axis of mandibular body) demonstrates thinning of the lingual bone (arrowhead, compare with the right side) and demineralization of the upper aspect of the mandibular nerve canal (arrow).

Box 15.1 Commonly Reported Microorganisms in Acute and Chronic Osteomyelitis

Actinomyces	*Lactobacillus*
Bacteroides	*Parvimonas*
Bacillus	*Peptostreptococcus*
Candida	*Porphyromonas*
Eikenella	*Prevotella*
Firmicutes	*Streptococcus*
Fusobacterium	*Selenomonas*
Haemophilus	*Staphylococcus*
Klebsiella	

Acute osteomyelitis is associated with *Streptococcus*, *Bacteroides*, *Peptostreptococcus*, and other opportunistic pathogens, whereas chronic osteomyelitis is based on origin of the infection. In chronic osteomyelitis that originates from odontogenic infections, microbacteria such as *Fusobacterium*, *Porphyromonas*, *Prevotella*, and *Parvimonas* are more common [10]. Overall, osteomyelitis of the jaw is not caused by a single organism. It consists of aerobic, anaerobic, gram-positive, gram-negative, and unculturable bacteria. Due to its polymicrobial nature, some of these bacteria may be difficult to culture [10].

Histologic Findings

In acute osteomyelitis, inflammatory exudate, decreased osteoblasts, and increased osteoclasts can be seen [9]. In chronic osteomyelitis, inflammatory cells such as lymphocytes and plasma cells may be seen [9]. Organisms may be difficult to identify due to the range of organism causing infection. This can also translate into different histologic findings [9]. Biopsy reports of chronic osteomyelitis show chronically inflamed fibrous connective tissue filling the intertrabecular space of bone [11] (Figure 15.7).

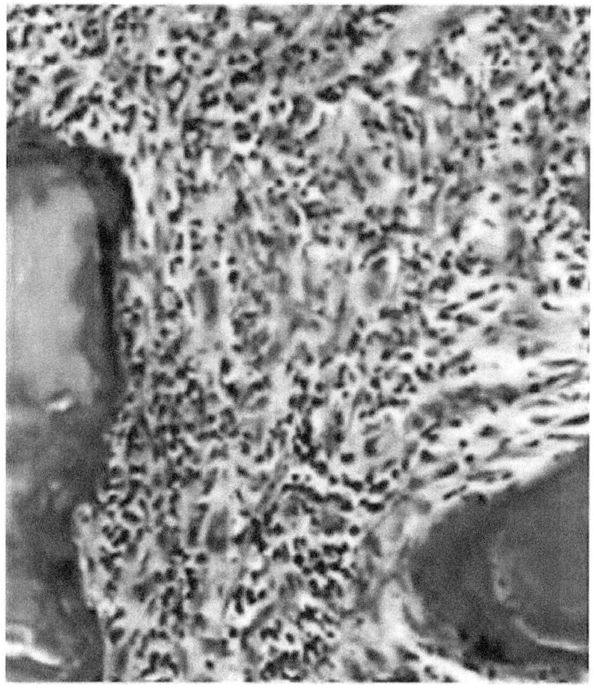

Figure 15.7 15 Photomicrograph showing chronically inflamed fibrous connective tissue filling the inter trabecular spaces of bone. Hematoxylin & eosin stain; original magnification × 100.

Treatment

Treatment of osteomyelitis includes medical and surgical interventions. The treatment consists of curettage, debridement, sequestrectomy, and systemic antibiotics via a peripherally inserted central catheter [10] (Box 15.2).

Antibiotic treatment should be guided by culture and sensitivity. Specimens should be sent to the lab for gram stain, culture, sensitivity, and histopathology. Preoperative antibiotics should be used with caution as they may interfere with an accurate culture and sensitivity. However, based on a gram stain, broad-spectrum empiric antibiotics should be started since culture and sensitivity may take several days. It is recommended to have an infectious disease specialist follow the patient with osteomyelitis as long-term intravenous antibiotics will be needed. Most commonly, the IV antibiotics are used for 6 weeks, but chronic osteomyelitis may require antibiotics for up to 6 months [10].

The most commonly used empiric antibiotic is penicillin. Other common antibiotics used are vancomycin 2–3 g/d, ertapenem 1 g/d, and ampicillin 1.5–3 g/d. Refractory organisms can be treated with many combinations such as clindamycin, metronidazole, clavulanic acid, cephalosporins, carbapenems, vancomycin, and fluoroquinolone [10] (Box 15.3).

Box 15.2 Principles of Treatment of Osteomyelitis

1. Early diagnosis
2. Elimination of the source of the infection
3. Establishment of surgical drainage
4. Bacteriologic identification and antibiotic sensitivity testing
5. Appropriate antibiotic coverage
6. Surgical debridement
7. Supportive care
8. Reconstruction

Source: Based on [10].

Box 15.3 Antibiotics Commonly Used in the Treatment of Acute and Chronic Osteomyelitis [10]

Augmentin	Penicillin
Carbapenems	Ticarcillin and clavulanic acid
Cephalosporins	Ampicillin
Clindamycin	Vancomycin in combination with other antibiotics
Doxycycline	
Ertapenem	
Fluoroquinolones	
Metronidazole	

Source: [10]/Elsevier.

Management of necrotic bone should involve surgical debridement [1, 12, 13]. Antibiotic therapy alone only provides palliative care and does not improve the outcome of osteomyelitis [1]. Conservative surgical management without any debridement and resection can lead to multiple recurrences [5]. However, aggressive management can result in uncomfortable morbidities and need for extensive reconstruction [5]. If choosing the conservative route, the suboptimal management of necrotic bone can result in prolonged treatment time and multiple surgeries, and may eventually require an aggressive surgical approach. Therefore, it is recommended to surgically remove the diseaseed segment to avoid recurrence and further surgical treatment [5].

Surgical treatment of osteomyelitis includes removal of lateral and inferior cortical plates for access to the medullary cavity [9]. Necrotic bone is removed until a 1–2 cm margin of vital bone is achieved [9]. It has been noted that removal of devitalized bone and soft tissue can shorten the extent of antibiotic therapy and decrease the risk of sequestra and abscess [14].

In the literature there are other adjuvant therapies such has platelet-rich plasma or hyperbaric oxygen therapy. However, these treatments lack the high-quality clinical studies to justify their use [6, 15].

Case Presentations

Osteomyelitis of the Maxilla

A 50-year-old female presented to the emergency department with a chief complaint of worsening pain and swelling of the right cheek for 3 weeks duration. The patient denied any generalized dental pain, headaches, nausea, vomiting, fever, chills, dyspnea, or dysphagia. She did complain of a low-grade chronic pain after she had a premolar removed from her upper right quadrant 6 weeks previously. She is now concerned about a bad taste and something showing in her mouth. Past medical and surgical histories, apart from tooth extraction, were benign. The patient was not taking any medications and denied any associated drug, food, or medication allergies. When initially interviewed, she was asked to discuss her social history, including history of alcohol, tobacco, or drug abuse.

Vital signs identified a blood pressure of 126/85 mmHg, a heart rate of 88 beats per minute, a normal respiratory rate of 16 breaths per minute, and afebrile with a temperature of 98.7 °F. Extraoral examination revealed a normal appearance with no facial swelling. There were no open wounds, abrasions, or contusions noted. Intraoral exam revealed multiple missing teeth and a dentition in poor repair. There was a region of erythema with exposed bone in the area of the upper right premolar area (see Figure 15.2). No neurosensory deficits were noted.

Radiologic imaging included a CT maxillofacial scan with and without contrast. Radiopacity of the maxillary sinuses wwas noted along with lytic lesions of the maxillary right premolar area (Figure 15.8).

The patient was admitted to the oral and maxillofacial surgery service with a diagnosis of rule-out osteomyelitis of right maxilla. Initial cultures were taken and she was

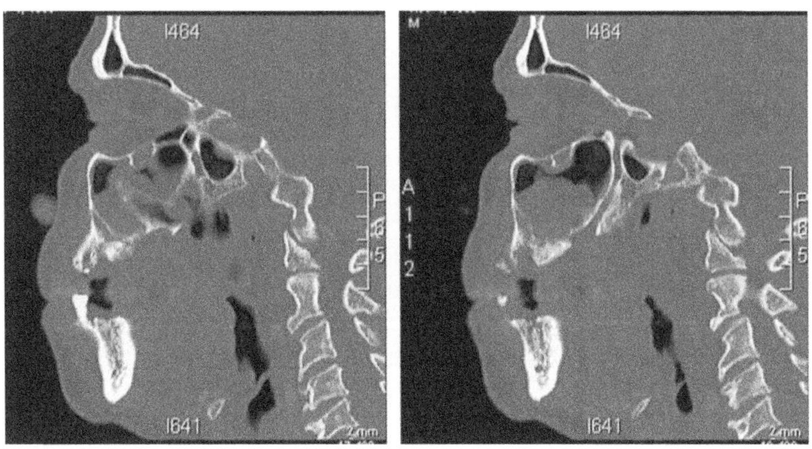

Figure 15.8 Preoperative view of the right maxilla. *Source:* Courtesy of H. Dym, DDS, Brooklyn, NY.

started empirically on IV clindamycin. Two days later, she was taken to the operating room for surgical debridement, sequestrectomy, and saucerization Under general anesthesia, debridement of the right maxilla was performed to remove all necrotic bone (Figures 15.9 and 15.10). Cultures were obtained for aerobic, anaerobic, and fungal specimens, as well as sensitivity for antibiotic therapy. Hard tissue specimens were submitted for histopathology. She was discharged the following day and the antibiotic was switched to amoxicillin/clavulanate 500 mg twice daily. The patient went home on antibiotics and did well after weekly follow-up. Postoperative pathology gave a definitive diagnosis of osteomyelitis of the right maxilla (Figures 15.11 and 15.12).

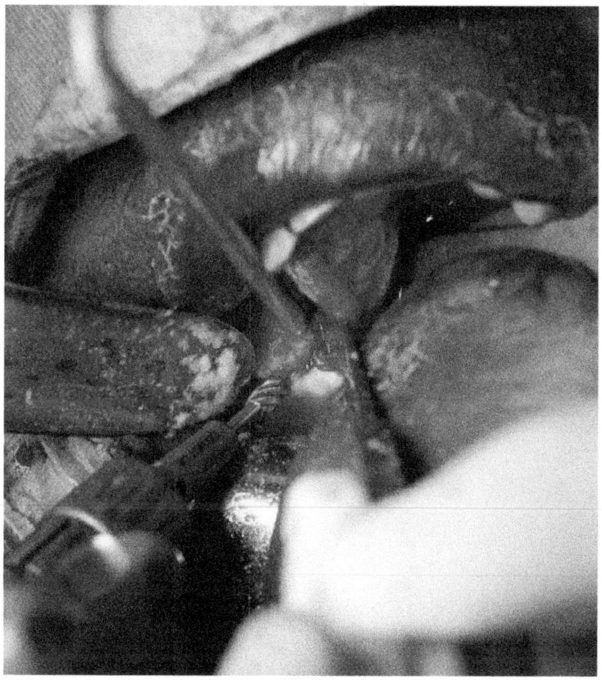

Figure 15.9 Debridement of the right maxilla. *Source:* Courtesy of H. Dym, DDS, Brooklyn, NY.

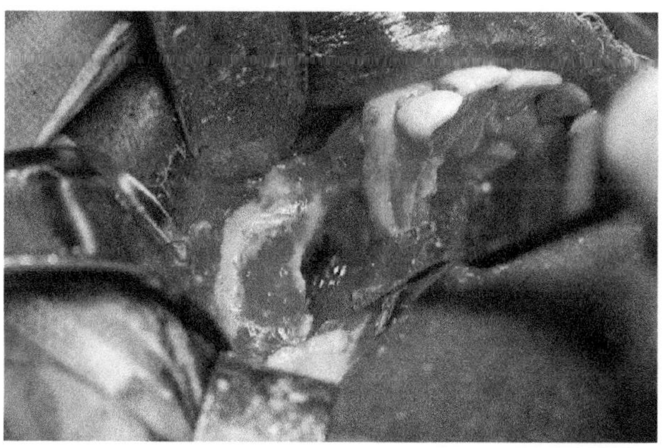

Figure 15.10 Completion of debridement of the right maxilla to healthy bleeding bone. *Source:* Courtesy of H. Dym, DDS, Brooklyn, NY.

Osteomyelitis of the Mandible

A 45-year-old homeless male with a significant past medical history of alcoholism presented to the emergency room with pain and swelling of his left parasymphysial region of 6 weeks duration. He stated that he went to a free clinic about 2 months previously where the dentist removed teeth #26, #27, and root tip of #28 at that time. He could not afford the prescribed antibiotics and never went back to the clinic.

Vital signs identified a blood pressure of 165/100 mmHg, slight tachycardia with a heart rate of 104 beats per minute, a normal respiratory rate of 12 breaths per minute, and a temperature of 99.8 °F. Extraoral examination revealed left-sided lower facial swelling which was induration. There were two draining cutaneous fistulae in the left parasympheal area. Minimal tenderness was appreciated upon palpation of the left lower face and upper lateral neck. Intraoral exam revealed a fetid odor upon opening with an

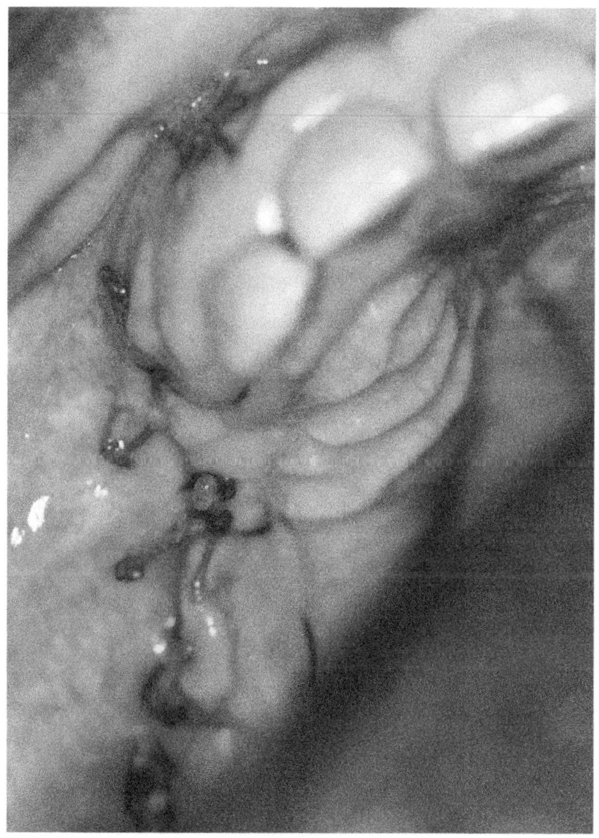

Figure 15.11 Right maxilla, 1 week postoperative. *Source:* Courtesy of H. Dym, DDS, Brooklyn, NY.

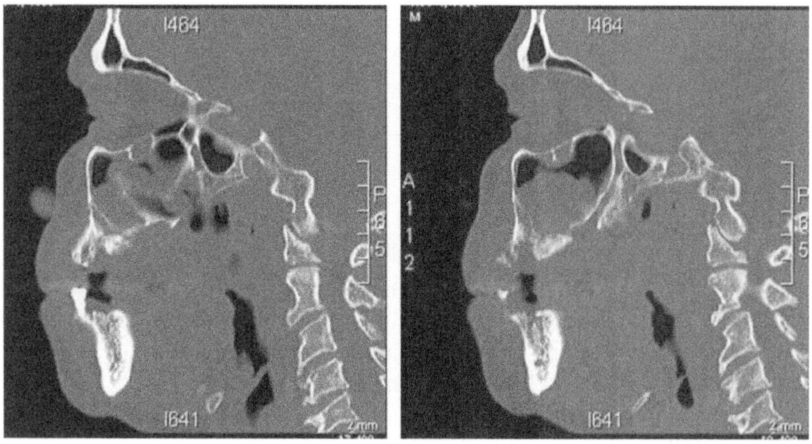

Figure 15.12 Postoperative sagittal view CT scan. *Source:* Courtesy of H. Dym, DDS, Brooklyn, NY.

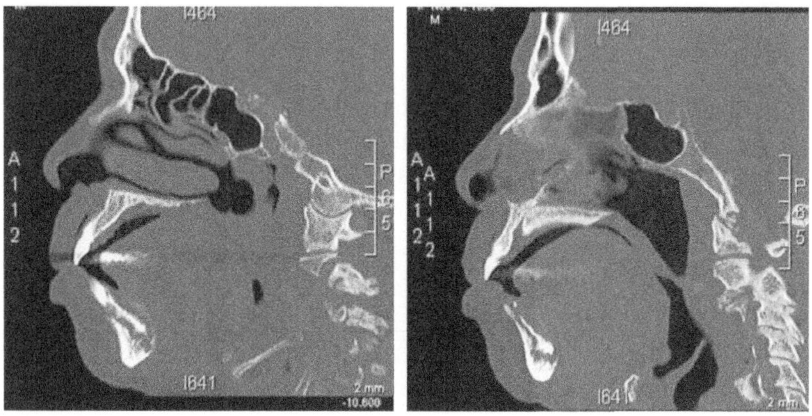

Figure 15.13 Preoperative sagittal view CT scan of the left mandible showing necrotic bone and sequestrum. *Source:* Courtesy of H. Dym, DDS, Brooklyn, NY.

interincisal opening of 38 mm without guarding. There was an ulcerated area with exposed bone in the edentulous region of teeth #27–28 (see Figure 15.1).

Laboratory values included a white blood cell count of 5800 per microliter. The CRP level was 9.0 mg/dL and ESR was 720 mm/h. With clinical findings of exposed bone and the elevation of both CRP and the ESR, a diagnosis of osteomyelitis was made.

Radiologic imaging included a CT maxillofacial scan with and without contrast. Maxillary sinuses were clear. Multiple views of the maxillofacial CT scan (Figure 15.13) revealed multifocal abscesses of the left submental region. The mandibular bone appeared necrotic with sequestra and soft tissue necrosis in the regions of interest.

The patient was scheduled for day of surgery admission (DOSA) in 3 days after imaging studies were completed when a planned debridement and sequestrectomy would be performed. On the day of surgery, he had the debridement, sequestrectomy, and saucerization performed under general anesthesia via a transbuccal approach (Figure 15.14a). Cultures were obtained for aerobic, anaerobic, and fungal specimens, as well as sensitivity for antibiotic therapy.

Bony tissue (Figure 15.15) returned a histopathologic diagnosis of chronic osteomyelitis of the left mandible. Culture showed a mixed anaerobic infection with *Actinomyces*, *Parvimonas*, and *Staphylococcus*. A consult was obtained from the Infectious Disease Service which recommended oral augmentin, 500 mg bid for 4–6 weeks. The patient went home with the recommended antibiotics and did well after 8 weeks of follow-up (Figures 15.16 and 15.17).

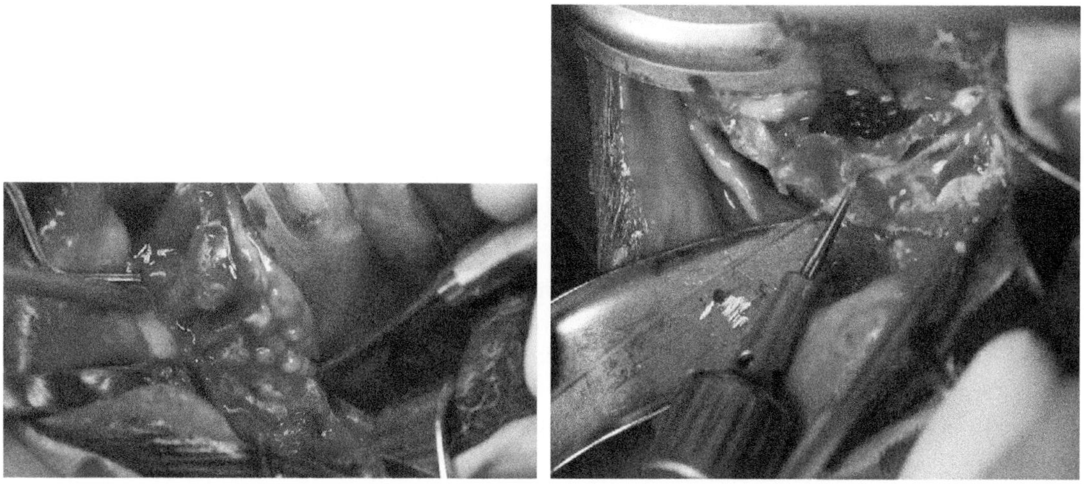

(a) (b)

Figures 15.14 (a) Ostectomy of the necrotic portion of the mandible. (b) Necrotic tissue and sequestrum. *Source:* Courtesy of H. Dym, DDS, Brooklyn, NY.

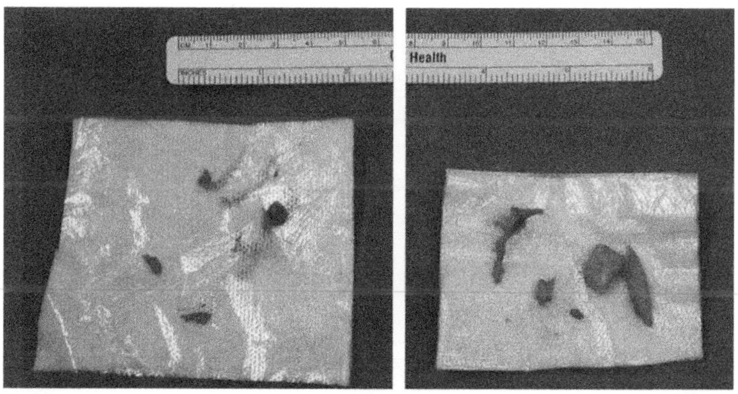

Figure 15.15 Specimens of necrotic bone removed during sequestrectomy.

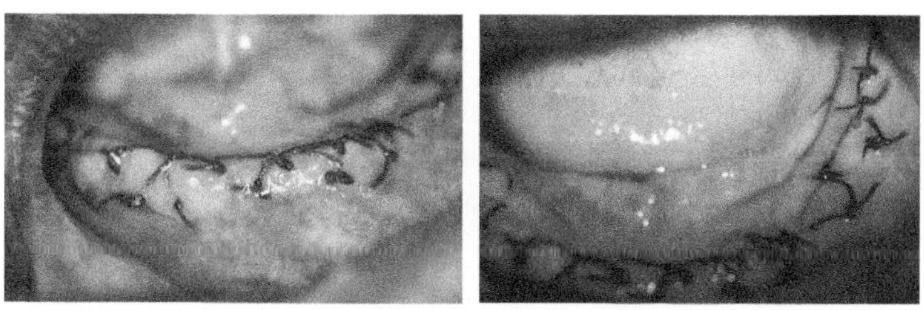

Figure 15.16 Mandible, 1 week postoperative. *Source:* Courtesy of H. Dym, DDS, Brooklyn, NY.

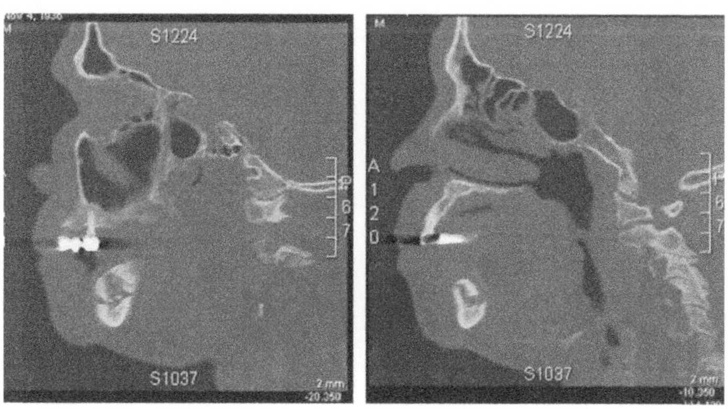

Figure 15.17 Postoperative sagittal view CT scan. *Source:* Courtesy of H. Dym, DDS, Brooklyn, NY.

References

1 Bauer, D.R., Altay, M.S., Flores-Hidalgo, A. et al. (2015). Chronic osteomyelitis of the mandible: diagnosis and management – an institution's experience over 7 years. *J. Oral. Maxillofac. Surg.* 73 (4): 655–665.

2 Bartensperger, M.M., Eyrich, G.K., and Marx, R.E. (ed.) (2009). *Osteomyelitis of the Jaws*, 315–320. New York: Springer Link.

3 Kim, S.G. and Jang, H.S. (2001). Treatment of chronic osteomyelitis in Korea. *Oral Surg. Oral Med. Oral Pathol. Oral Radiol. Endod.* 92: 394.

4 Tanaka, R. and Hayashi, T. (2008). Computed tomography findings of chronic osteomyelitis involving the mandible: correlation to histopathological findings. *Dentomaxillofac. Radiol.* 37: 94.

5 Bevin, C.R., Inwards, C.Y., and Keller, E.E. (2008). Surgical management of primary chronic osteomyelitis: a long-term retrospective analysis. *J. Oral Maxillofac. Surg.* 66 (3): 2073–2085.

6 Pincus, D.J., Armstrong, M.B., and Thaller, S.R. (2009). Osteomyelitis of the craniofacial skeleton. *Semin. Plast. Surg.* 23: 73–79.

7 Calderon, A.J. and Wener, M.H. (2012). Erythrocyte sedimentation rate and C-reactive protein. *Hosp. Med. Clin.* 1: e313–e337.

8 Ariji, Y., Izumi, M., Gotoh, M. et al. (2008). MRI features of mandibular osteomyelitis: practical criteria based on an association with conventional radiography features and clinical classification. *Oral Surg. Oral Med. Oral Pathol. Oral Radiol. Endod.* 105: 503–511.

9 Koorbusch, G.F., Deatherage, J.P., and Cure, J.K. (2011). How can we diagnose and treat osteomyelitis of the jaws as early as possible? *Oral Maxillofacial. Surg. Clin. North Am.* 23: 557–567.

10 Dym, H. and Zeiden, J. (2017). Microbiology of acute and chronic osteomyelitis and antibiotic treatment. *Dent. Clin. North Am.* 61: 271–282.

11 Kamran, A., Akram, A., and Akhtar, M.U. (2012). An unusual case of chronic suppurative osteomyelitis of the mandible. *Arch. Orofac. Sci.* 7 (1): 37–41.

12 Carlson, E.R. (2014). Management of antiresorptive osteonecrosis of the jaws with primary surgical resection. *J. Oral Maxillofac. Surg.* 72: 655.

13 Carlson, E.R. and Basile, J.D. (2009). The role of surgical resection in the management of bisphosphonate-related osteonecrosis of the jaws. *J. Oral Maxillofac. Surg.* 67 (Suppl): 85.

14 Topazian, R.G. (2002). Osteomyelitis of the jaws. In: *Oral and Maxillofacial Infections*, 4e (ed. R.G. Topazian, M.H. Goldberg and J.R. Hupp), 214–242. Philadelphia, PA: W.B. Saunders.

15 Fang, R.C. and Galiano, R.D. (2009). Adjunctive therapies in the treatment of osteomyelitis. *Semin. Plast. Surg.* 23: 141.

16

Obstructive Sleep Apnea

Orrett E. Ogle

Introduction

Obstructive sleep apnea (OSA) is a serious sleep disorder in which breathing repeatedly stops and starts during sleep and produces a significant decrease in airflow and oxygenation (apnea). It is the most common breathing disorder during sleep, affecting between 18 and 30 million adults over 18 in the US [1]. It is characterized by recurrent episodes of upper airway collapse during sleep that are associated with recurrent oxyhemoglobin desaturations and arousals from sleep [2]. Although the individual is not consciously awake, the frequent arousals cause fragmented sleep as the patient vacillates between wakefulness and sleep, making it difficult to achieve the necessary deeper stages of sleep. The arousal from sleep at times when there is hypopnea or apnea is believed to be an important protective mechanism for airway reopening [3]. Patients with OSA are less able to restore ventilation without cortical arousal [4]. In patients with severe OSA, these apneic periods may occur as often as 1–2 times per minute.

Etiology

The factors that predispose a patient to airway collapse are those that decrease intraluminal pressures (obstruction), increase external pressure (obesity, sleeping position), or decrease the resistance to collapse offered by the walls of the pharynx (collapsibility) [5]. During sleep, muscles of the jaws, tongue, and throat relax, allowing the tongue to fall back into the pharynx by gravitational collapsing effects, resulting in narrowing or total obstruction of the pharyngeal airway which causes substantially reduced or complete cessation of airflow despite ongoing breathing efforts. This produces periods of hypopnea or apnea depending on the amount of obstruction.

One significant mechanism believed to be important in the pathogenesis of OSA relates to the interaction between pharyngeal anatomy and a diminished ability of the person's genioglossus muscles to maintain a patent airway during sleep [6]

There are several anomalies of the upper airway which may produce intermittent obstructive breathing symptoms during sleep (Box 16.1). Also, facial, oral, and throat abnormalities occur in numerous congenital syndromes which can cause labored breathing and OSA (Box 16.2). Other major risk factors include obesity, male sex, and aging.

Obesity, in particular, is a key risk factor for the development of OSA. Deposition of fat around the pharyngeal airway increases the collapsibility of the pharyngeal airway. Obesity has also been associated with functional impairment in upper airway muscles [7]. OSA is more common in males than females. Imaging studies have shown that men have increased fat deposition around the pharyngeal airway and an increased length of the pharyngeal airway compared with women [8]. The frequency of apnea increases with aging but the increase in prevalence appears to plateau after 65 years [9]. There appears to be a preferential deposition of fat around the pharynx with aging, independent of systemic fat; deterioration of genioglossus reflexes and increased upper airway collapsibility are also common with aging [10, 11]. Studies have shown a familial basis to the development of OSA [12] (Box 16.3).

Oral and Maxillofacial Surgery, Medicine, and Pathology for the Clinician, First Edition. Edited by Harry Dym, Leslie R. Halpern, and Orrett E. Ogle.

Box 16.1 Anomalies That May Cause Obstructive Sleep Apnea

- Obesity (body mass index >30 kg/m^2)
- Enlarged neck circumference (men >43 cm [17 in]; women >37 cm [15 in])
- Increased Mallampati score
- Retrognathia or micrognathia
- Severe class 11 malocclusion
- High-arched hard palate
- Temporomandibular joint ankyloses with micrognathia in children
- Macroglossia
- Smoking

Box 16.2 Syndromes Associated with Obstructive Sleep Apnea

- Crouzon
- Apert
- Treacher–Collins
- Down
- Pierre Robin sequence

Box 16.3 Disorders Associated with Childhood Obstructive Sleep Apnea

- Adenotonsillar hypertrophy – the most common cause of OSA in children
- Chronic nasal obstruction
- Childhood morbid obesity
- Marfan syndrome
- Conditions involving neuromuscular weakness
- Cerebral palsy
- Sickle cell diseases: persons with sickle cell anemia have a tendency to obstructive apnea for reasons that are unclear

Symptoms

The most common and consistent symptom of OSA is loud and habitual snoring caused by narrowing or collapse in the upper airway during sleep. Pauses occur in the snoring when the individual stops breathing. Breathing usually resumes with a loud gasp, choking or snorting sound, often accompanied by body jerks. These arousals following the periods of breathing cessation do not lead to full alertness, but will disrupt sleep enough to prevent the person from getting a good night's sleep, leaving them groggy and waking up as tired as when they went to bed (Box 16.4). It should be noted, however, that snoring by itself does not mean that the person has OSA.

Box 16.4 Other Signs and Symptoms of Obstructive Sleep Apnea

- Witnessed apneas, which often interrupt the snoring and end with a snort
- Personality and mood changes
- Nocturia
- Daytime tiredness
- Constantly falling asleep during quiet activities (e.g., reading, watching television)
- In severe cases, patients will feel sleepy during activities that generally require alertness (e.g., school, work, driving)
- Cognitive deficits
- Morning headache, dry or sore throat
- Sexual dysfunction, including impotence and decreased libido

Pathophysiology and Related Health Issues

The human upper airway consists of collapsible soft tissue that extends from the posterior hard palate to the larynx. The cross-sectional area of the upper airway is reduced in patients with OSA compared with subjects without OSA [13]. Also, the arrangement of the surrounding soft tissues appears to be altered in patients with OSA in such a way that may put these individuals at risk for pharyngeal collapse during sleep [13].

Obstructive sleep apnea increases the heart rate and blood pressure, placing abnormal stress on the heart. This may be because apneas frequently reduce blood oxygen levels, activating the sympathetic nervous system and leading to increasing heart performance. In OSA patients, both sympathetic and parasympathetic nervous system control of the heart rate becomes unstable, with enhanced parasympathetic tone during the apneas and hypopneas punctuated with enhanced sympathetic nervous system activation subsequent to the apneic events [14]. In addition, levels of systemic inflammation rise. Such inflammation can damage the heart and blood vessels [15]. Many studies have reported that patients with OSA develop generalized systemic inflammation, with increased levels of inflammatory mediators, including intercellular adhesion molecules (ICAM), coagulation factors (factor VIII and tissue factor [TF]) and C-reactive protein (CRP), but not all studies have reported elevation of CRP in patients with

Box 16.5 Medical Problems Associated with Obstructive Sleep Apnea

- Systemic arterial hypertension: present in about 50% of obstructive sleep apnea cases
- Congestive heart failure
- Pulmonary hypertension
- Stroke
- Metabolic syndrome: a collection of risk factors linked to a higher risk of heart disease. The conditions that make up metabolic syndrome include high blood pressure, abnormal cholesterol, high blood sugar, and an increased waist circumference
- Type 2 diabetes mellitus: people with sleep apnea are more likely to develop insulin resistance and type 2 diabetes

OSA. An overexpression of interleukin (IL)-8 in human bronchial epithelial cells has been seen in response to a vibratory stimulus generated by snoring [16].

If left untreated, OSA can result in a significant number of health problems, including hypertension, increased risk of cerebrovascular accident (CVA), heart failure, cardiac arrhythmias – usually atrial fibrillation – and even heart attacks (Box 16.5). Several studies have shown an association between OSA and increased likelihood of premature death [17] because of the number of chronic medical conditions associated with OSA. Middle-aged men appear to be at greatest risk, with the cause of death most commonly related to cardiovascular disease.

Diagnosis and Classification

Obstructive sleep apnea is diagnosed when breathing stops more than five times per hour for longer than 10 seconds each time. The obstruction resolves when the person experiences a partial awakening, known as arousal. Currently, the only available tool for definitive diagnosis of OSA is an overnight polysomnographic evaluation in a sleep laboratory. The polysomnography should be performed overnight and during the individual's usual bedtime hours.

The classification is based on the Apnea/Hypopnea Index (AHI) which is # apneas + # hypopneas/sleep hours.

- AHI <5 normal
- AHI: 5–15 mild
- AHI 15–30 moderate
- AHI > 30 severe

The adult criteria usually used for the diagnosis of OSA do not apply to children. In the pediatric age range, abnormalities include:

- oxygen desaturation under 92%
- more than one obstructive apnea per hour
- elevations of end-tidal CO_2 measurement of more than 50 mmHg for more than 9% of sleep time or a peak level of greater than 53 mmHg.

AHI guidelines for children are related to treatment indications.

- An AHI of more than five events per hour represents an indication for treatment in children.
- An AHI <3 events per hour does not require any intervention.
- For >3 but <5 events per hour, the benefit of treatment is not determined.

Treatment

The following conservative measures may help to manage OSA.

- Avoid supine position during sleep.
- Sleeping in an upright position for markedly obese patients.
- Avoiding alcohol and other sedatives for 4–6 hours before bedtime.
- Weight loss.
- Smoking cessation.

Intraoral Devices

Oral appliances for OSA fall into two broad categories: mandibular advancement splints and tongue repositioning devices. The aim of the mandibular advancement devices is to keep the mandible forward during sleep so as to enlarge the upper airway and prevent it from collapsing. Similarly, tongue repositioning devices suction the tongue forward to prevent it from falling back and obstructing the airway during sleep.

Surgical Procedures

Uvulopalatopharyngoplasty (UPPP)

This is a procedure that removes excess tissue in the throat to make the oropharyngeal airspace wider. The aim is to allow air to move through the pharynx more easily during sleep, thus reducing the severity of OSA. It is currently the most common surgical procedure performed in the US for adults with OSA. Indications for UPPP are AHI of 15 or higher, oxyhemoglobin desaturation less than 90%, and/or cardiac arrhythmias associated with obstructions [18]. Patient selection is based on a staging system where stage 1 patients are the best candidates for surgery and stage 3 are not suitable for UPPP (Table 16.1).

Table 16.1 Staging of Patients for UPPP.

Criterion	Stage 1 Body mass index less than 40 kg/m^2	Stage 2 Body mass index less than 40 kg/m^2	Stage 3 Body mass index greater than 40 kg/m^2
Mallampati score	1 or 2	3 or 4	3 or 4
Brodsky tonsillar scale	3 or 4	3 or 4	3 or 4
Success rate for UPPP	80%	37%	8%

Surgical planning is based on the protocol established by the Stanford Sleep Disorders Center [19]. In this protocol, surgery is divided into two phases. Phase I is based on the level of airway obstruction. The type of surgery is dependent on patient's level of airway obstruction.

- Type 1 airway obstruction has a purely oropharyngeal (i.e., retropalatal) obstruction and is treated with uvulopalatopharyngoplasty.
- Type II airway obstruction has oropharyngeal and hypopharyngeal obstruction and is treated with UPPP, genioglossus advancement, and possible hyoid myotomy.
- Type III airway obstruction has hypopharyngeal obstruction alone and is treated with genioglossus advancement.

Phase II surgery consists of a maxillary-mandibular osteotomy and is indicated for patients who fail phase I.

Uvulopalatopharyngoplasty

Technique

1. After the induction of general endotracheal anesthesia, the oral tracheal tube is taped in the midline of the lower lip and a shoulder roll is placed.
2. 8–10 mg of intravenous dexamethasone is given.
3. Lidocaine with epi 1/100 000 is infiltrated along the posterior border of the soft palate.
4. A mouth prop with appropriate size tongue blade is placed (Davis–Boyle, Collis or Crowe–Davis).
5. Surgery begins with the bilateral removal of tonsillar tissue using the standard techniques for tonsillectomy.
6. Attention is then turned to the soft palate. The aim of this portion of the surgery is to resect the posterior portion of the soft palate along with the uvula in a beveled fashion, taking more oropharyngeal mucosa so that more nasopharyngeal mucosa will be preserved.
7. A horizontal incision is made along the soft palate mucosa just anterior (about 5–6 mm) to the uvula and connected to the anterior pillar mucosa incisions. The incision is carried down through the mucosa to the tensor veli palatini muscles. Beveled dissection proceeds toward the uvulae muscle and posterior border of soft palate until the redundant soft palate and lateral pharyngeal mucosa are resected [18]. Care should be taken not to remove excessive tissue from the posterior of the soft palate.
8. Cauterize all bleeding tissue using electrocautery. Use 2.0 Vicryl® horizontal mattress sutures to close the corners of the incision on the soft palate to bring the nasopharyngeal and oropharyngeal mucosa together in a single layer. The knot of the suture should be on the oropharyngeal surface. Care should be taken with the nasal mucosa as it tears very easily. Several interrupted stitches, running sutures, are then used to reapproximate the remainder of the soft palate mucosa. As the knots are tied, they will rotate the posterior edge anteriorly (Figure 16.1).

Tongue base reduction is a new procedure to further reduce redundant tissue in the pharynx.

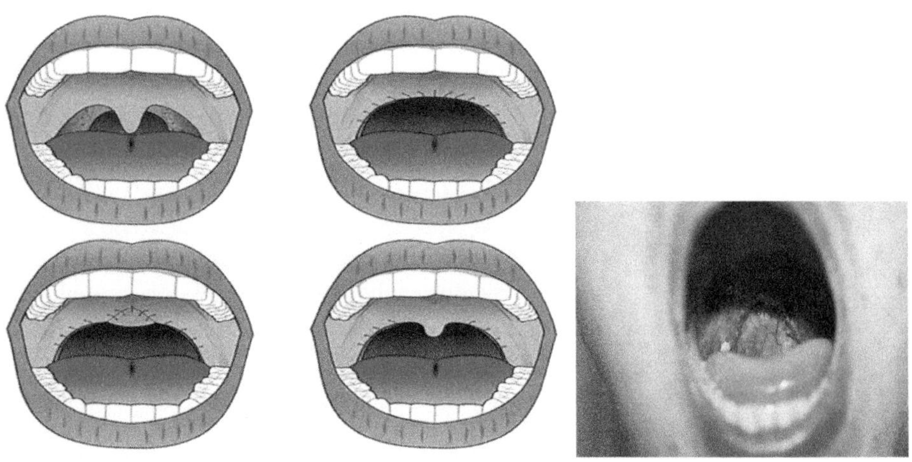

Figure 16.1 Uvulopalatopharyngoplasty (UPPP) preoperatively and postoperatively. *Source:* Dr M. Camacho – drcamachoen, 2015/ Wikimedia Commons/Licensed under CC BY 4.0.

Genial Tubercle Advancement

The purpose of this procedure is to advance the tongue by way of the genioglossus muscle away from the pharynx.

Technique

1. After the induction of general anesthesia using nasal intubation, a throat pack is placed. Lidocaine with epi 1/100 000 is infiltrated into the lower lip.
2. An incision is made from canine to canine inside the lower lip midway between the wet–dry line and the labial vestibule. The incision is made through the labial mucosa to include some fibers of the orbicularis oris muscle. Any fibers of the mental nerve that are encountered are isolated and retracted out of the field with a small vessel loop.
3. Using primarily blunt dissection, the mucosa and muscle fibers are elevated toward the bony chin. When the dissection gets to the bone, the periosteum is sharply incised. The chin muscle and other soft tissues are cleared away with a periosteal elevator to expose the central part of the mandible. About 5–7 mm of soft tissue should be left attached at the inferior border of the chin.
4. The apex of the lower incisors is identified, as well as the lower border of the chin. Using a small fissure bur, score a line 3 mm below the apices of the incisors from lateral to lateral incisor. Eight mm from the inferior border, score another line, parallel to the superior line and of the same length. Join the ends of the lines by scoring the bone vertically (Figure 16.2).
5. Drill a hole bicortically through one of the superior angles formed by the vertical and horizontal lines. Then drill another hole diagonal to the first. Introducing a reciprocal saw blade into the holes, make a rectangular cut to capture the area of attachment of the genioglossus muscle. The rectangular osteotomy should capture the entire genial tubercles to enable an adequate amount of the genioglossus muscle to be incorporated and advanced. Limited lateral extension of the osteotomy can result in a decreased incorporation of genioglossus muscle.
6. This rectangular segment of bone is moved forward and turned 6–90° to have the inner portion resting on the buccal cortical plate. A small contoured titanium plate or a screw is used to hold the bone fragment in place. If using a screw, be careful not to fracture off the bone at the cut edge.
7. The chin muscle and soft tissues are replaced, and Vicryl sutures are used to close the incision in the lip. No attempt is made to close the periosteum.
8. By advancing the rectangular block of bone, the chin will appear more pronounced. Any initial problem with swallowing should not be permanent.

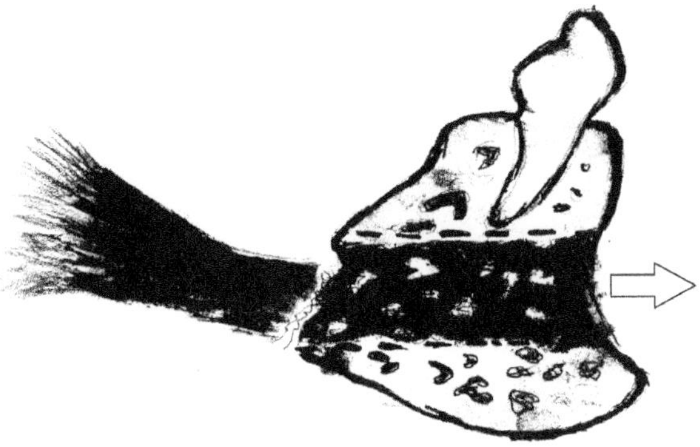

Figure 16.2 Area of chin with genioglossus muscle to be advanced.

Maxillary-Mandibular Advancement

With maxillary-mandibular advancement (MMA), the suprahyoid, genioglossus, and palatal muscles and lateral musculature of the pharynx are all advanced and tightened at once. This results in a significant increase in airway space and resolution of the OSA in 95% of cases [20].

A modification of the standard MMA technique where the maxilla has to be anteriorly repositioned up to 10 mm to resolve OSA was described by Sailer [21, 22]. With the conventional MMA procedure, the maxilla is advanced >10 mm [23, 24] which produces a very acute nasolabial angle, resulting in an unnatural appearance. The procedure described by Sailer is the bimaxillary "rotation advancement" (RA) procedure which produces a more natural and esthetic nasolabial angle. The esthetically important point is that the anterior–posterior position of the maxilla stays more or less the same when the RA technique is used, in contrast to the MMA technique where the maxilla has to be anteriorly repositioned up to 10 mm [22].

Technique

1. A standard LeFort 1 osteotomy is performed.
2. Reduction of the inferior turbinates can be done when the maxilla is down fractured.
3. The maxilla is advanced 2–3 mm and the posterior maxilla is rotated downwards about 4 mm, creating a gap in the posterior part of the zygomatic buttress. There should be adequate bony contact in the anterior.
4. This anticlockwise rotation (when viewed from the side) of the maxilla creates a new inclination angle of the occlusal and maxillary plane. This anticlockwise rotation of the occlusal plane will retroposition the mandible, allowing the mandible to be advanced by a greater distance anteriorly than with the conventional MMA procedure.

5. The maxilla is fixated with 2–3 L-shaped 2 mm plates on each side.
6. A long sagittal split of the mandible is performed and the mandible advanced into the appropriate occlusion.
7. The mandible may be fixated by 2.0 mm box-shaped plates or 2–4 bicortical screws on each side.
8. Maxillo-mandibular fixation is not absolutely necessary but patients should use maxillo-mandibular rubber bands for 4–6 weeks.

Maxillary-mandibular advancement will produce a significant enlargement of the posterior airway space [22]. The "tightening" effect on the lateral walls of the pharynx (which is composed of the aponeuroses and muscles of the hypopharynx) by the MMA procedure makes it more stable and significantly reduces collapsibility [25].

Distraction Osteogenesis

Mandibular retrognathism due to temporomandibular joint (TMJ) ankylosis is a cause of OSA encountered by oral and maxillofacial surgeons. TMJ ankylosis is often caused by high subcondylar fractures with bleeding into the joint space or by ear infections which spread to the TMJ. When TMJ ankylosis occurs in a young child, it leads to an underdeveloped retrognathic mandible. The relatively large tongue combined with narrowing of the upper airway space causes serious difficulties with breathing during sleep and results in apneic or hypopneic events during sleep.

Mandibular distraction osteogenesis (DO) is an effective method for expanding the pharyngeal airways in the pediatric patient [26]. It has been shown that mandibular DO results in significant increases in pharyngeal airway volume and a decrease in the AHI because more than half of upper pharyngeal airway obstructions occur at the base of the tongue [27–30].

Suggested Treatment Plan Sequencing of Procedures (Figure 16.3)

1. TMJ: coronoidectomy, release of ankylosis, costochondral graft.
2. Extensive physical therapy.
3. Osteogenesis distraction – mandible: bidirectional.
4. Inverted L osteotomy with bone graft/advancement genioplasty.

Conclusion

Obstructive sleep apnea is a potentially serious sleep disorder that affects the quality of sleep, general health, and the overall quality of life. It has been linked to hypertension, diabetes, heart disease, stroke, and work- and driving-related accidents. The risks of untreated OSA include heart attack, stroke, irregular heartbeat, high blood pressure, heart disease, and decreased libido. In addition, OSA causes daytime drowsiness that can result in accidents, lost productivity, and relationship problems [31]. Sleep apnea patients are at 30% higher risk of heart attack and heart-related death than those without the condition. Increased pulmonary pressures to the right side of the heart, a major concern in prolonged cases of OSA, can result in cor pulmonale, a very serious and dangerous form of congestive heart failure [32]. Available treatment options include lifestyle modification, continuous positive airway pressure, oral appliances, and surgical procedures aimed at increasing the size of the pharyngeal airspace.

References

1 Lattimore, J.D., Celermajer, D.S., Wilcox, I. et al. (2003). Obstructive sleep apnea and cardiovascular disease. *J. Am. Coll. Cardiol.* 41 (9): 1429–1437.

2 Guilleminault, C., Tilkian, A., and Dement, W.C. (1976). The sleep apnea syndromes. *Ann. Rev. Med.* 27: 465–484.

3 Remmers, J.E., deGroot, W.J., Sauerland, E.K., and Anch, A.M. (1978). Pathogenesis of upper airway occlusion during sleep. *J. Appl. Physiol.* 44 (6): 931–938.

4 Jordan, A.S., Wellman, A., Heinzer, R.C. et al. (2007). Mechanisms used to restore ventilation after partial upper airway collapse during sleep in humans. *Thorax* 62 (10): 861–867.

5 Abramson, Z.R., Susarla, S., Tagoni, J.R., and Kaban, L. (2010). Three-dimensional computed tomographic analysis of airway anatomy. *J. Oral Maxillofac. Surg.* 68 (2): 363–371.

6 Mezzanotte, W.S., Tangel, D.J., and White, D.P. (1992). Waking genioglossal electromyogram in sleep apnea patients versus normal controls (a neuromuscular compensatory mechanism). *J. Clin. Invest.* 89 (5): 1571–1579.

7 Carrera, M., Barbe, F., Sauleda, J. et al. (2004). Effects of obesity upon genioglossus structure and function in obstructive sleep apnoea. *Eur. Respir. J.* 23 (3): 425–429.

8 Eckert, D. and Malhotra, A. (2008). Pathophysiology of adult obstructive sleep apnea. *Proc. Am. Thorac. Soc.* 5 (2): 144–153.

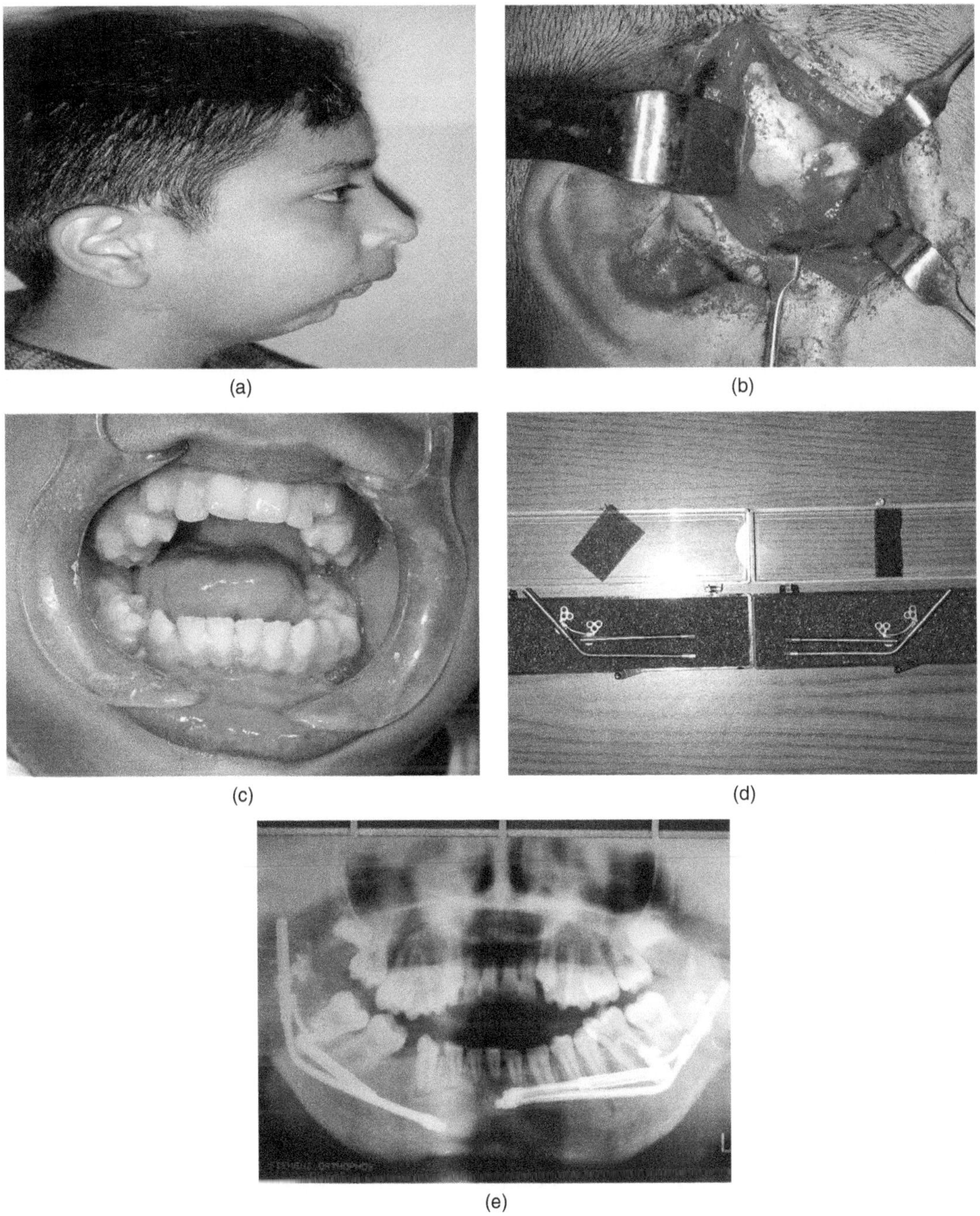

Figure 16.3 (a) Presurgical image of TMJ ankyloses and micronagthic mandible. (b) Bony ankyloses of TMJ. (c) Interincisal opening after release of TMJ ankyloses. (d) Bidirectional distractor by KLS-Martin. (e) Distractor in place. *Source:* Courtesy of Dr Orrett E. Ogle, Atlanta, GA.

9 Young, T., Skatrud, J., and Peppard, P.E. (2004). Risk factors for obstructive sleep apnea in adults. *JAMA* 291 (16): 2013–2016.

10 Malhotra, A., Huang, Y., Fogel, R. et al. (2006). Aging influences on pharyngeal anatomy and physiology: the predisposition to pharyngeal collapse. *Am. J. Med.* 119: 72.e9–72.e14.

11 Eikermann, M., Jordan, A.S., Chamberlin, N.L. et al. (2007). The influence of aging on pharyngeal collapsibility during sleep. *Chest* 131 (6O): 1702–1709.

12 Larkin, E.K., Patel, S.R., Redline, S. et al. (2006). Obstructive sleep apnea: evaluating whether a candidate gene explains a linkage peak. *Genet. Epidemiol.* 30 (2): 101–110.

13 Schwab, R.J., Gupta, K.B., Gefter, W.B. et al. (1995). Upper airway and soft tissue anatomy in normal subjects and patients with sleep-disordered breathing: significance of the lateral pharyngeal walls. *Am. J. Respir. Crit. Care Med.* 152 (5 pt 1): 1673–1689.

14 Belozeroff, V., Berry, R.B., and Khoo, M.C. (2003). Model-based assessment of autonomic control in obstructive sleep apnea syndrome. *Sleep* 26 (1): 65–73.

15 Dempsey, J.A., Veasey, S.C., Morgan, B.J., and O'Donnell, C.P. (2010). Pathophysiology of sleep apnea. *Physiol. Rev.* 90 (1): 47–112.

16 Nadeem, R., Molnar, J., Madbouly, E.M. et al. (2013). Serum inflammatory markers in obstructive sleep apnea: a meta-analysis. *J. Clin. Sleep Med.* 9 (10): 1003–1012.

17 Young, T., Finn, L., Peppard, P.E. et al. (2008). Sleep disordered breathing and mortality: eighteen-year follow-up of the Wisconsin sleep cohort. *Sleep* 31 (8): 1071–1078.

18 Adil EA, Meyers A. (2020) Uvulopalatopharyngoplasty. https://emedicine.medscape.com/article/1942134-overview

19 Riley, R.W., Powell, N.B., and Guilleminault, C. (1993). Obstructive sleep apnea syndrome: a review of 306 consecutively treated surgical patients. *Otolaryngol. Head Neck Surg.* 108 (2): 117–125.

20 Lye, K.W., Waite, P.D., Meara, D., and Wang, D. (2008). Quality of life evaluation of maxillomandibular advancement surgery for treatment of obstructive sleep apnea. *J. Oral Maxillofac. Surg.* 66 (5): 968–972.

21 Sailer, H.F. (2008). Rotation advancement of the face, for a new dimension of attractiveness, the reverse face lift, and the treatment of snoring and sleep apnea. *J. Craniomaxillofac. Surg.* 36 (Suppl. 1): 5.

22 Zinser, M.J., Zachow, S., and Sailer, H.F. (2013). Bimaxillary 'rotation advancement' procedures in patients with obstructive sleep apnea: a 3-dimensional airway analysis of morphological changes. *Int. J. Oral Maxillofac. Surg.* 42 (5): 569–578.

23 Lee, N.R., Givens, C.D. Jr., Wilson, J., and Robins, R.B. (1999). Staged surgical treatment of obstructive sleep apnea syndrome. *J. Oral Maxillofac. Surg.* 57 (4): 382–385.

24 Abramson, Z., Susarla, S., August, M. et al. (2010). Three-dimensional computed tomographic analysis of airway anatomy in patients with obstructive sleep apnea. *J. Oral Maxillofac. Surg.* 68 (2): 354–362.

25 Li, K.K., Guilleminault, C., Riley, R.W., and Powell, N.B. (2002). Obstructive sleep apnea and maxillomandibular advancement: an assessment of airway changes using radiographic and nasopharyngoscopic examinations. *J. Oral Maxillofac. Surg.* 60 (5): 526–530.

26 Yadav, R., Bhutia, O., Shukla, G., and Roychoudhury, A. (2014). Distraction osteogenesis for management of obstructive sleep apnoea in temporomandibular joint ankylosis patients before the release of joint. *J. Craniomaxillofac. Surg.* 42 (5): 588–594.

27 Tomonari, H., Takada, H., Hamada, T. et al. (2017). Micrognathia with temporomandibular joint ankylosis and obstructive sleep apnea treated with mandibular distraction osteogenesis using skeletal anchorage: a case report. *Head Face Med.* 13: 20.

28 Schneider, D., Kämmerer, P.W., and Bschorer R, S.G. (2015). A three-dimensional comparison of the pharyngeal airway after mandibular distraction osteogenesis and bilateral sagittal split osteotomy. *J. Craniomaxillofac. Surg.* 43 (8): 1632–1637.

29 Zanaty, O., El Metainy, S., Abo Alia, D., and Medra, A. (2016). Improvement in the airway after mandibular distraction osteogenesis surgery in children with temporomandibular joint ankylosis and mandibular hypoplasia. *Pediatr. Anesth.* 26 (4): 399–404.

30 Waite, P.D. (1998). Obstructive sleep apnea: a review of pathophysiology and surgical management. *Oral Surg. Oral Med. Oral Pathol. Oral Radiol. Endod.* 85 (4): 352–361.

31 American Association of Oral and Maxillofacial Surgeons. Obstructive sleep apnea. https://myoms.org/procedures/obstructive-sleep-apnea?gclid=EAIaIQobChMI64WEj6Sp2AIVFBuBCh3ryQVhEAAYAiAAEgLGLPD_BwE

32 American Sleep Association. Obstructive sleep apnea – research and treatments. www.sleepassociation.org/sleep-apnea/obstructive-sleep-apnea/

17

Temporomandibular Disorders: A Clinician's Guide for Nonsurgical and Surgical Interventions

Gary W. Lowder, David R. Adams and Leslie R. Halpern

Introduction

Temporomandibular disorders (TMD) comprise a group of anatomical and clinical problems involving the musculature of masticatory function, temporomandibular joint, associated neurologic structures, and surrounding musculature of the head and neck. Each unit can have an etiology unique to its structure, as well as by interactions during everyday physiological functioning of the patient. The common clinical presentations vary and include pain of the masticatory muscles, altered range of motion (ROM) during speech or eating, temporomandibular (TMJ) joint pain, pain in the myofascial musculature of the head and neck, clicking/popping and locking of the jaw joint with concomitant deviation upon opening during function, headaches, tinnitus, vertigo, and/or a combination of all.

The epidemiology of TMD can be classified with respect to gender and prevalence. TMD affects around 12% of the world population including 35 million people in the United States. Although TMD affects both men and women, the majority of those seeking care are women aged 19–49. In fact, TMD is diagnosed in women five times more frequently than in men [1, 2]. Women also tend to have more severe symptoms, with data showing women are nine times more likely to be diagnosed with major limitations in jaw movements and chronic, unremitting pain [1]. Women present with symptomatology that is more prevalent than their male cohorts.

A number of factors have been studied in relation to TMD, such as dental status, number of teeth, parafunctions, clicking and locking of the jaws, and a history of trauma. As such, it is difficult to characterize TMD as a uniform presentation owing to the large number of symptoms and signs, and the variation manifested in any one patient. A systematic review of clinical studies reported that age, gender, and psychological factors were associated with TMD. Another study on malocclusion and orthodontic treatment suggests that occlusion and prosthodontic treatment can influence symptomatology of TMD [2].

The complexity of TMD etiology(s) is significant and requires a stepwise algorithm in order to determine whether treatment can be accomplished in a nonsurgical manner. If nonsurgical treatment is unsuccessful, a variety of surgical options may be attempted that will provide relief, return to function, decreased pain, and an improved health-related quality of life.

The aims of this chapter are to provide the practitioner with well-received therapeutic options to treat the broad spectrum of both acute and chronic TMD. The pathophysiology of TMD will be described with an overview of nonsurgical and surgical modalities that are available to the patient population who present with TMD in clinical practice.

Classification and Diagnostic Evaluation

Classification

The criteria for classification of TMD are predicated upon location. In general, TMD can be categorized as articular (intracapsular) and nonarticular (extracapsular) disorders. Table 17.1 depicts both groups of which greater than 55–60% are of nonarticular origin, i.e., myofascial pain dysfunction (MFPD) [1, 2]. Nonarticular disorders are most often a result of parafunctional habits such as bruxism, clenching, nail biting, and chewing on objects. Myofascial pain involves

Oral and Maxillofacial Surgery, Medicine, and Pathology for the Clinician, First Edition. Edited by Harry Dym, Leslie R. Halpern, and Orrett E. Ogle.

Table 17.1 Disorders of TMD.

Articular disorders	Nonarticular disorders
Osteoarthritis	Myofascial pain dysfunction
Traumatic injuries	Acute muscle strain
Infectious/septic arthritis	Muscle spasms
Prior surgical intervention	Fibromyalgia
Gout/pseudogout; crystal arthropathies	Chronic pain
Rheumatoid arthritis (RA)/juvenile RA	Myotonic dystrophy
Psoriatic arthritis	Collagen diseases
Ankylosing spondylitis	

Source: Adapted from Ghali GE, Miloro M, Waite PD et al. (eds). Peterson's Principles of Oral and Maxillofacial surgery, 3rd edition. http://online.statref.com/document,aspx?fxod=100&docid=1212

discomfort or pain in the muscles of mastication that control jaw function (Figures 17.1 and 17.2).

The MFPD of these muscles is frequently associated/precipitated by emotional stress that leads to the degree of pain manifested (see section on diagnosis of nonarticular disorders and treatment modalities below). Positive responses to conservative, reversible, noninterventional therapy are often obtained and surgical intervention is of no value in these extracapsular disease presentations (see section on diagnosis and treatment for nonarticular disorders below).

Articular disorders, i.e., intracapsular dysfunction, present with similar clinical findings so the clinician must be careful in their diagnostic examination. The presentation is often characterized by localized preauricular pain and asymmetric opening during mandibular function. Ipsilateral deviation is observed on the affected side with restricted lateral excursions to the contralateral side. This is referred to as internal derangement and is defined as changes in the disc–condyle relationship [3].

The articular disorders are further characterized as either noninflammatory or inflammatory. Examples of noninflammatory include osteoarthritis, cartilage or bone diseases and previous surgical intervention as a result of trauma. The inflammatory disorders include immunocompromised diseases such as rheumatoid arthritis (RA) in adults or juvenile arthritis, psoriatic arthritis, ankylosing spondylitis, septic arthritis, gout or a variety of seronegative spondylopathies. All have their etiologies in an alteration of inflammatory cascades that can be genetic in origin, leading to a breakdown in inflammatory responses to tissue injury with resultant joint damage. Other signs include increased mobility of teeth and loss of periodontal bone support. Biomechanical activity during chewing and speech can exacerbate the degree of intracapsular cytokine secretions and can cause severe pain. Treating TMD from a dental perspective only may fall short due to undiagnosed anomalies caused by systemic disease that should be addressed concomitantly.

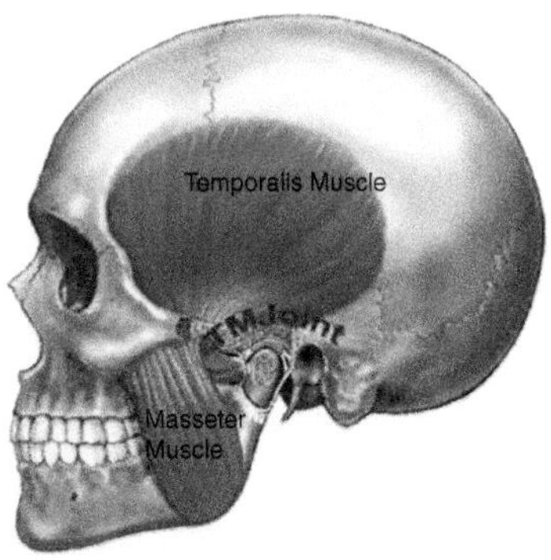

Figure 17.1 Lateral view of musculoskeletal structures of the temporomandibular apparatus.

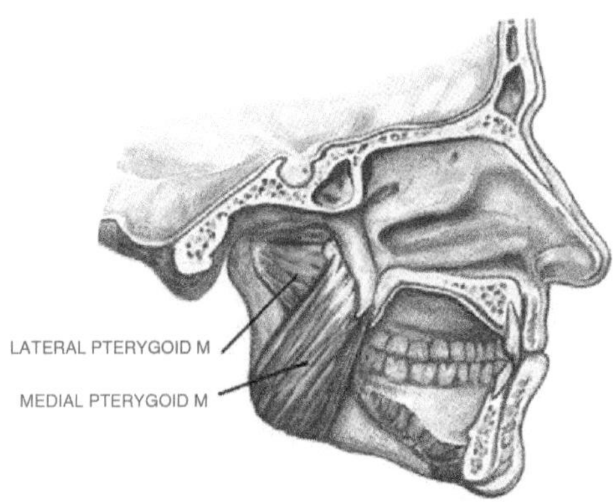

Figure 17.2 Sagittal medial view of the musculoskeletal apparatus.

Box 17.1 Wilkes staging criteria/treatment options

- Type I (early stage): painless click; Type 2 (early/intermediate): occasional pain and lock.
  - Similar to myofascial disorders: NSAIDs, anxiolytics/relaxers, "oral" hygiene and appliances if necessary for 4 weeks.
  - Radiographic: disc anteriorly positioned with normal bony contours.
  - Progression of symptoms may require surgical intervention.
  - Main goal is lysis of adhesions and repositioning of disc.
  - Arthrocentesis/arthroscopic/open joint surgery.
- Type 3 (intermediate): pain, joint tender, and displaced nonreducing disc.
  - Usually requires general anesthesia to mobilize jaw.
  - Aggressive medical and physical therapy is initiated, including a bite appliance.
  - Radiographic: anterior disc displacement with disc deformity.
  - If no improvement after 3 weeks, surgery is indicated to lyse adhesions and/or reposition disc via condylotomy or arthroscopy.
- Type 4 (intermediate/late): chronic pain/limited opening, bony changes.
  - Chronic pain, headaches, restricted movement, degenerative joint disease (DJD), remodeling of bone.
  - Radiographic: bony changes with a flattened eminence, condyle deformity, and osteosclerotic changes.
  - Open procedures: meniscus removal/reposition/fascia/fat/alloplastic materials.
- Type 5 (late): joint pain, crepitus and perforation or DJD of disc.
  - Crepitus, grinding, anterior displacement with perforation of disc, multiple adhesions.
  - Radiographic: disc perforation, gross deformities of bony structures, cartilage and progressive arthritic changes
  - Consider alloplastic/total joint replacement/fascia graft.

Source: Adapted from Bronstein S, Merrill B. Disorders of the TMJ. Oral Maxillofac Clin North Am 1989;7:16–24.

Internal derangement can be of two types: disc displacement with reduction and disc displacement without reduction. In a reducing disc displacement, during function the displaced disc generates a "click" followed by disc relocation anteriorly upon closing. Disc dislocation without reduction results in the condylar head being unable to completely move under the disc with a resultant decrease in opening during function [4]. Both disc dislocation with or without reduction can elicit pain. The articular disorders are classified according to the staging of the degree of internal derangement, referred to as the Wilkes staging classification for internal derangement of the TMJ [3]. There are five stages that satisfy several criteria, i.e., radiographic imaging, anatomic description, and clinical exam (Box 17.1).

Diagnostic Evaluation

The diagnosis of TMD requires a focused approach following a set of criteria that includes the history of the present illness and an in-depth physical examination. This begins with a head and neck exam, careful palpation of the muscles of mastication and muscles of neck and posterior occiput, and palpation of the preauricular areas. Occlusal analysis is required to address interfering tooth contacts during opening and lateral excursions, as well as protrusive mandibular movements. Parafunctional habit evaluation involves examination for wear facets and assessment of habit bite as compared to tooth contacts in a centric relation hinge axis position [1, 5]. Box 17.2 lists the modalities of imaging most often applied in diagnostic approaches to TMD.

Radiographic imaging includes periapical radiographs to evaluate localized pathology that may cause pain which may be referred throughout the head and neck.

Whether the etiology is trauma related, iatrogenic, or idiopathic in nature, the surgeon will usually conduct a history, exam, and diagnosis. With this accomplished, the appropriate care of the patient is directed toward conservative nonsurgical treatment that may include counseling, physical therapy, occlusal splint therapy, massage, manual therapy, and other low-risk and reversible forms of therapy. Ultimately, the goal is to achieve the maximum level of manageable patient comfort and stability. Of greatest importance is the emphasis on restoring orthopedic stability of the temporomandibular joint and associated masticatory muscles, and the reduction of the biologic burden on the masticatory system. When parafunctional habits and/or contributing malocclusions are detected, the dental standard of care generally calls for intraoral orthotic appliance (splint) therapy (a more detailed review of splint therapy is given in the Intraoral Orthotic/Splint Therapy section below) [6].

Box 17.2 Diagnostic imaging tools for TMD

- *Plain films* (orthopantogram) useful for initial screening, although largely replaced by MRI and CT.
- *Computed tomography*: best technique for bony pathology and 3D planning for surgical intervention.
  - Sagittal and coronal views for condylar remodeling/eminence/glenoid fossa relationships.
  - 3D reformatting for fabrication of total joints.
- *Magnetic resonance imaging*: best technique for joint space pathology: T1 and T2 weighting for joint effusions and disc displacements to determine reducing vs nonreducing discs.
- *Ultrasound*: Needle guided for localization of locules of purulence for specimens (septic arthritis of TMJ).

Box 17.3 Patient screening questionnaire and examination procedures for TMD

Recommended screening questionnaire

1. Do you have difficulty or pain, or both, when opening your mouth, as for instance, when yawning?
2. Does your jaw get "stuck," "locked," or "go out"?
3. Do you have difficulty or pain, or both, when chewing, talking, or using your jaws?
4. Are you aware of noises in the jaw joints?
5. Do you have pain in or about the ears, temples, or cheeks?
6. Does your bite feel uncomfortable or unusual?
7. Do you have frequent headaches?
8. Have you had a recent injury to your head, neck, or jaw?
9. Have you previously been treated for a jaw joint problem? If so, when?

Note: If any one of the first three questions is answered affirmatively, the clinician should complete a comprehensive history and examination; for questions 4 through 8, two should be answered affirmatively, and for question 9, a positive answer to two other questions (4–8) is required to warrant further evaluation.

Recommended examination procedures

1. Measure range of motion of the mandible on opening and right and left laterotrusion.
2. Palpate for preauricular TMJ tenderness.
3. Palpate or use stethoscope auscultation for TMJ crepitus.
4. Palpate or use stethoscope auscultation for TMJ clicking.
5. Palpate for tenderness in the masseter and temporalis muscles.
6. Note excessive occlusal wear, excessive tooth mobility, fremitus, or migration in the absence of periodontal disease, and soft tissue alterations, for example, buccal mucosal ridging, lateral tongue scalloping.
7. Inspect symmetry and alignment of the face, jaws, and dental arches.

Note: Any positive finding for procedures 1 through 3 warrants consideration for a comprehensive history and examination, whereas any two positive findings for procedures 4 through 6 suggest the same consideration; procedure 7 requires two other positive findings (4–6) to suggest the same consideration.

History

The diagnosis of TMD requires a focused approach following a set of criteria that includes the history of the present illness. It is noted that 70–80% of the diagnosis for TMD will be ascertained from taking a thorough history [6]. Etiology and initiation of symptoms, exacerbation of symptoms, intensity and duration, acute or chronic nature, etc. are all aspects of the history that provide evidence for an accurate diagnosis. Of the many possible patient screening and history forms available for the dentist treating TMD, the reader may find the questionaire in Box 17.3 to be useful.

Physical Exam

The physical exam is described above in the diagnostic evaluation of the patient.

Nonsurgical Treatment Approaches

Finding a dental provider who has training in nonsurgical management of TMD is important in accomplishing the successful outcomes needed for these patients, and should be the first avenue for care. Two major concepts must be considered in the evaluation and treatment of patients presenting with the chief complaint of TMD.

- Orthopedic stability of the masticatory system.
  - "A closed-pack relationship of the condyle, articular disc, and fossae as determined by the mandibular muscles during function" defines orthopedic stability of the masticatory system [7].
  - Dentally, orthopedic stability exists when the stable intercuspal position of the teeth is in harmony with the musculoskeletally stable position of the condyles in the fossae [6].
- Biologic burden: biologic burden consists of those factors that are imposed upon the masticatory system before, during, and after functional use. Assessing the degree of biologic burden is integral to diagnosis and treatment. A systematic review of research regarding TMD reports: "The neuromuscular system responsible for chewing function has a high potential to adapt to changing conditions. Only when the compensatory capabilities of the masticatory and the neuromuscular system are overstretched, dysfunction occurs resulting in clinical symptoms and manifests as pain, severe clicking, or limited mobility of the mandible, forcing the patient to seek help" [7].

Treatment is categorized into reversible (Box 17.4) and nonreversible (Box 17.5) methodologies. Each is discussed in terms of a flowchart of steps.

Methods of Therapy

When parafunctional habits and/or contributing malocclusions are detected, the dental standard of care primarily yields to intraoral orthotic appliance (splint) therapy. Since dentists are the only providers trained in the application of this form of therapy, an understanding of its design and application is crucial to the successful outcomes needed. Such therapy allows the dentist to create an artificial ideal bite relationship that allows for restoration of orthopedic stability in a reversible therapeutic modality. Once orthopedic stability is established, an occlusal analysis of the patient's dental interarch relationships can be accomplished in order to direct appropriate irreversible occlusal therapies for tooth relationships that will support this stability. These may include enamoplasty (dental occlusal equilibration), orthodontics, and a varied number of prosthodontic restorative procedures.

Splint Therapy

The primary objective of splint therapy is to eliminate occlusal imbalances in the natural dentition that may be contributing to TMD symptoms. A chairside fabrication device known as a "Lucia Jig" utilizes the proprioception of the mandibular incisors to deprogram the elevator muscles and eliminate all posterior occlusal prematurities and eccentric interferences. The Lucia jig is effective in deprogramming of muscle trismus-associated TMD symptoms.

Box 17.4 Reversible treatment options

Components of reversible treatment may include the following.

- Nontreatment, e.g., physical rest and minimal functional use allowing normal healing and recovery.
- Physical therapy, e.g., massage, soft diet, exercises, heat and cold, muscle stimulation, ultrasound, etc.
- Stress management counseling.
- Intraoral orthotic/splint therapy: utilizes an artificial, ideal occlusal support device designed to protect joints and masticatory muscles from malocclusion of the teeth that may predispose, initiate, or perpetuate symptoms.
- Any combination of the above.

Box 17.5 Nonreversible treatment options

Components of irreversible forms of therapy may include the following.

- Orthodontic correction of intra-arch and intraarch relationships of the teeth.
- Equilibration of occlusal contacts to provide for bilateral, simultaneous, and stable (BSS) interarch tooth contacts.
- Restorative crown and bridge therapy or restoration of edentulous, nonsupported interarch relationships.
- Surgical correction of skeletal and/or soft tissue conditions that inhibit orthopedic stability of the masticatory system.
- Any combination of the above required to establish or restore orthopedic stability.

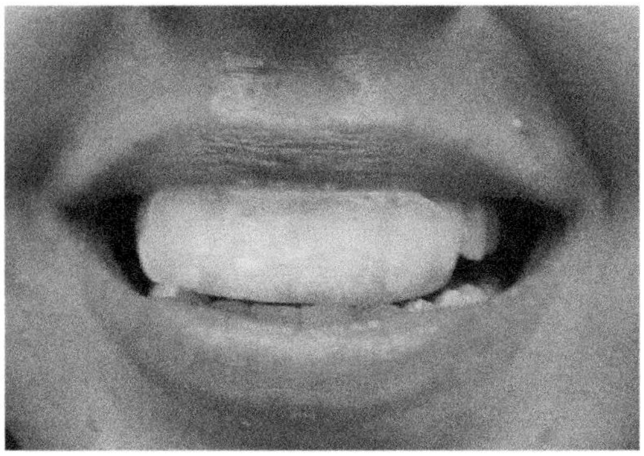

Figure 17.3 Lucia jig. *Source:* Courtesy of Gary W. Lowder.

The intent is that this device should only be employed on a temporary basis until a full arch intraoral orthotic appliance/splint can be fabricated in the lab (Figure 17.3). The splint becomes a more long-term stabilizing treatment device and establishes an artificial "ideal bite" acrylic appliance that covers the incisal and occlusal surfaces of one arch of teeth. The appliance is adjusted to provide for bilateral, simultaneous, and stable occlusal contacts of the opposing arch of teeth at the maximum intercuspation position (MIP) and establishes guidance planes on the acrylic to prevent posterior tooth contacts in protrusive, mediotrusive (balancing), and laterotrusive (working) eccentric mandibular movements. This is accomplished by designing canine-protected and incisal-guided inclines of acrylic in the splint that mimic incisal and canine guidance in the dentition (Figure 17.4).

It is believed that in patients who develop TMD, interfering functional tooth contacts contribute to orthopedic instability of the TMJ and associated masticatory muscles. These interferences may lead to clenching or bruxing patterns as the system seeks to eliminate tooth contact imbalances. Depending on frequency, intensity, and duration of clenching and bruxing habits (parafunctional habits), symptoms may develop that override the adaptability of the masticatory system. This creates a biologic burden to the system that leads to symptom development.

Splint therapy reduces the instability of the TMJ joint condyles to an orthopedically stable hinge axis position and muscle reprogramming to a normal functional state. The splint design and management must be such that it meets all the criteria of an ideal occlusal relationship. Otherwise, the dentist has introduced another form of occlusal imbalance for the masticatory system to deal with. Careful follow-up adjustments must be performed periodically to correct changes in occlusal contacts as the mandible assumes a corrected and orthopedically stable position at the hinge axis. This usually requires multiple adjustments at 2–3-week intervals until no further changes in occlusal contact patterns are required. At that point, it is assumed that the mandibular condyles are at the orthopedically stable position and further diagnostic evaluations can be performed to detect and correct any occlusal disharmony.

When a minimum of 50% improvement has occurred, an occlusal analysis with articulator-mounted diagnostic models of the teeth can then be evaluated for the best nonreversible treatment approach to correct an occlusal imbalance. If the patient has achieved a return to manageable comfort, the clinician may advise the patient to discontinue splint wear, wear the splint only while sleeping, or use the splint only as needed to control flare-ups.

Maxillary and Mandibular Full-Arch Splints

Full-arch splints (either maxillary or mandibular) incorporate all the features of ideal interarch occlusal contacts in order to achieve the desired results of functional orthopedic stability.

Other Reversible Therapeutic Options

Other forms of therapy include oral and injectable drug therapy and other physiotherapeutic techniques. All are often helpful and sometimes essential to the successful restoration of orthopedic stability. Any combination of the above may be employed in the effort to achieve symptom reduction and restoration of comfortable masticatory function [8].

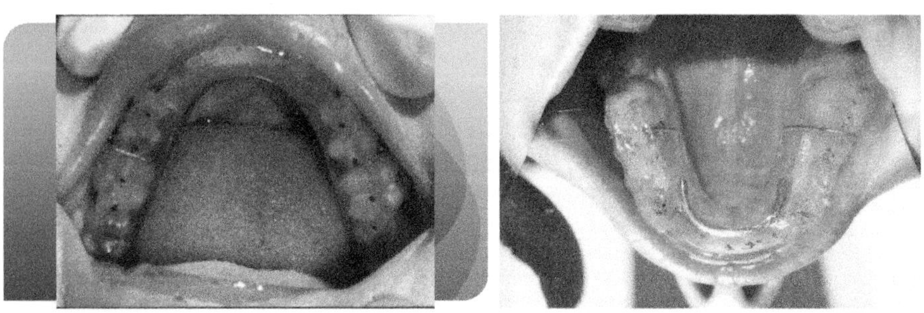

(a) (b)

Figure 17.4 (a) Mandibular splint with ideal occlusal contact design. (b) Maxillary splint with ideal occlusal contact design at centric and eccentric. *Source:* Courtesy of Gary W. Lowder.

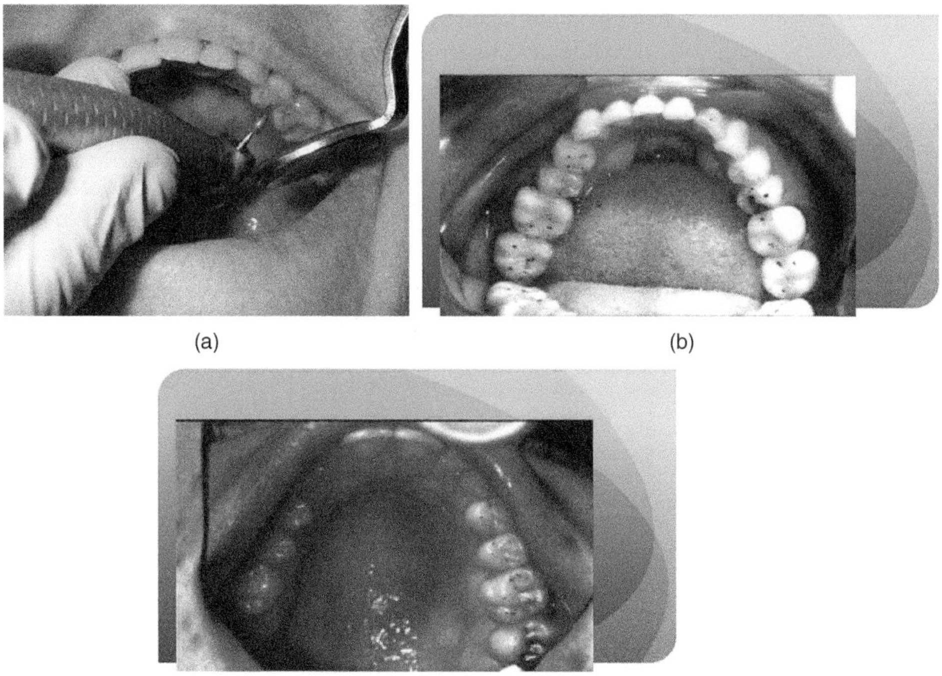

Figure 17.5 (a) Resculpting (enamoplasty) of teeth to eliminate interferences in eccentric mandibular movements. (b) Mandibular BSS occlusal contacts following equilibration procedure. (c) Maxillary BSS occlusal contacts following equilibration procedure. *Source:* Courtesy of Gary W. Lowder.

Integral to the success of therapy is the enrollment of the patient in taking an active and responsible role in improving their own health and well-being. Patient understanding of the complex nature of TMD and its negative effects on their day-to-day functions is a necessary part of healing. Successful therapeutic outcomes of TMD therapy, whether surgical or nonsurgical, depend on the patient's compliance with their recommended treatment.

Nonreversible General Dentistry Methods of Therapy

These varied forms of dental therapy must not be attempted if orthopedic stability of the joints and masticatory muscles has not been achieved. In the case of splint therapy, at least a 50% reduction in TMD symptoms must have been accomplished before irreversible forms of dental therapy are justified. These include:

- equilibration/resculpting of the teeth via odontoplasty (Figure 17.5)
- orthodontic tooth movement (Figure 17.6)
- prosthodontic procedures utilizing restorative materials or fixed prosthodontic treatments (Figure 17.7).

All of these are intended to restore functionally stable occlusal relationships that are in harmony with the orthopedically stabilized joints and masticatory muscles.

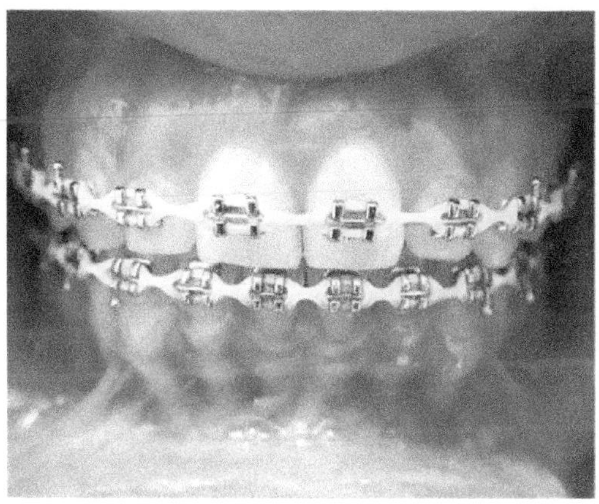

Figure 17.6 Typical orthodontic stabilization of interarch tooth contacts and alignment. *Source:* Courtesy of Gary W. Lowder.

Surgical Approaches

The clinician must understand that it does not necessarily follow that because nonsurgical efforts fail, then surgery will be the next option. Surgical intervention is a reasonable option when nonsurgical therapy has failed in relieving symptomatology, with continued disability and diminished health-related quality of life. Box 17.6 lists the general therapeutic goals of surgical therapy for TMD put forth by the American Association of Oral and Maxillofacial Surgeons (AAOMS) [5]. A discussion must

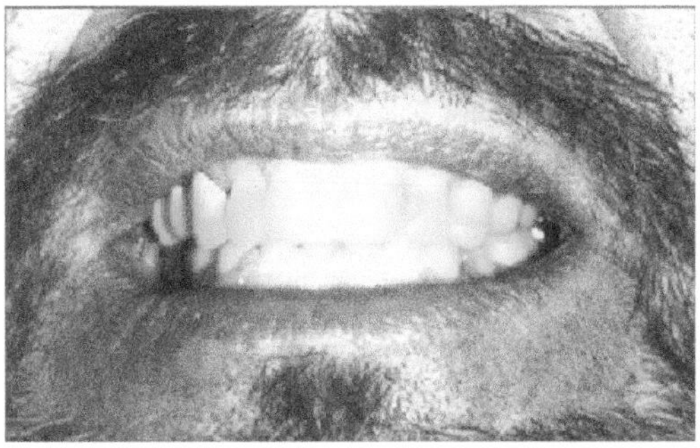

(a)

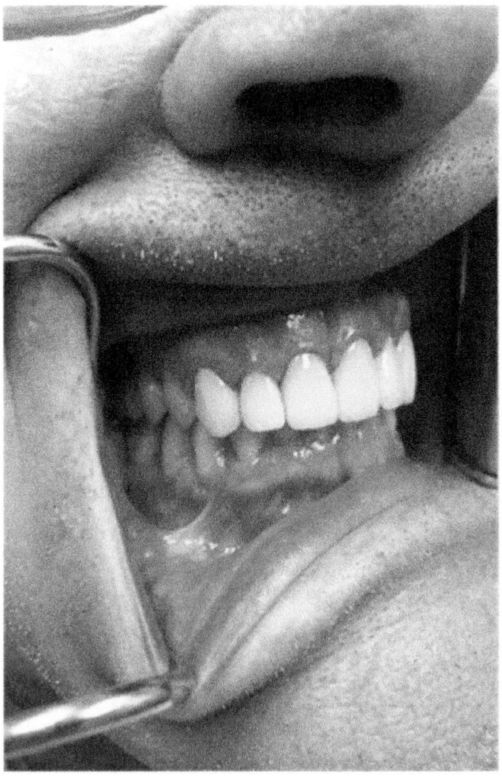

(b)

Figure 17.7 (a) Anterior guidance, vertical dimension and BSS occlusal contacts restored via composite resin bonding. (b) Anterior guidance, vertical dimension and BSS occlusal contacts restored via fixed prosthodontic treatment. *Source:* Courtesy of Gary W. Lowder.

be undertaken by the clinician to address the risk-to-benefit ratio of surgical intervention. Aspects for consideration include identifiable pathology amenable to surgical therapy, biomechanical disruption during speech and nutrition, degree of pain, and risk for multiple surgical interventions if further procedures are warranted. Regardless of the surgical approach, the clinician and patient must appreciate the varied predictability as to the progression of TMD with or without active treatment since the disease may self-correct or progress whether or not surgical intervention is undertaken [6, 9].

The surgical procedures that can be considered range from chairside, minimally invasive arthrocentesis with manipulation of the mandible, to arthroscopy. Maximal surgical intervention includes; condylotomy, arthrotomy, orthognathic surgery, and total replacement of the condylar ramal TMJ apparatus (Box 17.7).

Minimally Invasive Approaches

Intraarticular Injections Several pharmacologic solutions can be injected into the TMJ to allow for relief of inflammation and joint degeneration. The most common approach is to inject into the superior joint space above the disc. Injections can also be applied to the inferior joint space, which is more difficult but can be successful in providing pain relief and resolution of mouth opening. Common solutions include hyaluronic acid and corticosteroids. Table 17.2 compares these agents with respect to risks/benefits and efficacy [4].

Complications of intraarticular injections must be considered. Risk of mechanical nerve trauma during injection has been reported, although the chance of permanent paresthesia is minimal.

Nerve damage and risk of neuroma formation have been reported, as well as hematoma formation and injury to adjacent structures at the site of injection. Systemic side-effects can occur due to intravascular compromise which can be minimal with aspiration techniques. The latter can be exacerbated if patients are on pharmacologic management of other major systemic illnesses, i.e., cardiovascular disease requiring anticoagulants and antiplatelet medications (the

Box 17.6 Therapeutic goals for temporomandibular joint surgery

- Improve function and form
- Limited period of disability
- Improved range of jaw motion and/or function
- Appropriate understanding by patient (family) of treatment options and acceptance of treatment plan
- Appropriate understanding and acceptance by patient (family) of favorable outcomes and known risks and complications
- Reduction in pain
- Improved quality of life

Box 17.7 Surgical approaches for temporomandibular joint surgery

Minimally invasive
- Intraarticular injections
- Arthrocentesis
- Arthroscopy

Maximal surgery
- Condylotomy
- Arthrotomy
- Hypermobility procedures
- Total joint replacement

Table 17.2 Comparison of agents for intraarticular TMJ treatment.

	Hyaluronic acid	*Corticocosteroids*
Benefits	A natural ingredient of synovial fluid: lubricatant	Decrease inflammation/immune activity
Adverse effects	Mild pain/swelling at injection site; transient	Infection Erode articular cartilage Avoid repeat injection
Efficacy	Improvement in symptoms over time but imaging may not show anatomical improvement	Same overall improvement as hyaluronic acid

Source: Adapted from: Liu F, Steinkeler A [4].

reader is referred to Chapter 20 in this book for further interest).

Arthrocentesis and Arthroscopy McCain and colleagues blazed a trail for the use of minimally invasive technology in order for the oral and maxillofacial surgeon to allow the naked eye an alternative technique to perform micro- and macroscopic surgical intervention beyond boundaries that were previously exposed only with large incisions [10]. Oral clinicians can be trained to apply this technology in an effort to decrease patient postsurgical consequences, providing bloodless surgery and little trauma to surrounding anatomy. Access for intervention is smaller and distant to the area of interest and therefore less likely to cause injuries seen with larger access. Microinstrumentation under higher magnification has made endoscopy more appealing and well accepted by both practitioner and patient. Advantages include minimal morbidity, shorter hospital stay, quicker return to more normal function, and less postoperative discomfort [10].

Arthrocentesis Arthrocentesis is an office-based procedure that is easy to perform and involves the placement of two needles into the superior joint space for the purpose of applying hydraulic pressure followed by lavage of the joint space with Ringer's lactate. The technique itself involves the continual flushing of the superior joint space with a minimum of 100 cc of lactated Ringer's or normal saline solution. Patients who present with an acute "closed lock" or painful self-reducing disc displacement disorder benefit from this approach due to the lysis of intracapsular adhesions, lavage and mobilization of the TMJ disc, and removal of painful inflammatory mediators. Numerous algorithms for TMJ therapy suggest that arthrocentesis should be attempted before performing any open surgical intervention [5]. The procedure is completed with the injection of a corticosteroid.

Postoperative instructions should include pharmacotherapy, continued occlusal splint therapy, and physical therapy during recovery. Patients who will benefit from this procedure are most often those with early stages of internal derangement [5].

Arthroscopy Arthroscopy requires a steeper learning curve and is done in the hospital outpatient setting. Most arthroscopic procedures are used for diagnosis, lysis of adhesions and lavage of debris due to inflammatory cytokines within the superior joint space. A thin fiberoptic device (typically 1.9–2.7 mm diameter) attached to a high-intensity light source and camera is inserted through a 3 mm cannula into the superior joint space (Figure 17.8).

This technique allows a direct view, displayed on a video monitor, of all tissues in the joint space. Using a second cannula, special surgical instruments are inserted under

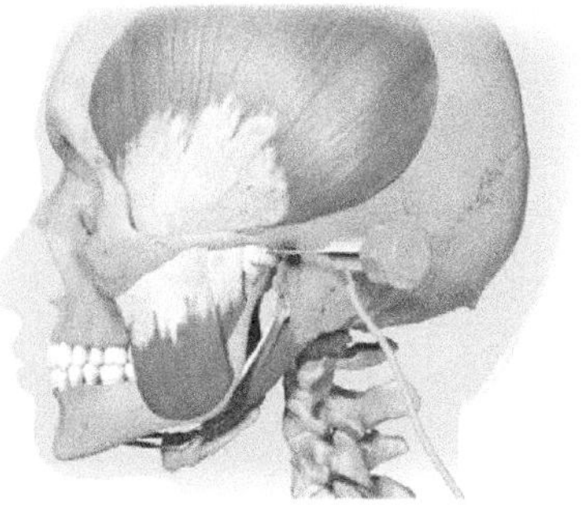

Figure 17.8 Sagittal view of arthroscopic instrumentation within the left TMJ joint space. *Source:* Courtesy of NEXUS CMF Corporation, with permission.

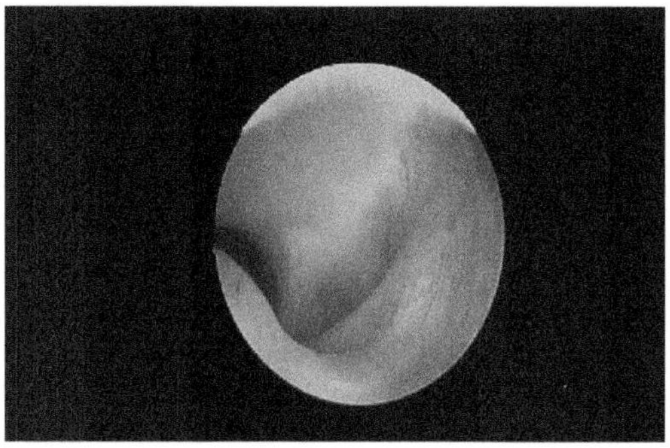

Figure 17.9 Arthroscopic view of the left temporomandibular joint superior joint space. *Source:* Courtesy of NEXUS CMF Corporation, with permission.

direct arthroscopic visualization to treat pathology. Surgical manipulation can allow the operator to remove adhesions from the disc and reposition it either by passive or active plication of synovial tissues (Figures 17.9 and 17.10).

Treatment goals include a reduction in pain and improved biomechanical function, as well as formulation of an accurate diagnosis for treatment of hypermobility, synovitis, hypomobility, and early osteoarthritis.

Complications of arthroscopy are uncommon but may include injury to the external acoustic meatus, middle ear, and tympanic membrane which can result in hearing loss due to ear infection and sensorineural hearing loss. Additional possible complications include auricular temporal nerve damage, invasion of the middle cranial fossa and Frey syndrome as a result of violation of the parotid capsule.

Risks and benefits of treatment must be discussed with the patient so that proper informed consent can be gained. Patients who may not be considered for this technique include those with infections of tissues outside and within the TMJ proper, bony ankylosis and patients who have a previous history of arthrotomy of the joint. The latter may be considered if arthroscopy has not been successful in relieving symptomatology [10].

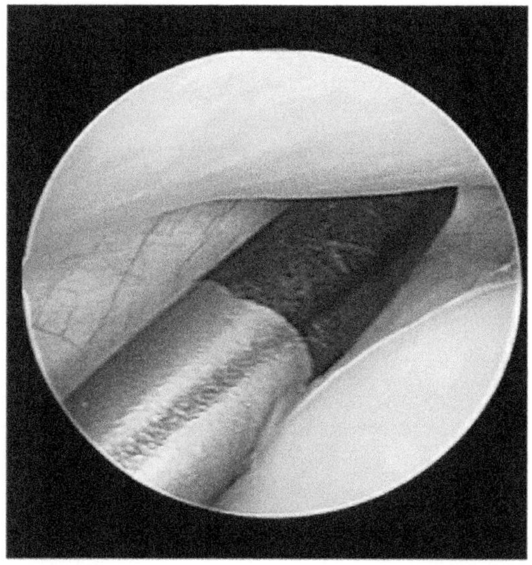

Figure 17.10 Arthroscopic view of triangulating instrument removing adhesions from the superior aspect of the left temporomandibular joint superior to the disc. *Source:* Courtesy of NEXUS CMF Corporation, with permission.

Maximal Surgery

Condylotomy The primary indication for a condylotomy approach is a chronic, painful, TMJ disc displacement. The Wilkes criteria staging for this is usually Wilkes II and III internal derangement with a nonself-reducing disc displacement [3]. This procedure is also advocated for recurrent temporomandibular joint dislocation. Hall et al. modified the condylotomy for the treatment of painful temporomandibular joint with reducing discs [11]. Their technique has withstood the evidence-based assumptions for reducing disc resolution as a result of a "condylar sag."

This procedure is performed with a modified intraoral vertical ramus osteotomy (IVRO). This will alter the condylar/disc/glenoid fossa relationship, resulting in a "sag" that provides space for repositioning of the disc (Figure 17.11). The osteotomy is completed and the patient is placed into maxillomandibular fixation to allow the proximal condylar segment to heal laterally against the distal ramus segment. After 2 weeks, the patient is placed into elastics to allow their occlusion to settle into the postoperative position. Elastics are maintained for 3–4 weeks. Most patients gain relief without further reoperation [11].

Complications of the procedure include possible inferior alveolar nerve damage, masseteric artery violation, and malocclusion.

Arthrotomy/Arthroplasty Arthrotomy is an umbrella term for a procedure that requires surgical opening of a joint and directly identifying the abnormality to be treated. An incision is made over the TMJ joint via a variety of approaches – preauricular, postauricular, or endaural (Figure 17.12a).

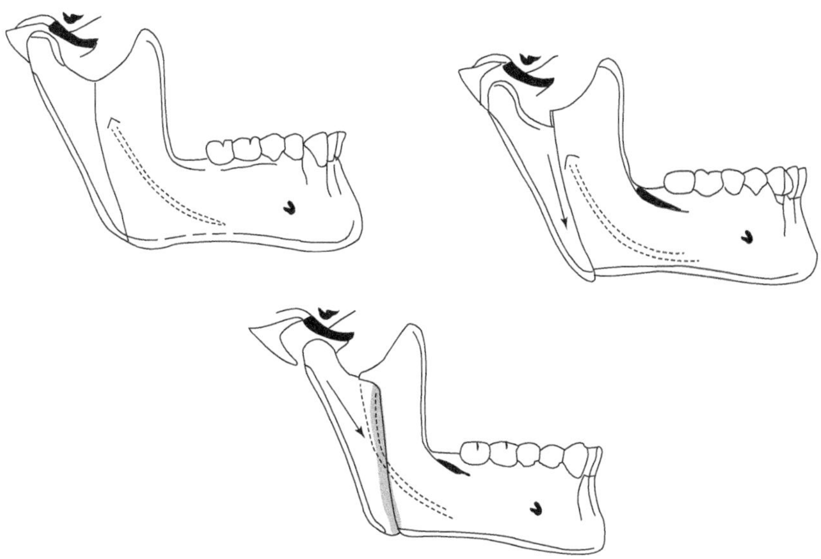

Figure 17.11 Modified condylotomy procedure for the temporomandibular joint.

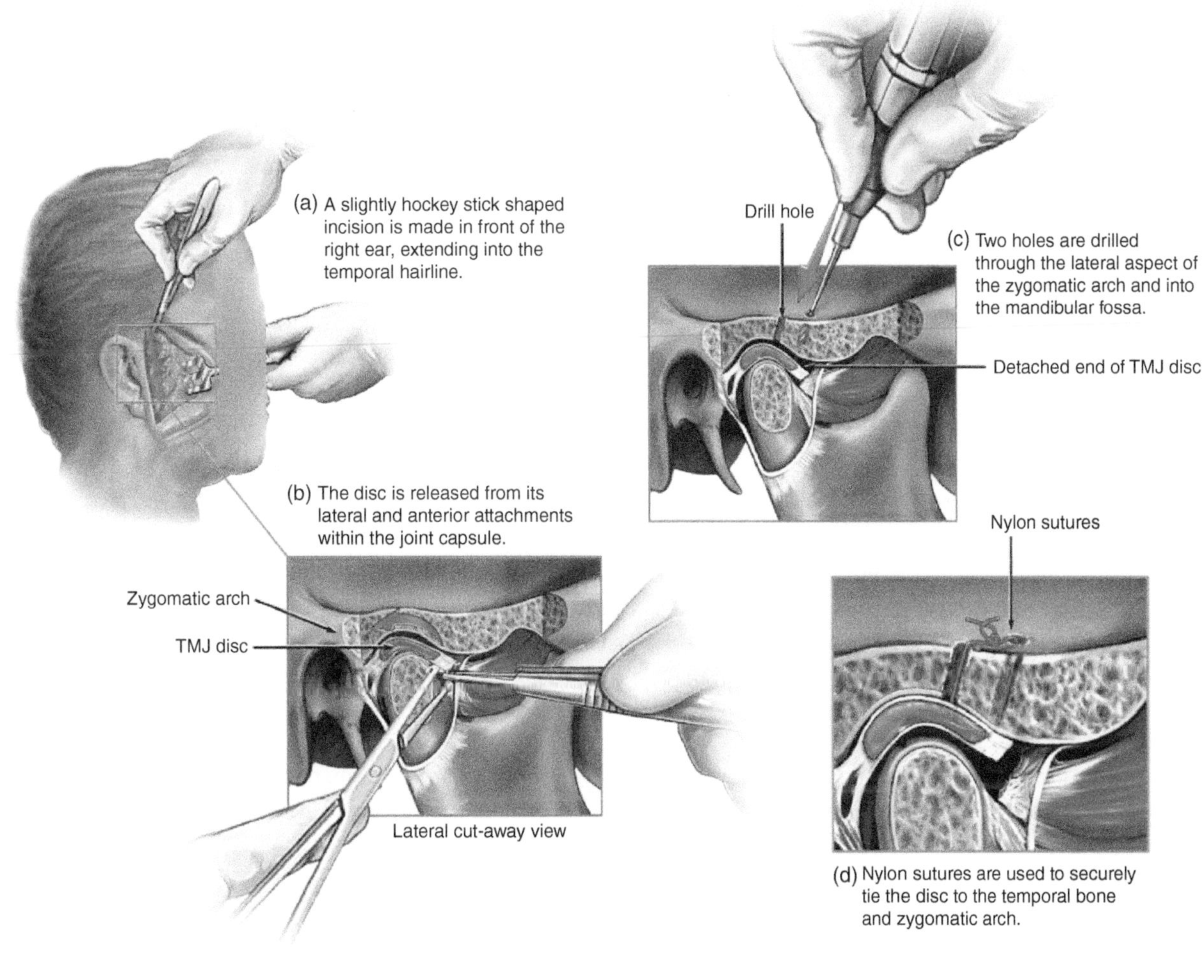

(a) A slightly hockey stick shaped incision is made in front of the right ear, extending into the temporal hairline.
Drill hole
(c) Two holes are drilled through the lateral aspect of the zygomatic arch and into the mandibular fossa.
Detached end of TMJ disc
(b) The disc is released from its lateral and anterior attachments within the joint capsule.
Nylon sutures
Zygomatic arch
TMJ disc
Lateral cut-away view
(d) Nylon sutures are used to securely tie the disc to the temporal bone and zygomatic arch.

Figure 17.12 Preauricular approach to the right temporomandibular joint.

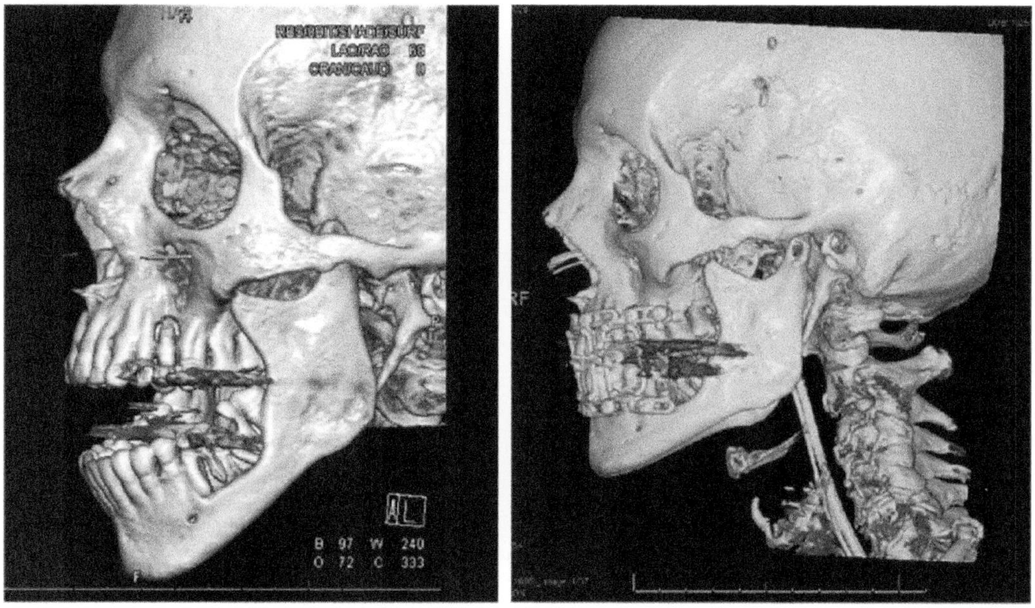

(a) (b)

Figure 17.13 (a) Chronic dislocated mandibular condyle resulting in an open bite. (b) Chronic dislocated mandible that was repaired with removal of fibrotic tissue and reposition of condylar heads in the glenoid fossae. *Source:* Courtesy of Leslie R. Halpern and David R. Adams.

The criteria for an arthrotomy include patients with progressive internal derangement that does not respond to nonsurgical or minimally invasive therapies. Examples of disease states that require this open procedure include articular disc degeneration and displacement, the treatment of pathologic entities such as condylar hyperplasia, septic arthritis, chronic dislocation, and the formation of bony ankylosis due to placement of alloplastic implants into the joint cavity.

Arthroplasty is an open joint procedure in which the articular surface of the condylar head is remodeled/reshaped to remove bony pathology that is due to severe disc pathology or other pathologic conditions of the cartilage and bone. Many patients present with severe disc perforations, degeneration, and displacement that require removal of the disc followed by arthroplasty. Examples of arthroplasty procedures include high condylar shaves and condylectomy, resulting in the formation of a gap that increases the joint space and interface between the condylar head and glenoid fossa.

TMJ Disc Repositioning The most common TMJ pathologic disease is anterior-medial displacement of the articular disc, which can lead to TMJ-related symptoms. The disc can be surgically repositioned into its normal anatomic position to relieve a painful locking TMJ. The indication for disc repositioning surgery is irreversible TMJ damage associated with temporomandibular pain. The anterior or medially displaced disc can often be manually reduced into a more anatomically active position with retrodiscal relief which can lead to improvement in symptoms (Figure 17.13). This procedure is best undertaken with a disc that is firm, white, and minimally displaced [4, 12]. Discal tissue repair can be accomplished at the same time with sutures that provide tension-free primary closure.

TMJ Discectomy without Grafting When a disc is damaged beyond repair, it is extirpated by a menisectomy (discectomy). The severe pathology of the disc can interfere with the biomechanics of TMJ function since it precipitates/exacerbates the hard tissue changes exhibited by the condylar head. Once the discal tissue is removed, a decision must be made as to the maintenance of "normal anatomy" of the underlying cartilage/bone since the removal of discal and osseous pathology will increase the joint space and the condyles' relationship with the glenoid fossa. Arthroplasty can be performed to alleviate the pain associated with disc perforations and possible osteophyte formation. The size of gap formed by the arthroplasty will determine whether a graft is needed.

TMJ Discectomy with Replacement of a Graft The prevention of fibrous and bony union requires the placement of a graft that will protect the joint from further degeneration, as well as providing a soft tissue interface between the condylar head and glenoid fossa during range of motion. There is no consensus as to the type of replacement material that can be applied over the condylar head or whether it is necessary in order to prevent fibrous and bony ankyloses. The choices of grafting materials available can vary from autogenous to alloplastic in nature. Examples of autogenous material include articular cartilage, temporalis fascial grafting, and/or dermal fat [13, 14]. The grafting of fascia has been shown to be a very reliable technique, especially when tensile strength is required. Fascia is much more predictable than fat, with respect to retaining anatomic characteristics. Fascia, however, lacks bulk which limits its use in soft tissue augmentation [13, 14].

Transplanted nonvascularized muscle almost always loses its anatomic form and is partially replaced by fibrous tissue. As such, free muscle grafts therefore have very limited application in TMJ discectomy procedures [3, 13]. The use of autogenous dermal fat has the potential for superior clinical outcomes with respect to range of motion, decreased pain, and increased health-related quality of life [13, 14]. More recent studies have supported the use of autogenous full-thickness skin-subcutaneous fat graft as an interpositional material following discectomy and ankylosis release [13, 14]. The overall findings agreed that autogenous grafts do not prevent remodeling of the condylar head but do reduce crepitus and other painful sequelae in the postoperative functioning of the TMJ following discectomy.

Hypermobility Hypermobility in the most simple terms is a condition where the condyle translates beyond its normal position/range in relation to the articular eminence. The hypermobile TMJ is thus prone to a traumatic subluxation or dislocation that may be difficult to reduce back to a normal position and function. Subluxation is characterized by an incomplete dislocation whereby the condyle translates beyond the articular eminence upon opening, and may be manipulated back into the glenoid fossa by the patient.

Dislocation is a more significant mechanical event, usually due to a hypermobile TMJ. The condyle will advance anterior to the articular eminence with a resultant "open lock" that cannot be manipulated back into the fossa by the patient. The latter will require surgical intervention. Dislocation of the mandibular condyle (MC) is an uncommon event with an incidence around 3% in the overall population and a slight female predominance [1]. There are several causes for this condition, with trauma being the most common. Etiologies of dislocation/subluxation include trauma, laxity of the TMJ capsule due to connective tissue diseases, degenerative joint disease, internal derangement, accidental trauma or iatrogenic injury from health procedures such as endotracheal intubation or dental extractions [15].

Most cases of acute hypermobility of the TMJ can be corrected by manual reduction and stabilization with either wires on arch bars or loops to maintain the jaw position for at least 2 weeks [12, 15]. This is followed by placement of light elastics with instructions to open and close in a way that avoids certain triggers for hypermobility, i.e., opening the mouth wide when yawning.

Surgical correction of TMJ hypermobility is reserved for cases that cannot be manually manipulated back in cases of chronic dislocation or a dislocation that has not been corrected for an extended period of time. Both can affect the patient's health-related quality of life. Surgical correction of hypermobility can be further divided into two groups: mobility that limits the range of condylar movement and a "blocking" of surrounding anatomy that prevents the condyle from returning to its normal position. Surgical interventions include eminectomy by performing an osteotomy over the articular eminence that will flatten and prevent biomechanical blocking of the condyle during movement; down-fracturing of a portion of the zygomatic arch (LeClerc procedure) to prevent excessive translation of the condyle; capsular plication; condylotomy, and sclerosing agents to enhance fibrotic scar formation that will limit condylar movement [15].

The intramuscular injection of botulinum neurotoxin into the inferior head of the lateral pterygoid either intraorally or transcutaneously is highly effective and safe for treating patients with recurrent TMJ dislocation. This method should be the first choice in patients for whom surgical procedures are contraindicated [16].

Long-term chronic traumatic dislocation of the condyle has been reported in the medical literature with the potential to erode the middle fossa, resulting in severe complications. Clinical features are similar to the usual dislocation of the MC such as open bite, limitation of mouth opening, and pain. Additional complications can arise including dural tears, cerebrospinal fluid leak, pneumocephalus, intracranial hemorrhage, brain contusion, hearing loss, facial palsy, and chronic TMJ degenerative changes and dysfunction. This must be treated more invasively with exposure by a coronal approach and debridement of fibrotic tissue to allow condylar repositioning into the fossa and stabilization of the occlusion and postoperative care as stated above (Figure 17.13).

Total Joint Reconstruction Reconstruction of the TMJ may be required for a number of reasons when more conservative or less invasive procedures are either not indicated or have failed to treat significant TMJ-related pathologies.

Box 17.8 Indications for TMJ total joint replacement.

- Chronic, recurrent or worsening joint ankylosis
- Congenital or developmental disorders (e.g., Treacher–Collins syndrome, Pierre Robin syndrome, hemifacial microsomia)
- Avascular necrosis
- Neoplasia of the TMJ requiring resection
- Severe degenerative joint disease including connective tissue and autoimmune diseases (osteoarthritis, rheumatoid arthritis, traumatic arthritis, scleroderma, lupus, etc.)
- Irreparable severe condylar fracture
- Revision procedure after failed previous surgeries (>2 previous surgeries) and after removal of failed alloplastic implants
- Significant maxillofacial deformities requiring surgical repositioning with symptomatic, unstable TMJs
- Significant maxillofacial deformities with severely hypoplastic TMJs
- Post resection of the condyle or the condyle with additional adjacent portions of the mandible

Source: Based on [14,15].

The indications for total joint replacement are shown in Box 17.8.

In years past, autogenous tissue grafts such as costochondral, sternoclavicular, temporalis fascia, auricular cartilage, dermis, dermal fat, and sliding ramus osteotomies have been advocated for TMJ reconstruction. However, many of these have unpredictable results, are susceptible to the conditions which caused the original joint conditions, and have a high incidence of graft failure [14]. Many of these pathologic conditions significantly alter the anatomy and function of not only the TMJ but also the jaws and supporting structures. Beginning in the 1960s, various versions of fossa prostheses were developed in different sizes. Later, stock condylar prostheses were developed with varying success rates and failures. Many of these, though using common orthopedic materials, were not extensively clinically tested. Earlier versions consisted of just a fossa or just a condyle [13, 14].

The advantages of the stock prosthesis include lower costs, immediate availability, less planning, greater availability in countries where custom prostheses are not available. Disadvantages include the recipient site usually has to be modified, the stock sizes and configurations have limited adaptability and may not fit, the function may be compromised because of incorrect angulation, the hospital may need to stock various sizes, there is very limited adaptability if additional corrective jaw surgery is concomitantly anticipated or if large or unusual defects are involved [14, 17].

During the latter part of the 1980s, custom-made TMJ total joint replacement prostheses became available. With virtual surgical planning, there are many advantages of the custom patient-fitted prosthesis. They can be made to accommodate a wide range of deformities and defects. Surgical cutting guides can be used in order to ensure that the surgical osteotomies very closely follow the anticipated procedure and that the custom prosthesis fits accurately. When combined with orthognathic surgery, virtually designed, customized prosthetic joints are essential for accurate results. The screw placements are designed to make optimum use of available bone and to avoid critical structures such as the inferior alveolar nerve and vessels [13, 14, 18, 19]. Long-term follow-up studies of custom TMJ prostheses (Techmedica/TMJ Concepts) have shown overall good function and low failure rates [13, 14].

The design process of a custom-made TMJ prosthesis begins with a CT scan following the prosthesis company guidelines. Using the CT data, a 3D printed skull model is used to design and manufacture a patient-specific condyle and fossa prosthesis using the protocol described above [13, 14].

Case Presentation

A 65-year-old male was referred to the University of Utah OMS clinic with a chief complaint of severe limitation of opening. The history of the presenting symptoms revealed 12-year history of intermittent left jaw swelling every 3–6 months. Multiple consultations with ENT and OMS specialists, including CT scans, biopsies and cultures, failed to result in a diagnosis. Two years prior to presenting at our clinic, he had a symptomatic left mandibular molar removed. For the following 2 years, he experienced a gradual decrease in his mandibular opening and ROM but no recurrence of swelling. His past medical history and review of systems were unremarkable except for some arthritic joint pain, especially in his knees which was treated with arthroscopic surgery.

His TMJ physical exam showed an interincisal opening of 2 mm which could be stretched to 3 mm. His lateral movements were 2 mm. Palpation of the jaws elicited mild-to-moderate pain over the left TMJ and very little muscle pain. CBCT imaging showed significant ankylosis of the left TMJ (Figures 17.14 and 17.15).

A temporal bone/glenoid fossa ostectomy and mandibular condylectomy with total joint prosthesis reconstruction was planned with the prosthesis design through TMJ Concepts®. Following the TMJ design protocols of TMJ Concepts, the CBCT files for a 3-D stereolithic model were produced and sent to the surgeons. In conjunction with the technical specialists, the surgeons planned and mapped the proposed surgery on the model which was returned to the company. The model was prepared to duplicate the planned surgery. The prosthesis was designed in wax-up form and returned to the surgeons for final approval. It was returned to the company for final prosthesis production (Figure 17.16). The final prosthesis was then sent in sterile packaging to the hospital with the nonsterile 3D model showing the planned surgery osteotomies.

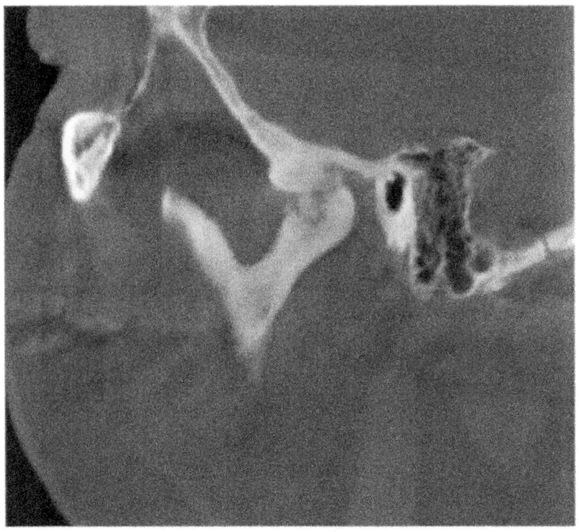

Figure 17.14 CBCT sagittal view showing bony ankylosis of left TMJ. *Source:* Courtesy of Leslie R. Halpern and David R. Adams.

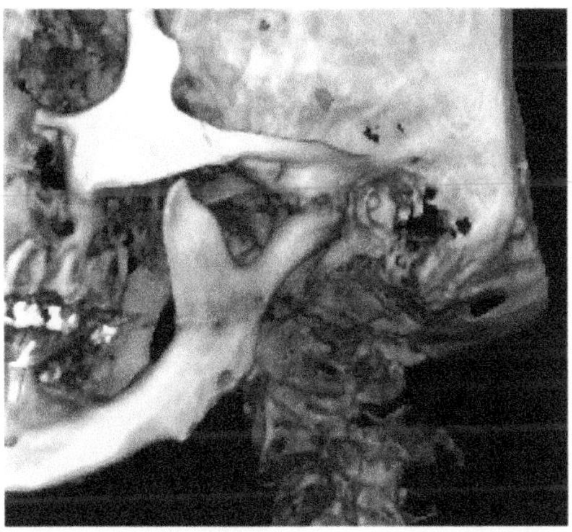

Figure 17.15 CBCT 3D view of bony ankylosis of left TMJ. *Source:* Courtesy of Leslie R. Halpern and David R. Adams.

In the operating room, the patient was given general anesthesia and nasal-tracheal intubation. The mouth was prepped and hybrid arch bars were placed. The left preauricular and submandibular areas were prepped and draped. Through a preauricular approach, the bony ankylosis, condyle, and coronoid notch were surgically exposed. Osteotomies in the glenoid fossa area and condylar neck were made closely following the surgical plan on the 3D model and the diseased bony segments were removed, allowing the mandible to be mobile. The glenoid fossa was contoured following the surgical guide and the fossa prosthesis was placed and secured with bone screws. Through a submandibular incision, the lateral mandible ramus was exposed and the dissection was connected to the preauricular dissection (Figure 17.17). The surgical areas were covered with sterile drapes, the mouth was entered and the jaws were placed into intermaxillary fixation. The surgical sites were uncovered after gowns and gloves were changed. The mandibular/condyle prosthesis was placed through the inferior incision and articulated with the fossa prosthesis. Following the guide, the mandibular prosthesis was screwed into place.

The incisions were irrigated and sutured. The intermaxillary wires were cut and the arch bars removed. The mandibular opening was measured at 35 mm. The patient was treated by physical therapy for a few months postoperatively and was given homecare stretching exercises. He has been able to maintain an opening of greater than 30 mm and is able to chew without problems (Figure 17.18).

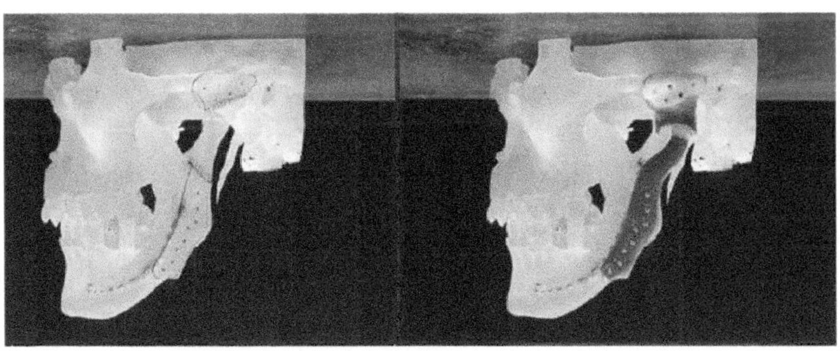

Figure 17.16 Stereolithic models. (Left) The surgeon-proposed osteotomy cuts and technician-proposed implant positions. (Right) Wax-up of the prosthesis. *Source:* Courtesy of Leslie R. Halpern and David R. Adams.

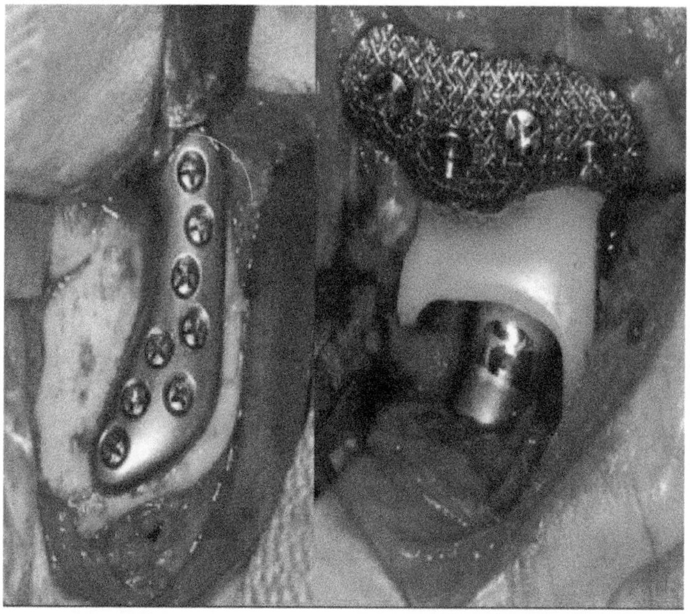

Figure 17.17 Final prosthesis in place. (Left) Ramus/condyle as seen through the submandibular incision. (Right) Fossa prosthesis with the condylar head in position as seen through the preauricular incision. *Source:* Courtesy of Leslie R. Halpern and David R. Adams.

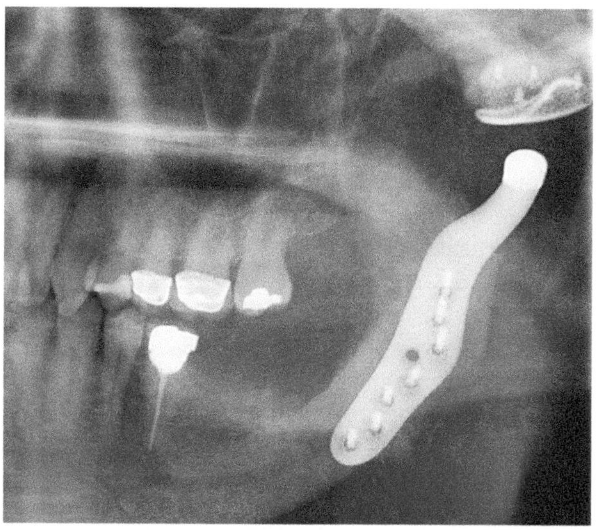

Figure 17.18 Panoramic view of total joint prosthesis in place. *Source:* Courtesy of Leslie R. Halpern and David R. Adams.

Conclusion

The authors of this chapter have presented a multidisciplinary team algorithm to manage TMD. The clinician should understand that a stepwise approach is essential regardless of whether a nonsurgical or surgical therapy is chosen. The main objective is the long-term care and health-related quality of life in patients who suffer from TMD. This begins with a thorough patient assessment, a carefully derived diagnosis and, most important, a solid therapeutic alliance between clinician and patient. The treatment rendered must be specifically tailored to each patient. Appropriate case selection must be considered when surgery is recommended with a thorough discussion of risks and benefits and the clinician needs to identify patients who will be compliant with the regimen chosen and will not harbor unrealistic expectations for treatment outcomes.

References

1 National Institute of Dental and Craniofacial Research. TMJ Disorders. www.nidcr.nih.gov/health-info/tmd.

2 Bagis, B., Ayaz, E.A., Turgut, S. et al. (2012). Gender difference in prevalence of signs and symptoms of temporomandibular joint disorders: a retrospective study on 243 consecutive patients. *Int. J. Med. Sci.* 9 (7): 539–544.

3 Wilkes, C.H. (1978). Structural and functional alterations of the temporomandibular joint. *Northwest Dent.* 57 (5): 287–294.

4 Liu, F. and Steinkeler, A. (2013). Epidemiology, diagnosis, and treatment of temporomandibular disorders. *Dent. Clin. North Am.* 57: 465–479.

5 Miloro, M., Basi, D., Halpern, L., and Kang, D. (2017). Patient assessment. *J. Oral Maxillofac. Surg.* 75: e12–e33.

6 Okeson, J.P. (2013). *Management of Temporomandibular Disorders and Occlusion*, 7e. St Louis, MO: Mosby.

7 McNeill, C., Mohl, N., Rugh, J., and Tanaka, T. (1990). Temporomandibular Disorders: Diagnosis, Management, Education, and Research. *J. Am. Dent. Assoc.* 120 (3): 253, 255, 257 passim.

8 Wieckiewicz, M., Boening, K., Wiland, P. et al. (2015). Reported concepts for the treatment modalities and pain management of temporomandibular disorders. *J. Headache Pain.* 16: 106.

9 Schiffman, E., Ohrbach, R., Truelove, E. et al. (2014). Diagnostic criteria for temporomandibular disorders (DC/TMD) for clinical and research applications: recommendations of the International RDC/TMD Consortium Network and Orofacial Pain Special Interest Group. *J. Oral Facial Pain Headache* 28 (1): 6–27.

10 Pedroletti, F., Johnson, B.S., and McCain, J.P. (2010). Endoscopic techniques in oral and maxillofacial surgery. *Oral Maxillofac. Clin. North Am.* 22: 169–182.

11 Hall, D.H., Nickerson, J.W., and McKenna, S.J. (1993). Modified condylotomy for the treatment of the painful temporomandibular joint with a reducing disc. *JOMS* 51 (2): 133–142.

12 Baker, G.I. (1999). Surgical considerations in the management of temporomandibular joint and masticatory muscle disorders. *I Orofacial Pain* 13: 307–312.

13 Mercuri, L.F. (2012). Alloplastic TMJ replacement: Rationale for custom devices. *Int. J. Oral Maxillofac. surg.* 41: 1033–1039.

14 Wolford, L., Mercuri, L., Schneiderman, E.D. et al. (2015). Twenty-year follow-up study on a patient-fitted temporomandibular joint prosthesis: the Techmedica/TMJ Concepts device. *J. Oral Maxillofac. Surg.* 73 (5): 952–960.

15 Monteiro, J.J., Almeida de Arrudea, J., de Melo, A.R. et al. (2019). Updated review of traumatic dislocation of the mandibular condyle into the middle cranial fossa. *J. Oral Maxillofac. Surg.* 77 (1): 132.e1–132.e16.

16 Yuan-fu, K., Chen, H.M., Sun, Z.P. et al. (2010). Long-term efficacy of botulinum toxin type A for the treatment of habitual dislocation of the temporomandibular joint. *Br. J. Oral Maxillofac. Surg.* 48: 281–284.

17 Quinn, P. and Granquist, E. (ed.) (2015). *Atlas of Temporomandibular Joint Surgery*, 2e. Oxford: Wiley.

18 Movahed, R. and Wolford, L.M. (2015). Protocol for concomitant temporomandibular joint custom-fitted total joint reconstruction and orthognathic surgery using computer-assisted surgical simulation. *Oral Maxillofac. Surg. Clin. North Am.* 27 (1): 37–46.

19 Dimitroulis, G. (2018). Management of temporomandibular joint disorders: a surgeon's perspective. *Australian Dent. J.* 63 (1 Suppl): S79–S90.

18

Postoperative Complications in Oral Surgery

Junaid Mundiya and Feiyi Sun

Complications in oral surgery can be divided into two majors parts: those that occur during a procedure and those that occur after a procedure. Complications that occur during the procedure include extraction of the wrong tooth, damage to adjacent tooth or soft tissue, root displacement and root tip fracture, oroantral communication, aspiration, and nerve injury [1, 2]. Complications occurring after a procedure include infection, pain, swelling, trismus, postoperative bleeding, and alveolar osteitis, also known as dry socket [1, 2]. Some of these complications can be avoided with good surgical and anatomic knowledge, patient selection, and operator skill and experience. However, even in the hands of knowledgeable and skillful surgeons, complications may still arise [1].

Complications Arising During the Procedure

Extraction of the Wrong Tooth

Extraction of the wrong tooth might sound like a rare complication, but the most common malpractice lawsuits are for wrongful tooth extraction [1]. Extraction of the wrong tooth can be due to miscommunication between a specialist and the referring dentist, mislabeled or outdated radiographs, distractions during the surgical procedure, or human error.

To better avoid wrongful tooth extraction, the surgeon and referring dentist should communicate via written referral. The clinical and radiographic exam should be complete and up to date. If there are any disagreement between the clinicians, they should discuss their findings [2]. A proper time out where the clinician and assistant are aware of the correct tooth that needs to be removed is a technique that can prevent this completion. The radiograph exam should also indicate which tooth is to be removed by marking it (Figure 18.1). Also there should be no disturbance while the surgery is taking place.

If the wrong tooth is extracted, it should be reimplanted into the socket and stabilized by a splint. The patient and referring dentist should be made aware of the complication. Most importantly, the event needs proper documentation supported by radiographs [1].

Teeth Splint Technique

Splinting technique can be used for a traumatic injury to the tooth or if the tooth is wrongfully extracted [3]. Splinting stabilizes the teeth and prevents damage to surrounding periodntal tissue [3]. The splint should be slightly flexiblle to allow for physiologic mobility to accelerate healing [3]. The splint should be maintained for 7–10 days. Acid-etched resin splints are most commonly used due to ease of use and esthetics [3].

The labial surface is cleaned of blood and debris, the teeth are air dried, and 35% phosphoric acid gel is applied to the incisal/buccal surface for 20 seconds [3]. The acid-etch gel is removed with water spray and air dried. The composite resin is placed on the teeth and light cured. At least two teeth mesial and distal to the luxuated tooth should be used as anchorage for support [3]. A modification to this technique is to use a 28 gauge wire to provide semi-rigid fixation [3]. The wire id placed at the site of interest and stabilized by composite. Occlusion should be checked afterwards to make sure there are no interferences [3]. Postoperative instructions include not eating hard, chewy, sticky food as it may dislodge the splint. Oral hygiene is important to promote healing and possibly to avoid any infection [3].

Oral and Maxillofacial Surgery, Medicine, and Pathology for the Clinician, First Edition. Edited by Harry Dym, Leslie R. Halpern, and Orrett E. Ogle.

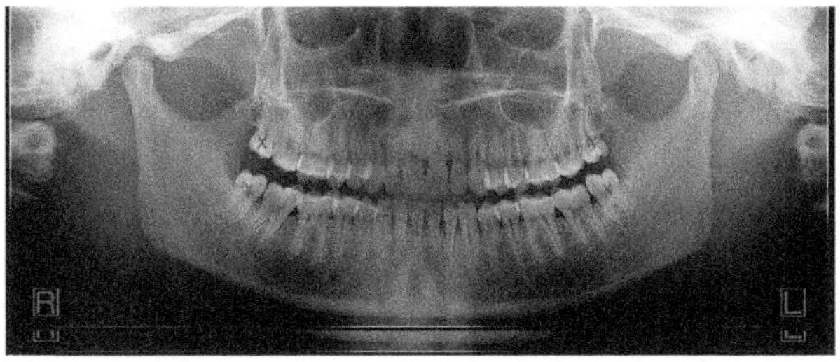

Figure 18.1 Dental panoramic radiograph showing four third molars marked with X for removal.

Damage to Adjacent Tooth or Structures

Damage to adjacent structures is a common risk of any oral surgery. It can consist of subluxation of adjacent tooth, unintentional removal of crown, fracture of adjacent tooth, fracture of restoration present in an adjacent tooth, and soft tissue injury. Thorough examination prior to starting the procedure, with a special focus on adjacent crowns or large restorations, should be documented [2]. The patient should be made aware of the increased risk of injury to adjacent structures if there is a large restoration or crown. Soft tissue injury includes torn flaps, burns, puncture wounds, and abrasion. If there is any form of injury to adjacent soft tissue or teeth, the patient should be made aware. If a tooth is damaged, the referring dentist should be made aware of the complication [2]. The patient may require temporalization of the tooth, replacement of dental crown, or soft tissue closure if there is a laceration. The complication should be well documented in the chart, and explained to the patient [1, 2].

Root Fracture and Displacement

The root of a tooth can fracture even with good surgical technique. There are many reasons why a root fracture might occur. It can be due to previous endodontic treatment which can make the root brittle, or an anatomic variant such as dilacerated or divergent root [1]. Poor surgical technique includes improper buccal lingual movement of the tooth or poor sectioning of the tooth while using the handpiece. If the root tip is less than 2 mm and next to a vital structure such as nerve bundle or maxillary sinus, the patient should be made aware and a clinical decision can be made to leave the root. There should be proper radiograph and documentation [2]. If there is periapical pathology associated with the fractured root, it is recommended to remove it due to the possible chance of infection [2] (Figure 18.2).

Displacement of root is a rare event but it may occur with an inexperienced surgeon with improper technique and use of excessive force. The area of displacement of

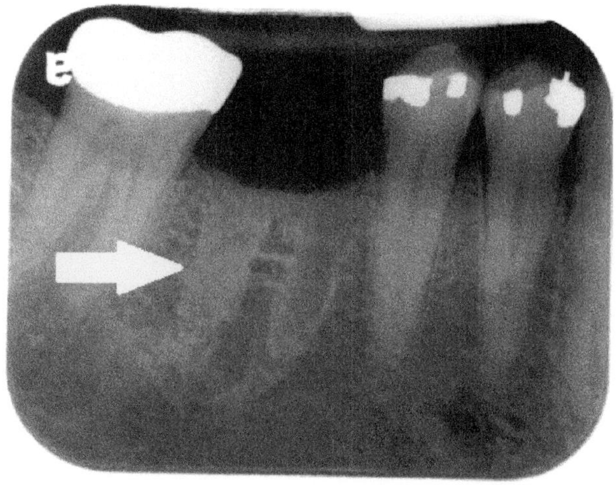

Figure 18.2 Periapical radiograph pointing toward distal root of lower first molar retained in the socket.

maxillary teeth includes the maxillary sinus and infratemporal space. The area of displacement with mandibular teeth includes the submandibular space [1, 2].

When working on maxillary teeth with pneumatized sinus, care should be taken not to apply apical force to remove the root. If the root is displaced into the sinus, attempts should be made to retrieve it with suction. If this is not possible, a radiograph should be taken. If CBCT is available, it should be the first choice, otherwise a panoramic image (Figure 18.3). After the root has been localized, Caldwell–Luc technique should be used to remove the root from the sinus [1, 2].

The most common tooth or root to be displaced into the infratemporal space is the maxillary third molar. The displacement can be due to improper surgical technique, no distal stop, or poor apical pressure. If the tooth is displaced into the infratemporal space, a radiograph should be taken to localize it [2]. If the tooth/root is accessible, it should be removed. If it is not, research recommends no surgical intervention if the patient is asymptomatic during routine close follow-up [1].

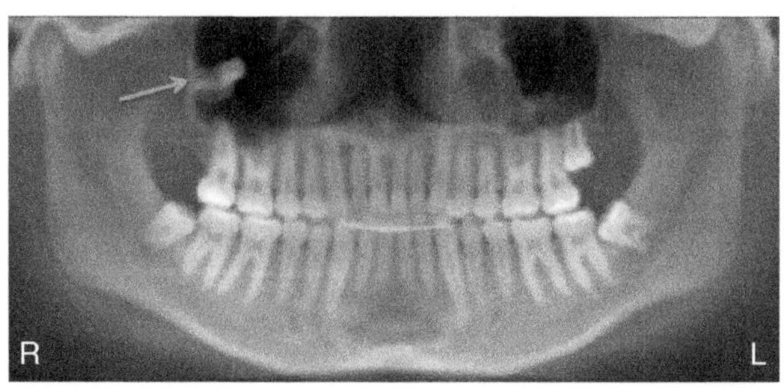

Figure 18.3 Dental panoramic radiograph showing third molar displaced into right maxillary sinus.

Displacement of root into the sublingual space is a rare occurrence. The mandibular molar roots can be displaced into the sublingual space due to thin lingual cortex bone and lingual pressure with a dental elevator [2, 4]. If the root is displaced into the sublingual space, the lingual aspect should be palpated, and an attempt made to retrieve the root with manual pressure. If retrieval is unsuccessful, then a lingual flap should be raised, and the mylohyoid muscle is dissected to facilitate removal of the displaced object [1, 2, 4].

Oroantral Communication

Oroantral communication is one of the well-known complications with extraction of maxillary molars [2]. This is an important complication and it should always be discussed with the patient before extraction of maxillary teeth as part of informed consent. Close attention should be paid to a radiograph which shows pneumatized sinus, large bulbous roots, and dilacerated roots. In cases where roots are dilacerated or in close proximity to the sinus, sectioning the tooth should be considered and apical pressure must be avoided while extracting the tooth [2].

If maxillary sinus perforation is suspected, probing the site or using a curette is not recommended. A small perforation of less than 2 mm does not need any surgical intervention. The patient should be advised about sinus precautions such as no sneezing, blowing of the nose, using a straw, or smoking [2].

When the perforation size is between 2 and 6 mm, a collagen plug or absorbable gelatin sponge (Gelfoam®) can be placed in the socket and figure-of-eight style sutures can be used to retain the packing. A good blood clot will help heal the perforated membrane [2]. Along with sinus precautions, patient should also receive antibiotics and nasal decongestants. The recommended antibiotic for sinus-related pathology is augmentin [2]. If the patient is allergic to antibiotics in the penicillin family, then clindamycin can be prescribed. The patient should be followed up to monitor the healing process (Figure 18.4).

If the perforation is greater than 6 mm, then primary closure is required [2]. There are many different techniques for closing a large communication such as buccal or lingual rotational flap, buccal fat pad advancement, or three-layer closer as described by Dr Harry Dym [5]. Composite three-layer oroantral communication is performed with a Caldwell–Luc procedure [5]. The bony window from the Caldwell–Luc is then press fit over the bony oroantral communication defect, and soft tissue closure is achieved using the buccal fat pad flap and buccal mucosal advancement flap [5]. Refer to Weinstock et al. for detailed description [5]. A close follow-up, antibiotics, and sinus precautions are needed.

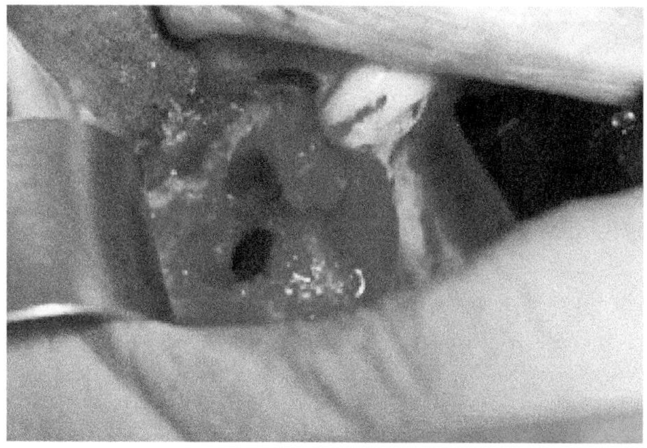

Figure 18.4 Clinical picture of oroantral communication that will require repair.

Aspiration of Teeth, Instruments, Restoration, or Dental Crowns

When working in the oral cavity with instruments or foreign bodies, there is a chance of aspiration [2]. Therefore, a throat curtain is strongly recommended. A fully opened piece of 4×4 gauze will protect the posterior pharynx from aspiration or swallowing [2].

If a patient does swallow any foreign body, they should be sent to a hospital for chest radiograph to localize it. If the patient aspirates a foreign body, then the Heimlich maneuver is recommended to remove it. If an attempt to remove the foreign body is unsuccessful and the patient is unconscious, use a laryngoscope and McGill forceps to remove the foreign body. If the foreign body is not visualized, then it mostly likely entered the right mainstem bronchus or right lung [2]. The patient will require surgical intervention to have the foreign body removed in the hospital setting. One must activate an emergency response when such complication occurs to have the patient transported to hospital. A detailed record must also be kept of the events that occurred.

Nerve Injury

The most common nerve to be injured in dentistry is the mandibular branch of the trigeminal nerve. The inferior alveolar nerve, lingual nerve, and mental nerve are also damaged [6]. The injury can occur during extraction, aggressive curettage of a pathology, improper implant placement, or iatrogenic injury. Temporary or permanent sensory nerve disturbance can occur anywhere from 0.4% to 2% of the time [2]. Before any surgical procedure, the clinician should obtain an informed consent, and explain the risk of possible nerve injury to the patient [7]. During the removal of mandibular third molars, it should be an important part of discussion [2, 7]. Third molar removal is a common procedure and many factors such as root proximity, anatomic location, and age of the patient should be discussed during the consultation [6] (Figure 18.5). If the third molars are close to the inferior alveolar canal, intentional partial odontectomy should be consider [2, 7].

Neurosensory alteration can be due to hemorrhage in the area, causing compression on the inferior alveolar canal; this type of neurosensory alteration is usually temporary but it can also be permanent [6]. Injury to the lingual nerve can occur if poor technique is used to elevate a lingual flap, perforation or fracture of lingual cortex. Care must be taken especially during third molar surgery to protect the lingual nerve [2].

Even though rare, mental nerve injury can occur during extraction of premolars, apicoectomies, implant placement, or during removal of apical cyst in the vicinity (Figure 18.6). Care must be taken while approaching the area [2].

If CBCT is available, a diagnostic image should be taken after a questionable panoramic radiograph to better plan the surgical approach for extractions, pathology removal, or implant placement. If there is a nerve injury, proper follow-up and documentation are needed. The patient should also be referred to a neuromicrosurgeon if there is no improvement, and nerve repair is required [2].

There are two common classifications of nerve injury. Seddon includes neurapraxia, axonotmesis, and neurotmesis [8] whereas Sunderland includes first, second, third, fourth, and fifth degree. Neurapraxia or first degree is described as conduction block from transient anoxia owing to acute epineurial/endoneurial vascular interruption resulting from mild nerve manipulation (traction or compression) with rapid and complete recovery of sensation and no axonal degeneration. Damage is confined within the endoneurium [8]. First-degree Sunderland is further divided into types I, II, and III. Type I is mild nerve manipulation with rapid return of sensation. Type II is moderate traction or compression with formation of transudate or exudate fluid and intrafascicular edema, return to sensation in days [8]. Type III is severe nerve manipulation that may result in segmental demyelination; recovery occurs in days to weeks.

Axonotmesis correlates with second, third, and fourth degree with the difference being degree of axonal damage. Second degree is injuries from traction or compression resulting in ischemia, intrafascicular edema, or demyelination [8]. Recovery is slow and may take weeks to month, and complete recovery may not be achieved. Third degree is significant neural trauma with intrafascicular disruption and damage extending to the perineurium. Recovery is variable. Fourth degree is damage to entire fascicle extending through the perineurium to the epineurium. Spontaneous recovery is unlikely. Neurotmesis or fifth-degree injuries result from complete or near complete transection of the nerve with epineurial discontinuity and likely neuroma formation [8].

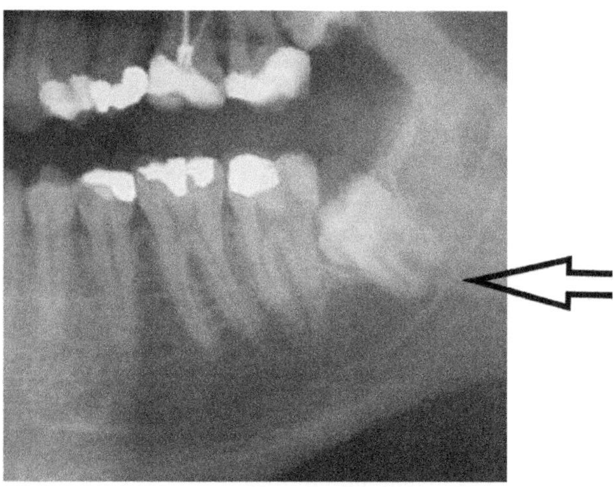

Figure 18.5 Radiograph showing close proximity of third molar roots to the inferior alveolar nerve canal.

Complications after Oral Surgery

Alveolar Osteitis (Dry Socket)

Alveolar osteitis (dry socket) is a common complication seen after dental extraction. Dry sockets are rare in the maxilla and more common in the mandible [6]. The cause of dry socket is unknown but it is hypothesized that a disturbance in blood clot formation by smoking, oral contraceptive, difficulty of extraction, poor oral hygiene, and surgeon experience can contribute to it [7].

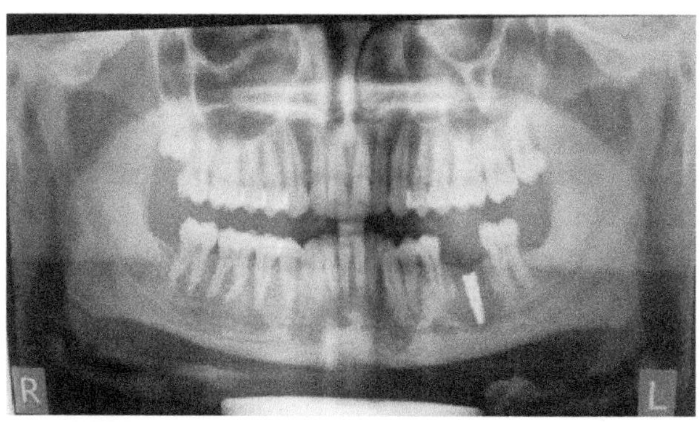

Figure 18.6 Dental panoramic radiograph showing dental implant at site of first molar. The implant is in close proximity to the inferior alveolar nerve canal.

Symptoms of dry socket usually appear on the third or fourth day after surgery, and presents as dull pain that radiates to ear and head. It can be mistaken for earache or headache. Narcotics do not provide relief compared to NSAIDs. Clinically, there is no sign of infection, no erythema, and no edema [6]. The extraction site is open and socket walls are visible (Figure 18.7). There might be odor and food debris in the socket [7].

Since it is delayed healing, there is no treatment for dry socket. However, the clinician can help alleviate the pain. The site should be irrigated with saline solution, or chlorhexidine, and dry socket paste can be placed into the socket. Dry socket paste contains eugenol which provides comfort to the patient (Figure 18.8). Some clinicians place Gelfoam or radiographic opaque dressing into the socket. Patients may return in 2 days to replace the dressing and for more dry socket paste. The healing process usually takes 3 weeks. If the pain persists, then radiographs should be taken to rule out different causes.

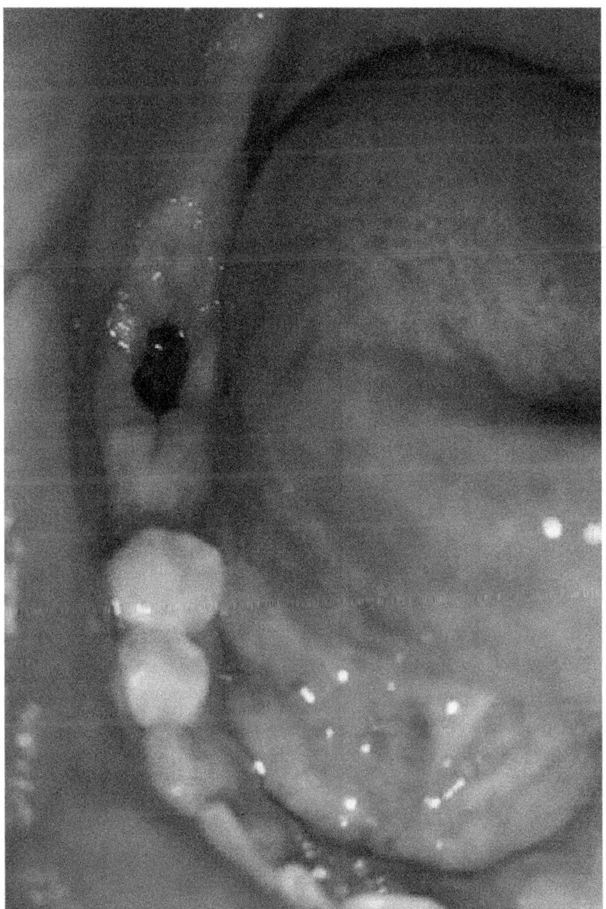

Figure 18.7 Delayed healing of extraction socket with exposed bone.

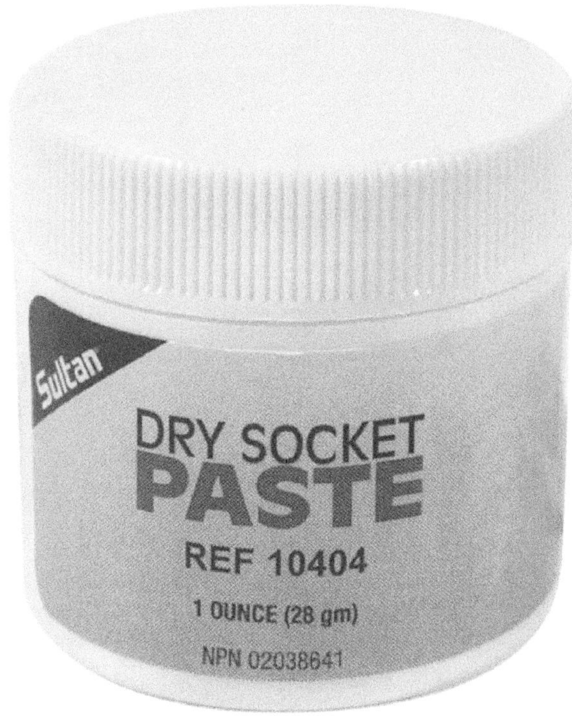

Figure 18.8 Dry socket paste.

Infection

Infections after oral surgery can occur even with the most experienced surgeon. Most infections manifest 2–4 days after the surgical procedure. Sign and symptoms include swelling, trismus, tenderness, temperature, and purulence [1, 9].

Poor oral hygiene, immunocompromised status, and difficulty of extraction are factors that can lead to postoperative dental infection. The most common bacteria seen are streptococci species. Antibiotics such as penicillin and amoxicillin are used frequently for oral bacteria [1]. If the patient is allergic to penicillin, then clindamycin is usually prescribed. Use of prophylactic antibiotics for a routine procedure is a controversial topic with many different opinions [9] (Figure 18.9).

For a minor infection, antibiotics may be enough and surgical intervention is not required. If the infection is spreading to the vestibular space, then incision and drainage is recommended. In rare and severe cases, if the infection spreads to fascial spaces, the patient requires an admission to hospital, incision and drainage, IV antibiotics, and infectious disease consult [1] (Table 18.1).

Infections can be minimized by following good surgical techniques such as irrigation during the procedure, good oral hygiene, and postoperative instructions after the procedure [1, 2, 8].

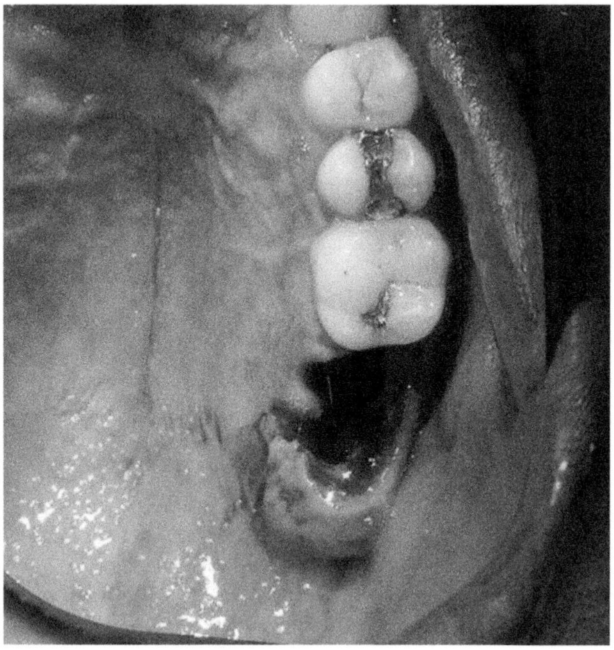

Figure 18.9 Fracture of left tuberosity with palatal tissue tear. *Source:* Medscape Drugs & Diseases.

Pain, Swelling, and Trismus

Pain and swelling are common postoperative complications. Most swelling occurs in the first 24–48 hours, and then gradually decreases. Swelling is attributed to inflammatory mediators such as prostaglandins, leukotrienes, and thromboxane A2 [2, 10]. Factors that contribute to swelling include the complexity of extraction, length of procedure, retraction of soft tissue, and surgeon experience [10].

Trismus is due to inflammation of the muscles of mastication. It can be caused by surgical procedure, length of opening the mouth, and local anesthesia in the area. Use of NSAIDs and steroids can help with postoperative pain, swelling, and trismus. If trismus, pain, and swelling last for more than 5–7 days then radiograph and clinical exam are warranted to rule out different causes [2, 10].

Bleeding

Bleeding can occur during or after any surgical intervention. If there is a history of coagulopathy or anticoagulants, a careful history should be taken and prothrombin time (PT), partial thromboplastin time (PTT), and international normalized ratio (INR) should be ordered [2]. The recommended range of coumadin is less than 3.0 [11]. However, some clinicians may choose to operate well above the limit. If there is no history of coagulopathy, and there is bleeding, then a local source needs to be identified [8].

Intraoperative bleeding can be due to bone bleed, injury to soft tissue, or in rare cases injury to vessels [7]. Bone bleed is controlled by burnishing the bone or placing bone wax to the area. If a vessel is the source of bleeding, it should be ligated or cauterized. Hemostatic agents such as absorbable gelatin sponges (Gelfoam), oxidized regenerated cellulose (Surgicel®), microfibrillar collagen (Avitene®), absorbable collagen dressing (Collatape®) or topical thrombin can be used [2, 8, 11] (Table 18.2).

Fracture of Bony Structures

Fracture of bony structures is seen commonly with extraction of teeth by a novice surgeon. If the buccal plate is fractured,

Table 18.1 Antibiotics commonly used for oral infections.

Medication	Indication	Coverage	Adult dose/route of administration	Pediatric dose/route of administration
Penicillin VK	First line for odontogenic infections	Streptococci, oral anaerobes	250–500 mg by mouth every 6 hours for 7 days	25–50 mg/kg/d every 6–12 hours for 7 days
Cephalexin, cephadroxil	Bacteriocidal broader coverage	Gram-positive cocci, some gram-negative rods, oral anaerobes	250–500 mg by mouth every 6 hours for 7 days. 225–500 mg/kg/d divided every 12 hours for 7 days. Severe infections 100 mg/kg/d	
Amoxicillin	Broad-spectrum infection >3 days	Gram-positive cocci, *Escherichia coli*, *Haemophilus influenzae*, oral anaerobes	250–500 mg by mouth every 8 hours or 500–875 by mouth every 12 hours for 7 days	40 mg/kg/day by mouth divided every 9 hours or 45 mg/kg/day every 12 hours for 7 days
Clindamycin	Broad spectrum, oral anaerobes, penicillin-allergic patients	Gram- positive cocci, anaerobes	150–450 mg by mouth every 6 hours for 7 days	8–25 mg/kg/day suspension by mouth divided every 8 hours or 6 hours for 7 days

Source: Joseph E. Pierse et al., 2012/With permission of Elsevier.

Table 18.2 Local Hemostatic Agents for Oral Bleeding.

Name	Source	Action	Application
Avitene	Microfibrillar collagen	Stimulates platelet adherence and stabilizes clot; dissolves in 4–6 weeks	Mix fine powder with saline to desired consistency, and place in Site
Collaplug®	Preshaped, highly cross-linked collagen plugs	Stimulates platelet adherence and stabilizes clot; dissolves in 4–6 weeks	Place into extraction site
Collatape	Highly cross-linked collagen	Stimulates platelet adherence and stabilizes clot; dissolves in 4–6 weeks	Place ribbon into extraction site
Gelfoam	Absorbable gelatin sponge	Scaffold for blod clot formation	Place into socket and retain with suture
Surgicel	Oxidized regenerated methylcellulose	Binds platelets and chemically precipitates fibrin through low pH	Place into socket (do not mix with thrombin)
Thrombin	Bovine thrombin	Causes cleavage of fibrinogen to fibrin and positive feedback to coagulation cascade	Mix fine powder with $CaCl_2$ and spray into area

Source: Adapted from Moghadam H, Caminiti MF. Life threatening hemorrhage after extraction of third molars. Case report and management protocol. J. Can. Dent. Assoc., 2002;68(11):670–674.

localized alveoloplasty is recommended to smooth the bone and provide proper soft tissue closure. Maxillary tuberosity and palatal tissue tear is another complication seen with extractions of maxillary third molars [2, 8] (Figure 18.10). To avoid fracture of the maxillary tuberosity, careful dissection of soft tissue and release of periodontal ligament fibers is necessary, then using the dental elevator, care must be taken to elevate the tooth. Palatal tissue tear coincides with tuberosity fracture and should be closed with sutures [1, 8].

Extraction of mandibular molars can result in mandible fracture [7] (Figure 18.11). If the fracture is nondisplaced, closed reduction maxillary mandibular fixation is recommended. If the fracture is displaced and cannot be reduced by closed reduction, then the patient should be hospitalized for open reduction internal fixation [8].

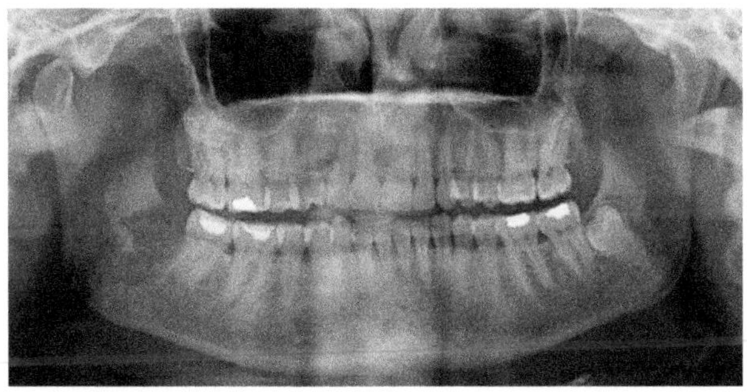

Figure 18.10 Fracture of right angle of the mandible associated with extraction of lower right third molar. *Source:* Ivyspring International Publisher.

References

1 Lieblich, S., Kleiman, M., and Zak, M. (2012). Dentoalveolar surgery. *J. Oral Maxillofac. Surg.* 70 (11 Suppl 3): e50–e71.

2 Fonseca, R.J., Marciani, R.D., and Turvey, T.A. (2009). *Oral and Maxillofacial Surgery*. St Louis, MO: Saunders/Elsevier.

3 Fonseca, R.J. (2013). *Oral and Maxillofacial Trauma*. St Louis, MO: Elsevier/Saunders.

4 Ehrl, P. (1980). Oroantral communication. Epicritical study of 175 patients, with special concern to secondary operative closure. *Int. J. Oral Surg.* 9 (5): 351–358.

5 Weinstock, R., Nikoyan, L., and Dym, H. (2014). Composite three-layer closure of oral antral communication with 10 months follow-up-a case study. *J. Oral Maxillofac. Surg.* 72 (2): 266.e1–266.e7.

6 Haug, R., Perrott, D., Gonzalez, M., and Talwar, R. (2005). The American Association of Oral and Maxillofacial Surgeons age-related third molar study. *J. Oral Maxillofac. Surg.* 63 (8): 1106–1114.

7 Bui, C., Seldin, E., and Dodson, T. (2003). Types, frequencies, and risk factors for complications after third molar extraction. *J. Oral Maxillofac. Surg.* 61 (12): 1379–1389.

8 Miloro, M., Ghali, G.E., Larsen, P.E., and Waite, P. (2012). *Peterson's Principles of Oral and Maxillofacial Surgery*. Shelton, CT: People's Medical Publishing House.

9 Gill, Y. and Scully, C. (1988). The microbiology and management of acute dentoalveolar abscess: views of British oral and maxillofacial surgeons. *Br. J. Oral Maxillofac. Surg.* 26 (6): 452–457.

10 Benediktsdóttir, I., Wenzel, A., Petersen, J., and Hintze, H. (2004). Mandibular third molar removal: risk indicators for extended operation time, postoperative pain, and complications. *Oral Surg. Oral Med. Oral Pathol. Oral Radiol. Endod.* 97 (4): 438–446.

11 Alexander, R. (2000). Dental extraction wound management: a case against medicating postextraction sockets. *J. Oral Maxillofac. Surg.* 58 (5): 538–551.

19

Odontogenic Infections: Anatomy, Etiology, and Treatment

Orrett E. Ogle and Leslie R. Halpern

Introduction

Odontogenic infection has plagued human populations for thousands of years, and is possibly the most common bacterial infection around the world. According to the World Health Organization, oral diseases are major public health problems due to their high incidence and prevalence across the globe, with the disadvantaged affected more than other socioeconomic groups [1].

Although deaths from odontogenic infection are rare today, it was one of the leading causes of death up to about 300 years ago. When the London, England, Bills of Mortality began listing the causes of death in 1665, "teeth" were continually listed as the fifth or sixth leading cause of death [2]. Between 2000 and 2008, there were more than 61 000 hospitalizations in the United States for periapical abscesses, and of the 61 000-plus admissions, 66 patients died [3]. Today, with sophisticated diagnostic modalities, advanced oral surgical techniques, and modern antibiotic therapy, the complications from spread of odontogenic infections havd been greatly reduced.

Definition

An odontogenic infection is an infection of the alveolus, jaws, or face that originates from a tooth or its supporting structures. The most common causes are dental caries, failed root canal treatment, pericoronitis, and periodontal disease. Bacteria from untreated dental caries can invade the root canal system and infect the periradicular tissues, as the latter is an extension of the former. Once the microorganisms enter the periapical tissues via the apical foramen, they induce an inflammatory reaction which can lead to the formation of an abscess. In the majority of cases, the infection will remain localized to the region where it started, but it can spread into adjacent or distant areas depending on the virulence of the bacteria, the local anatomy, and host resistance factors.

Pericoronitis and periodontal disease are soft tissue infections that can also lead to abscess formation. Pericoronitis, which occurs around the mandibular third molar, will be in close proximity to the pharynx and airway obstruction becomes a very strong possibility with spread of the infection. Table 19.1 depicts the stages of an odontogenic soft and hard tissue infection.

Microbiology

Odontogenic infections are polymicrobial, consisting of various facultative anaerobes, such as the viridans streptococci group, the *Streptococcus anginosus* group, and strict anaerobes, such as anaerobic cocci, *Prevotella*, and *Fusobacterium* species [4, 5]. Overall, anaerobes tend to be the predominant organisms involved in almost all dental infections. Less than 5% of odontogenic infections are caused solely by aerobic bacteria [6]. Dental abscesses caused solely by strict anaerobes occur in only about 20% of cases. Anaerobic infections are characterized by abscess formation, foul-smelling pus, and tissue destruction. The majority of infections are mixed but strict anaerobes outnumber facultative by a ratio which varies between 1.5 and 3:1 [7]. In the early stages of dental infections (3–4 days). the facultative streptococci will predominate but gram-negative obligate anaerobes appear in increasing numbers as time passes without treatment (>4 days).

It is not only the type of bacteria that is significant in the clinical picture and in the management of odontogenic infections, but also the bacterial load. A high bacterial load

Oral and Maxillofacial Surgery, Medicine, and Pathology for the Clinician, First Edition. Edited by Harry Dym, Leslie R. Halpern, and Orrett E. Ogle.

Table 19.1 Stages of an odontogenic infection.

Stage	Bacteria	Presentation
Inoculation	Aerobe	Occurs over 0–3 days
Cellulitis	Mixed	Occurs over 1–5 days
Abscess	Anaerobe	Occurs over 4–7 days
Facial spread, rupture, pus	Anaerobe/dead cells	Spreads over path of least resistance

may overwhelm the host defense mechanisms and make the clinical presentation much worse. Interventions such as tooth extraction, root canal therapy, incision and drainage, mechanical debridement, and copious irrigation of the infected area are all methods of decreasing the total bacterial load and thus reducing the infectious bioburden on the individual. Table 19.2 depicts the type of bacterial flora seen in odontogenic infections.

Table 19.2 Most Common pathogens identified in orofacial infections.

Microorganisms	Percentage
Prevotella spp.	74
Streptococcus milleri group	65
Peptostreptococcus spp.	65
Fusobacterium spp.	52
Porphyromonas spp.	17
Other anaerobic streptococci	9

SPP are members of the oral, vaginal, and gut microbiota. *Source:* Data from: Sakamoto H, Kato H, Sato T et al. Semiquantitative bacteriology of closed odontogenic abscesses. Bull. Tokyo Dent. Coll., 1998;39(2):103–107.

Clinical Presentation

The clinical presentation of an odontogenic infection is highly variable, depending on the source of the infection (anterior teeth vs posterior teeth; maxillary vs mandibular teeth), whether the infection is localized or if it has become disseminated (Table 19.3, Figure 19.1). The potential pathways of spread of odontogenic infections within the head and neck regions are depicted in Figure 19.1. The presenting symptoms will be pain/tenderness, erythema, and edema. Patients with superficial dental infections will present with localized pain, cellulitis, and sensitivity to tooth percussion and temperature. On the other hand, patients with deep infections or abscesses that spread along the fascial planes may present with swelling, fever, and sometimes difficulty swallowing, opening the mouth, or breathing [8].

Clinical Work-Up

Physical Examination

The clinical work-up of an odontogenic infection, whether superficial or deep, begins with a physical examination involving patient's vital signs – blood pressure, temperature, pulse rate, and respiratory rate – plus timing of

Table 19.3 Clinical presentation of odontogenic infections by location.

Type of infection	Clinical presentation
Dentoalveolar infection	Swelling of the alveolar ridge with periodontal, periapical, and subperiosteal abscess
Submental space infection	Firm midline swelling beneath the chin. Due to infection from the mandibular incisors
Submandibular space infection	Swelling of the submandibular triangle of the neck around the angle of the mandible. Infection is caused by mandibular molar infections. Trismus is typical
Sublingual space infection	Swelling of the floor of the mouth with possible elevation of the tongue and dysphagia
Retropharyngeal space infection	Stiff neck, sore throat, dysphagia, raspy voice. These infections are due to infections of the molars (the retropharyngeal space infection has a high potential to spread to the mediastinum)
Buccal space infection	Swelling of the cheek. Due to infection of premolar or molar tooth
Masticator space infection	Swelling on either side of the mandibular ramus and is due to infection of the mandibular third molar. Trismus will be present
Pterygomandibular	Trismus, swelling medial to mandibular ramus
Masseteric	Trismus, swelling of the mandibular ramus
Temporal	Trismus, swelling above zygomatic arch; orbit (late)
Canine space infection	Swelling of the anterior cheek with loss of the nasolabial fold and possible extension to the infraorbital region

Source: Ogle OE. Odontogenic infections. Dent. Clin. North Am., 2017;61(2):235–252, with permission.

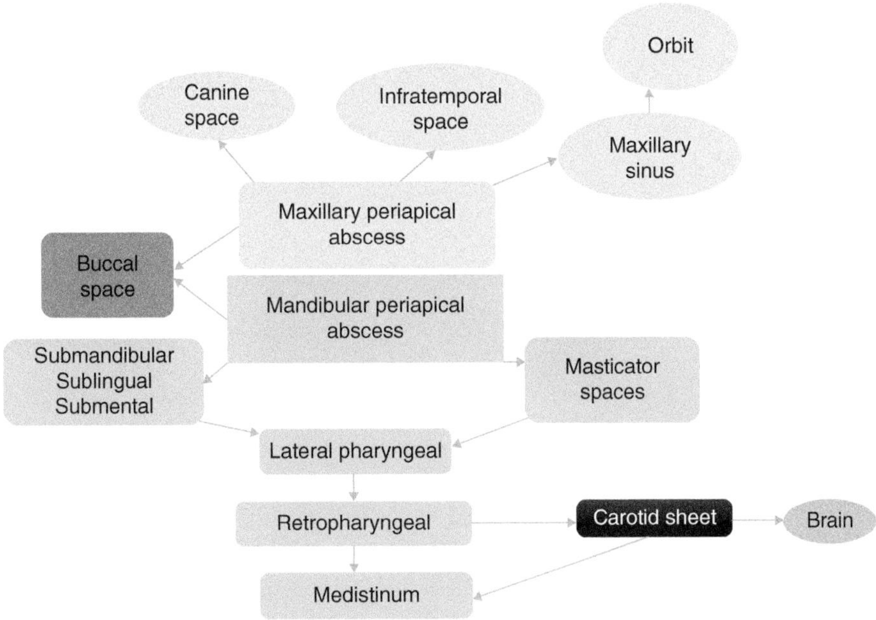

Figure 19.1 Potential extension of odontogenic infections into deep fascial space infections of the head and neck.

appearance, ability to open the mouth, whether dysphagia, dysphonia, or difficulty breathing exists, as well as a history of fever, dehydration, and presence of lymphadenopathy. This presentation characterizes the patient as presenting in a "toxic state." Clinical palpation follows to check for tenderness, local warmth/heat, consistency of edema, i.e. doughy, indurated, or fluctuant. This is followed by an intraoral exam if the patient can open their mouth to determine the site of odontogenic infective etiology. The latter clinical finding will then provide information on the stage of infection as depicted in Table 19.1. The distinction between an inoculate, cellulitis, and abscess will determine whether this is an acute or chronic presentation which will give the practitioner a sense of the host's resistance to the infection [9]. Although the presence of purulence indicates a walling off by the body, the presence of a cellulitis can mask deeper extension into the fascial planes that will require a more aggressive approach for infective resolution other than just performing an incision and drainage of a local locule of purulence.

Radiographic Imaging

Radiographic imaging should begin with a panoramic X-ray (Figure 19.2) since this provides the location(s) of the offending tooth/teeth. Periapical radiographs provide help in locating periapical pathology (see arrow, Figure 19.3).

Although superficial and deep fascial plane infections require the above protocols, computed tomography (CT) provides a highly specific modality for visualizing deep and

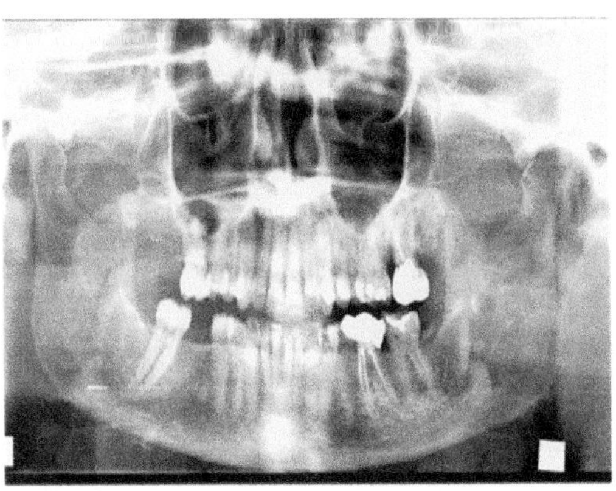

Figure 19.2 Panoramic radiograph of maxillofacial area.

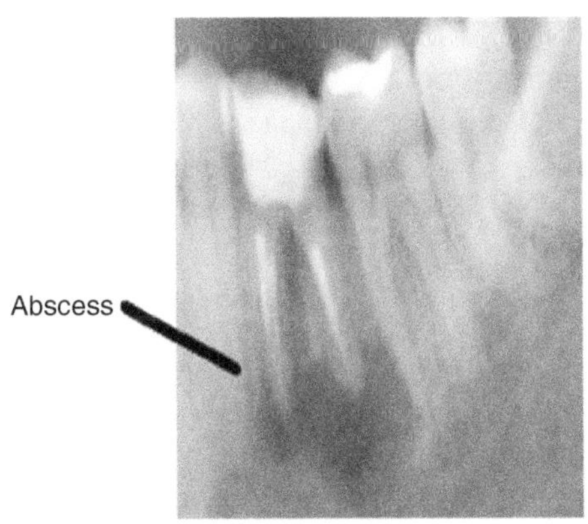

Figure 19.3 Periapical radiographs provide help in locating periapical pathology.

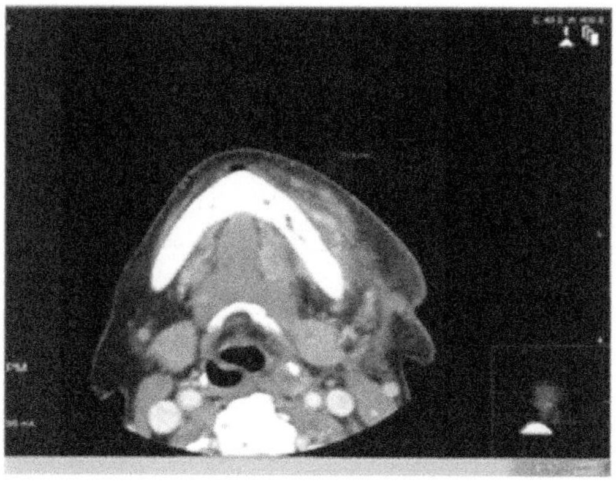

Figure 19.4 Soft tissue axial view of submandibular abscess.

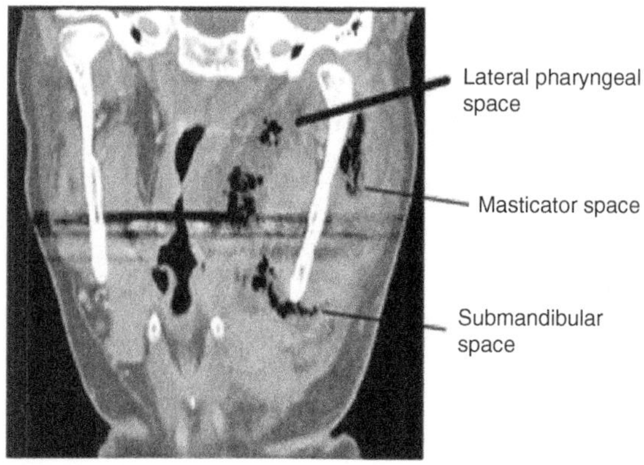

Figure 19.5 CT soft tissue coronal view of lateral pharyngeal, masticator, and submandibular spaces infection.

potential life-threatening infective spread. A patient presenting with trismus, respiratory stridor, and difficulty swallowing is a candidate for CT imaging to determine the location of locules of pus to be drained and where the infection has spread in a three-dimensional boundary. Many argue, however, that imaging results in a harmful delay to emergent/urgent intervention. Well-accepted radiographic criteria require contrast dye to determine areas of ring enhancement of drainable collections. Numerous prospective, and retrospective studies confirm that CT is highly specific in diagnosing the spread of infections and is thus the superior tool to augment the clinical exam. Figures 19.4 and 19.5 provide examples of locations within the submandibular, masticator, and lateral pharyngeal spaces that were determined by CT to require exploration and drainage.

Procurement of Cultures

An understanding of the microbiology (discussed above) of head and neck infections and antibiotic susceptibility is paramount to avoid life-threatening infections. Although there is no compelling evidence for routine cultures, infections that spread to adjacent fascial planes, especially in medically compromised patients, require "sterile" culturing of the site(s) to isolate aerobic, anaerobic, and fungal organisms. Swabs can be used as well. Figure 19.6 depicts the use of a 10 cc syringe with an 18 gauge needle extraorally to obtain samples of purulent drainage for culture. It is important to apply this approach with respect to the percentages of resistant bacteria that may be highly variable and dependent upon the patient population. The cohort sampling may demonstrate bacterial cultural resistance to the empiric antibiotic therapy usually started and based upon the narrow spectrum of odontogenic bacteria normally associated with the infections seen (see section 19.9 below).

Pain Control

In the presence of an odontogenic infection, pain control for the surgical procedure can be a challenge. Adequate pain control can be achieved fairly successfully when the origin of the infection is a mandibular tooth. Regional block can be performed using the traditional Halstead technique if trismus is not present. When the patient is unable to fully open their mouth, the Vazirani–Akinosi technique should be used. The inferior alveolar nerve block will produce adequate anesthesia for the incision and drainage but may be inadequate for extraction and particularly for endodontic intervention where pulpal anesthesia may not be obtained. Alternatively, there are several supplemental injection techniques available to help the surgeon achieve anesthesia for tooth extraction. Intraligamental injection is usually successful. Supplemental injection should only be used after attaining a clinically successful inferior alveolar nerve block.

Infection arising from a maxillary tooth and presenting as a vestibular abscess, buccal/canine space abscess or in the anterior maxilla will decrease the efficacy of dental

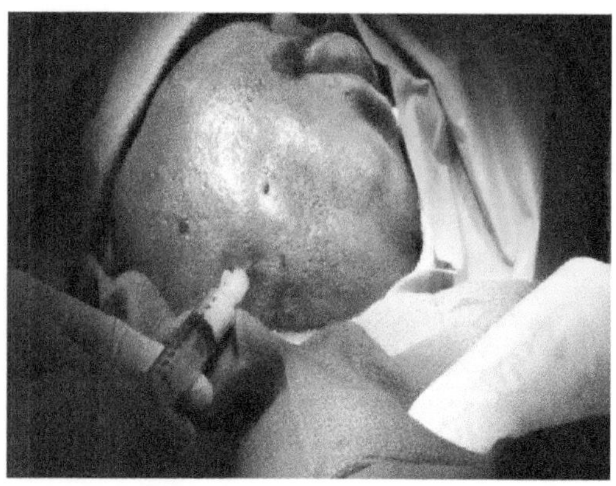

Figure 19.6 Aspiration of purulence from right masticator space.

local anesthetics. Inflammatory acidosis is most frequently cited as the cause of this clinical phenomenon. Most local anesthetics are weak bases with a pKa in the range of 7.9–8.4. As the extracellular pH gets lower in infected tissue, the nonionized fraction of the local anesthetic is significantly reduced, resulting in inadequate membrane penetration with delayed onset and decreased intensity of local anesthesia. Mepivacaine, with a pKa of 7.6, is a good anesthetic to use in an infected patient since it has the closest pKa to infected tissue [10]. It is best administered without the vasoconstrictor in order to help overcome the acidity created by the infection. Using a larger amount of local anesthetic to "flood" the area will allow a greater concentration of the unionized form to penetrate the tissue. A needle that penetrates into the abscess cavity should be discarded and a new needle used for other injections if necessary.

Injecting a large volume of fluid into the inflamed area will be very painful. It would be preferred if nitrous oxide or IV sedation could be used concurrently. If not available, the dentist should advise the patient about the pain and try to get cooperation from the individual.

Treatment Techniques

The treatment of an odontogenic infection will always involve a dental procedure to remove the source of the infection and, more importantly, its spread as evidenced by purulent and/or "cellulitis" drainage. This may consist of tooth extraction, endodontic intervention, curettage of deep periodontal pockets, and incision and drainage of an abscess. The dental procedure can then be followed by antibiotic therapy (see below). Antibiotics should rarely be considered as the first-line therapy for a dental infection.

The type of dental intervention will most often be based on patient preference. Some patients will just want to have the offending tooth removed while others will prefer to avoid extractions at all costs and would opt for an endodontic treatment. Other options include tooth extraction and later replacement with implants and there are an increasing number of dentists who think implants may offer better results than root canal treatment [9].

Odontogenic infections are usually mild and are generally confined to the alveolar ridge or tissues in close proximity, i.e., the buccal, labial or lingual vestibule. However, the infection can go beyond the localized muscle attachments and spread into fascial spaces, resulting in more severe infections. In the case of an acute abscess, incision and drainage to remove accumulated pus (purulence) which contains bacterial biofilm and necrotic tissue will be required.

The focus of this section will be surgical techniques to treat intraoral and extraoral odontogenic infections most commonly encountered in the head and neck.

Alveolar/Vestibular/Palatal Abscess

Figures 19.7 and 19.8 depict the intraoral locations of abscesses that present with swelling and require surgical drainage from a transbuccal approach. Infections involving the space of the body of the mandible, the buccal space, canine space, anterior vestibule, and pterygomandibular space should be drained intraorally. The abscess should be drained at the same time that the dental procedure is performed if fluctuant, and before it ruptures spontaneously. Maxillary infected teeth with the root apex below the origin of the buccinator muscle, and mandibular infected teeth with the apex above the insertion of the buccinator will have the abscess pointing in the labial vestibule. Anterior teeth of both maxilla and mandible will most frequently have the abscess pointing in the labial vestibule between the apex of the involved tooth and the elevators of the upper lip or depressors of the lower lip. The vast majority of these abscesses will be superficial.

Method

1. Using a #15 Bard-Parker® blade, make a 1 cm sharp incision at the most dependent site of exudate collection, through both mucosal and submucosal tissue layers.

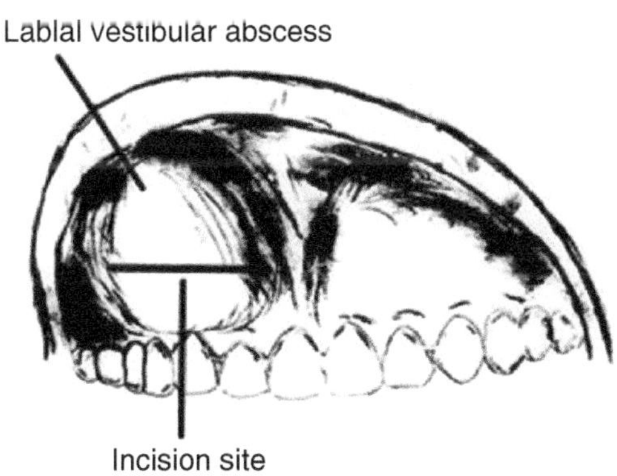

Figure 19.7 Abscess in vestibule upper anterior. *Source:* Kymbree Ogle-Forbes/With permission of Kymbree Ogle-Forbes.

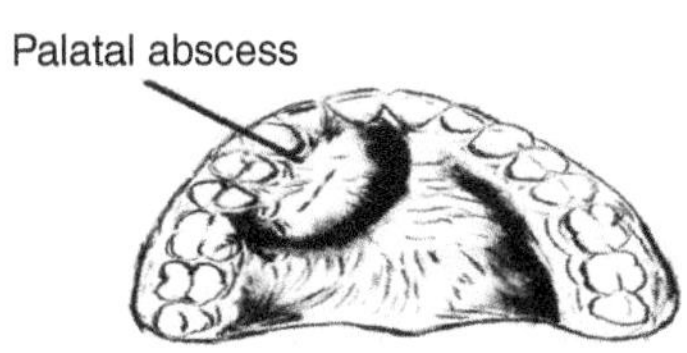

Figure 19.8 Palatal abscess. *Source:* Kymbree Ogle-Forbes/With permission of Kymbree Ogle-Forbes.

A 1 cm length will allow adequate drainage and room to use a hemostat and provide good access for irrigation. Do not incise over the mental nerve between the two lower premolars or at the maxillary frenulum. Contents of the abscess may project out of the abscess when it is incised, especially if a large volume of local anesthetic was injected into the abscess. The surgeon should be wearing the standard Universal Precaution materials (gown, gloves, protective eyewear) to avoid self-contamination.

2. Use a mosquito hemostat to gently perform blunt dissection into the lesion to break up loculations. Enter the wound with the beaks of the hemostats in a "closed" position, spread and then withdraw in an opened position. Probing with the hemostat should also be done toward the apex of the infected tooth.
3. Using a syringe, copiously irrigate the wound with about 50 cc of sterile saline solution while maintaining constant suction to avoid aspiration.
4. If necessary, insert a rubber drain of adequate length into the surgical site and secure it to the mucosa using a 3.0 silk suture to allow for residual drainage. The purpose of the drain is to keep the incision site opened. Not placing a drain may allow the wound to close early and cause the abscess to redevelop. The drain should be removed or changed after 48 hours.
5. Along with incision and drainage of an abscess, the practitioner can perform an extraction or endodontics if they feel that the tooth can be salvaged.

Palatal Abscess

A palatal abscess (see Figure 19.8) is usually the result of periapical infection arising from a nonvital lateral incisor or the palatal root of an upper first or second molar and is usually lateral to the midline. Large palatal abscesses arising from the apex of the lateral incisor can sometimes be seen in the midline. A palatal abscess can be confused with a salivary gland tumor in the palate. The abscess will produce pain while benign salivary gland tumors of the palate are usually asymptomatic. Dental radiographs and clinical exam will easily differentiate between the two.

Method

1. The incision is oriented parallel to the course of the greater palatine artery and is carried only through the mucosa and submucosa. The incision should never be taken directly to the bony palate because it may lacerate the greater palatine artery or vein which runs on the surface of the palatal shelf.
2. After the incision, open the area for continuous drainage with a hemostat. Spread the beaks of the hemostat anterior–posterior to avoid injury to the underlying vessels and resultant bleeding.
3. Irrigate with a large volume of saline, place drain and secure it with a 3-0 silk suture. The drain can be changed or removed within 48–72 hours.

Submandibular/Submental Abscess

Dental infection from a mandibular tooth is one of the most common causes of a submandibular abscess (Figures 19.9 and 19.10). The mandibular third molar is the most commonly offending tooth, followed by the mandibular second molar because their root apices lie inferior to the mylohyoid muscle [11]. The submental space, located below the chin, is bounded below by the skin, above by the mentalis muscles, and laterally by the anterior bellies of the digastric muscles (Figure 19.11). Infection in this area is either directly from a mandibular incisor or an extension from the submandibular space. Surgical access for drainage of these abscesses may either be intraoral or extraoral, but the extraoral approach is preferred since dependent drainage

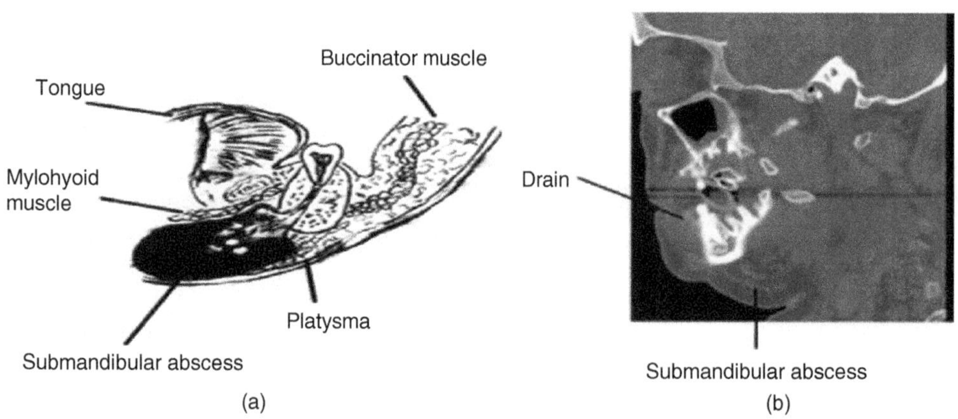

Figure 19.9 (a) Depiction of submandibular abscess. *Source:* Kymbree Ogle-Forbes/With permission of Kymbree Ogle-Forbes. (b) Sagittal CT view showing intraoral drains.

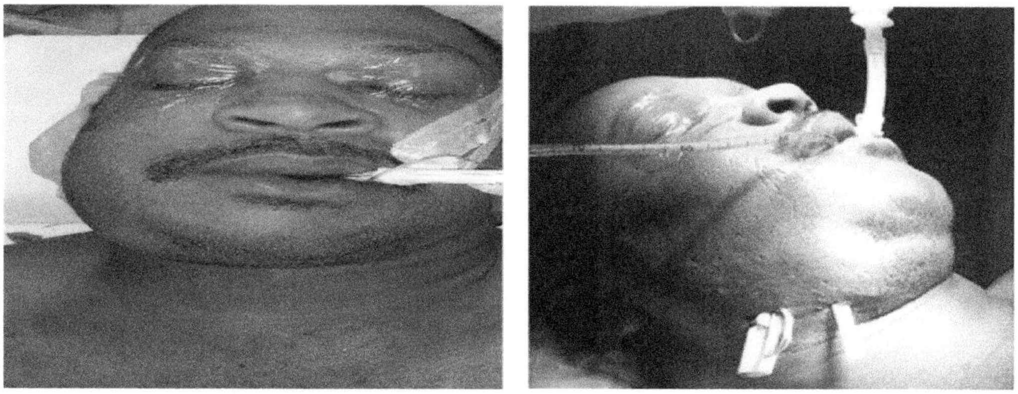

(a) (b)

Figure 19.10 (a) Submandibular abscess right side. (b) Drains in place.

cannot be established from an intraoral approach. Trismus is usually not associated with infection of these fascial spaces.

Method

1. Prep the surface of the abscess and surrounding skin with povidone-iodine or chlorhexidine solution. If not available, alcohol-based solutions can be used. Painting the skin with povidone antiseptic paint is also acceptable. Do not blot or wipe off the paint solution. Allow prepping solution to dry completely (Box 19.1).
2. Perform a field block by infiltrating local anesthetic around and under the tissue surrounding the abscess. Lidocaine with epinephrine is ideal. Allow adequate time for the anesthetic to take effect and to achieve adequate hemostasis. Avoid injecting directly into the abscess cavity.
3. For drainage of a submental abscess, make a horizontal incision in the most inferior portion of the chin in a natural skin crease to make for an acceptable scar. This incision should only be through skin and the immediate subcutaneous layer.

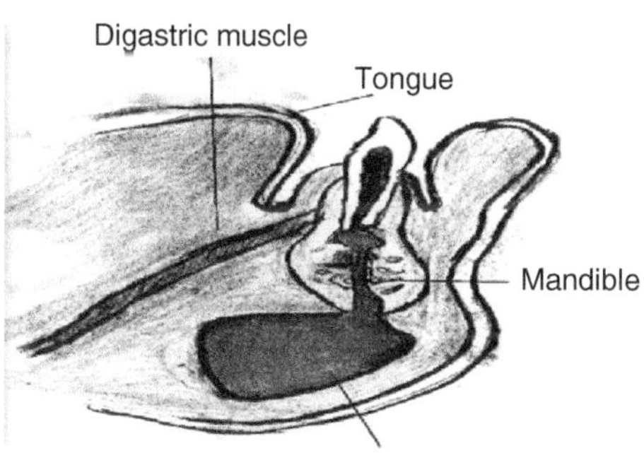

Figure 19.11 Submental abscess. *Source:* Kymbree Ogle-Forbes/With permission of Kymbree Ogle-Forbes.

4. For a submandibular abscess, make a horizontal skin incision at the level of the hyoid to avoid transecting the marginal mandibular nerve. This incision should be through healthy skin and not directly over the abscess. Carry the incision through the platysma muscle using blunt dissection with a hemostat until the dissection falls into the abscess cavity.
5. Puncture through the incision into the cavity of the abscess with a hemostat, which is inserted with closed beaks.
6. Open the beaks of the hemostat to obtain drainage, then withdraw with open beaks.
7. Steps 2 and 3 are repeated several times to break up loculations within the abscess cavity.
8. Irrigate thoroughly with sterile saline.
9. Place a rubber drain and secure with a suture one side of the incision, so as to keep the incision open for continuous drainage.
10. Make a gauze "fluff" with a 2 × 2 gauze pad and place directly over the rubber drain.

Box 19.1 Guidelines for skin prep of surgical site

- Use lint-free sponges.
- Prep from planned incision site outwards.
- Do not dip a sponge that has been used into the antiseptic solution. Discard the sponge and use another sterile sponge.
- Do not "back track" with the same sponge over an area that has already been prepped.
- Prep an area wide enough to provide an adequate working space.
- Do not blot or wipe the area. Antibacterial solution kills by contact.

11. Fold a 4 × 4 gauze pad and place over the fluff. Secure with nylon or paper tape.
12. The dressing can be left in place for up to 2 days if there is not a lot of drainage from the wound. However, once the dressing is soaked, it mut be changed. The patient should be advised to return if they note that the dressing is soaked.

Sublingual Abscess

The sublingual space is separated from the submandibular space by the mylohyoid muscle (Figure 19.12). Infection of this space generally originates from mandibular anterior teeth because their root apices lie above the mylohyoid muscle. Clinically, an abscess in this space will appear as an indurated, erythematous, tender swelling in the floor of the mouth. It extends from close to the mandible and spreads toward the midline or posteriorly above the mylohyoid muscle. Some elevation of the tongue may be noted.

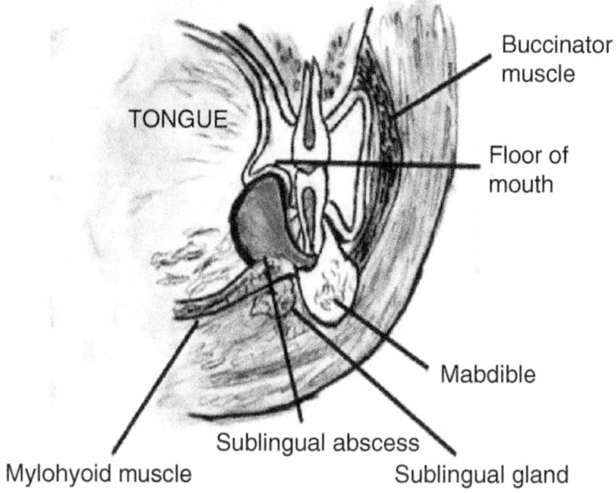

Figure 19.12 Sublingual abscess. *Source:* Kymbree Ogle-Forbes/With permission of Kymbree Ogle-Forbes.

Method

1. An inferior alveolar nerve block is carried out.
2. The incision is made through the mucosa parallel to Wharton's duct, taking into consideration the position of the lingual nerve. The lingual nerve courses close to the medial surface of the mandibular ramus before entering the floor of the mouth opposite to the posterior root of the lower third molar. Here it is very superficial, covered only by the mucosa of the floor of the mouth. As it travels forwards toward the tongue, it usually passes lateral to the submandibular duct, goes below it in the vicinity of the first molar/second premolar, and then courses upwards and forwards on the medial side of the duct to enter the tongue. It is recommended that anterior to the second premolar, the mucosal incision should be lateral to the duct, while posterior to the first molar, it should be closer to the base of the tongue medial to the duct.
3. Using a curved hemostat, dissect bluntly toward the swelling, taking care not to injure the lingual nerve or the submandibular ducts.
4. Lightly irrigate the cavity after all the pus has been drained with sterile saline. A high-speed suction should be available to prevent aspiration.
5. Place a wide rubber drain. The bulk of the tongue will allow the wound to close very quickly.

Buccal and Midfacial Abscess

The buccal space is located between the fascia of the skin and the fascia overlying the buccinator muscle (Figure 19.13). The anterior extent is the labial musculature, posteriorly the pterygomandibular raphe, superiorly the zygomatic arch, and inferiorly the lower border of the mandible. A buccal space abscess originates from carious maxillary or mandibular bicuspid and molar teeth.

Midfacial abscesses involve the canine space and can precipitate an orbital cellulitis. A canine space infection is usually caused by maxillary canine infection that perforates the lateral cortex of the maxilla above the insertion of the levator anguli oris muscle of the upper lip. If infection stays below the insertion of the levator muscle, it will present as a vestibular abscess in the labial sulcus of the

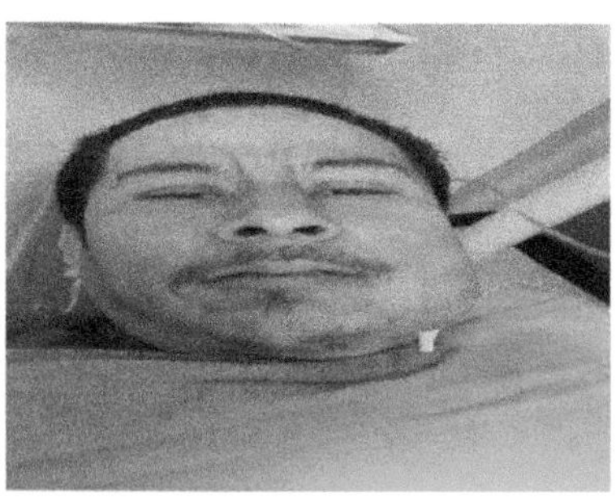

(a)

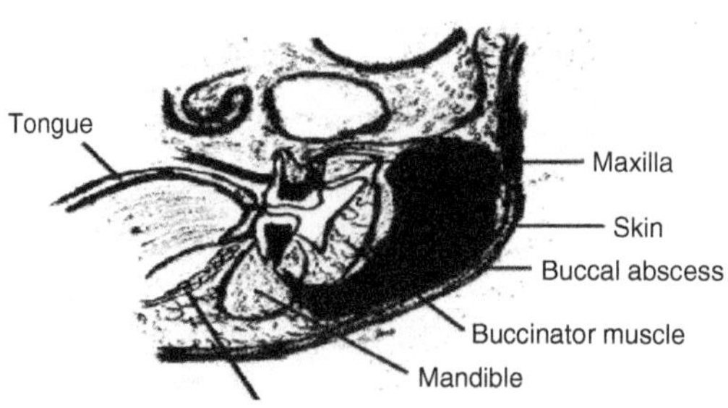

(b)

Figure 19.13 (a) Clinical view of buccal space abscess. (b) Schematic of buccal space abscess.

maxilla. The canine space infection may cause marked cellulitis of the eyelids. A canine space abscess can lead to a cavernous sinus thrombosis (Box 19.2) (see Figure 19.14b for vascular pathway of spread). The clinical pathologic sign is nonfunctioning of the lateral rectus muscle on the same side as the infection.

Method

Buccal abscess This should be drained intraorally to avoid a facial scar and possible injury to the terminal branches of the facial nerve. The intraoral approach, however, does not allow for dependent drainage. There are several options as to where to place the incision: (i) just inferior to the point of fluctuance; (ii) just inferior to the opening of the parotid duct; or (iii) in the mandibular and/or maxillary vestibules.

1. Blunt dissection is undertaken only to the periphery of the space to avoid possible injury to branches of the facial nerve.
2. For incisions placed in the vestibule, it will be necessary to dissect bluntly through the buccinator muscle into the abscess.

Canine space The canine space, like the buccal space, is drained from an intraoral approach.

1. The incision is placed at the depth of the maxillary labial vestibule, cutting toward the bone.
2. Using a small curved hemostat, dissect superiorly through the levator anguli oris muscle, staying close to the facial aspect of the anterior maxilla to avoid injury to the infraorbital nerve.
3. After the abscess is drained, irrigate and place a rubber drain which should be removed after 48 hours.

Box 19.2 Eye Findings of cavernous sinus thrombosis (eye findings are nearly universal in 90%)

Periorbital edema (initially unilateral then typically bilateral)
Lid erythema
Chemosis, ptosis, proptosis (due to impaired venous drainage of the orbit)
Restricted or painful eye movement
Diminished pupillary reflex
Sixth cranial neuropathy with limited eye abduction
Most cases will progress rapidly to complete external ophthalmoplegia from third, fourth, and sixth cranial neuropathy if not treated early

Masticator Space

The masticator space is a potential fascial space encased by the superficial layer of the deep cervical fascia that splits into lateral and medial slings at the inferior border of the mandible to enclose the masseter muscle, part of the temporalis muscle, and the medial and lateral pterygoid muscles before attaching to the zygomatic arch and base of the skull (Figure 19.15) [12]. The masticator space can be further subdivided into the submasseteric space, pterygomandibular space, and superficial and deep temporal spaces.

Infection of the masticator space is generally from the mandibular third molar (Figure 19.16). The infection may be localized to only one of the masticator subcompartments but may spread to another or all the compartments. Patients with any of the masticator space infections will generally present with pain and moderate-to-severe trismus. The surgical approach to drainage of each compartment will be unique to the particular space.

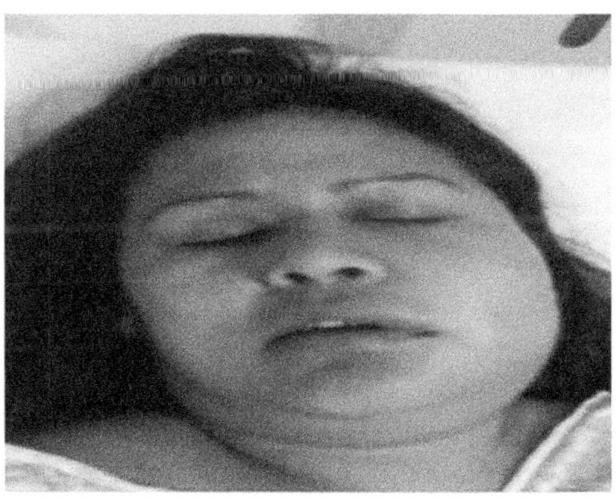

(a)

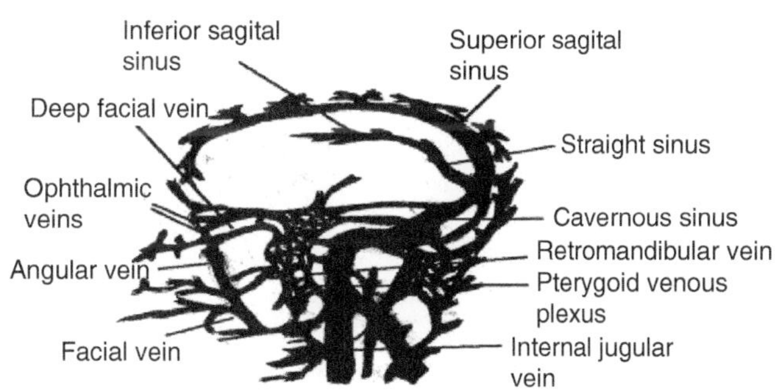

(b)

Figure 19.14 (a) Canine space abscess. (b) Vascular pathways for spread to cavernous sinus. *Source:* Kymbree Ogle-Forbes/With permission of Kymbree Ogle-Forbes.

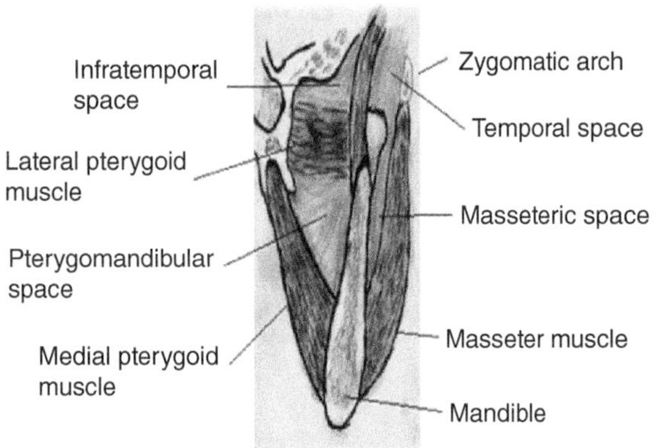

Figure 19.15 Anatomical drawing of masticator space. *Source:* Kymbree Ogle-Forbes/With permission of Kymbree Ogle-Forbes.

Submasseteric Space

The submasseteric space is located between the lateral aspect of the mandibular ramus and the medial aspect of the investing fascia of the masseter muscle. Since the submasseteric space is deep, the clinical presentation will be a firm, nonfluctuant swelling, with pain and severe trismus.

Methods

Intraoral Approach If an intraoral approach is to be used, an inferior alveolar nerve block should be done utilizing the Vazirani–Akinosi technique.

1. A Molt mouth gag (prop) may be required to fully open the mouth. Opening the mouth with a ratchet mouth prop can be very painful. Conscious sedation with midazolam or nitrous oxide analgesia would be very helpful. A useful technique is to start opening the mouth with tongue blades until it is possible to introduce the Molt mouth prop between the premolars on the contralateral side. Once the mouth prop is securely in place on the surfaces of the premolars, slowly squeeze the mouth prop one tooth of the rack every 15–20 seconds. Do not try to fully open the mouth all at once. This technique will get the mouth open with the least amount of pain.
2. Make a vertical incision along the anterior ramus or the external oblique ridge.
3. Use blunt dissection lateral to the mandibular ramus and medial/deep to the masseter muscle to reach the abscess cavity. The beak of the hemostat should always be able to touch the lateral ramus.
4. Irrigate copiously with a syringe.
5. Using the hemostat, place a rubber drain and secure with 3-0 silk suture.
6. The offending tooth should be removed at a subsequent visit.

Transcutaneous Approach

1. For a transcutaneous approach, make a skin incision about 2 cm below the angle of the mandible and parallel to the inferior border. Avoid cutting at the region of the antegonial notch of the mandible in order to avoid violation of the facial artery.
2. After cutting through the skin and subcutaneous tissue, use a curved hemostat to dissect upwards through the platysma to touch the inferior border of the mandible.
3. After touching the inferior border of the mandible, step off laterally and puncture through the pterygomandibular sling, staying close to the lateral wall of the mandibular ramus, to enter the submasseteric space.
4. After all the exudate has been expressed, irrigate and place a drain.
5. Place fluff and a gauze and secure with nylon or paper tape.

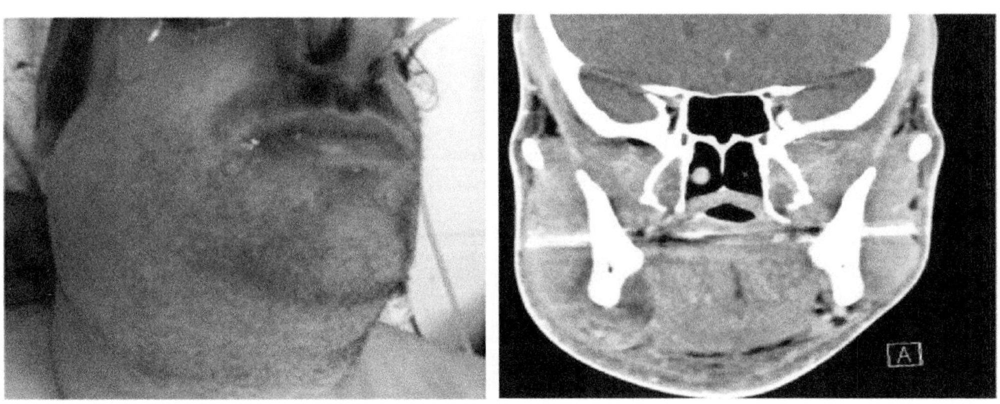

(a) (b)

Figure 19.16 (a) Masticator space abscess. (b) CT of masticator space abscess.

Pterygomandibular Space

The pterygomandibular space is located between the fascia of the medial pterygoid muscle and the medial surface of the mandibular ramus (see Figure 19.15). It contains the inferior alveolar nerve, artery and vein, the lingual nerve, and the nerve to the mylohyoid muscle. Infection of this space commonly originates from a carious mandibular third molar tooth, following third molar surgery or from sagittal split osteotomy of the mandibular ramus for orthognathic surgery. It is also fairly common following inferior alveolar nerve blocks. Pain, trismus, and difficulty swallowing are the common presenting signs and symptoms.

Although intraoral incision and drainage is possible under general anesthesia in an operating room, it will be very difficult under local anesthesia in a dental chair because of the trismus and inability to achieve profound anesthesia.

Method

The approach would be similar to that used for the submasseteric abscess except that after touching the inferior border of the mandible, step off medially and advance the closed beaks of the hemostat superiorly on the medial side of the mandible to enter the pterygomandibular space.

For an intraoral approach, the mucosal incision would be the same as that used for the submasseteric abscess except that the dissection is on the medial wall of the mandibular ramus.

Temporal Spaces

The temporal spaces are compartments of the masticator space which lies between the temporalis fascia and the periosteum of the temporal bone. The temporalis muscle divides the space into deep and superficial compartments. The superficial compartment is a continuation of the submasseteric space and extends superiorly to the pericranium, lateral to the temporalis muscle and medial to the temporo parietal fascia. The deep compartment is separated from the pterygomandibular space by the lateral pterygoid muscle (see Figure 19.15) and extends superiorly to the attachment of the temporalis muscle to the inferior temporal crest.

Temporal space infections from odontogenic causes are rare but can originate from infected mandibular or maxillary molars, with the majority being from maxillary molars. Infections involving the superficial and deep temporal spaces will present as swelling in the temporal areas, superior to the zygomatic arch and posterior to the lateral orbital rim. Because of the tight attachment of the deep cervical fascia to the zygomatic arch, a temporal space infection which occurs as an extension from the submasseteric space may appear as two separate swellings on frontal view. Infratemporal space infection usually originates from a maxillary third molar tooth. Clinically, there will be significant trismus and pain, but only a slight swelling will be noted.

The standard surgical management of the temporal space abscess requires extraoral temporal incision.

Method

1. Drainage is done in the operating room with general anesthesia.
2. Shave the hair at the planned site of incision.
3. Inject lidocaine with epinephrine for hemostasis.
4. Place the incision at the most fluctuant location. Incision should be at about a 45° angle to the zygomatic arch and behind the superficial temporal artery.
5. Incise through the scalp to the superficial temporal fascia.
6. Puncture through the thick fascia with a hemostat or make a small incision in the fascia, then undermine it before widening it.
7. Explore the abscess cavity in multiple directions.
8. Place drains.
9. Dress in standard fashion.

Ludwig Angina

Ludwig angina is a very serious and potentially life-threatening necrotizing cellulitis affecting the sublingual, submental, and submandibular spaces (Figure 19.17). Clinically, it presents as a firm board-like swelling with edema in the floor of the mouth, elevation of the tongue, dysphagia, trismus, drooling, and airway obstruction (Table 19.4). Signs of airway obstruction include hoarseness, stridor, labored breathing, and a "sniffing" position. The cause of infection in most cases is infected lower second or third molars or pericoronitis. There is generally no abscess formation.

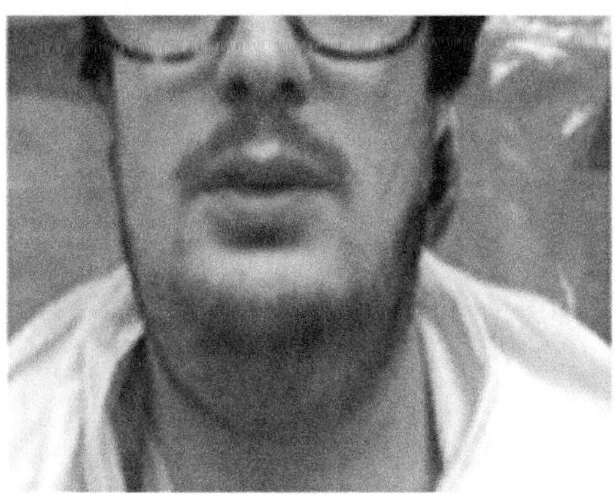

Figure 19.17 Ludwig angina. Note bilateral submandibular and submental swelling.

Table 19.4 Signs and Symptoms of Ludwig Angina.

Rapid swelling of the sublingual, submandibular, and submental regions
Fetid breath
Trismus
Drooling
Unusual speech
Tongue swelling or protrusion of the tongue out of the mouth
Difficulty swallowing
Neck pain
Fever
Breathing difficulty

Treatment of Ludwig Angina

Securing an airway is the initial objective. One should have a low threshold for performing an awake tracheostomy under local anesthesia to secure the airway before inducing anesthesia. Transoral intubation may be hazardous and is often unsuccessful. Fiberoptic intubation requires skill and experience and may cause nasal/nasopharyngeal bleeding. Nebulized adrenaline (1 mL 1:1000 adrenaline diluted to 5 mL with 0.9% saline) and intravenous dexamethasone (controversial) has been suggested to create more controlled conditions for flexible nasotracheal intubation. It is important to note that after incision and drainage, there is often even more swelling which may compromise the airway on day 1–2 after the surgery.

One of the main controversies in management of Ludwig angina is whether surgical drainage is always indicated in the earlier stages of the infection. In the authors' experience, a more aggressive surgical approach should be followed in all cases, i.e., early tracheostomy and empiric placement of drains in the affected spaces. Drainage may be intraoral and/or external depending on the spaces involved. The submandibular spaces are drained externally. If sepsis extends both above and below the mylohyoid muscle, through-and-through drains extending between the oral cavity and the skin of the neck may be inserted.

Pericoronitis

Pericoronitis is another common cause of odontogenic infection. The primary etiology is the accumulation of bacteria and food debris that gets trapped in the space between the overlapping gum of a partially exposed (erupted) mandibular third molar and the crown of the tooth (Figure 19.18). The majority of cases are chronic and

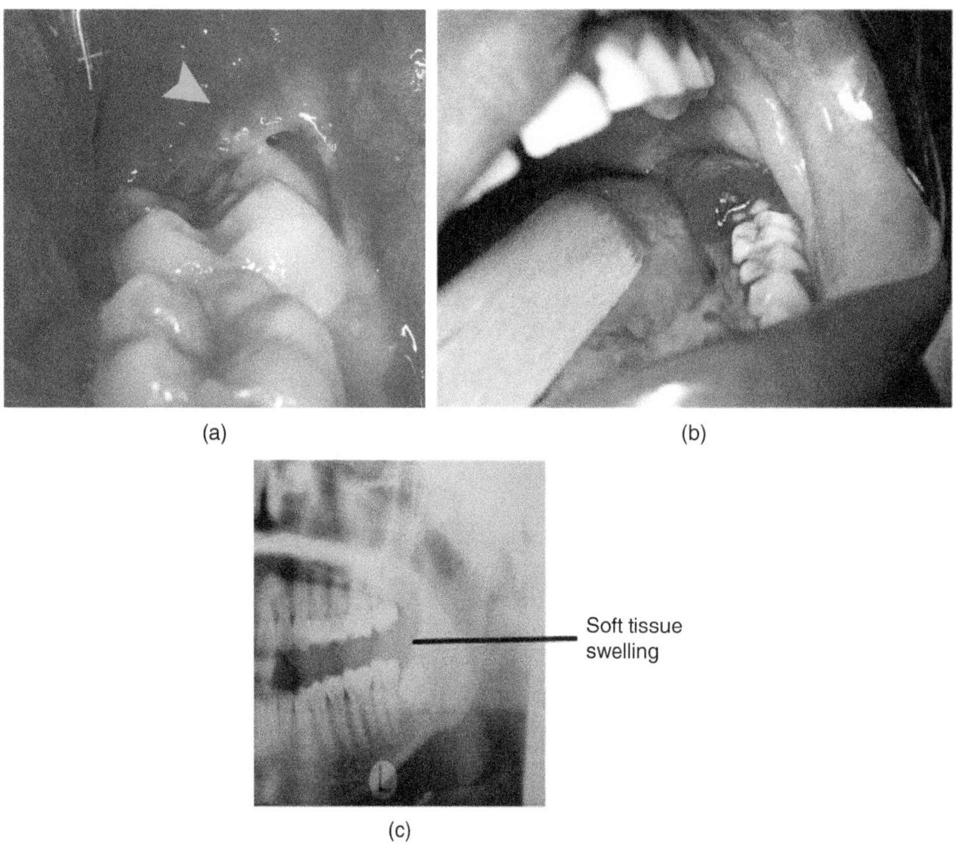

Figure 19.18 (a) A simple pericoronitis. *Source:* Coronation Dental Specialty Group/Wikimedia Commons/CC BY 3.0. (b) Severe pericoronitis. Operculum traumatized by upper tooth. (c) Radiograph showing soft tissue swelling.

consist of a mild persistent inflammation of the mandibular third molar area. Pericoronitis can, however, become a serious infection associated with fever, swelling, and an abscess which has the ability to spread if left untreated. On occasion, the symptoms can become severe due to the rapid spread of infection, requiring that the patient be hospitalized for intravenous antibiotics and possibly tooth extraction in an operating room under general anesthesia. Because of the close proximity to the pharynx, airway obstruction becomes a very strong possibility.

The treatment of pericoronitis consists of irrigation using salt water, diluted hydrogen peroxide or 0.12% chlorhexidine under the flap with subsequent removal of the third molar. An alternative approach is extraction of the maxillary third molar that if erupted may be traumatizing (biting) on the flap surface.

Table 19.5 Common Orally Administered Antibiotics for Odontogenic Infections.

- *Penicillin*: gram-positive aerobes and anaerobes commonly found in alveolar abscesses
- *Amoxicillin*: broader spectrum gram-positive and gram-negative aerobes/anaerobes
- *Clindamycin*: penicillin-allergic choice and penicillin-resistant organisms
- *Metronidazole*: good for anaerobic bacteria and combined with penicillin for excellent coverage in deep space infections
- *Azithromycin/clarithromycin*: aerobic, facultative aerobes: *Staphylococcus/Strep* species and atypical pyogenic bacteria. Good for sinus infections and for pediatric infections due to short duration of therapy
- *Moxifloxacin*: broad spectrum
- *Fluoroquinolone*: good for *Eikinella* sp., *Bacteroides* sp., *Prevotella* sp. and beta-lactamase-positive bacteria. Not good for children <18 years due to effects on bone and joints

Source: Based on [13].

Antibiotic Therapy

The resolution of an odontogenic infection must be based upon an approach that not only removes the causative agents but prevents further spread and chronic recurrences. Chemotherapeutic antibiotic therapy is an adjunct to complete surgical exploration, drainage, and obtainment of cultures so that the therapy is successful. Antibiotic therapy is never a substitution for invasive dental and surgical intervention. Often initial therapy involves empiric antibiotics that are narrow spectrum since the pathogens for odontogenic infections are susceptible to these agents. Table 19.5 lists the most common antibiotics administered and Table 19.6 depicts regimens of antibiotic therapy for odontogenic infections.

Table 19.6 Antibiotic regimens for odontogenic infections.

Antibiotic	Route/mechanism	Dosage/frequency	Indication
Penicillins			
Penicillin G	IM or IV/Bactericidal	600 000–1.2 million units/12–24h	Drug for most infections
Penicillin VK	PO/Bactericidal	250–500 q6h	As above/bacterial endocarditis
Amoxicillin	PO/Bactericidal	1 g initial/500 q6h	*Staphylococcus* sp.
Cloxacillin	PO/Bactericidal	250–500 mg q6h	Drug for serious infection
Dicloxacillin	PO/Bactericidal	125–250 mg q6h	High risk infection
Piperacillin/tazobactam	IV/IM/Bactericidal	IV 3–4 g/dose – 24 g max/24 h IM 2–3 g/dose/q4–6h	High risk infection
Meropenem	IV/Bactericidal	IV 500 mg–1 g q8h	

(Continued)

Table 19.6 (Continued)

Antibiotic	Route/mechanism	Dosage/frequency	Indication
Cephalosporins			
Cefaclor	PO/Bactericidal	250–500 q8h	Broard spectrum
Cefadroxil	PO/Bactericidal	500 mg –1 g q1224h	Broad spectrum
Cephalexin	PO/Bactericidal	250–500 mg q6h	Broad spectrum
Macrolides			
Erythromycin	PO/Bacteriostatic	250–500 mg q6h	Mild infection/ penicillinallergic
Azithromycin	PO/Bacteriostatic	10 mg/kg to 500 mg/5 mg/kg to 250 mg 5 days	Broad spectrum
Clarithromycin	PO/Bacteriostatic	250–500 mg/bid Peds 7.5 mg/kg PO bid	Broad spectrum
Clindamycin	PO/IV/Bacteriostatic	150 mg q6h, 300–600 mg IV or Bactericidal (300 mg q8h, 900 mg IV q8h	Serious infections
Tetracyclines			
Doxycycline	PO/Bacteriostatic	100 mg initial q24h or 50 mg q12h	Mild; periodontal
Oxytetracycline	IM/Bacteriostatic	250 mg q24h	Periodontal
Tetracycline	PO/Bacteriostatic	500 mg q6h	Periodontal
Metronidazole	IV/PO/Bactericidal	500 mg q6h Second line for odontogenic/HIV	Periodontitis
Vancomycin	IV/Bactericidal	1 g infused 1 h prior to surgery	High risk/resistant
Aminoglycosides			
Gentamicin	IM/IV/Bactericidal	3 mg/kg/day q8h/blood levels	High risk/resistant

HIV, human immunodeficiency virus; IM, intramuscular; IV, intravenous; PO, by mouth.

References

1 WHO. Oral Health. www.who.int/news-roo.m/fact-sheets/detail/oral-health

2 Clarke, J.H. (1999). Toothaches and death. *J. Hist. Dent.* 47 (1): 11–13.

3 Cortes J. Anyone can die of a toothache. www.politifact.com/florida/statements/2016/jan/26/john-cortes/ignoring-toothache-really-could-potentially-kill-y.

4 Nair, P.N. (2004). Pathogenesis of apical periodontitis and the causes of endodontic failures. *Crit. Rev. Oral Biol. Med.* 15 (6): 348–381.

5 Robertson, D. and Smith, A.J. (2009). The microbiology of the acute dental abscess. *J. Med. Microbiol.* 58 (2): 155–162.

6 Mohanty, S. (2006). Spread of oral infections. In: *Textbook of Oral Pathology* (ed. S. Saraf), 190. New Delhi: Jaypee Brothers Medical Publishers.

7 Khemaleelakul, S., Baumgartner, J.C., and Pruksakorn, S. (2002). Identification of bacteria in acute endodontic infections and their antimicrobial susceptibility. *Oral Surg. Oral Med. Oral Pathol. Oral Radiol. Endod.* 94 (6): 746–755.

8 Ogle, O.E. (2017). Odontogenic infections. *Dent. Clin. North Am.* 61 (2): 235–252.

9 Flynn, T.R. and Halpern, L.R. (2003). Antibiotic selection in head and neck infections. *Oral Maxillofac. Surg. Clin. North Am.* 15 (1): 17–38.

10 Setzer, F.C. and Kim, S. (2014). Comparison of long-term survival of implants and endodontically treated teeth. *J. Dent. Res.* 93 (1): 19–26.

11 Becker, D.E. and Reed, K.L. (2006). Essentials of local anesthetic pharmacology. *Anesth. Prog.* 53 (3): 98–109.

12 Bahl, R., Sandhu, S., Singh, K. et al. (2014). Odontogenic infections: microbiology and management. *Contemp. Clin. Dent.* 5 (3): 307–311.

13 Free Medical Dictionary. https://medical-dictionary.thefreedictionary.com/masticator+space

Part VI

Pain Control

20

Approaches to the Management of Facial Pain

Leslie R. Halpern

Introduction

The definition of pain according to the International Association for the Study of Pain is "an unpleasant sensory and emotional experience associated with actual or potential tissue damage, or described in terms of such damage" [1–3]. Pain is a universal experience that has profound effects on the physiology, psychology, and sociology of the population. The World Health Organization (WHO) has estimated that over one-third of the population suffers from some form of acute or chronic pain [1, 2]. Within the United States, the healthcare costs of diagnoses and treatment of pain exceed several billion dollars annually [1].

Orofacial pain (OFP) refers to pain in the head and neck regions – soft and hard tissues, as well as both extraorally and intraorally. Okeson divides orofacial pain into physical (Axis 1) and psychological (Axis 2) conditions [3]. Chronic orofacial pain, i.e., atypical odontalgia, burning mouth syndrome (BMS), and idiopathic facial pain, is often regarded as a diagnosis of exclusion and as such remains challenging both for a definitive diagnosis and therapeutic solution. Physical conditions comprise disorders of the temporomandibular joint (TMJ) and disorders of the musculoskeletal structures (e.g., masticatory muscles and cervical spine); intraoral dental and pulpal pain of somatic origin; neuropathic pains, which include episodic (e.g., trigeminal neuralgia [TN]) and continuous (e.g., peripheral/centralized mediated) characteristics, and neurovascular disorders/headaches (e.g., migraine and temporal arteritis).

In addition, OFP can often be a presenting symptom for systemic illnesses such as chronic pain seen in fibromyalgia, gastroesophageal reflux disease (GERD)/irritable bowel disease, posttraumatic stress disorder (PTSD)/other psychological disorders, myocardial ischemia, and cancerous lesions in other parts of the body [4].

Since the evaluation of patients presenting with OFP accounts for a wide range of diagnostic possibilities, the oral healthcare clinician must be judicious in diagnosing clinical presentations as odontogenic and other dental conditions as a primary versus secondary cause of orofacial pain [4–6]. A careful deciphering of signs and symptoms for an accurate diagnosis will set the foundation for specific treatment to improve long-term prognosis and resolution of the majority of OFP syndromes.

The aim of this chapter is to provide the practitioner with therapeutic options to treat a broad spectrum of both acute and chronic orofacial pain syndromes. The epidemiology and neurophysiology/pathophysiology of facial pain will be introduced with respect to the most common treated areas of the head and neck followed by the latest in nonsurgical (pharmacologic management) and surgical strategies that the oral healthcare physician can utilize to treat this population of patients.

Epidemiology

Demographic studies have determined that greater than 39 million people, which is 22% of US citizens, report pain in the orofacial region [5, 7, 8]. Eighty percent of patients presenting with orofacial pain symptomatology have concomitant systemic pain, e.g., fibromyalgia, panic disorders, multiple chemical sensitivities, and PTSD [1, 4, 5, 7]. Evidence-based studies have been published at a greater pace over the past decade in the field of orofacial pain but there are still many questions unanswered with respect to the dynamics of this disease process [1, 7]. The latest experimental evidence demonstrates gender/sex differences in

Oral and Maxillofacial Surgery, Medicine, and Pathology for the Clinician, First Edition. Edited by Harry Dym, Leslie R. Halpern, and Orrett E. Ogle.

etiologies and clinical presentation of pain, such as pharmacogenetic specific responses to different analgesics and other medications used to treat orofacial pain. Clinical case series suggest a preponderance of middle-aged/older women as those most affected by chronic orofacial pain.

Neurophysiology of Orofacial Pain

Orofacial pain can arise from different regions and etiologies within the head and neck. Therefor, the clinician must have a clear understanding of the neuroanatomy/physiology of these regions. Most of these pathways communicate with cranial nerve (CN) V that forms the trigeminal nociceptive system [9]. Figure 20.1 depicts pathways for innervation by the trigeminal sensory system. This complex network of reflex arcs functions based on the properties of trigeminal afferents innervating distinct target tissues. Most are transmitted by somatic, motor, and autonomic nerve networks. These target tissue interactions with trigeminal neuron terminals contribute to the awareness and degree of pain perceived.

Trigeminal pain conditions can arise from injury secondary to dental procedures, infection, neoplasia, or other diseases/dysfunction within the peripheral and/or central nervous system. Neurovascular disorders, such as primary headaches, can present as chronic orofacial pain, such as in the case of facial migraine, where the pain is localized in the second and third division of the trigeminal nerve. Cranial nerves [6, 8, 9] also contribute to afferent input of the head and neck, precipitating and/or exacerbating

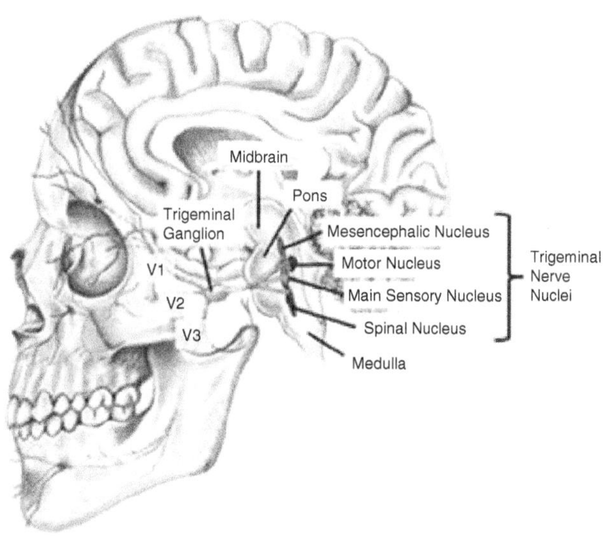

Figure 20.1 Sagittal view of brain depicting the trigeminal nerve pathway and circuits to higher centers of the cerebral cortices.

orofacial pain. Their afferent pathways converge on the trigeminal system at the level of the brainstem. This complex network can cause dilemmas with respect to determining the origin of pain. The clinician must differentiate heterotopic pain (source of pain not localized at site of pain) from referred pain (pain at one area that is supplied by afferents from another source of nociception). This explains why a patient complains of shoulder and neck pain when describing intraoral pain .

The trigeminal system of pain sensation and response is a complex network of sensory fibers that transmit conduction to interneurons via synaptic connections which process incoming information from the three divisions of the trigeminal nerve. This afferent information not only innervates the trigeminal system but also shares innervation from the facial, glossopharyngeal and vagus nerves, as well as the cervical nerve plexus. It is the latter that provides mechanistic causation in facial pain and headaches.

Nerve fibers of the trigeminal complex are both sensory and motor: sensory innervation to the anterior face, teeth mucosa, conjunctiva, dura mater intracranial and extracranial vasculature and motor to the muscles of mastication (see Figure 20.1). This neurosensory pathway has provided a model for studying how pharmacologic therapy contributes to the resolution of inflammatory cascades and their effect on pain pathways [7, 10, 11]. Studies on chronic trigeminal myofascial pain syndromes demonstrate that sex/gender and exposure to sex steroids are risk predictors for developing chronic orofacial pain conditions [11–13]. Additional studies have characterized morphologic changes in trigeminal neurons exposed to injury-induced inflammatory insult to tissue innervated by afferents from peripheral and central pathways that are further modulated by the sex steroids prolactin and estradiol [7, 11–13] (for further interest the reader is referred to reference #13)

Diagnostic Approach to Facial Pain Patients

Pain in the orofacial region is a common presenting symptom seen every day and so the physical exam should include paradigms based upon anatomic and physiologic correlations. The history of the present illness (HPI) will give the practitioner an accurate diagnosis 90% of the time, and so it is essential to allow the patient to describe their symptomatology. The common algorithm of chief complaint/HPI/medical history, physical examination, radiologic images, and a psychosocial profile will enable the practitioner to rule out certain pathology and home in on specific patterns, leading to a reasonable differential and definitive diagnosis (Tables 20.1 and 20.2).

Table 20.1 Differential diagnosis of orofacial pain.

Intraoral pain	*Temporomandibular disorder (TMD)*	*Intracranial pain*
Dental caries	Myofascial pain	Intracranial hemorrhage
Dental abscess	Internal derangement of TM joints	Aneurysm
Dentin sensitivity	Muscles of mastication	Tumor/cyst
Dry socket	Eagle syndrome	Abscess
Periodontal disease		
Pericoronitis		
Cracked tooth		
Neuropathic pain	***Headaches***	***Cervical pain***
Trigeminal neuralgia	Migraine	Myalgia
Glossopharyngeal neuralgia	Tension type headache	Neck
Postherpetic neuralgia	Cluster headache	Degenerative joint disease
Atypical odontalgia	Paroxysmal hemicrania	
Burning mouth syndrome	Temporal arteritis	
Atypical facial pain	Trigeminal autonomic	
Referred pain		
Cardiac		
Renal		
Gastrointestinal		
Jaw		

A complete head, neck, and facial exam should include extraoral and intraoral evaluations. Along with these, there should be a thorough visual inspection for lumps and bumps, unusual discoloration, and lesions that have not healed. The neurologic exam includes both CN VII and trigeminal V3 distribution along the skin, as well as intraoral V2 and V3 distribution along the mucosa. Sensory evaluation should be characterized using two-point discrimination, directional sense, pressure, cold and heat sensation, as well as sharp and light touch along the above dermatomes. Intraoral neurosensory evaluation should include taste. Reflex evaluation includes lid and gag stimulation. Both muscles of mastication and muscles of VII nerve expression should be documented. Cranial nerve evaluation should also include CN I (smell), CN II (visual acuity), and CN VIII (balance and hearing). The neck exam should include evaluation of the cervical plexus along the scalp, lateral neck and angle of the jaw in order to assess trigger points of pain, muscle hypertrophy, and wasting, as well as TMJ function (Table 20.2).

Table 20.2 Typical clinical presentation of patients with orofacial pain.

- Acute presentation due to trauma or disease, trigger points
- Delayed/chronic occurrence over days/months; trigger points
- Pain described as burning, lancinating, sharp, dull, episodic or unremitting
- Local pathophysiology due to invasive procedures; abnormal nerve
- healing
- Paresthesia, dysesthesia, hypesthesia, allodynia, phantom tooth pain
- Neurosensory loss; anesthesia dolorosa; hypoesthesia
- Parafunctional habits: bruxism, clenching
- Facial nerve weakness; loss of taste to anterior 2/3 of tongue
- Headaches, tinnitus, vertigo, photophobia, phonophobia, dysgeusia
- Psychosocial issues; referred pain; heterotopic pain

There is a vast range of causation for intraoral pain and so the oral healthcare provider should be vigilant when examining the oral cavity. Etiologies include periodontal, oral mucosal, odontogenic, and/or a combination of all (see below). Hard tissue examination includes evidence for parafunctional habits, bony destruction and nonhealed white/red lesions, and painful tongue. Diagnostic imaging can provide an adjunct for determination of neurosensory deficits along the mandible or maxilla. Methods using panoramic, plain films or computed tomography (CT) are methods that will give a 2–3-dimensional approach to rule out certain diseases. CT with 3D reconstruction can help to determine the boundaries of disease and isolate regions of causation. Magnetic resonance imaging (MRI) allows greater specificity for ruling in pathology of intraparenchymal brain and vascular formations, as well as orofacial paresthesia of unknown cause. Infection, degenerative disease, and neoplasms can be identified and characterized for aggressiveness using bone scanning with technetium-99m, and angiography can be an adjunct to determine tumor growth and metabolism [14].

Along with physical presentation, the symptomatology of pain needs to be evaluated from a psychosocial perspective. There are well-researched questionnaires that are valid and reliable in discerning psychosocial causation [15]. Comprehensive measurements of these impacts are commonly captured using quality-of-ife instruments [15]. Orofacial pain is also known to have a negative impact on the person experiencing it and oral health-related quality of life (OHRQoL) is an acknowledged and widely used method for measuring this impact [15]. These tools have the potential to decipher causation and support treatment strategies for a variety of pain disorders and may involve an interdisciplinary approach that consists of oral healthcare, neurology, neurosurgery, and other subspecialties to assist in the treatment of OFP.

Grouping of Oral Facial Pain

Acute Facial Pain

Pain presenting acutely is often relatively easy to diagnose definitively and manage effectively . Causation includes odontogenic, periodontal oral mucosa, hard tissue or a combination of these. Odontogenic pain is often short and sharp that progresses to a dull ache depending upon whether there exists a reversible or nonreversible pulpitis. Pain within the mucosa presents as raw, aching, and burning. Periodontal disease also presents as a continuous ache or one that occurs intermittently.

Other etiologies include maxillary sinusitis and salivary gland disorders. The former may or may not have pain associated with etiologies such as oroantral communications and bacterial/viral disease. Salivary diseases are often due to blockage of ducts with resultant infection. Pain pathways from the trigeminal system will not only act at the site but refer to other areas of the head and neck. Imaging/ultrasound will allow for localization and determination as to whether surgical intervention is needed (the reader is referred to Chapter 13 for a detailed description of surgical intervention).

Neuropathic Pain

Neuropathic pain (NP) is defined as pain caused by a lesion or disease of the somatosensory nervous system. NP is diagnosed quite commonly, with up to 25–35% presenting to facial pain centers across the US and Europe [16–18]. Etiologies of NP include trauma, infection, chemotherapy, surgery, neurotoxins, inflammation, and tumor infiltration. Studies have equated NP with a dysfunctional pain due to afferent stimulation that can be both spontaneous and stimulus dependent [16]. The trigger can be perioral stimuli and/or environmental such as cold and touch. Table 20.2 lists the clinical presentation/features exhibited by patients who present with orofacial NP. NP most often presents on the face in relation to the dermatome of the trigeminal nerve.

Further classification separates NP into episodic and continuous. Episodic is characterized by sudden electric-like, shooting pains that can last for seconds to minutes. Continuous NP is pain originating in neural structures which is constant and varies in intensity without total remission. Episodic disorders include trigeminal neuralgia and glossopharyngeal neuralgia whereas continuous pain disorders can arise from injury of nerves in both the peripheral and central nervous system, such as neuromas and atypical odontalgia [16–18].

An understanding of the pathophysiology of episodic and continuous neuropathic pain provides the clinician with a strong rationale for choices of pharmacologic therapy. Table 20.3 lists the majority of agents broken into three main tiers that vary in mechanism of action by site of neurologic innervation – synapses, membrane stabilizing agents, and receptor agonists/antagonists. Each agent can be administered either by topical application or systemically. All agents may be preceded by the use of local anesthesia to localize peripheral versus central origin [18–21].

In general, analgesic drugs are usually the number 1 choice for relief in patients suffering from neuropathic pain [21, 22]. Morphine, for example, can interact with endorphins, the natural opioid of CNS. Tricyclic antidepressants act to increase catecholiminergic analogs that travel systemically to targets for relief by acting as membrane stabilizers and transsynaptic effects [16, 17]. The salicylates can act as antiinflammatory agents that inhibit cyclooxygenase pathways with inhibition of prostaglandins. The anticonvulsant medications can act as membrane stabilizers because they suppress hyperexcitability of the axonal membrane [22].

The clinician must apply careful dosing regardless of drug type administered due to side-effects, allergic

Table 20.3 Pharmacologic agents by location/etiology of drug action.

Synaptic cleft
Benzodiazepines
Clonidine
Tricyclic antidepressants:
Amitriptyline
Nortriptyline
Imipramine
Serotonin reuptake inhibitors/norepinephrine selective reuptake inhibitors:
Venlafaxine
Duloxetine
Trazodone
Milnacipran
Membrane-stabilizing drugs
Anticonvulsants
Carbamazepine
Oxcarbazepine
Phenytoin
Gabapentin
Pregabalin
Lamotrigine
Valproic acid
Tolpiramate
Tiagabine
Zonisamide
Other drugs
Opioids
Local anesthetics
Corticosteroids
Nonsteroidal antiinflammatory drugs (NSAIDs)
Aspirin
Acetaminophen
Antifungal agents
Antiviral agents
BOTOX
Antioxidants: alpha-lipoic acid
Salivary stimulants: pilocarpine, cevimiline
Topical agents
Lidocaine patches
Proparaciane
Streptomycin/lidocaine
Capsaicin
Topical NSAIDs
Antidepressants
Anticonvulsants
Botulinum toxins

reactions, and risk of drug dependence. Pharmacotherapy is eclectic based upon a diversity of analgesics whose dosing and concentrations vary with the type of neuropathic pain being treated.

Episodic Neuropathic Pain

Trigeminal Neuralgia (TN)

Trigeminal neuralgia is an episodic, unilateral pain that consists of brief shocking pains that can be sudden in onset and termination, that originate from one or more divisions of CN V, usually V2 and V3. There are pain-free periods between attacks. The most common trigger zone(s) of the face is the ala of nose and commissure of lip, both innervated by V2 and V3 divisions of CN V. The pain can refer to the teeth, making diagnosis difficult. Many clinicians have treated teeth with endodontic therapy without considering a neuropathic origin such as TN [1, 5, 7].

The etiologic mechanism is often a result of vascular compression and focal demyelination both peripherally and centrally. MRI is usually a reliable imaging strategy since these findings may also be related to a neoplasm/tumor impinging on the nerve [5]. Vascular brainstem lesions, angiomas, or AV malformations are further causes of TN [21, 22]; 15–20% of patients also exhibit a sensory loss along the distribution of CN V2/V3 [22]. The differential for demyelination should also include multiple sclerosis (MS) since symptomatology and demographics are within this patient population [21, 22].

The pharmacological paradigm for TN typically consist of first, second, and third line therapy [8, 14, 18, 20].

Anticonvulsive Agents First-line therapy consists of antiepileptic medications such as carbamazepine, oxcarbazepine, and gabapentin [23–26]. Systematic reviews have supported the use of carbamazepine (200–1200 mg/day) as a prognostic marker for definitive therapy since when it eliminates the symptoms, the clinician has successfully diagnosed TN [22]. Carbamazepine inactivates voltage-gated sodium channels and depresses postsynaptic reflex arcs in the spinal cord. Although it is very effective in resolving pain, it does not address the etiology of this neuralgia. The use of carbamazepine requires judicious dosing since this medicine has numerous side-effects, including leukopenia, agranulocytosis, aplastic anemia, drowsiness, and ataxia. Therapeutic levels must be followed to avoid adverse events, especially thrombocytopenia. Oxcarbazepine is a newer agent that has fewer side-effects and has become the drug of choice for treating TN unless it fails.

Another group of anticonvulsive agents, gabapentin and pregabalin, are now being used to treat neuropathic pain with even fewer side-effects [27]. The mechanism of action resides in their ability to increase gamma-amino butyric acid (GABA) in the central nervous system (CNS) and therefore increase the inhibition of pain sensors [28]. The main side-effect of this group is drowsiness. Baclofen and lamotrigine are two other agents that have fewer side-effects and are used for treatment of TN. Baclofen has less of an effect on blood cells but does have gastrointestinal (GI) sequelae, including vomiting and cramping. Lamotrigine is a phenothiazine derivative and also acts by stabilizing sodium channels and inhibiting release of neurotransmitters [22, 27]. Caution must be exercised when this agent is chosen since it can elicit Stevens–Johnson syndrome. It must be discontinued at a tapering dose.

Topiramate is another agent that can act at the voltage-sensitive sodium channels, as well as modulating GABA. It is derived from the sulfonamide group and has side-effects such as nephrolithiasis, somnolence, anxiety, and drowsiness. This agent must also be tapered if discontinuing its use. Table 20.4 depicts the dosing and daily administration of the anticonvulsant medications for TN.

Antidepressants Use of the tricyclic antidepressants (TCAs) in NP treatment has met with some debate due to their anticholinergic and cardiac side-effects, which include xerostomia, constipation, urinary retention, and anesthetic drug interactions. Amitriptyline has been used at doses that elicit a membrane-stabilizing effect [21, 22, 28]. A 10 mg dose of this agent can have a profound effect due to its mechanism of increasing the load of biogenic serotonin and norepinephrine at the synaptic cleft. TCAs act to relieve tension headaches and NP. In addition, they are first-line agents in the treatment of musculoskeletal pain associated with fibromyalgia [22, 28].

More recently, the selective serotonin reuptake inhibitors (SSRIs) have been applied for treatment of NP and other OFP syndromes such as chronic pain [22, 29]. SSRIs (fluoxetine and paroxetine) as well as serotonin and norepinephrine reuptake inhibitors (SRNIs) (duloxetine/milnacipran) have been successfully used for fibromyalgia and other centrally mediated pain syndromes (see section on Neurovascular Pain below). Table 20.4 lists the dosing schedule for the antidepressants.

The benzodiazepines have been used in combination with the above groups of agents for TN (see list of references for further information on benzodiazepine therapy for neuropathic pain).

Glossopharyngeal Neuralgia (GPN)

Glossopharyngeal neuralgia is another episodic form of NP. It is unilateral with electric shock-like episodes localized to the tongue, throat, and ear and under the mandible. It is usually provoked with swallowing or speech and can occur concurrently in 10% of patients with TN [22, 24]. Its incidence rate is 0.2/100 000 patients seen yearly and is also seen in patients suffering from MS. Often there are other symptoms such as syncope and cardiac arrhythmias as well as poor nutrition since swallowing food or liquids precipitates severe attacks. Pharmacologic therapeutics are similar to TN. First-line therapy is carbamazepine or oxcarbazepine with second-line use of local anesthetics to direct sites of pain. If medical treatment is unsuccessful then surgical procedures are warranted [21, 24, 30].

Occipital Neuralgia (OP)

Occipital neuralgia presents as a unilateral pain in the posterior scalp area innervated by the greater and lesser occipital nerves. It must be distinguished from referred pain from the neck. It is treated with corticosteroids and local anesthesia [31].

Continuous NP

As stated above, continuous NP has its causation in central neural regions and is manifested by pain that is constant in awareness and unremitting. There may be refractory periods but it never totally resolves. In Okeson's classification of facial pain, Axis 1 maps the three types of continuous NP: centrally mediated, peripherally mediated, and metabolic polyneuropathies (the reader is referred to reference #23 for a full explanation of these three presentations). Several examples are described below.

Peripheral Trigeminal Neuritis

This type of neuritis is a unilateral facial/orofacial pain that manifests as a burning sensation following trauma of the trigeminal nerve. The latency period is about 3–6 months and is preceded by allodynia and hyperalgesia. The etiology is often exposure to dental work like a root canal or dentoalveolar trauma. Chronic pain will persist in 5% of patients who report this event [32]. Diagnostic blocks with local anesthetics can be applied as immediate relief followed by topical medicaments (discussed below) to both alleviate pain and reduce adverse systemic events [16, 33].

Pharmacologic management consists of antidepressant therapy and anticonvulsants to control explosive periods of burning and stabbing in the area traumatized. In addition, capsaicin at a concentration of 0.05% with benzocaine 20% can be applied on a stent [33]. Other topical agents have compounded several drugs such as ketamine, NSAIDs, and anticonvulsants for relief (see below).

Peripheral Neuritis

Peripheral neuritis describes neuropathy secondary to inflammation usually mediated by the production of cytokines. Perineural inflammation occurs in the orofacial cavity due to dental procedures such as implant placement. Other etiologies include chronic sinusitis, TMJ joint degeneration, and malignant neoplasms that spread on the nerve trunk [16, 24, 33]. Pharmacologic intervention consists of antiinflammatory agents such as NSAIDs, corticosteroids, and topical agents [16, 34].

Table 20.4 Pharmacologic agents for neuropathic pain (episodic: trigeminal neuralgia/glossopharyngeal neuralgia/occipital neuralgia): dosing schedule.

Drug/Condition	Dosing
First line	
• Carbamazepine	200–1200 mg/d
• Oxcarbazepine	600–1800 mg/d
Second line	
• Combination of first line +	400 mg/d
• Lamotrigine	40–80 mg/day
• Baclofen	15 mg TID then 50–60 mg/day
Third line	
Phenytoin	
Gabapentin	300–1600 mg/day; mg dosing varies depending on side effects
Pregabalin	25–300 mg/day; start with 25 mg at night and then increase by 25 mg over 7 days to 3 times/day
Valproate	800–1500 mg/day
Tizanidine	
Tocainide	
Local anesthetics	
Continuous neuropathic pain	
Peripheral neuritis/ postherpetic neuralgia	
NSAIDs	
Corticosteroids	
Atypical odontalgia	
Antivirals	
Acetaminophen	
NSAIDs	
Opioids	
Tricyclic antidepressants (TCAs)	
Anticonvulsants	
Burning mouth syndrome	
Benzodiazepines	
Clonazepam	0.5–2 mg/day
Chlordiazepoxide	10–30 mg/day
Anticonvulsants	
Gabapentin	300–1600 mg/day; mg dosing varies depending upon side-effects seen. Can start with 100 mg at night and increase to 3×/day
Pregabalin	25–300 mg/day: start with 25 mg at night and then increase by 25 mg over 7 days to 3×/day

(Continued)

Table 20.4 (Continued)

Drug/Condition	Dosing
Antidepressants	
Amitriptyline	10–150 mg/day: 10 mg at night and increase by 10 mg over 7 days not exceeding 4×/day
Nortriptyline	10–150 mg /day: 10 mg at night and increase as needed 10/day over 7 days not exceeding 4×/day
Selective serotonin reuptake inhibitors	
Paroxetine	20–50 mg/day
Sertraline	50–200 mg/day: 50 mg initially and can increase by 25 mg every 7 days; max 200 mg/day
Trazodone	100–400 mg/day: 5–0 mg initially and increase by 50 mg 4–7 days; max 400 mg/day
Selective norepinephrine reuptake inhibitors	
Milnacipran	100 mg/day: 50 mg bid; 12.5 initially then bid; max 200 mg/day
Duloxetine	60–120 mg/day; PO qid
Antioxidants	
Alpha-lipoic acid	600–1200 mg/day; 300–600 mg bid

Herpes Zoster (HZ)/Postherpetic Neuralgia (PHN)

Postherpetic neuralgia occurs after an outbreak of herpes zoster virus. The virus undergoes a dormant period within the dorsal root ganglia – 55% of the time in the thoracic spine and associated with the cranial nerves, most often CN V and CN VII [18, 35]; 10–15% of cases are localized to CN V3 and 80% are recorded in CN V1. The incidence of disease is greater in the elderly and begins with significant prodromal symptomatology including headache, malaise, abnormal skin sensation, and fever. Once reactivated, the condition is referred to as "shingles."

The goals of pharmacologic management are to eliminate pain and accelerate healing. A number of prescribed modalities exist to address these concerns (refer to Table 20.4 for dosing schedule): medication groupings are as follows.

- *Antivirals*: these agents are applied within several days of symptomatology in order to decrease the rash and pain severity. Examples are aciclovir, valaciclovir, and famciclovir.

- *Opioids*: used for severe pain.
- *Nonopioids*: acetaminophen or NSAIDs to control inflammation, pain, and fevers.
- *Corticosteroids* added to antivirals to relieve pain.
- *Antidepressants*: amitriptyline, despiramine, and nortriptyline are often used in small doses and the gabapentin group has been recently approved by the FDA to treat PHN [36].

Both HZ and PHN are preventable with vaccinations. The Centers for Disease Control recommends patients 60 years or older receive vaccinations regardless of exposure risk (the reader is referred to reference #21 for further information).

Atypical Odontalgia/Nonodontogenic Toothache

Atypical odontalgia is a centralized trigeminal neuropathy characterized by an idiopathic pain that is throbbing or burning and misdiagnosed as dental in origin, resulting in unnecessary treatment. The age range is usually from 25 to 65 years and the most common tooth is the molar followed by the premolar followed by the incisor, with the maxilla as site of origin more often than the mandible. Diagnostic imaging shows no pathology but the teeth can elicit a hyperesthetic response to percussion. Diagnostic blocks with local anesthetics may either relieve the pain temporarily or exhibit an equivocal response. Associated symptomatology includes depression, oral dysesthesia, and problems with oral hygiene [3, 6, 20, 22]. Studies have suggested that vascular mechanisms as well as sympathetic system imbalance may play a role in the neuropathology of atypical odontalgia. The patient will be frustrated since they may want the specific tooth to be treated in a case of nonodontogenic toothache [22, 37, 38].

Pharmacologic therapy is challenging since both central and peripheral mechanisms are "misaligned" [37, 38]. The TCAs are first-line agents since at low doses they exhibit their analgesic action: 25–50 mg/day. The reuptake inhibition of serotonin and norepinephrine increases the effectiveness of inhibitory pathways of pain perception [22, 38]. The anticonvulsant gabapentin at a moderate dosing of 3600 mg/day is effective, with drowsiness as a side-effect. Pregabalin can also be used to relieve continuous NP [22, 38]. Peripheral components of atypical odontalgia may be treated with topical agents that are placed in a stent. Benzocaine mixed with carbamazepine and/or ketamine may also provide a true benefit in pain relief. Topical agents dosed in patches are now being studied to reduce the symptoms of continuous neuropathic pain (see section below on pharmacology of topical agents).

Burning Mouth Syndrome (BMS)

Burning mouth syndrome presents as burning sensations within the oral cavity, i.e., tongue, lips, and oral mucosa, that are continuous with an increase in intensity throughout the day [39–41]. The epidemiology of BMS varies from 1% to 3%. Women are predisposed (6:1 male) to BMS during the perimenopausal to postmenopausal years and up to 50% report a concomitant xerostomia and dysgeusia [22, 40]. The greatest frequency of BMS occurs on the anterior one-third of the tongue followed by the gingiva and palate. It is most often a diagnosis of exclusion. As to a definitive etiology, an in-depth HPI is essential prior to management since BMS can manifest in a variety of systemic diseases – GERD, diabetes, and autoimmune diseases. Deficiencies in certain vitamins including iron, vitamin B12, and folic acid can exacerbate BMS-induced xerostomia and the clinician may consider saliva flow studies as a prerequisite to treating BMS [1, 42].

Pharmacologic strategies for treatment must begin with establishing a definitive diagnosis, followed by a well-tailored treatment schedule that accounts for the multifactorial risk factors. Treatment can be palliative, symptomatic, or a combination of both in order to reach a therapeutic range of pain relief. It is judicious for the clinician to explain why therapy is complex so patient compliance can be achieved. The mainstay of treatment is the use of topical medications. Randomized control trials have established that clonazepam should be considered first at a dose of 0.25 mg–2 mg/day in wafer or oral disintegrating tablet forms [43, 44]. Other topical agents are capsaicin (1:2 dilutions), doxepin (5% cream), and 2% viscous lidocaine, every 4–6hours or prn. Additional choices include artificial sweeteners providing mucosal relief, antimicrobials such as lactoperoxidase rinses tid, and antifungal medications when candidiasis is the etiology [43, 44].

Systemic medications are the next choice of pharmacotherapy. As with neuropathic pain management, the TCAs amitriptyline and nortriptyline can be administered at doses of 10–150 mg maximum (due to side-effects) over 5–7 days [44–46]. The use of the SSRIs paroxetine and sertraline, trazodone, and the anticonvulsants pregabalin and gabapentin as combination therapy has demonstrated variable success in population studies [45–47] (see Table 20.4 for a summary of pharmacologic agents for BMS). Studies of clinical outcomes in large populations conclude that only 3–5% of patients achieve complete resolution of their symptoms [47].

Although the management of BMS is quite challenging, better strategies for definitive diagnoses will aid clinicians in choosing more efficacious pharmacology in order to better manage patients presenting with BMS [48, 49].

Neurovascular Pain

Neurovascular pain is episodic and based upon disturbance(s) of the trigeminovascular system and often presents clinically as a headache in patients with OFP [50]. The WHO characterizes headache disorders as the 10th disability in women and the cost of care exceeds 27 billion dollars globally [22, 51, 52]. The International Headache Society (HIS) divides primary headaches into four categories: (i) migraines, (ii) tension type headaches (TTH), cluster headaches and paroxysmal hemicranias; (iii) trigeminal autonomic cephalgias, and (iv) other headaches. The reader is referred to the bibliography for further interest [50–52].

Topical Medications for Orofacial Pain

Topical medications offer distinct advantages over systemic agents: greater safety, rapid onset of action, and low side-effect profile [53, 54]. Complete cessation of pain on application of topical anesthetic may not, however, be possible, as some of the neuronal changes may be central or due to neuropathic changes not easily reached by most topical anesthetics. Nevertheless, topical medications are useful for neuropathic pain due to peripheral nerve sensitization, as well as for centralized neuropathy that is accompanied by local allodynia. In the latter situation, the topical medication is used over the trigger site to reduce the ongoing neural stimulation that maintains the central sensitization. In cases of mild-to-moderate pain, local therapy might be the sole intervention. For moderate-to-severe pain, the use of systemic medications as well as local topical medications is more appropriate. A locally applied medication can offer faster relief while a centrally acting medication can be titrated up to effective levels [53–55].

Clinicians can manage OFP by applying topical medications that are formulated according to accepted clinical indications, i.e., the composition can be modified for individual patient requirements. These medications should be compounded by a pharmacy known to have high standards of quality, manufacturing technique, and reproducibility of compounded products. Topical medications can be applied directly to mucosa and skin, as well as indirectly utilizing a custom-made, stable intraoral carrier referred to as a neurosensory stent to ensure adequate drug delivery at the site of neuropathic pain. Examples of the most commonly used medicaments are discussed below.

Topical Anesthetics

Lidocaine Patches

The 5% lidocaine transdermal patch (Lidoderm®) is currently FDA approved for the treatment of pain associated with PHN [55, 56]. The patch is 10–14 cm in area and contains 700 mg of lidocaine, although only about 3% of this dose is absorbed, resulting in peak blood levels of 130 ng/mL during the recommended 12-hour application. This is slightly more than that achieved following an injection of one-half cartridge of 2% lidocaine with epinephrine [57, 58]. According to the manufacturer, the patch can be cut into smaller sizes with scissors before removal from the release liner. In addition to placebo-controlled trials in PHN, the drug has also proven efficacious in other neuropathic pain states, including in patients who have chronic lower back pain and osteoarthritis [59–61].

The systemic absorption of lidocaine from the patch is minimal in healthy adults even when four patches are applied for up to 24 hours per day, and lidocaine absorption is even lower among PHN patients than healthy adults at the currently recommended dose. Because of its proven efficacy and safety profile, the lidocaine patch 5% has been recommended as a first-line therapy for the treatment of the neuropathic pain of PHN [62].

Proparacaine

The benefit of the topical anesthetic proparacaine in trigeminal neuralgia was investigated in a randomized double-blind placebo-controlled trial of 47 patients [63]. Subjects were assigned randomly to either two drops of 0.5% proparacaine or buffered saline into the eye on the side of the TN. The results showed no benefit from proparacaine delivered in this way. Further studies are in progress to determine a proper dose, as well as combination therapeutic alternative in this group of agents.

Streptomycin and Lidocaine

Seventeen patients with TN were entered into a randomized double-blind study involving weekly injections of 2 mL of 2% lidocaine with or without 1 g streptomycin [64]. The authors concluded that although effective initially, streptomycin is not responsible for any pain relief in the long term.

Vanilloid Compounds (Capsaicin)

Capsaicin is a derivative of the chili pepper. Its proposed mechanism of action involves depletion of substance P and calcitonin gene-related peptide from peripheral afferent nerve endings. Several randomized double-blind trials in osteoarthritis and neuropathic pain have demonstrated efficacy in these chronic pain populations [53, 65–67].

The recently characterized capsaicin receptor is known as the transient receptor potential channel–vanilloid subfamily 1 (TRPV1) whose activation is believed to be necessary for the release of these inflammatory and pain-provoking compounds [53, 67]. Although the use of topical capsaicin has been proposed in patients who have TMD, surprisingly there are no clinical trials or even case-controlled studies evaluating its therapeutic effect in the TMD population [53, 67].

From a safety profile viewpoint, topical application of the drug is devoid of systemic toxicity, although patients must be counseled to expect a burning feeling during the initial applications of the drug; with continued application, this unpleasant feeling will dissipate. Combining capsaicin with a topical anesthetic, such as benzocaine 20% in pluronic lecithin organogel, may help reduce this burning sensation [67].

Capsaicin is probably best used as an adjunct to NSAIDs, benzodiazepines, or other systemic modalities.

Topical NSAIDs

Ketoprofen

Ketoprofen (Topofen®) is a fast-acting transdermal gel NSAID that possesses analgesic, antipyretic, and antiinflammatory properties. Topical application of the active ingredient is locally effective and at the same time minimizes the risk of systemic adverse events. A study at the University of Zagreb, in Croatia, evaluated the use of topical ketoprofen (called Fastum gel in Croatia) with the concurrent use of physical therapy for the treatment of TMD in 32 patients over an 8-month period [68]. The authors found that in comparing asymptomatic subjects, their active mouth opening was greater post medication administration than in placebo-treated controls ($p < 0.0001$) [68].

Diclofenac

In patients with painful TMD, topical diclofenac (Voltaren® Gel 1%) was as effective as 100 mg oral diclofenac in reducing symptoms. Di Rienzo Businco et al. reported that topically applied diclofenac and oral diclofenac are equally effective in the treatment of TMD symptoms, but topical Diclofenac did not have untoward effects on the gastric apparatus seen with oral diclofenac [69].

Antidepressants

Topical amitriptyline alone or combined with ketamine relieves peripheral neuropathic pain [70, 71]. Topical application of doxepin significantly relieves chronic neuropathic pain and when mixed with capsaicin, the effect was observed significantly earlier. TCAs have been used for their central analgesic effect. While it is known that there are serotonin receptors in peripheral nerves outside the CNS, it is unclear if this fact is important to the topical effect of TCAs, which are known to block the reuptake of serotonin. Additionally, cyclobenzaprine, a TCA analog, is used as a muscle relaxant. It has been used for peripheral application for muscle trismus and spasm, but adequate studies supporting this use as a standard of care are lacking.

Sympathomimetic Agents

Sympathomimetic agents may be useful in some forms of chronic neuropathic pain where nocioceptor activity is being stimulated by sympathetic fiber release of norepinephrine in the periphery. It has been shown that injured C fibers express alpha-1 receptors on their peripheral membranes. Sympathetic activity then would excite the C fibers, signaling pain. Clonidine, an alpha-2-adrenergic agonist, is thought to relieve pain by decreasing the abnormal excitability of these functional nociceptors. Clonidine is available as a transdermal patch for extraoral use. For intraoral use, it is better to have clonidine compounded into a transdermal penetrating cream and dispensed in a calibrated syringe so that the dose can be better controlled.

NMDA-Blocking Agents

Recent studies have shown that NMDA receptor antagonists may be useful in the treatment of neurogenic pain [72]. Several studies have been conducted in which orally administered ketamine, a NMDA antagonist, has shown effectiveness in alleviating refractory neuropathic pain. Although this medication has promise for the treatment of neuropathies, it can cause adverse effects such as hallucinations and dysphoria. Topical ketamine may be useful but specific studies are needed to evaluate this therapeutic alternative. As with clonidine, this medication would be best compounded into a transdermal penetrating cream and dispensed in a calibrated syringe.

Botulinum A Toxin

Botulinum A toxin is produced by *Clostridium botulinum* which affects the presynaptic membrane of the neuromuscular junction where it prevents acetylcholine release and therefore muscle contraction. Inactivation persists until collaterals form in junction plates on new areas of muscle cell walls.

Botulinum toxin has been applied as a strategy for pain management whose mechanism of action is a reduction in spasticity in both dystonias and migraines [73]. BOTOX A® injections have been shown to be effective in the prevention of migraines. Headaches must be greater than or equal to 15 days per month with headache lasting 4 hours a day or longer. The BOTOX A is administered via 31 injections into seven specific head and neck sites [74, 75]. When injected at labeled doses in recommended areas, it is expected to produce results lasting up to 3 months depending on the individual patients. Side-effects of botulinum toxin include pain, erythema, and unintended paralysis of nearby muscles.

There has been an increase in the number of studies investigating the use of BOTOX A to treat TMDs and bruxism, but it is not considered a first-line treatment option. Prior to employing BOTOX A as a treatment modality for bruxism, it is imperative that a definitive diagnosis of bruxism be made and that all other noninvasive and commonly validated methodologies are utilized in an attempt to manage the condition. The possible clinical effects of BOTOX A in the treatment of bruxism and TMDs at first appear attractive. Soares et al. in a Cochrane review on the long-term efficacy of BOTOX A concluded there was not enough evidence to support its use for myofascial pain syndrome and that more RCTs are needed [74].

Surgical Treatment Strategies for OFP

Facial pain whether acute or chronic can often be recalcitrant to pharmacotherapy. The pharmacologic approaches although efficacious can elicit adverse effects due to co-morbid conditions, as well as contraindications with other drug therapy. Drug overuse in the treatment of facial pain can also diminish a medication's prophylactic capabilities and lead to a "chronification" or transformation of episodic pain into chronic pain that is refractory to any pharmacologic management.

Minimally invasive surgical therapy can be a viable option for treatment based upon a patient's age, co-morbid medical conditions, the anatomical pathways involved, as well as the quality of pain perceived. The following can be administered in the oral healthcare office setting:

Injection Therapy

Injection therapy for peripheral and central nerve blockade is often a viable alternative for patients with facial pain that is refractory to medical therapy [74]. Peripheral nerve blockade has its basis in the use of low concentrations of local anesthetics which specifically block sensory fibers in mixed nerves which then converge on neural networks outside the immediate vicinity to relieve pain in other areas of the head, face, and neck. The duration of action is often predicated upon the pharmacokinetics of the local anesthetic administered. Local anesthetics in the amide groups are well tolerated since many formulations are hypoallergenic in the patient population. The choices most utilized in practice are 1% lidocaine, 3% mepivacaine, and 0.25% bupivacaine with increasing duration from 2 to 8 hours, respectively [74]. Epinephrine additives are not often needed for duration of action.

The following are the common target sites for peripheral nerve blocks in head and face pain syndromes.

- *Supraorbital/supratrochlear nerve block*: the supraorbital and supratrochlear nerves are branches of the ophthalmic division (V1) of the trigeminal nerve. The supraorbital nerve is often a source of facial pain as a result of herpes zoster in the V1 distribution. Figure 20.2 depicts the anatomic locations for injecting local anesthesia. The patient is positioned in supine or seated and the supraorbital notch is palpated. The area is prepped, and a 25 gauge needle is placed at the notch and advanced medially at 15° to avoid direct placement into the notch; 2–3 mL of anesthetic solution is injected. To access the supraorbital nerve, the injection is applied 2 cm lateral to the supratrochlear nerve (see Figure 20.2). A gauze is placed on the upper eyelid with pressure to avoid extirpation of anesthetic fluid into the loose areolar tissue. If the target is the supratrochlear area, the approach involves palpation of the bridge of the nose and supraorbital ridge. The supratrochlear nerve is injected above the medial border of the eyebrow (Figure 20.2) using 1–2 cc of lidocaine or bupivacaine [75].
- *Infraorbital nerve block*: the infraorbital nerve branches off V2 and innervates skin between the upper lip and lower eyelid on the ipsilateral side of the face. The infraorbital nerve is often a source of pain due to herpes zoster in the V2 distribution, infraorbital neuralgia, facial bone fractures, and malignancies. Figure 20.3 depicts the

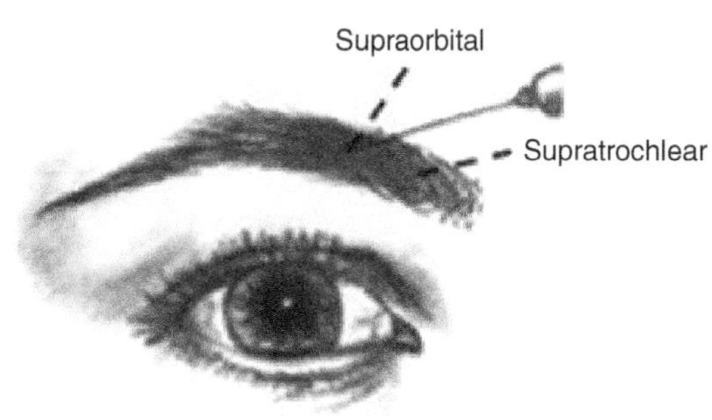

Figure 20.2 A diagrammatic approach for a supratrochlear nerve injection.

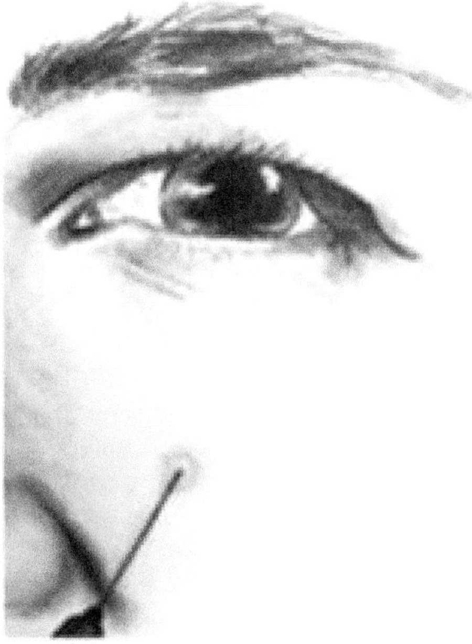

Figure 20.3 An extraoral approach for an infraorbital injection.

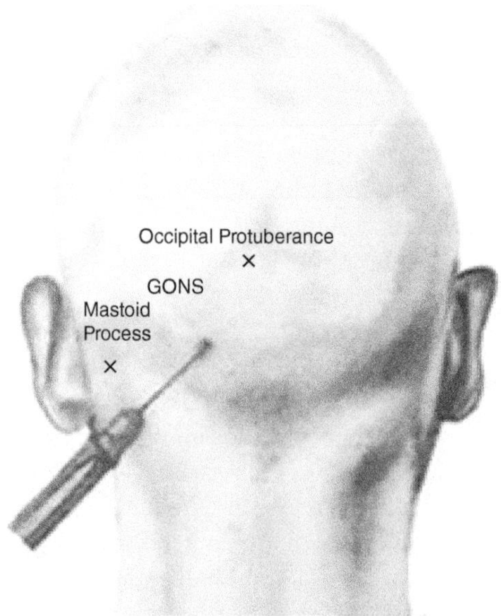

Figure 20.4 A diagrammatic approach for an occipital nerve block.

location which is 5 and 8 mm inferior to the infraorbital region and 2.5 cm lateral to the facial midline. The patient is placed in a seated position followed by palpation of the infraorbital notch. After prepping with an antibacterial, a 25 gauge 1.5 in. needle is advanced at a 15° angle followed by 2–3 mL of anesthetic solution administered in a fan-like fashion. A gauze is applied with pressure at the lower eyelid to avoid seepage into the loose areolar tissues of the lid.

- *Greater occipital nerve block*: the greater occipital nerve is the primary branch of the cervical root (C2) and innervates the scalp (Figure 20.4). Two conditions treated with this block are occipital neuralgia and cervicogenic headaches. The landmark for injection is 3 cm from the midline and 2 cm below the occipital protuberance. The local anesthetic amount injected is usually 2 mL [74, 75].
- *Auriculotemporal nerve block*: the auriculotemporal nerve is a branch of V3 of the trigeminal nerve and is sensory to the ear and temporalis muscle. The nerve block is accomplished by injecting 2–3 cc of lidocaine or bupivacaine superior to the posterior area of the zygoma that is just anterior to the tragus of the ear (Figure 20.5). Many patients feel relief from pain due to neuralgias as well as TMDs.

Complications of Injection Therapy

Local anesthetic injection therapy, although advantageous, does have the risk of complications and adverse events. Risk of mechanical nerve trauma during injection has been reported, although permanent paresthesia is minimal. Nerve damage and risk of neuroma formation have been reported, as well as hematoma formation and injury to adjacent structures at the site of injection. Systemic side-effects can occur due to intravascular compromise which can be minimal with aspiration techniques. The latter can be exacerbated if patients are on pharmacologic management of other major systemic illnesses, i.e., cardiovascular disease requiring anticoagulants and antiplatelet medications, as well as hepatic and renal disease that can

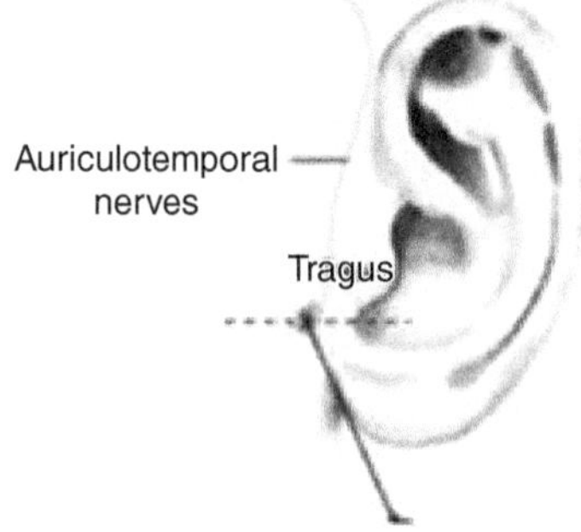

Figure 20.5 A diagrammatic approach for an auricular temporal nerve block.

Table 20.5 Complications and contraindications for injection therapy.

Anatomic complications

- Abscess or cellulitis in a fascial plane of the head and neck
- Open defect in the bony skull since anesthetic can diffuse into cranial compartment
- Altered anatomy due to trauma/infection/obesity

Physiologic complications

- Pregnancy; a relative contraindication since FDA drug category for lidocaine is B and bupivacaine is C
- Allergic reactions to local anesthetics
- Use of drugs that elicit bleeding dyscrasias, i.e., anticoagulant and antiplatelet therapy

Behavioral complications

- Syncopal vasovagal events
- Patients who are poor with respect to cooperation/anxiety and can indirectly injure the physician during injections

compromise the mechanism of action of the local anesthetic agents administered. Table 20.5 lists common contraindications and complications and the reader is referred to references #75 and #76 for further interest.

Summary and Future Directions

Orofacial pain comprises an extensive spectrum of pain disorders due to their unique anatomic/physiologic and biochemical components. The oral healthcare clinician must be systematic in eliciting a differential diagnosis on a case-specific basis. Once a definitive diagnosis is obtained, the primary approach of pain management is through rational pharmacotherapy, both invasive and noninvasive.

Future directions include innovations in routes of minimally invasive surgical skills and pharmacotherapy that will not only augment the efficacy of medication, but, in addition, allow for combination therapy with fewer adverse effects and greater prolongation of relief. Future directions will also involve evidence-based interprofessional collaborations that provide both nonsurgical and surgical paradigms for optimal treatment success. These therapeutic options will encourage greater choices for oral healthcare practitioners with respect to patient-centered care of orofacial pain syndromes.

References

1 De Rossi, S.S. (2013). Orofacial pain: a primer. *Dent. Clin. North Am.* 57 (3): 383–392.

2 Melzack, R. and Wall, P.D. (1965). Pain mechanisms: a new theory. *Science* 150 (3699): 971–979.

3 Okeson, J.P. (2008). The classification of orofacial pain. *Oral Maxillofac. Surg. Clin. North Am.* 20 (2): 133–144.

4 Lipton, J.A., Ship, J.A., and Larach-Robinson, D. (1993). Estimated prevalence and distribution of reported orofacial pain in the United States. *J. Am. Dent. Assoc.* 124 (10): 115–121.

5 Lancer, P. and Gesell, S. (2001). Pain management: the fifth vital sign. *Healthc. Benchmarks* 8 (6): 68–70.

6 De Leeuw, R. (2008). *Orofacial Pain: Guidelines for Assessment, Classification, and Management*, 4e. Chicago, IL: Quintessence Publishing.

7 Hargreaves, K.M. (2011). Orofacial pain. *Pain* 152: S25–S32.

8 Shinal, R.M. and Fillingim, R.B. (2007). Overview of orofacial pain: epidemiology and gender differences in orofacial pain. *Dent. Clin. North Am.* 51 (1): 1–18.

9 Bereiter, D.A., Hargreaves, K.M., and Hu, J.W. (2008). Trigeminal mechanisms of nociception: peripheral and brainstem organization. In: *The Senses: A Comprehensive Reference* (ed. A.L. Basbaum, A. Kaneko, G.M. Sheperd, et al.), 435–460. San Diego, CA: Academic Press.

10 Cooper, S.A. and Desjardins, P.J. (2010). The value of the dental impaction pain model in drug development. *Methods Mol. Biol.* 617: 175–190.

11 Kim, H., Ramsay, E., Lee, H. et al. (2009). Genome-wide association study of acute post-surgical pain in humans. *Pharmacogenomics* 10: 171–179.

12 LeResche, L., Mancl, L.A., Drangsholt, M.T. et al. (2007). Predictors of onset of facial pain and temporomandibular disorders in early adolescence. *Pain* 129: 269–278.

13 Schaefer, J., Holland, N., Whelan, J.S. et al. (2013). Pain and temporomandibular disorders: a pharmaco-gender dilemma. *Dent. Clin. North Am.* 57 (2): 233–262.

14 Ohba, S., Yoshimura, H., Matsuda, S. et al. (2014). Diagnostic role of magnetic resonance imaging in assessing orofacial pain and paresthesia. *J. Craniofac. Surg.* 25 (5): 1748–1751.

15 Shueb, S.S., Nixdorf, D.R., John, M.T. et al. (2015). What is the impact of acute and chronic orofacial pain on quality of life? *J. Dent.* 43: 1203–1210.

16 Romeo-Reyes, M. and Uyanik, J.M. (2014). Orofacial pain management: current perspectives. *J. Pain Res.* 7: 99–115.

17 Costigan, M., Scholz, J., and Woolf, C.J. (2009). Neuropathic pain: a maladaptive response of the nervous system to damage. *Ann Rec Neurosci* 31: 1–32.

18 Spencer, C.J. and Gremillion, H.A. (2007). Neuropathic orofacial pain: proposed mechanisms, diagnosis, and treatment considerations. *Dent. Clin. North Am.* 51: 209–224.
19 Katusic, S., Williams, D.B., Beard, C.M. et al. (1991). Incidence and clinical features of glossopharyngeal neuralgia. Rochester, MN, 1945–1984. *Neuroepidemiology* 10 (5–6): 266–275.
20 Balasubramaniam, R. and Klasser, G.D. (2014). Orofacial pain syndromes: evaluation and management. *Med. Clin. North Am.* 98: 1385–1405.
21 Stacey, B.R. (2005). Management of peripheral neuropathic pain. *Am. J. Phys. Med. Rehabil.* 84 (Suppl): S4–S16.
22 Okeson, J.P. (2014). General considerations in managing oral and facial pain. In: *Bell's Oral and Facial Pain*, 7e (ed. J.P. Okeson), 181–232. Hanover Park, IL: Quintessence Publishing.
23 Mueller, D., Obermann, M., Yoon, M.S. et al. (2011). Prevalence of trigeminal neuralgia and persistent idiopathic facial pain: a population based study. *Cephalalgia* 31 (15): 1542–1548.
24 Rozen, T.D. (2004). Trigeminal neuralgia and glossopharyngeal neuralgia. *Neurol. Clin. North Am.* 22: 185–206.
25 Zakrzewska, J.M. (2010). Medical management of trigeminal neuropathic pains. *Expert. Opin. Pharmacother.* 11 (8): 1239–1254.
26 Reisner, L. and Pettengill, C.A. (2001). The use of anticonvulsants in orofacial pain. *Oral Surg. Oral Med. Oral Pathol. Oral Radiol. Endod.* 91 (1): 2–7.
27 Attal, N., Crucco, G., Baron, R. et al. (2010). EFNS guidelines on the pharmacological treatment of neuropathic pain: 2010 revision. *Eur. J. Neurol.* 17: 1113–e88.
28 Saarto, T. and Wiffen, P.J. (2005). Antidepressants for neuropathic pain. *Cochrane Database Syst. Rev.* (3): CD005454.
29 Lee, Y.C. and Chen, P.P. (2010). A review of SSRIs and SNRIs in neuropathic pain. *Expert. Opin. Pharmacother.* 11: 2813–2825.
30 Stieber, V.W., Bourland, J.D., and Ellis, T.L. (2005). Glossopharyngeal neuralgia treated with gamma knife surgery: treatment outcome and failure analysis case report. *J. Neurosurg.* 102 (Suppl): 155–157.
31 Vanelderen, P., Lataster, A., Levy, R. et al. (2010). Occipital neuralgia. *Pain Pract.* 10 (2): 137–144.
32 Polycarpou, N., Ng, Y.L., Canavan, D. et al. (2005). Prevalence of persistent pain after endodontic treatment and factors affecting its occurrence in cases with complete radiographic healing. *Int. Endod. J.* 38 (3): 169–178.
33 Bramwell, B.L. (2010). Topical orofacial medications for neuropathic pain. *Int. J. Pharm. Compd.* 14 (3): 200–203.
34 Benoliel, R. and Sharav, Y. (2010). Chronic orofacial pain. *Curr. Pain Headache Rep.* 14: 33–40.
35 Kennedy, P.G. (2002). Varicella-zoster virus latency in human ganglia. *Rev. Med. Virol.* 12: 327–334.
36 Scheinfeld, N. (2003). The role of gabapentin in treating diseases with cutaneous manifestations and pain. *Int. J. Dermatol.* 42: 491–495.
37 Rees, R.T. and Harris, M. (1978). Atypical odontalgia: differential diagnoses and treatment. *Br. J. Oral Surg.* 16: 212–218.
38 Graff-Radford, S.B. and Solberg, W.K. (1992). Atypical odontalgia. *J. Craniomandib. Disord.* 6: 260–265.
39 Rhodus, N.L., Carlson, C.R., and Miller, C.S. (2003). Burning mouth syndrome (disorder). *Quintessence Int.* 34: 587–593.
40 Danhauer, S.C., Miller, C.S., Rhodus, N.L. et al. (2002). Impact of criteria-based diagnosis of burning mouth syndrome on treatment outcome. *J. Orofac. Pain* 16: 305–311.
41 Rodriguez-de Rivera-Campillo, E. and Lopez-Lopez, J. (2013). Evaluation of the response to treatment and clinical evolution in patients with burning mouth syndrome. *Med. Oral Patol. Oral Cir. Bucal.* 18: e403–e410.
42 Sreebny, L.M., Yu, A., Green, A. et al. (1992). Xerostomia in diabetes mellitus. *Diabetes Care* 15: 900–904.
43 Heckmann, S.M., Kirchner, E., Grushka, M. et al. (2012). A double-blind study on clonazepam in patients with burning mouth syndrome. *Laryngoscope* 122 (4): 813–816.
44 Thoppay, J.R., DeRossi, S.S., and Ciarrocca, K.N. (2013). Burning mouth syndrome. *Dent. Clin. North Am.* 57 (3): 497–512.
45 Patton, L.L., Siegel, M.A., Benoliel, R. et al. (2007). Management of burning mouth syndrome: systematic review and management recommendations. *Oral Surg. Oral Med. Oral Pathol. Oral Radiol.* 103 (Suppl): S39.e1-13.
46 deMorales, M., do Amaral Bezerra, B.A., da Rocha Neto, P.C. et al. (2012). Randomized trials for the treatment of burning mouth syndrome: an evidence-based review of the literature. *J. Oral Pathol. Med.* 41 (4): 281–287.
47 Gorsky, M., Silverman, S. Jr., and Chinn, H. (1991). Clinical characteristics and management outcome in the burning mouth syndrome. An open study of 130 patients. *Oral Surg. Oral Med. Oral Pathol.* 72: 192–195.
48 Klasser, G.D., Epstein, J.B., Villines, D. et al. (2011). Burning mouth syndrome: a challenge for dental practitioners and patients. *Gen. Dent.* 59 (3): 210–220.
49 Sardella, A., Lodi, G., Demarosi, F. et al. (2006). Burning mouth syndrome: a retrospective study investigating

spontaneous remission and response to treatments. *Oral Dis.* 12 (2): 152–155.

50 Franco, A.L., Goncalves, D.A., Castanharo, S.M. et al. (2010). Migraine is the most prevalent primary headache in individuals with temporomandibular disorders. *J. Orofac. Pain* 24 (3): 287–292.

51 Olesen, J. (2013). The International Classification of Headache Disorders, 3rd editon (beta version). *Cephalalgia* 33: 629–808.

52 Hu, X.H., Markson, L.E., Lipton, R.B. et al. (1999). Burden of migraine in the United States: disability and economic costs. *Arch. Intern. Med.* 159: 813–818.

53 Padilla, M., Clark, G.T., and Merrill, R.L. (2000). Topical medications for orofacial neuropathic pain: a review. *J. Am. Dent. Assoc.* 131 (2): 184–195.

54 Heir, G., Karolchek, S., Kalladka, M. et al. (2008). Use of topical medication in orofacial neuropathic pain: a retrospective study. *Oral Surg. Oral Med. Oral Pathol. Oral Radiol. Endod.* 105 (4): 466–469.

55 Comer, A.M. and Lamb, H.M. (2000). Lidocaine patch 5%. *Drugs* 59 (2): 245–249.

56 Campbell, B.J., Rowbotham, M., Davies, P.S. et al. (2002). Systemic absorption of topical lidocaine in normal volunteers, patients with post-herpetic neuralgia, and patients with acute herpes zoster. *J. Pharm. Sci.* 91 (5): 1343–1350.

57 Rowbotham, M.C., Davies, P.S., Verkempinck, C. et al. (1996). Lidocaine patch: double-blind controlled study of a new treatment method for post-herpetic neuralgia. *Pain* 65 (1): 39–44.

58 Galer, B.S., Rowbotham, M.C., Perander, J. et al. (1999). Topical lidocaine patch relieves post herpetic neuralgia more effectively than a vehicle topical patch: results of an enriched enrollment study. *Pain* 80 (3): 533–538.

59 Galer, B.S., Jensen, M.P., Ma, T. et al. (2002). The lidocaine patch 5% effectively treats all neuropathic pain qualities: results of a randomized, double-blind, vehicle-controlled, 3-week efficacy study with use of the neuropathic pain scale. *Clin. J. Pain* 18 (5): 297–301.

60 Galer, B.S., Gammaitoni, A.R., Oleka, N. et al. (2004). Use of the lidocaine patch 5% in reducing intensity of various pain qualities reported by patients with low-back pain. *Curr. Med. Res. Opin.* 20 (Suppl 2): S5–S12.

61 Galer, B.S., Sheldon, E., Patel, N. et al. (2004). Topical lidocaine patch 5% may target a novel underlying pain mechanism in osteoarthritis. *Curr. Med. Res. Opin.* 20 (9): 1455.

62 Davies, P.S. and Galer, B.S. (2004). Review of lidocaine patch 5% studies in the treatment of postherpetic neuralgia. *Drugs* 64: 937–947.

63 Kondziolka, T., Lemley, J.R., Kestle, L.D. et al. (1994). The effect of single-application topical ophthalmic anesthesia in patients with trigeminal neuralgia: a randomized double-blind placebo-controlled trial. *J. Neurosurg.* 80: 993–997.

64 Stajcic, Z., Juniper, R.P., and Todorovic, L. (1990). Peripheral streptomycin/lidocaine injections versus lidocaine alone in the treatment of idiopathic trigeminal neuralgia: a double blind controlled trial. *J. Craniomaxillofac. Surg.* 18: 243–246.

65 Kopp, S. (1998). The influence of neuropeptides, serotonin, and interleukin 1ß on temporomandibular joint pain and inflammation. *J. Oral Maxillofac. Surg.* 56: 189–191.

66 Sato, J., Segami, N., Yoshitake, Y. et al. (2005). Expression of capsaicin receptor TRPV-1 in synovial tissues of patients with symptomatic internal derangement of the temporomandibular joint and joint pain. *Oral Surg. Oral Med. Oral Pathol. Oral Radiol. Endod.* 100: 674–681.

67 Epstein, J.B. and Marcoe, J.H. (1994). Topical application of capsaicin for treatment of oral neuropathic pain and trigeminal neuralgia. *Oral Surg. Oral Med. Oral Pathol.* 77: 135–140.

68 Badel, T., Krapac, L., Pavičin, I.S. et al. (2013). Physical therapy with topical ketoprofen and anxiety related to temporomandibular joint pain treatment. *Fiz. Rehabil. Med.* 25 (1–2): 6–16.

69 Di Rienzo Businco, L., Di Rienzo Businco, A., D'Emilia, M. et al. (2004). Topical versus systemic diclofenac in the treatment of temporomandibular joint dysfunction symptoms. *Acta Otorhinolaryngol. Ital.* 24 (5): 279–283.

70 Lynch, M.E., Clark, A.J., and Sawynok, J. (2003). A pilot study examining topical amitriptyline, ketamine, and a combination of both in the treatment of neuropathic pain. *Clin. J. Pain* 19: 323–328.

71 Lynch, M.E., Clark, A.J., Sawynok, J., and M.J. (2005). Sullivan topical amitriptyline and ketamine in neuropathic pain syndromes: an open-label study. *J. Pain* 6: 644–649.

72 Mathisen, L.C., Skjelbred, P., Skoglund, L.A., and Oye, I. (1995). Effect of ketamine, an NMDA receptor inhibitor, in acute and chronic orofacial pain. *Pain* 61: 215–220.

73 Soares, A., Andriolo, R.B., Atallah, A.N., and da Silva, E.M.K. (2012). Botulinum toxin for myofascial pain syndromes in adults. *Cochrane Database Syst. Rev.* (4): CD007533.

74 Kleen, J.K. and Levin, M. (2016). Injection therapy for headache and facial pain. *Oral Maxillofac. Clin. North Am.* 28: 423–434.

75 Levin, M. (2010). Nerve blocks in the treatment of headaches. *Neurotherapeutics* 7: 197–203.

21

Local Anesthesia: Agents and Techniques

Orrett E. Ogle and Ricardo Boyce

No other scientific development has advanced the practice of modern-day dentistry more than the introduction of local anesthesia. The invention of the hollow-bore needle and hypodermic syringe in 1853 [1], the use of cocaine for local anesthesia by Carl Koller in 1884 [2], and the introduction of procaine (more commonly known as novocaine) in 1904 [3] were the foundations that made invasive oral procedures possible. Today, local anesthetics are the most commonly used drugs in dentistry. Without good pain control, very few surgical or other dental procedures would have developed and the current number of specialties would not have existed. Local anesthesia has also made the office practice of dentistry possible and safe. As patients do not require general anesthesia, the operator can perform the surgery in a careful and unhurried fashion where the patient will be comfortable and cooperative. Excellent pain control is the key to a successful surgical practice.

Dentoalveolar surgery and other minor oral surgical procedures performed in the ambulatory setting rely overwhelmingly on good local anesthesia, even when IV sedation is being used. Today, there are several techniques for administering local anesthesia, and different devices and anesthetic agents which are safe, effective, nonirritating to oral mucosa and of low allergenic risk. Successful local anesthesia will involve proper injection technique, familiarity with the neuroanatomy of the region, knowledge of the pharmacology of the local anesthetics being used, and a thorough understanding of the physiology of nerve conduction. Improper identification of anatomic landmarks and poor injection techniques will lead to anesthetic failure. The proper selection of the appropriate local anesthetic is important to the success of local anesthesia.

This chapter will present techniques for nerve block anesthesia, adjunctive techniques, and a brief review of local anesthetics used in oral surgery.

Local Anesthetics

Local anesthesia is defined as a loss of sensation to a specific area of the body that causes a depression of excitatory nerve endings and/or an inhibition of the conduction process in peripheral nerves [4]. The drugs used cause reversible absence of pain sensation along specific nerve pathways from specific areas. These drugs fall into one of two classes: aminoamide and aminoester local anesthetics (Table 21.1). All amide local anesthetics contain an "I" in the name. For example, lidocaine, mepivacaine, prilocaine, bupivacaine, ropivacaine, and levo-bupivacaine contain the "i" before the "-vacaine." Esters such as procaine, chloroprocaine, and tetracaine do not contain an "i" before the "-caine" [5]. Infiltration anesthesia and regional nerve blocks are commonly used for tooth extractions and other oral surgical procedures

Apart from their chemical classification as amides or esters, local anesthetics are further classified according to their duration of action as short-, intermediate-, or long-acting agents.

Table 21.1 Chemical Structures of Commonly Used Local Anesthetics.

Ester anesthetics	Amide anesthetics
Procaine[a]	Lidocaine
Chloroprocaine	Mepivacaine
Cocaine	Bupivacaine
	Etidocaine
	Articaine
	Prilocaine

a) Procaine is no longer used in dentistry because of a high incidence of allergic reactions.

Oral and Maxillofacial Surgery, Medicine, and Pathology for the Clinician, First Edition. Edited by Harry Dym, Leslie R. Halpern, and Orrett E. Ogle.

- Short acting: <2 hours
- Intermediate acting: 2–4 hours
- Long acting: 4–18 hours

The duration of the planned surgical procedure along with the anticipated need for postoperative pain control guide the surgeon on which agent to select (Table 21.2). Long-acting anesthetic agents offer the surgeon the option of long-term control to obliterate postoperative pain. This would be desirable, for example, for the removal of full bony impacted third molars [6].

Nerve Block Techniques

Nerve blocks are a type of regional anesthesia in which the anesthetic solution is deposited close to a specific nerve trunk to interrupt pain sensations from a specific area of the body. Nerve blocks usually last longer than anesthesia administered by local infiltration. Some of the techniques that will be described here are methods that will not be used routinely, but should be in the armamentarium of the oral surgeon since there may be situations in which their application may be needed despite the fact that general anesthesia is always an option. General anesthesia, however, whether in the office or a hospital, poses a greater overall risk, is more expensive and requires longer and more intense postanesthesia care coupled with risk of postoperative nausea or vomiting. A nerve block with sedation enables faster postoperative recovery than general anesthesia, offers better pain relief and faster discharge

Maxillary Nerve Blocks

Maxillary nerve block is rarely ever necessary in routine intraoral surgery but will be useful if there is a need to obtain anesthesia of the mucosa of the maxillary sinus, the maxillary teeth, and the oral soft tissues all at once. The few specific indications for maxillary nerve block anesthesia are listed in Box 21.1.

Anatomy (Figure 21.1)

The maxillary nerves leave the cranium via the foramen rotundum on the greater wing of the sphenoid to enter the pterygopalatine fossa. The nerve has three divisions: the pterygopalatine nerve, the infraorbital nerve, and the zygomatic nerve. The pterygopalatine nerve has several divisions, but the most significant one in oral surgery would be the anterior palatine nerve. The anterior palatine nerve enters the oral cavity through the greater palatine foramen where it splits into several branches that spread fanwise anteriorly as the greater palatine nerve to supply the mucosa of the hard palate up to the canine line [7]. The infraorbital nerve releases three branches before it emerges at the infraorbital foramen: the anterior superior alveolar nerve, which innervates the maxillary alveoli, gingivae, and periodontal tissues of the central and lateral incisors and the canines; the middle superior alveolar nerve, which innervates the maxillary alveoli, gingivae, and periodontal tissues of the maxillary premolar area; and the posterior superior alveolar nerve which innervates the molar areas. In the base of the alveolar process, these nerves form a plexus called the superior dental plexus. These dental nerves are the ones anesthetized by infiltration of local anesthesia [7]. The terminal branch of the

Table 21.2 Common Local Anesthetics.

Local anesthetic agent	Duration for nerve block anesthesia	Maximum adult dose
Lidocaine 2%	30 min–1 h	300 mg, 8 cartridges
Prilocaine HCL	30 min–1.5 h	600 mg, 8 cartridges
Mepivacaine 3%	45 min–1.5 h	400 mg, 7 cartridges
Articaine 4% w epi 1/100 000	1–2 h	500 mg, 7 cartridges
Lidocaine 2% w epi 1/100 000	2–4 h	500 mg, 12 cartridges
Mepivacaine 2% w neocobefrin 1/20 000	2–4 h	400 mg, 11 cartridges
Bupivacaine 0.5% w epi 1/200 000	3–7 h	90 mg, 10 cartridges
Etidocaine 1.5% w epi 1/200 000	3–7 h	400 mg, 14 cartridges
Chloroprocaine 2%	30 mn–1 h	800 mg, 12 cartridges
Procaine 2%	30 min–1.5 h	200 mg, 6 cartridges

Box 21.1 Indications for Maxillary Nerve Block

- Procedures requiring anesthesia of multiple teeth and surrounding areas where it would require the injection of multiple cartridges of the anesthetic and then run the risk of exceeding the toxic dose.
- Failure of local infiltration as a result of infection or abscess formation requiring a maxillary nerve block administered away from the site of infection.
- Chronic maxillary pain of unknown etiology that has not responded to systemic analgesics (pain management by anesthesiologist).

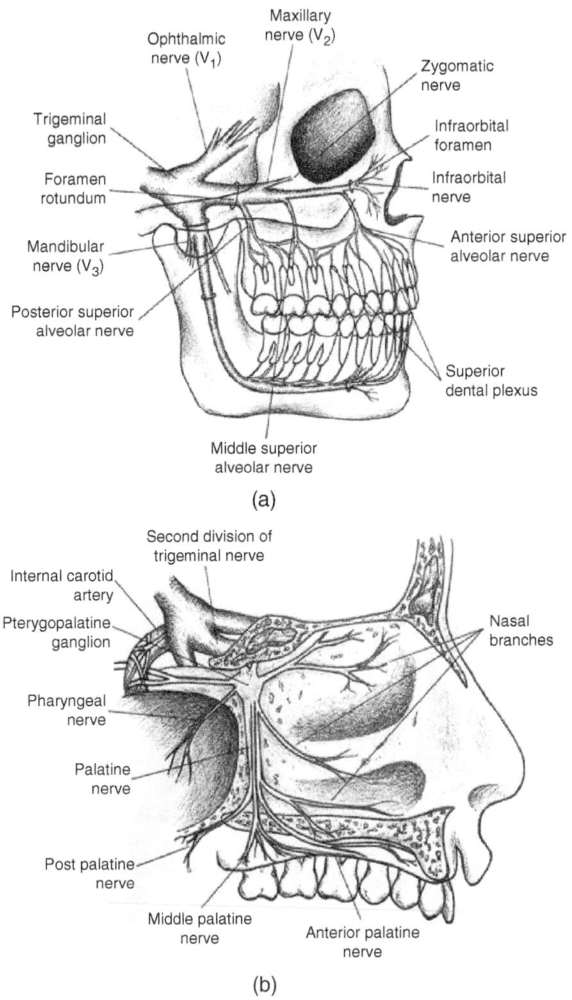

Figure 21.1 (a) Maxillary nerve showing alveolar nerves and infra-orbital nerve. (b) Pterygopalatine nerve and anterior palatine nerve. *Source:* Ogle O, 2001/With permission of Elsevier.

infraorbital nerve spreads fanwise from the infraorbital foramen to supply the eyelid, the skin on the nose, and the upper lip and labial mucosa.

A successful block of the maxillary nerve will provide anesthetic effect to the teeth, palatal and gingival mucosa, skin of the midface, maxillary sinus, and nasal cavity.

Maxillary nerve block can be achieved by the following approaches.

- Greater palatine canal approach
- High tuberosity approach
- Sigmoid notch approach

Greater Palatine Approach

The greater palatine approach attempts to block the maxillary nerve as it travels through the pterygopalatine fossa. It is the most frequently used approach and has a high rate of success but sometimes it can be difficult to located or negotiate the canal.

The greater palatine foramen is located at the junction of the alveolus and the bony palate just medial to the third molar tooth. It can be located by applying pressure on a cotton swab at the junction of the hard palate and the maxillary alveolar process until the depression caused by the foramen is noted.

Technique

1. Attach a 27 gauge long dental needle to the standard dental anesthetic syringe containing a 1.8 mL cartridge of local anesthesia. The length of the long dental anesthesia needle is usually about 32 mm (1.5 in.) from hub to tip, but this may vary slightly by manufacturer. Be sure that the needle is 32 mm. Never insert the needle to the hub.
2. Deposit about 1/8 of a carpule of local anesthetic in the area of the greater palatine foramen to obtain surface anesthesia.
3. When the area is numb (about 3 minutes), hold the syringe like a pen at about a 60° angle and probe the anticipated area of the greater palatine canal in a stepwise fashion with the tip of the needle until the bony canal is located.
4. When the needle enters the canal, advance it about 30 mm. If the needle advances with little or no resistance, slowly inject 1.8 mL of local anesthetic after it is confirmed that no blood is aspirated. If resistance is encountered, the needle is redirected and reinserted at a different angle. If the canal cannot be negotiated, this approach should be terminated. If the needle advances too easily and with no resistance, it has possibly gone beyond the posterior border of the bony palate and into the soft palate. Aspiration may produce air bubbles. When successful, anesthesia effect should be noted in 5–15 minutes.

The length of the canal may vary and a short canal may lead to serious complications. For more precise determination of the length of the canal, cone beam computed tomography (CBCT) is indicated prior to the procedure to analyze its length. If anesthesia fails, the canal is most likely longer than 30 mm. According to Das, the length of the greater palatine canal varies between 27 and 44 mm with a mean of 32 mm [8].

High Tuberosity Approach

The high tuberosity approach blocks the nerve as it courses along the pterygopalatine fossa. The posterior superior alveolar nerve may be blocked before it enters the bony canal located on the zygomatic aspect of the maxilla above the third molar [9]

Technique (Figure 21.2)

1. Open the mouth about 15–20 mm and retract the cheek.
2. The puncture is made high in the mucobuccal fold above the distobuccal root of the second molar.
3. The needle is directed upward and inward to a depth of about 20 mm, keeping the point of the needle close to the periosteum of the tuberosity at all times. This will minimize the risk of entering the pterygoid venous plexus.
4. Aspirate for blood, and if negative, slowly inject 1.8 mL of local anesthetic.

Sigmoid Notch Approach

This technique will require a 22 gauge 3.5 in. spinal needle and a 10 cc syringe. This procedure is best performed under imaging guidance.

Technique

1. Using a marking pen, draw the inferior border of the zygomatic arch on the external skin. With the mouth closed, identify the coronoid process and mark it on the skin. Next, have the patient open and close the mouth and palpate in front of and below the tragus to identify the condyle. Mark the condyle. The sigmoid notch will be between the condyle and the coronoid process. At the midpoint, the deepest part of the notch is about 8–10 mm below the zygomatic arch when the mouth is closed.
2. Determine the entry point, wipe it with alcohol and make a wheal with local anesthesia.
3. With the mouth closed, penetrate the skin at the center of the coronoid notch below the zygomatic arch, trying to stay close to the depth of the notch.
4. Slowly advance the needle perpendicular to the skin until bone is encountered at about a depth of 4–5 cm (1.5–2 in. or about half of the length of the needle). This will be the lateral pterygoid plate.

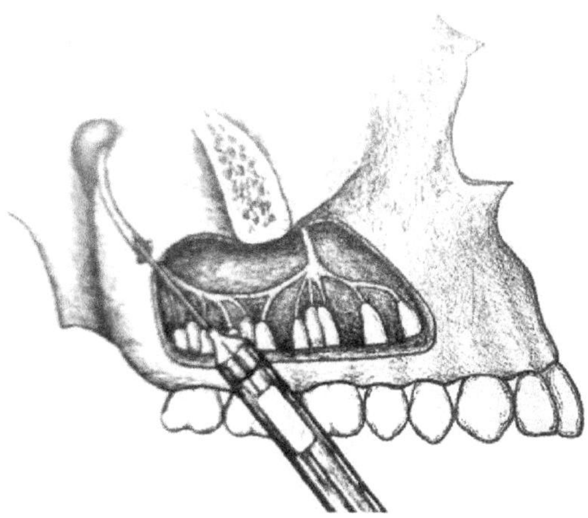

Figure 21.2 Technique for blocking the posterior superior alveolar nerve close to the ptereygomaxillary fissure. *Source:* Ogle O, 2001/With permission of Elsevier.

5. Withdraw the needle slightly, then redirect it anteriorly and superiorly, and advance it another 1 cm. If the needle has been properly directed, the point will now be in the pterygopalatine fossa.
6. During the entire process, aspiration should be done a few times. In the pterygopalatine fossa, aspirate before injecting. If aspiration is negative, slowly deposit about 5–10 mL of the anesthetic solution.

Contraindications and complications for maxillary nerve block are detailed in Boxes 21.2 and 21.3.

Mandibular Nerve Block

Unlike maxillary nerve block which is rarely indicated, the mandibular nerve block is the most common type of nerve block used for oral surgical procedures. The majority of surgical procedures performed on the lower jaw will require anesthesia of the inferior alveolar, lingual, and buccal nerves. These nerves are accessible in the pterygomandibular space (Figure 21.3). A nerve block in the pterygomandibular space will anesthetize the following.

- All mandibular teeth
- Gingivae on the buccal/labial and lingual surfaces of the mandible
- The floor of the mouth
- The body of the mandible and lower portion of the ramus
- The anterior two-thirds of the tongue
- Mucosa and skin of the lower lip and chin

Box 21.2 Contraindications to maxillary nerve block

- Infection over the point of injection
- Patients with bleeding disorders or those who are taking anticoagulant medications

Box 21.3 Reported complications of maxillary nerve block

- Diplopia is the most common (35.6%) [10], resulting from accidental block of the abducens nerve which innervates the lateral rectus muscle by dissemination of the anesthetic through the superior orbital fissure
- Transient ophthalmoplegia
- Ptosis
- Infraorbital nerve injury
- Temporary blindness from vasoconstriction of the ophthalmic artery or block of the optic nerve
- Retrobulbar hematoma
- Needle track infection

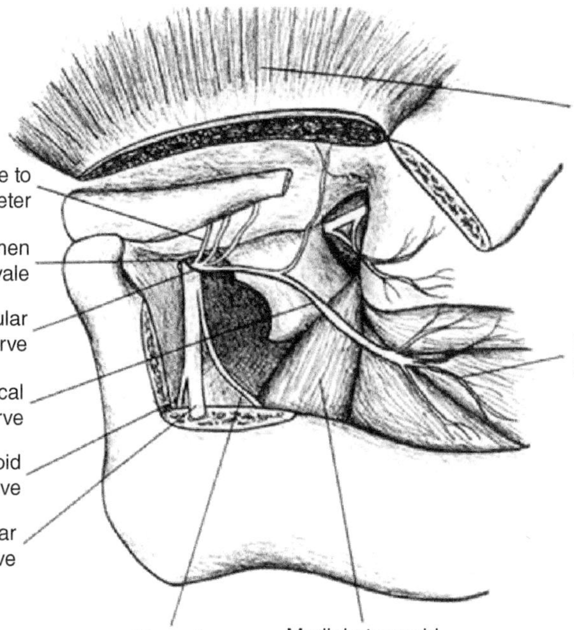

Figure 21.3 Pterygomandibular space. *Source:* Ogle O, 2001/With permission of Elsevier.

Inferior alveolar nerve block can be achieved by the following techniques.

- Halstead method
- Akinosi technique
- Gow-Gates technique.

Halstead Method

This is the most common method used in the United States [11] and is generally referred to as the "traditional method." With this technique, the inferior alveolar nerve (IAN) is approached via an intraoral route and is blocked just before the nerve enters the mandibular canal at the lingual. This method of blocking the IAN has a success rate of 71–87% [12] and incomplete anesthesia is not uncommon.

Technique 1 (Figure 21.4)

1. Place the thumb of the noninjecting hand in the deepest portion of the concavity of the ramus between the external and internal ridges of the mandible.
2. Place the other four fingers extraorally on the posterior border of the ramus. The foramen of the mandibular canal will be approximately midway between the internal oblique ridge and the posterior border of the mandible along a line that bisects the thumb [6].
3. Orient the syringe so that the barrel is in the opposite corner of the mouth over the premolars with the needle directed parallel to the occlusal plane of the mandibular teeth, bisecting the thumb, and is aimed at the midpoint of the ramus located between the thumb and the extraorally placed fingers. The puncture should be made through the pterygomandibular raphe and the needle advanced to touch the medial surface of the mandible. If the needle does not contact the bone, reorient the barrel of the syringe more posteriorly and repeat attempt. Once contact is made with the bone, the needle is then withdrawn 2 mm, aspirated, and the local anesthetic solution is slowly deposited.
4. The lingual nerve can be anesthetized by depositing a small amount of the anesthetic solution as the needle is being withdrawn.

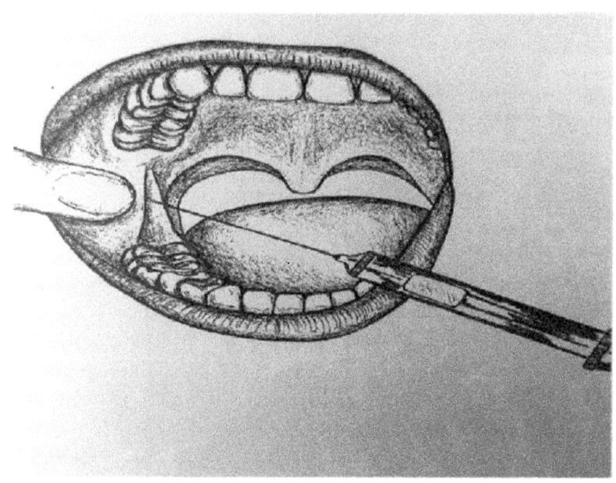

Figure 21.4 Halstead technique method 1. *Source:* Ogle O, 2001/With permission of Elsevier.

5. The buccal nerve will not be anesthetized by this technique. It will require a few drops of the solution to be placed over the external oblique ridge in the vicinity of the third molar about 5–7 mm above the occlusal plane.

Technique 2 (Figure 21.5)

1. The patient's mouth is opened to the maximum. Use the middle finger and thumb to determine the width of the ramus in its anterior–posterior dimension. The mandibular foramen lies in the middle of the ramus in this dimension.
2. The index figure of the noninjecting hand is placed on the occlusal surface of the last molar with the nail facing upward [6].
3. The barrel of the syringe is placed over the ipsilateral lateral incisor and the penetration is made right above the nail of the index finger. The needle should first touch the internal oblique ridge, and then be advanced along the medial aspect of the ramus to a point located in the mid ramus or about 14–15 mm beyond the internal ridge. The average width of the ramus, including the thickness of the soft tissue, is approximately 35 mm [13]. The average "long" dental needle is about 32 mm, so advancing it about half the length should be close to the lingual.
4. After aspiration, the local anesthetic is slowly deposited. As in technique 1, the lingual and buccal nerves are anesthetized in a similar fashion.

Akinosi Technique (Figure 21.6)

This technique uses a more superior injection level and anesthetizes the inferior alveolar, lingual, and buccal nerves by a single injection. It is useful in patients with limited jaw opening, particularly those with trismus from infection and in fearful individuals who will not fully open their mouth for administration of traditional block techniques [6].

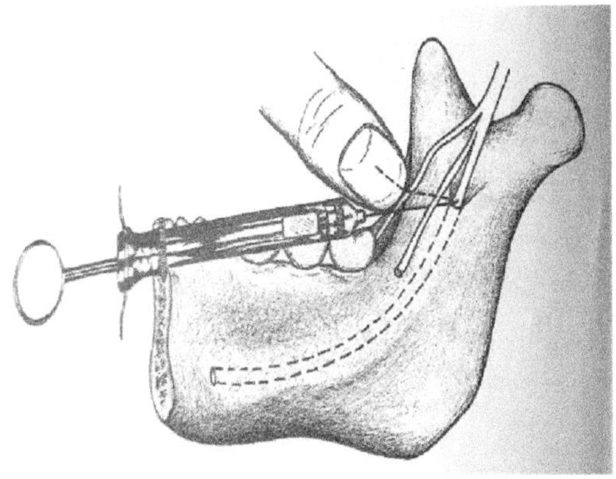

Figure 21.5 Halstead technique method 2. *Source:* Ogle O, 2001/With permission of Elsevier.

1. Technique The injection is given with the mouth closed. The thumb of the noninjecting hand is used to reflect the cheek laterally and to identify the coronoid process.
2. Place the syringe parallel to the occlusal plane at the level of the mucogingival junction adjacent to the maxillary third molar. The needle is aligned with the mucogingival line of the upper third molar and penetrates the mucosa just medial to the ramus. It is very important that as the needle advances, it stays close to the medial aspect of the ramus. A more medial course may place the needle medial to the sphenomandibular ligament and result in failure.
3. Advance the needle about 25 mm or a bit more than three-quarters of the needle. Aspirate and deposit the solution. It should be noted that with this technique, the posterior portion of the mouth will become anesthetized before the anterior. The classic sign of tingling of the lower lip will be delayed.

Gow-Gates Technique (Figure 21.7)

This technique uses external landmarks that direct the needle to a higher puncture point. One landmark is a line

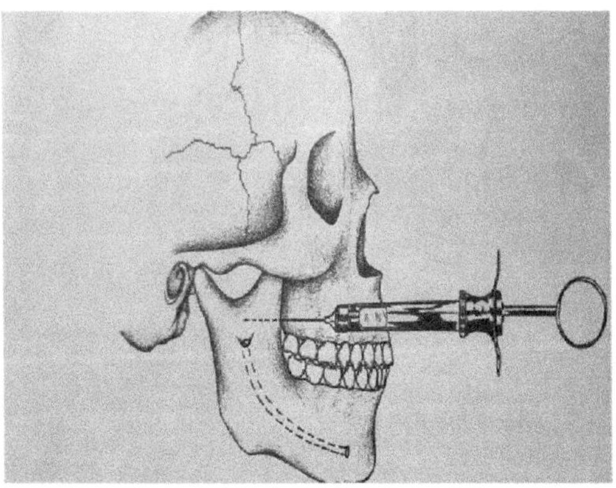

Figure 21.6 Akinosi technique. *Source:* Ogle O, 2001/With permission of Elsevier.

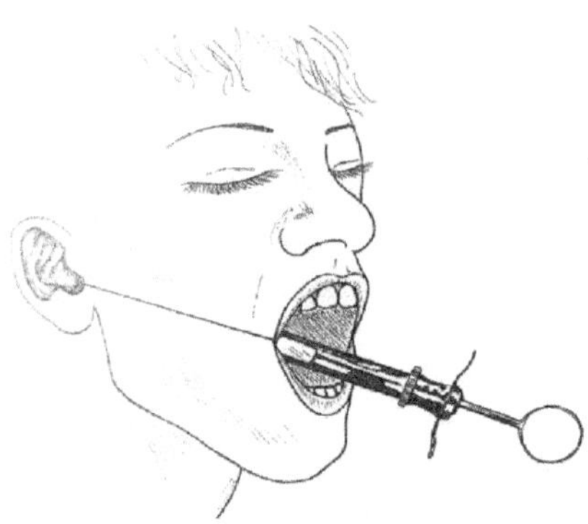

Figure 21.7 Gow-Gates technique. *Source:* Ogle O, 2001/With permission of Elsevier.

and the other a point. The following two extraoral landmarks are used.

- A line that identifies the desired direction for aiming the syringe. This line is from the lower border of the tragal notch of the ear to the commissure of the lips.
- A point that identifies the landmark to which the needle is directed. This point is 5 mm anterior to the tragus of the ear.

1. Technique The head is placed against the headrest of the chair with the chin elevated so that the commissure–tragal line is almost horizontal.
2. The patient is asked to open the mouth as widely as possible so that the condyle will be more anterior and will be in closer proximity to the mandibular nerve. A rubber bite block should be placed between the molar teeth on the contralateral side to keep the mouth opened and fixed.
3. The anterior border of the ramus is palpated, and the desired puncture point that would allow the syringe to be positioned along the commissure–tragal line is identified. With this alignment, the syringe will usually be over the tip of the canine on the opposite side but may vary to either side depending on the divergence of the ramus.
4. Place the index finger of the noninjecting hand extraorally over the head of the condyle. (The patient can be asked to relieve the biting pressure on the bite block and move the jaw to the injection side to help identify the head of the condyle.) The penetration is made as close as possible to the anterior border of the mandible, staying away from the internal oblique ridge. Aim the needle toward the posterior border of the tragus where the finger is located extraorally and advance it about 25 mm until it touches the bone at the base of the condyle. If it does not touch the bone after 25 mm, it could mean that the needle has been placed too far posteriorly and has entered the sigmoid notch or that the syringe was too far anteriorly and has gone past the medial-posterior portion of the mandible. Once the needle touches bone and it is ascertained that the needle is in the desired position, withdraw 1 mm, aspirate, and inject. The mouth must be kept open for 20–30 seconds after the injection so that the straightened mandibular nerve will be adequately bathed in the anesthetic solution. Simply leaving the bite block in place for the 20–30 seconds will achieve this goal.

Complications of mandibular nerve block are detailed in Box 21.4.

Auxilliary/Supplemental Techniques

Auxilliary/supplemental techniques discussed here will not be suitable for the majority of oral surgical procedures but may occasionally be necessary when anesthesia from conventional injections is inadequate and the pain is too severe for the dental procedure to proceed.

There are a few theories as to why nerve block techniques may not provide profound anesthesia.

- The anesthetic solution did not diffuse into the nerve trunk to reach all the nerves to produce an adequate block even if deposited at the correct site [14].
- Preoperative pain is a risk factor for incomplete local anesthesia.
- Altered membrane excitability of peripheral nociceptors from inflamed tissue altering the resting potential and decreasing the excitability threshold [14].

Box 21.4 Reported complications of mandibular nerve block

Idiosyncratic reactions to the local anesthetic
Toxicity – overdose
Syncopy
Trismus
Infection at the injection site
Prolonged pain at the injection site
Neurologic complications
Intravascular injection
Broken needle (see Figure 21.8)
Injection into the parotid gland with facial nerve paralysis
Visual disturbance
Lip biting in children

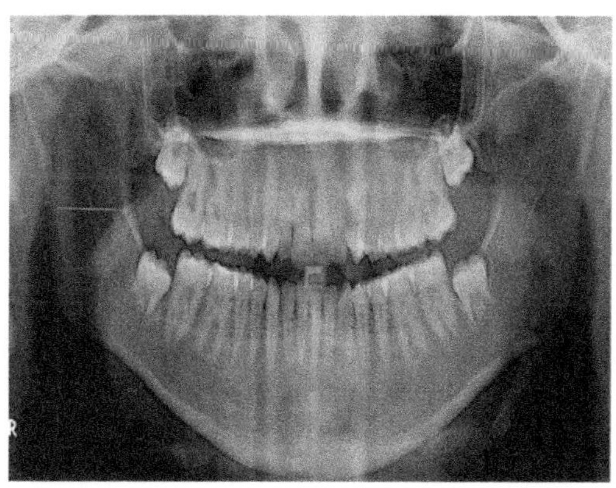

Figure 21.8 Broken needle while performing inferior alveolar nerve block.

- Tetrodotoxin-resistant channels (TTXr) sodium channels are resistant to the action of local anesthesia. TTXr channels represent a mechanism for local anesthetic failures. These channels are relatively resistant to lidocaine and are expressed only by small-diameter sensory neurons in adult dorsal root and trigeminal ganglia [15]. Increased sensitization may amplify incoming signals from sensory nerves. Under conditions of central sensitization, there is an exaggerated response to peripheral stimuli and under these conditions the inferior alveolar nerve block may permit for sufficient signaling to occur to lead to the perception of pain. Thus the central sensitization may contribute to local anesthetic failures [14].

Supplemental anesthetic techniques include injections into the:

- periodontal ligament
- intracrestal, intraseptal, intraosseous
- intrapulpal
- intrasulcular infusion.

Intrasulcular Infusion

Intrasucular infusion, first described by Boyce [16], is the process by which a blunted (not sharp) delivery tip is used to infuse, rather than inject, a variety of anesthetics into the sulcus for minor dental treatment (i.e., scaling and root planing, restorations, etc.), that can be managed without the use of a needle. Intrasulcular infusion can be used as a first-line anesthetic, for the patient who is phobic of needles or children or in deep periodontal pockets. If the patient cannot be managed via the infusions, then the dentist may resort to administering an infiltration or block.

The NumBee® (Novoject) consists of a plastic hub which fits all standard dental syringes attached to a plastic blade that is thinner than most toothpicks, and only needs to be placed into the gingival sulcus (Figures 21.9 and 21.10). A smaller and thinner blade intended for children was recently introduced (see Figure 21.9b). Children and phobic dental patients can appreciate that there is no piercing of any tissue because there is *no sharp tip*. The plastic blade encases a rounded-tip steel cannula which allows the *infusion* of the anesthetic through the blade. At the tip of the NumBee, a small tip achieves a superior seal between the device and the ligament, which in turn makes it easier to deliver the anesthetic under pressure.

Other intrasulcular anesthetic agent include the following.

1. *HurriPAK*™ (Beutilich Pharmaceuticals) is an anesthetic liquid that contains 20% benzocaine which comes in multiple flavors. This product is used with a plastic syringe (3 mL) and disposable periodontal irrigation tips (Figure 21.11). It is marketed as a needle-free periodontal anesthetic kit. The plastic tip is placed deep into the gingival sulcus, while the liquid is *infused* into the gingiva. The onset is 30 seconds and duration is 15 minutes. Fifteen minutes duration will not provide adequate anesthesia for a routine dental visit on an adult patient so multiple administration of the liquid anesthetic may be needed.
2. *Cetacaine*® (Cetylite Industries) is a liquid anesthetic that contains 14% benzocaine, 2% butamben, and 2% tertracaine hydrochloride. It is marketed as a clinical kit that includes liquid bottle, delivery syringes, and microcapillary delivery tips for *infusion* into periodontal pockets. Cetacaine should *never* be injected. It can also be applied topically using a cotton swab or microbrush (Figure 21.12). It is indicated for topical pain control of all accessible mucous membrane, except the eyes.
3. *Oraqix*® (Dentsply Pharmaceutical) has a unique dispenser (Figure 21.13) and is marketed as a periodontal anesthetic, which contains 2.5% lidocaine and 2.5%

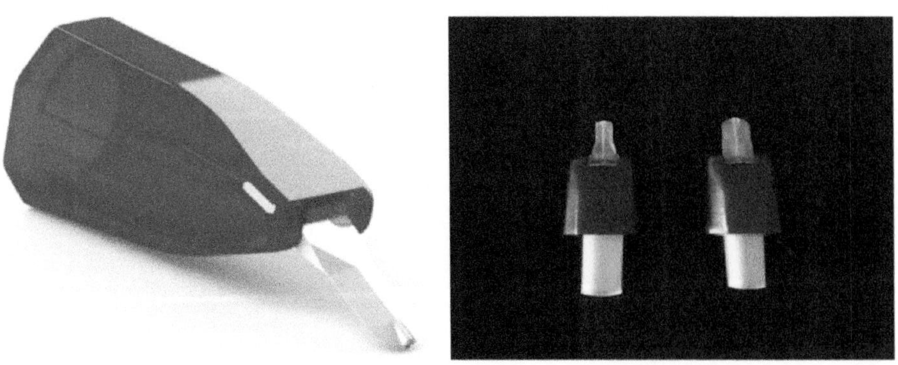

(a) (b)

Figure 21.9 (a) NumBee from Novoject. The Numbee device has the ability to move the plastic blade into different angulations. (b) The smaller thin blade (left) and the regular traditional (right). *Source:* Courtesy of Novoject USA LLC, Austin, TX; with permission.

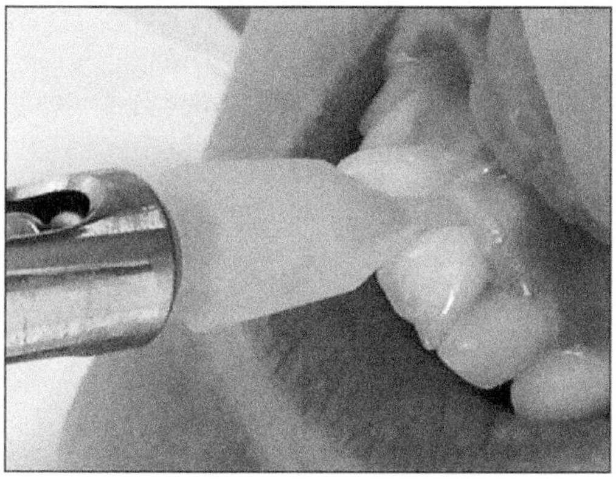

Figure 21.10 Numbee's plastic blade in the gingival sulcus for proper delivery of intrasulcular infiltration. *Source:* Novoject USA LLC, Austin, TX; with permission.

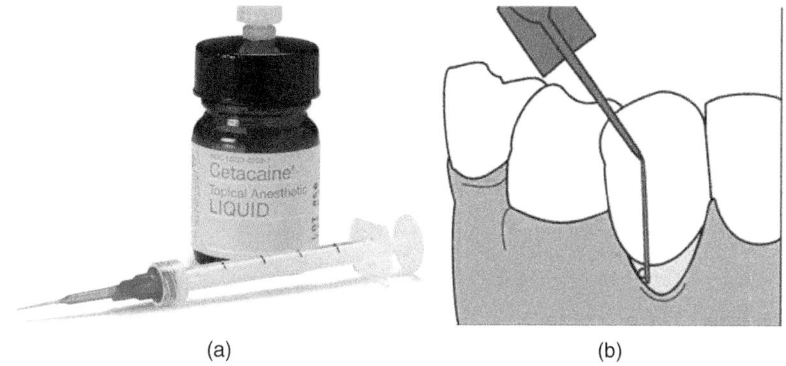

Figure 21.12 Cetacaine contains 14% benzocaine, 2% butamen, and 2% tetracaine HCL. It is indicated for topical pain control of all accessible mucous membranes. It can be applied topically using a microbrush. *Source:* Courtesy of Cetylite Industries, Inc.

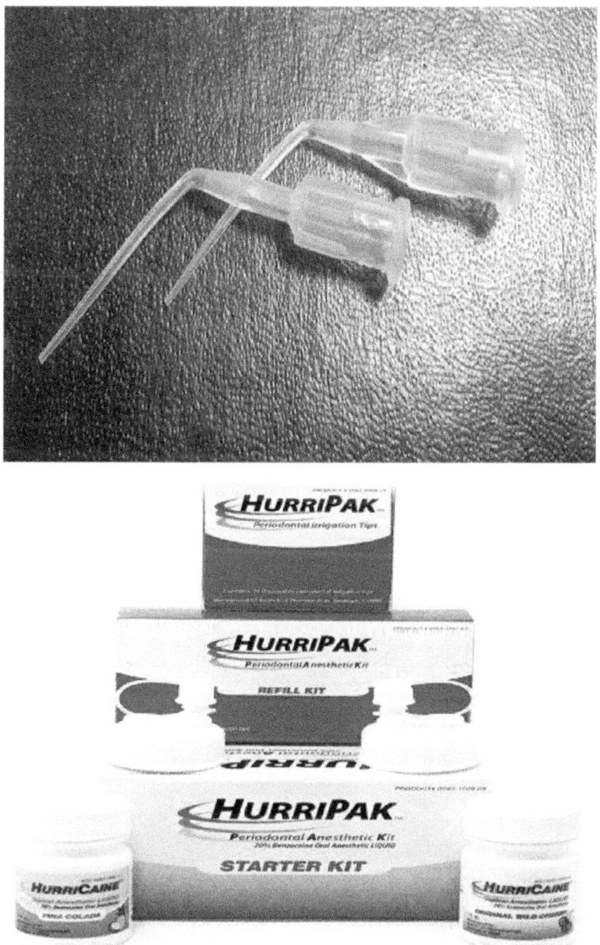

Figure 21.11 The HurriCaine solution of 20% benzocaine as an anesthetic liquid and gel (which comes in multiple flavors) along with a plastic syringe (3 mL) and intrasulcular tip for use with the syringe. *Source:* Courtesy of Beutlich Pharmaceuticals, LLC, Waukegan, IL.

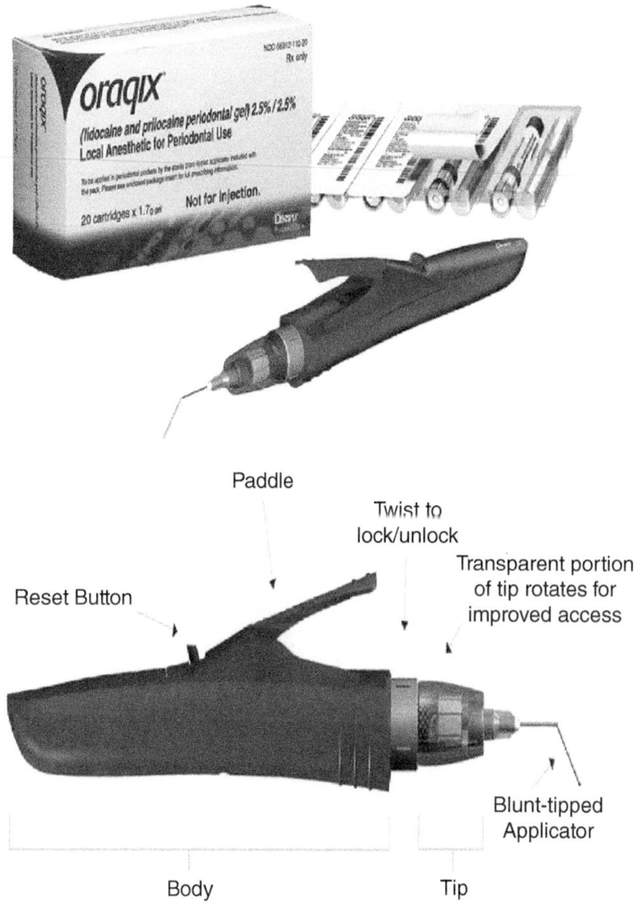

Figure 21.13 Oraqix contains 2.5% lidocaine and 2.5% prilocaine. It comes with a unique dispenser.

prilocaine. Inside the package are 20 cartridges and "blunted" tips to be assembled by the clinician. Oraqix should *not* be injected, instead, it should be *infused* into periodontal pockets during scaling and root planing. It is contraindicated in patients with a known allergy or hypersensitivity to amide-type LA. Oraqix should *not* be used in patients with known deficiency of glucose-6-phosphate dehydrogenase (G6PD) or methemoglobinemia (congenital, idiopathic). Clinicians should be very cautious when using Oraqix in combination with other local anesthetics.

Intraosseous Injection

Intraosseous injection is when a local anesthetic is deposited in bone between two teeth via a guide sleeve and needle (27 gauge) [17]. The brand names that are popular in North America are Stabident and X-tip® (Figure 21.14 shows the X-Tip by Dentsply). Both systems have specific manufacturer instructions that should be reviewed prior to using the device. This technique is perfect for the classic "hot tooth" when attempting to carry out root canal therapy.

The injection site should be at least 2–4 mm apical to the crest of the alveolar bone and a good bitewing and periapical radiograph should be used to evaluate the area of planned injection to prevent perforation or injury to adjacent root structures. The cortical plate should be perforated with the drill (X-tip) or perforator (Stabident), distal to the tooth to be anesthetized, taking care to avoid injury to root structure. The guide sleeve is removed at the end of the endodontic procedure.

Trigger Point Injections

Myofascial pain is sometimes associated with trigger point pain. Trigger point pain can be defined as any cutaneous or muscular areas that, when stimulated, causes an acute neuralgic or referred musculoskeletal pain [16, 18]. The common presentation of myofascial trigger point pain is that it is steady, deep and painful. It is almost never

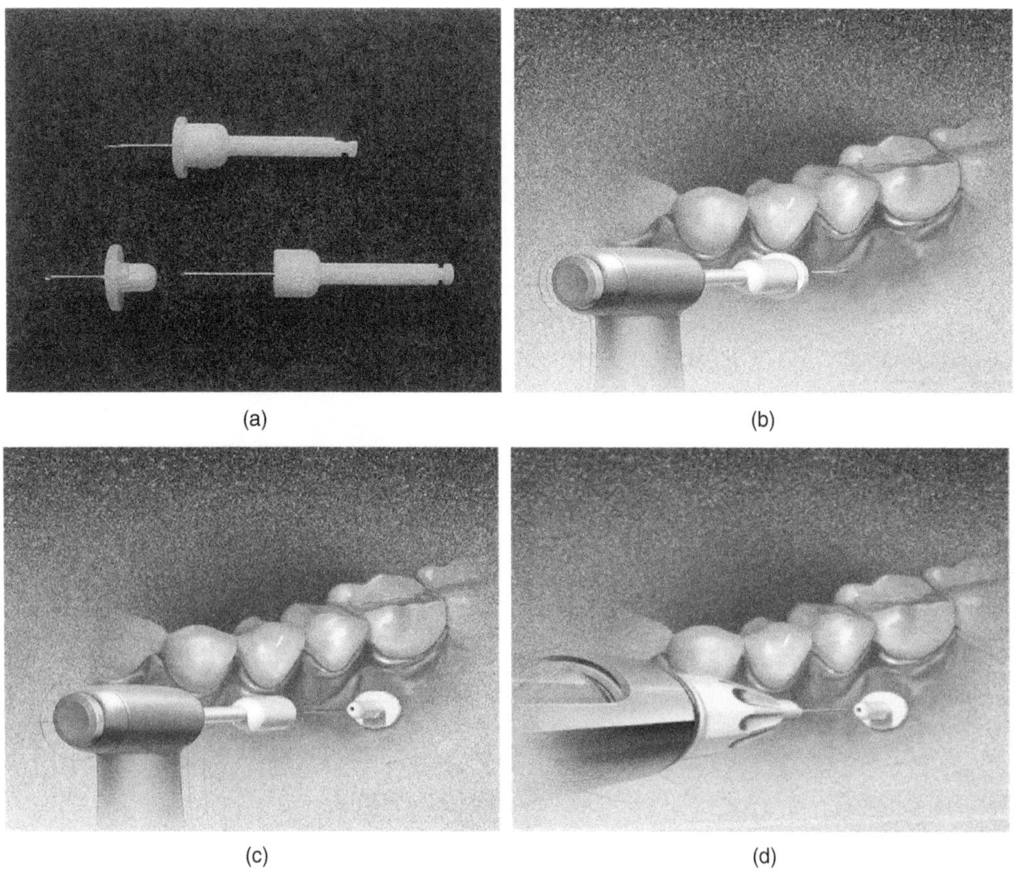

(a) (b) (c) (d)

Figure 21.14 (a) Perforator for penetrating the buccal cortical plate. The image shows the ability to separate the drill and guide sleeve prior to administration of the local anesthetic. (b) Step 1: The drill and handpiece in position to drill distal to tooth #20, while making sure not to perforate the root surface of the adjacent tooth. (c) Step 2: Note the careful separation of the drill and guide sleeve. (d) Step 3: The guide sleeve (white) is left in place for insertion and administration of LA. *Source:* Courtesy of Dentsply Maillefer, Ballaigues, Switzerland; with permission.

present as a burning sensation. Some factors that may trigger the pain are heavy activity of the muscle (usually temporalis or masseter), pressure being applied at the trigger point, and emotional stress. Successful discovery of the trigger point on palpation will elicit a high level of sensitivity [19].

When persistent trigger points are resistant to coolants and stretching manipulations, they should be treated with direct injections. Trigger point injections should only be used, however, after other modalities have failed to achieve a lasting effect. Trigger point injections usually involve injecting dilute solutions of vasoconstrictor-free anesthetic into the trigger point [19]. The choice of local anesthetic is 2% lidocaine (without vasoconstrictor), which is favored due to its low toxicity into the muscle. If properly administered, the injection(s) will decrease or eliminate the pain associated with the trigger point area, as well as any referred pain [19, 20].

This technique, which involves the injection of a local anesthetic into the muscle causing the pain, will not be the end result of treatment. In fact, patients often times need multimodal therapy (i.e., NSAIDs, night guard, muscle relaxants, physical therapy, and acupuncture) in order to alleviate the trigger point.

Nasal Spray

There is an agent that can provide needle-free pulpal anesthesia for restorative treatment on teeth #5–12 via nasal spray. Kovanaze™ (St Renatus) (Figure 21.15) is a nasally administered local anesthetic, containing tetracaine HCL and oxymetazoline HCL. Tetracaine is an ester-type local anesthetic and oxymetazoline is a vasoconstrictor, the same active ingredient as in nasal decongestant spray. While there is 96% efficacy in the treatment of teeth #5–12, the US Food and Drug Administration has approved it for the treatment of teeth between #4–1 (permanent teeth) to tooth # 3 and A-J (deciduous). The child must weigh >40 lbs. There are too few studies to inform any risks in pregnant women but tetracaine by itself is contraindicated in the gravid patient and maybe this agent should not be used. The side-effects include runny nose (52%), nasal congestion (32%), nasal discomfort (26%), and watery eyes (23%).

The clinician should thoroughly review the precautions and warnings from the manufacturers in patients with hypertension, thyroid disease, methemoglobinemia, dysphagia, and a history of epistaxis. The allergic reactions associated with Kovanaze are characterized by urticaria, angioedema, bronchospasm, and shock. If an allergic reaction occurs, the manufacturers recommend seeking emergency help immediately.

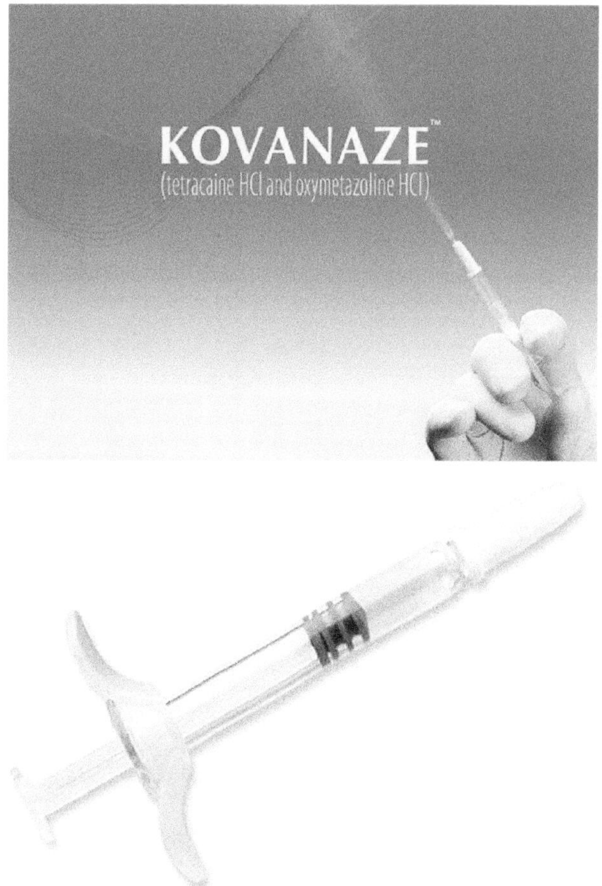

Figure 21.15 Kovanaze (tetracaine HCL and oxymetazoline HCL). A nasally administered local anesthetic, used for restorative treatment on teeth #5–12. *Source:* Courtesy of St Renatus, LLC, Fort Collins, CO.

Reversal of Local Anesthesia

Phentolamine mesylate (PM) (OraVerse™, Septodont) (Figure 21.16) functions to antagonize the vasoconstrictor effect of sympathomimetic amines and reverse or decrease prolonged anesthesia in a patient who is at risk for soft tissue injury. The manufacturers *do not* recommend PM in children under 6 years old or weighing less than 15 kg (33 lb) and its dosage is dependent on the number of cartridges administered [21]. The clinician will administer PM in the same quadrant/working area of the initial LA given [22]. PM can minimize lip biting or cheek biting which occurs commonly in pediatric, physically disabled, or mentally disabled patients. It can also be used to benefit that patient who may have a speaking engagement or needs to return to work without the feeling of "numbness."

Some basic guidelines for the safe use of local anesthetics are outlined in Box 21.5.

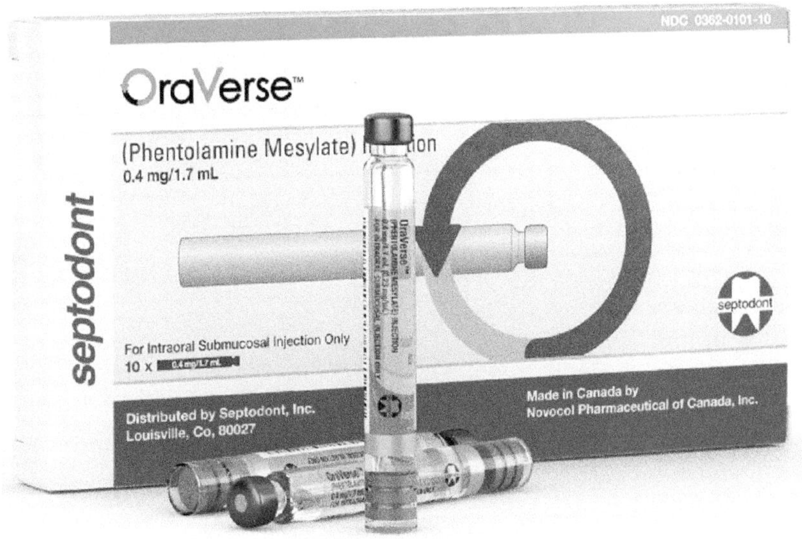

Figure 21.16 Phentolamine mesylate (OraVerse) is used to reverse prolonged anesthesia in patients who are prone to lip or cheek biting (i.e., pediatric, physically or mentally disabled patients).

Box 21.5 Take-home points regarding the use of local anesthetics

- Objectively test the treatment tooth for profound pulpal anesthesia after administering LA.
- Local anesthetics are absorbed into the cardiovascular system.
- Be aware of the *low safety margin* in children that can lead to LA overdose.
- The first signs and/or symptoms of LA overdose include drowsiness which can lead to loss of consciousness and respiratory arrest.
- Avoid epinephrine in patients with angina and those within 6 months of an acute MI.
- Minimize the use of epinephrine in patients with hyperthyroidism.
- Minimize the use of epinephrine in patients on tricyclic antidepressants.
- Minimize the use of epinephrine in patients taking nonselective beta-adrenoreceptor blockers, cocaine, and alpha-adrenergic blockers [23].
- Articaine should not be used for inferior alveolar nerve block.
- Local anesthesia should not be administered to a patient with <50 000 platelets, unless replacement therapy has been planned.
- Always consider the use of supplemental or auxilliary techniques.
- When the intraosseous technique is used, always remember to remove the guide sleeve prior to dismissal of the patient.
- Bupivacaine can be given for postoperative pain management and patient comfort.
- Bupivacaine should not be given to children and special needs patients, in order to avoid trauma from lip/cheek biting.

References

1 Calthorpe, N. (2004). The history of spinal needles: getting to the point. *Anaesthesia* 59 (12): 1155–1275.

2 Goerig, M., Bacon, D., and van Zundert, A. (2012). Carl Koller, cocaine, and local anesthesia: some less known and forgotten facts. *Reg. Anesth. Pain Med.* 37 (3): 318–324.

3 Prichard D. A Brief History of Dental Anesthesia. Spear Education. www.speareducation.com/spear-review/2013/08/a-brief-history-of-dental-anesthesia.

4 Covino, B.G. and Vassallo, H.G. (1976). *Local Anesthetics: Mechanism of Action and Clinical Use*. New York: Grune & Stratton.

5 Local anesthetics. https://emedicine.medscape.com/article/873879-overview#a3.

6 Ogle, O. (2001). Local anesthesia. In: *Atlas of Minor Oral Surgery* (ed. H. Dym and O. Ogle), 30–40. Philadelphia, PA: WB Saunders.

7 Ogle, O. (2001). Regional surgical anatomy. In: *Atlas of Minor Oral Surgery* (ed. H. Dym and O. Ogle), 22–29. Philadelphia, PA: WB Saunders.

8 Das, S., Kim, D., Cannon, T.Y. et al. (2006). High-resolution computed tomography analysis of the greater palatine canal. *Am. J. Rhinol.* 20 (6): 603–608.

9 (1947). *Manual of Local Anesthesia in General Dentistry*, p12. New York: Cook-Waite Laboratories.

10 Douglas, R. and Wormald, P.J. (2006). Pterygopalatine fossa infiltration through the greater palatine foramen: where to bend the needle. *Laryngoscope* 116 (7): 1255–1257.

11 Malamed, S.F. (2013). Techniques of mandibular anesthesia. In: *Handbook of Local Anesthesia*, 6e. St Louis, MO: Mosby.

12 Kaufman, E., Weinstein, P., and Milgrom, P. (1984). Difficulties in achieving local anesthesia. *J. Am. Dent. Assoc.* 108 (2): 205–208.

13 Gaum, L.I. and Moon, A.C. (1997). The "ART" mandibular nerve block: a new approach to accomplishing regional anesthesia. *J. Can. Dent. Assoc.* 63 (6): 454–459.

14 Boopathi, T., Sebeena, M., and Sivakumar, K. (2013). Supplemental pulpal anesthesia for mandibular teeth. *J. Pharm. Bioallied Sci.* 5 (Suppl 1): 103–108.

15 Sorensen, H., Skidmore, L., Rzasa, R. et al. (2004). Comparison of pulpal sodium channel density in normal teeth to diseased teeth with severe spontaneous pain. *J. Endod.* 30 (4): 287–291.

16 Boyce, R.A., Kirpalani, T., and Mohan, N. (2016). Updates of topical and local anesthesia agents. *Dent. Clin. North Am.* 60 (2): 445–471.

17 Cassamani, F. (1924). Une nouvelle technique d'anesthesia intraligamentarie: la seringue. PhD thesis. PERI Press, Paris.

18 Unverzagt, C., Berglund, K., and Thomas, J.J. (2015). Dry needling for myofascial trigger point pain: a clinical CommentarY. *Int. J. Sports Phys. Ther.* 10 (3): 402–418.

19 Ogle, O. and Hertz, M. (2000). Myofascial pain. *Oral Maxillofac. Clin. North Am.* 12 (2): 217–231.

20 Travell, J.G. and Simons, D.G. (1983). *Myofascial Pain and Dysfunction: The Trigger Point Manual*, 63–158. Baltimore, MD: Williams and Wilkins.

21 (2015). *OraVerse Prescribing Information*. San Diego, CA: Novalar Pharmaceuticals.

22 Frutos, J.C., Rojo, R., Gonzalez-Serrano, J. et al. (2015). Phentolamine mesylate to reverse oral soft-tissue local anesthesia: a systematic review and meta-analysis. *J. Am. Dent. Assoc.* 146 (10): 751–759.

23 Moore, P.A. and Hersh, E.V. (2010). Local anesthetics: pharmacology and toxicity. *Dent. Clin. North Am.* 54 (4): 587–599.

22

Nitrous Oxide

Lester Woo, DDS

History

Nitrous oxide is colorless nonflammable gas, with a slightly sweet odor and taste. Joseph Priestley has been credited with the discovery of oxygen and nitrous oxide gas in 1772. In 1799, Sir Humphrey Davy was the first person to inhale nitrous oxide (N_2O) and discover that the experience was very pleasurable and euphoric. He thus used the term "laughing gas" to describe N_2O. Between the years 1800 and 1844, N_2O was mainly used recreationally at social gatherings and sideshows for entertainment. The medical community, however, largely ignored it as an anesthetic. In 1844, Horace Wells, a dentist, discovered the analgesic properties of nitrous oxide when he had it administered to himself during a tooth extraction. When he later recovered from the effects of the gas, Wells could not recall any pain or the details of the procedure [1, 2].

For the next century, nitrous oxide along with ether and chloroform supplied most of the anesthesia for surgery. It has been administered to billions of patients as part of general anesthesia, sedation for diagnostic and therapeutic procedures, obstetrics analgesia, and trauma analgesia. It remains one of the most widely available and widely used anesthetic agents [2].

Properties

Administration of N_2O is simple and painless. It has a rapid onset and a short duration of action, and its effects are analgesic, anxiolytic, and sedative. N_2O is the only inhaled anesthetic that possesses analgesic properties at a subanesthetic concentration [3]. Its euphoric effect is induced by dopamine release and the activation of dopaminergic neurons [4].

Although the mechanism underlying the analgesic action of nitrous oxide is still unclear, there is evidence it involves the interaction between the endogenous opioid system and the descending noradrenergic system. Its noncompetitive inhibition of N-methyl-D-aspartate (NMDA) receptors leads to hypothalamic release of corticotropin-releasing hormone and activation of opioidergic neurons in the periaqueductal gray matter. This N_2O-induced release of endogenous opioids causes disinhibition of brainstem noradrenergic neurons, which release norepinephrine into the spinal cord and inhibit pain signaling [4, 5].

Use and Administration

Although nitrous oxxide is not very potent, it significantly reduces the anesthetic requirements of anesthetic agents required to produce hypnosis. The minimum alveolar concentration (MAC) of nitrous oxide is 104% and it is not used alone to produce general anesthesia. Commonly, nitrous oxide is administered as 50–75% of the anesthetic gas admixture. The concentration of N_2O required to prevent response to command in 50% of patients is 60–70%. A mixture of 70%, N_2O and 30% O_2 alone will render the majority of patients amnestic and provide moderate analgesia [2, 6].

In a study which delivered N_2O via nasal hood to children, there was no difference in the level of sedation or number of adverse events between children administered greater than 50% N_2O and those administered equal to or less than 50% N_2O. However, the incidence of adverse effects was higher when N_2O was administered for more than 15 minutes. In another study carried out at a US dental school, an average patient required 30–40% N_2O to achieve ideal sedation. The study also revealed that some

Oral and Maxillofacial Surgery, Medicine, and Pathology for the Clinician, First Edition. Edited by Harry Dym, Leslie R. Halpern, and Orrett E. Ogle.

patients responded well to lower concentrations of N_2O whereas others required higher concentrations to achieve the same level of sedation. Finally, N_2O at 70% delivered by full facemask has been shown to be more effective than 50% at reducing venipuncture pain in children [2, 7].

Risks and Concerns

One of the more common concerns in the anesthesia literature regarding N_2O is its potential to cause postoperative nausea and vomiting. The effect, which is dose and duration dependent, is less than that related to opioids or volatile anesthetic agents and can be prevented by titration of the gas and administration of antiemetic agents. One large study found that there was no association between preprocedural fasting and emesis in children receiving nitrous oxide [8–10].

Several of the undesired effects of nitrous oxide are caused by its inhibition of methionine synthetase. This enzyme is linked to vitamin B12 metabolism and vitamin B12 is necessary for DNA production and subsequent cellular reproduction. Although generally of limited consequence for the patient who receives a one-time administration for procedural sedation, concern has been expressed regarding the chronic exposure of healthcare workers to N_2O. These adverse effects include bone marrow suppression and central nervous system depression, but there also has been concern that chronic exposure may lead to issues with infertility or increased rates of spontaneous abortion. It has been shown that in high concentration and with long exposure (greater than 24 hours), N_2O has an effect on fetal development in rats [1, 11–13].

Nitrous oxide-induced infertility has not been demonstrated at exposures of 1000 ppm, but there have been reports of infertility in some species at 5000 ppm. These levels exceed the occupational exposure limits for N_2O in both the United States and the United Kingdom by a factor of 5–10. Despite this, two studies in 1992 and 1996 involving the use of questionnaires suggested that high occupational exposure to N_2O may have increased incidence of decreased fertility and abortions, but the evidence was limited. A metaanalysis including 19 studies performed between 1971 and 1995 reported a relative risk of spontaneous abortion with N_2O exposure of 1.48%. However, other studies and surveys have provided conflicting results [2, 11].

In 1995, a worldwide literature search on the topic of biohazards associated with nitrous oxide use was conducted. This research became the impetus for a meeting of interested parties representing dentistry, government, and manufacturing. A result of the September 1995 meeting, sponsored by the American Dental Association's Council of Scientific Affairs and Council of Dental Practice, was the formal position statement that a maximum nitrous oxide exposure limit in parts per million has not been determined. The exposure limits suggested by the National Institute for Occupational Safety and Health (NIOSH) and Occupational Safety and Health Administration (OSHA) are largely based on what concentrations could be achieved in clinical practice with routine use of waste gas scavenging rather than what limits are reasonable. It is likely that the levels usually found in operating rooms and the maximum exposure limits as recommended by NIOSH (less than 25 ppm) have no untoward effect [11, 12].

Currently, there are limited data in the literature to clearly substantiate concerns about the reproductive toxicity of occupational exposure to N_2O at levels below the currently recommended and accepted guidelines. There appears to be no risk associated with brief acute exposures as might occur during anesthesia. However, appropriate scavenging of gases is recommended to ensure that excessive occupational exposure does not occur. Proper use of scavenging equipment, effective mask fit on the patient, functioning delivery equipment with no leaks, and adequate room venting are several methods used to reduce environmental pollution and exposure to N_2O [2, 11].

Another concern is the abuse of nitrous oxide by healthcare professionals. Nitrous oxide causes euphoria and therefore has a potential for abuse. This abuse is usually not as addictive as some drugs, but nonetheless can cause incapacitation of the affected person. When chronically abused, nitrous oxide can have serious health consequences, including various neuropathies. This is particularly concerning if resulting loss of tactile sensation interferes with their occupation, i.e., dentists [11].

Contraindications

There are few contraindications for the use of nitrous oxide sedation. Relative contraindications include patients with psychiatric disorders, drug and alcohol abuse, chronic obstructive pulmonary disorder (COPD), pregnancy, and bowel obstruction [11, 12, 14].

When administered alone and in the absence of comorbid diseases, N_2O generally has limited effects on ventilatory and cardiovascular function. The more clinically significant respiratory effect of N_2O on ventilatory function is a dose-dependent depression of the ventilatory response to hypoxemia than to hypercapnia. As little as 0.1 MAC N_2O can depress the hypoxemic drive by 50%. Therefore, should respiratory depression occur, N_2O blunts the body's normal response to hypoxemia more than to hypercarbia. Normally, respiratory drive is directly related to the $PaCO_2$, but patients with chronic respiratory disorders such as COPD rely almost entirely on hypoxemic drive [2, 12, 14].

Absolute contraindications include patients who are unable to use a nasal mask (i.e., nasal obstruction to airflow), recent middle ear surgery, pneumothorax, and patient refusal [15].

Interactions with Other Sedatives

Synergistic respiratory depression has been demonstrated clinically in the pediatric population when N_2O is administered with either oral chloral hydrate or midazolam. In addition to its central ventilatory effects, upper airway obstruction has been reported especially in children with tonsillar hypertrophy. The potential for synergistic effects of N_2O on respiratory function when administered with other sedative agents is further emphasized by reports reviewing the database of the US Food and Drug Administration of adverse sedation events in children. Nitrous oxide when administered with any other sedative agent has been identified as an independent risk factor for adverse events. An additional effect that may impact on ventilatory function is depression of the diaphragmatic strength of contraction [2].

Delivery

The technique for administration of nitrous oxide-oxygen inhalation sedation has changed little in recent decades. One of the most important safety features associated with the technique is the ability of the dentist or dental hygienist to administer to a patient the precise amount of nitrous oxide required to provide the desired level of sedation. This ability to titrate is an important safety feature to minimize side-effects and is necessary to carry out a successful sedation. Unpleasant side-effects, such as nausea, vomiting, and bizarre behavior, are more likely to occur when titration is not performed [11].

In the precooperative pediatric patient (younger than 5 years old), acceptance of the nasal hood is not likely. When a child is screaming or combative, it is difficult to employ inhalation sedation and the practitioner may need to gently restrain the patient and apply the mask. Also, a screaming/crying patient is primarily breathing through their mouth and sedation is less likely to be successful. If this is the case, an acceptable technique is placement of the nasal hood over the mouth of the patient. In this manner, the crying patient will have increased intake of N_2O, which eventually willlead to the patient calming down, at which time the nasal hood is repositioned over the nose and treatment can be commenced. This procedure is repeated as often as needed [11].

In general, a tight seal should be provided to deliver N_2O without entrainment of room air so that the delivered concentration can be close to the set concentration. An effective seal will also minimize environmental contamination and permit effective scavenging of exhaled gases. When N_2O is used for sedation during dental procedures, a nasal hood is commonly used [2].

One of the more commonly discussed respiratory effects of N_2O is diffusion hypoxia. Elimination of nitrous oxide is so rapid that alveolar oxygen and carbon dioxide are diluted. The resulting diffusion hypoxia is prevented by administering 100% oxygen for 5–10 minutes after discontinuing nitrous oxide [2].

Safety Mechanisms

Although the technique of nitrous oxide-oxygen delivery has changed little, during recent decades the inhalation sedation machine has undergone considerable revision. Before the introduction of local anesthetics, nitrous oxide was administered as the sole agent in general anesthesia. This administration of 100% nitrous oxide produced what is called "anoxic anesthesia." It was not until the 1940s, with the introduction of lidocaine hydrochloride, that the need for nitrous oxide as the sole anesthetic disappeared. Since there was a better method of providing pain-free treatment, anoxic delivery of N_2O became a potential liability [11].

The American Dental Association's Council on Dental Materials, Instruments, and Equipment adopted an Acceptance Program for inhalation sedation units that mandated safety features on units being considered for purchase. Safety features on the N_2O delivery systems should include mechanisms to guard against the delivery of a hypoxic mixture, including an in-line FiO_2 monitor, a "fail-safe" device that cuts off N_2O flow if the oxygen supply fails, and a proportioning mechanism to regulate the ratio of the flow rates of the oxygen and nitrous oxide so that no more than 70% N_2O can be delivered. These safety features are mandated for commercial devices delivering N_2O but may not be present on "home-made" devices. In 1997, the American Dental Association published recommendations for responsible maintenance and monitoring of nitrous oxide and its equipment [2].

Today, it is below the standard of care not to have a scavenging nasal hood. The scavenging nasal hood is a double mask made up of an inner mask contained within a slightly larger outer mask. The inner mask receives a fresh supply of nitrous oxide-oxygen through tubing from the delivery unit and delivers gas to the nose of the patient. The outer larger mask connects to slightly smaller tubes that connect with the vacuum system. Exhaled gases are vented into the outer nasal hood and then carried away via vacuum.

Two of the most common causes of nitrous contamination in the office are from patients talking and mouth breathing. The clinician should make talking and interaction with the patient as brief and concise as possible [1].

Monitoring

Nitrous oxide delivered at a concentration <50% with no other sedative or analgesic medication is accepted as a minimal sedation drug by the American Society of Anesthesiologists (ASA) whereas a concentration ≤50% is considered minimal sedation by the American Academy of Pediatrics (AAP). According to the most recent guidelines, children intended to remain in a minimally sedated state require no more than observation and intermittent assessment of their level of sedation. In concentrations >50%, however, the AAP cautions that the likelihood for moderate or deep sedation increases. Children intended to reach a level of moderate sedation require continuous monitoring of oxygen saturation and heart rate and intermittent recording of respiratory rate and arterial blood pressure. Therefore, use of pulse oximetry is not mandated to monitor O_2 saturation in minimal sedation, but it is required for moderate sedation according to the ASA Practice Guidelines for Non-Anesthesiologists [1].

During N_2O/O_2 sedation, it is necessary to continuously monitor the patient. The ASA Task Force, the ADA, and the AAP/AAPD recommend that monitoring the patient should include evaluating level of consciousness, pulmonary ventilation, oxygenation, and circulation/hemodynamics [1].

Regulation

Certification (sedation permit) by the Dental Board is required when conscious (moderate) sedation is intended. Nitrous oxide sedation, however, when used as the sole agent, does not require a special permit from the Dental Board. The ADA, in its guidelines for teaching pain control and sedation to dentists and dental students, states that competency in nitrous oxide sedation can be accomplished at the predoctoral level provided the course fulfills the clinical and didactic requirements (14 hours of didactic and clinical exposure). However, each state may have its own set of regulations. The administration of nitrous oxide-oxygen inhalation sedation by trained dental hygienists is permitted by some state dental boards [1].

References

1. Clark, M. and Brunick, A. *Handbook of Nitrous Oxide and Oxygen Sedation*, 4e. Amsterdam: Elsevier.
2. Tobias, J.D. (2013). Applications of nitrous oxide for procedural sedation in the pediatric population. *Pediatr. Emerg. Care* 29 (2): 245–265.
3. Tomi, K., Mashimo, T., Tashiro, C. et al. (1993). Alterations in pain threshold and psychomotor response associated with subanaesthetic concentrations of inhalation anaesthetics in humans. *Br. J. Anaesth.* 70 (6): 684–686.
4. Pedersen, R.S., Bayat, A., Steen, N.P., and Jacobsson, M.L. (2013). Nitrous oxide provides safe and effective analgesia for minor paediatric procedures – a systematic review. *Dan. Med. J.* 60 (6): A4627.
5. Sawamura, S., Obara, M., Takeda, K. et al. (2003). Corticotropin-releasing factor mediates the antinociceptive action of nitrous oxide in rats. *Anesthesiology* 99 (3): 708–715.
6. Babl, F.E., Oakley, E., Seaman, C. et al. (2008). High-concentration nitrous oxide for procedural sedation in children: adverse events and depth of sedation. *Pediatrics* 121 (3): e528–e532.
7. Zier, J.L., Tarrago, R., and Liu, M. (2010). Level of sedation with nitrous oxide for pediatric medical procedures. *Anesth. Analg.* 110 (5): 1399–1405.
8. Babl, F.E., Puspitadewi, A., Barnett, P. et al. (2005). Preprocedural fasting state and adverse events in children receiving nitrous oxide for procedural sedation and analgesia. *Pediatr. Emerg. Care* 21 (11): 736–743.
9. Fernández-Guisasola, J., Gómez-Arnau, J.I., Cabrera, Y., and del Valle, S.G. (2010). Association between nitrous oxide and the incidence of postoperative nausea and vomiting in adults: a systematic review and meta-analysis. *Anaesthesia* 65 (4): 379–387.
10. Pasarón, R., Burnweit, C., Zerpa, J. et al. (2015). Nitrous oxide procedural sedation in non-fasting pediatric

patients undergoing minor surgery: a 12-year experience with 1,058 patients. *Pediatr. Surg. Int.* 31 (2): 173–180.

11 Malamed, S.F. and Clark, M.S. (2003). Nitrous oxide-oxygen: a new look at a very old technique. *J. Calif. Dent. Assoc.* 31 (5): 397–403. Erratum in: J Calif Dent Assoc. 2003 Jun;31(6):458.

12 Butterworth, J.F.,. M.D.,. W.J. (2013). *Morgan & Mikhail's Clinical Anesthesiology*. New York: McGraw-Hill.

13 Ohara, A., Mashimo, T., Zhang, P. et al. (1997). A comparative study of the antinociceptive action of xenon and nitrous oxide in rats. *Anesth. Analg.* 85 (4): 931–936.

14 Murray, M. (2014). *Faust's Anesthesiology Review*, 4e. St Louis, MO: Elsevier.

15 Krall, B. (2011). *Nitrous Oxide Manual*. Loma Linda, CA: Loma Linda University.

Part VII

Oral Medicine

23

Antibiotic Prophylaxis in Oral and Maxillofacial Surgery: Recent Trends in Therapeutic Applications

David R. Adams and Andrew R. Rahn

Introduction

The prophylactic use of antibiotics in oral and maxillofacial surgery to prevent infection and improve outcomes continues to be studied and debated. The evidence-based data for prescribing practices range from metaanalyses and systematic reviews of multiple randomized controlled trials (RCT) to expert opinions, practice guidelines, and/or experimental laboratory research as depicted in Table 23.1 [1].

In oral and maxillofacial surgery, there is no evidence-based consensus beyond the guidelines developed by the American Heart Association for endocarditis antibiotic prophylaxis in dental and oral and maxillofacial procedures. This chapter is an examination and summarization of the current literature relating to evidence-based antibiotic prophylaxis practices and recommendations in the following clinical categories of oral and maxillofacial surgery.

- Endocarditis and other cardiovascular risks
- Prosthetic joint replacements
- Medically and/or immunologically compromised patients
- Impacted third molars and other extractions
- Orthognathic surgery
- Cleft lip and palate
- Dental implants
- Sinus lift bone grafts
- Facial trauma

Rationale for Antibiotic Prophylaxis

The historical rationale for pretreatment antibiotic prophylaxis is based on the observation that the oral cavity contains a high concentration of potentially pathologic organisms and that certain surgical and dental procedures create a seeding or bacteremia of these organisms into the bloodstream. These circulating organisms can then colonize implanted surgical hardware, grafts, or other areas of traumatized tissue. Several studies have shown that, especially in individuals with periodontal disease, normal activities such as brushing, flossing or even chewing can cause bacteremia [2, 3].

The challenge is to show with a high level of evidence that a given bacteremia as a result of an invasive oral procedure has a significant chance to cause an infection at a distant site and that a prescribed prophylactic antibiotic has a high probability of preventing that infection. Another significant consideration is in certain situations such as endocarditis, as even though the statistical chance for a resulting infection after a bacteremia is very small, the resulting infection can have severe consequences. However, there is no clear evidence to support an association between

Table 23.1 Research Evidence Levels.

Evidence level	Type of research
1a	Metaanalyses and systematic reviews of multiple randomized clinical trials (RCT)
1b	Individual RCTs
2	Quasi-experimental research: cohort studies, low-quality RCTs, outcomes research
3	Case–control studies
4	Case series
5	Expert opinion, practice guidelines, experimental laboratory research

Source: Flynn, Thomas, 2011/With permission of Elsevier.

Oral and Maxillofacial Surgery, Medicine, and Pathology for the Clinician, First Edition. Edited by Harry Dym, Leslie R. Halpern, and Orrett E. Ogle.

bacteremia resulting from dental treatment and the incidence of infective endocarditis.

In oral and maxillofacial surgery, prophylactic administration of oral antibiotics may be indicated in some cases but the data and literature to support their use are often inconsistent. Regarding surgical site infection or alveolar osteitis, many recent studies have demonstrated that neither preoperative nor postoperative prophylactic administration of antibiotics has shown any statistically significant benefit over patients who did not receive antibiotic prophylaxis [4]. For example in the treatment of the immunocompromised patient, prophylactic antibiotics may be indicated as well. Patients with poorly controlled diabetes, chronic steroid users, and patients with immune deficiency diseases (e.g., HIV1) may benefit from preoperative antibiotic prophylaxis before surgical procedures. But as mentioned before, preoperative antibiotic prophylaxis in other patients is not well supported by current literature [5].

Shamo and Shafer characterized several general principles of effective antibiotic prophylaxis in both pediatric and adult patient populations (Tables 23.2 and 23.3) [6, 7].

Many practitioners are faced with the decision to empirically use prophylactic antibiotics rather than consider the risks and benefits of not using them [4]. Many practitioners are concerned about liability issues if an infection does develop when no prophylactic antibiotics were given. The use of antibiotics is widely perceived to be benign but there is a risk of adverse reactions to antibiotic prophylactic administration [8]. Medically and immunologically compromised patients are at increased risk of infection resulting from surgical procedures. While the incidence of adverse reactions for many antibiotics is low, for others there is a risk of significant reactions or even death. Thornhill et al. in a 10-year retrospective study showed the use of clindamycin prophylaxis was associated with significant rates of fatal and nonfatal adverse drug reactions associated with *C. difficile* infections [9].

With the above considerations, however, antibiotic prophylaxis must be considered in cases when the benefits will outweigh the risks. Among the variables which should be considered are: (i) the extent of the infective agent or bacteremia; (ii) species of bacteria; (iii) host susceptibility; (iv) presence of comorbidities; (v) type of implanted devices; (vi) grafts or tissue injury; (vii) antibiotic type; (viii) dosage and timing; (ix) bacteria response to the antibiotic; (x) nature

Table 23.2 Prophylactic Antibiotic Principles.

1) Prophylactic antibiotics should be effective against the organisms most frequently associated with infections seen with particular surgical procedures or anatomic sites
2) The prophylactic antibiotic dosage should be 3–4 times the minimal inhibitory concentration for the predicted potential infection-causing organisms
3) Most antibiotics should be given 60 minutes before incision; if given more than 2 hours before, they are unlikely to be effective. Because of longer administration times, vancomycin and fluoroquinolones are started 2 hours before surgery
4) Effective antibiotic tissue concentrations should be maintained throughout the surgical procedure. If procedures last more than two half-lives of the antibiotic or if there is excessive bleeding, another dose of antibiotic should be given
5) Local patterns of antibiotic resistance should be considered
6) The routine use of broad-spectrum antibiotic prophylaxis should be avoided

Source: Adapted from Shamo R, Shafer D. Prophylatic and perioperative antibiotics. In: Mizukawa M, McKenna S, Vega L (eds) Anesthesia Considerations for Oral and Maxillofacial Surgeons. Quintessence Publishing, Chicago, 2017; pp. 49–62.

Table 23.3 Recommended Dosages for Common Prophylactic Antibiotic Dosages, Half-Life, and Redosing Intervals.

Antibiotic	Recommended dose for adults	Recommended dose for children	Half-life in adults with normal renal function (h)	Recommended redosing interval from beginning of preop dose (h)
Ampicillin-sulbactam	3 g (ampicillin 2 g, sulbactam 1 g)	50 mg/kg of the ampicillin component	0.8–1.3	2
Cefazolin	2 g (3 g for pts weighing ≥120 kg)	30 mg/kg	1.2–2.2	4
Cefurozime	1.5 g	50 mg/kg	1–2	4
Clindamycin	900 mg	10 mg/kg	2–4	6
Metronidazole	500 mg	15 mg/kg (neonates weighing <1200 g should receive a single 7.5 mg/kg dose)	6–8	NA

Source: Adapted from Shamo R, Shafer D. Prophylatic and perioperative antibiotics. In: Mizukawa M, McKenna S, Vega L (eds) Anesthesia Considerations for Oral and Maxillofacial Surgeons. Quintessence Publishing, Chicago, 2017; pp. 49–62.

and extent of surgical procedures [4]. Incorrectly prescribed antibiotics also contribute to the promotion of resistant bacteria. Studies have shown that treatment indication, choice of agent, or duration of antibiotic therapy is incorrect in 30–50% of cases. Incorrectly prescribed antibiotics have questionable therapeutic benefit and expose patients to potential complications of antibiotic therapy [8]. Worldwide, there is continuing emergence of resistant bacteria which is endangering the efficacy of our current antibiotics.

The Problem with Biofilms

Almost all the infections related to oral and maxillofacial surgery are caused by bacteria which are organized into biofilms [4, 10]. Many of these infections begin as planktonic "normal oral flora" that become attached to a surface and develop into a biofilm, which is a complex, highly communicative, and interactive grouping of usually multi-species bacteria surrounded by a polymetric matrix [4, 10]. Biofilm populations adhere to each other and/or to surfaces or interfaces such as bone, endothelial linings, teeth, and inert implanted devices [3, 4]. Treatment of these types of infections with traditional antibiotics alone is ineffective [10]. While free-floating or planktonic bacteria may be susceptible to conventional antibiotics, the bacteria imbedded within biofilms are protected by a physical barrier and by molecular interactions between the different species in the matrix which results in additional resistance to antibiotics. Many of the more deeply imbedded bacteria may be dormant, which makes them especially resistant to antibiotics that are effective only against bacteria in their growth phase [10]. The prevention of infections caused by organisms associated with or imbedded within biofilms is both critical and challenging.

The remainder of this chapter contains the current evidence-based recommendations for oral healthcare providers for antibiotic prophylaxis in the following categories.

Infective Endocarditis

The most recent literature from the American Dental Association and the American Heart Association concludes that: "there are currently relatively few patient subpopulations for whom antibiotic prophylaxis may be indicated prior to certain dental procedures" [11]. This is based on a review of scientific evidence, which showed that the risk of adverse reactions to antibiotics generally outweighs the benefits of prophylaxis for many patients who would have been considered eligible for prophylaxis in previous versions of the guidelines. Concern about the development of drug-resistant bacteria also was a factor. Infective endocarditis prophylaxis for dental procedures should be recommended only for patients with underlying cardiac conditions associated with the highest risk of adverse outcome from infective endocarditis (IE) (Box 23.1) [11].

Dental Procedures for Which Endocarditis Prophylaxis is Recommended

For patients with these underlying cardiac conditions, prophylaxis is recommended for all *dental procedures that involve manipulation of gingival tissue or the periapical region of teeth or perforation of the oral mucosa* (Table 23.4).

The procedures and events that do not need prophylaxis are routine anesthetic injections through noninfected tissue, taking dental radiographs, placement of removable prosthodontic or orthodontic appliances, adjustment of

Box 23.1 American heart association prevention of infective endocarditis

Cardiac conditions associated with the highest risk of adverse outcome from endocarditis for which prophylaxis with dental procedures is recommended:

- Prosthetic cardiac valve
- Previous IE
- Congenital heart disease (CHD)[a]
- Unrepaired cyanotic CHD, including palliative shunts and conduits

Completely repaired congenital heart defect with prosthetic material or device, whether placed by surgery or by catheter intervention, during the first 6 months after the procedure[b]

Repaired CHD with residual defects at the site or adjacent to the site of a prosthetic patch or prosthetic device (which inhibits endothelialization)

Cardiac transplantation recipients who develop cardiac valvulopathy

a) Except for the conditions listed above, antibiotic prophylaxis is no longer recommended for any other form of CHD.

b) Prophylaxis is recommended because endothelialization of prosthetic material occurs within six months after the procedure [12].

Table 23.4 Regimens for Dental Procedure Prophylaxis.

Regimen: single dose 30–60 min before procedure			
Situation	**Agent**	**Adults**	**Children**
Oral	Amoxicillin	2 g	50 mg/kg
Unable to take oral medication	Ampicillin	2 g IM or IV	50 mg/kg IM or IV
	OR		
	Cefazolin or Ceftriaxone	1 g IM or IV	50 mg/kg IM or IV
Allergic to Penicillin or Ampicillin – oral	Cephalexin[a,b]	2 g	50 mg/kg
	OR		
	Doxycycline	100 mg	<45 kg, 2.2 mg/kg, >45 kg, 100 mg
	OR		
	Azithromycin or Clarithromycin	500 mg	15 mg/kg
Allergic to Penicillin or Ampicillin	Cefazolin or Ceftriaxone[b]	1 g IM or IV	50 mg/kg IM or IV
and unable to take oral medication	OR		

IM, intramuscular; IV, intravenous.
[a] Or other first- or second-generation oral cephalosporin in equivalent adult or pediatric dosage.
[b] Cephalosporins should not be used in an individual with a history of anaphylaxis, angioedema, or urticaria with penicillins or ampicillin.
Source: Wilson W et al./Reproduced with permission of Wolters Kluwer Health, Inc.
Clindamycin is no longer recommended for antibiotic prophylaxis for dental procedures.
Source: Adapted from [38].

orthodontic appliances, placement of orthodontic brackets, shedding of deciduous teeth, and bleeding from trauma to the lips or oral mucosa.

Additional Considerations about Infective Endocarditis Antibiotic Prophylaxis (When Indicated)

Wilson et al. discussed a recommendation for patients who forget to premedicate before their appointments. The recommendation is that for patients with an indication for antibiotic prophylaxis, the antibiotic be administered before the procedure in order for it to reach adequate blood levels. However, the guidelines on prevention of IE state: "If the dosage of antibiotic is inadvertently not administered before the procedure, the dosage may be administered up to 2 hours after the procedure" [13]. For a patient with an indication for prophylaxis who appropriately received antibiotic premedication prior to a dental procedure one day and is then scheduled the following day for a dental procedure also warranting premedication (e.g., dental prophylaxis), the antibiotic prophylaxis regimen should be repeated prior to the second appointment.

Another concern that dentists have expressed involves patients who require prophylaxis but are already taking antibiotics for another condition. In these cases, the guidelines for IE recommend that the dentist select an antibiotic from a different class than the one the patient is already taking. For example, if the patient is taking amoxicillin, the dentist should select doxycycline, azithromycin, or clarithromycin for prophylaxis [13, 14].

Prosthetic Joint Replacements

There is no evidence-based consensus on the use of prophylactic antibiotics associated with dental procedures on patients with prosthetic joints. Based on extensive reviews by the American Academy of Orthopedic Surgeons and the American Dental Association in 2012, 2013 and again reviewed in 2015, the recommendations in Box 23.2 were made.

Immunologically Compromised Patients

Patients with compromised immune systems may be at great risk for infections resulting from bacteremia. At-risk patients include those with poorly controlled diabetes, undergoing chemotherapy or with other immunologically suppressed conditions. In these patient groups, if invasive oral surgical procedures are indicated, the surgeon should consider the prophylactic use of antibiotics even though the patient may not normally be considered at risk for IE [4]. In immunocompetent patients, most infections of the oral cavity are localized infections of odontogenic origin caused by bacteria. In severely immunocompromised patients, many of the oral infections are fungal or viral. As reported by Palmason et al., infections in this population can present in an unusual fashion, can spread rapidly to other organs in the body, and are more frequently resistant to therapies [15]. In these patients, such as those undergoing allogeneic hematopoietic cell transplantation (HCT), the risk of infection is not only significantly increased but infections in these patients may present with unusual patterns, resolve slowly despite prolonged and intensive therapy, and in some cases become life-threatening [15].

Box 23.2 Management of patients with prosthetic joints undergoing dental procedures

Clinical recommendation

For most patients with prosthetic joint implants, prophylactic antibiotics are *not* required prior to dental procedures to prevent prosthetic joint infection.

For patients with a history of complications associated with their joint replacement surgery who are undergoing dental procedures that include gingival manipulation or mucosal incision, prophylactic antibiotics should only be considered after consultation with the patient and orthopedic surgeon. The orthopedic surgeon should recommend and write the prescription for the antibiotic regimen deemed necessary. To assess a patient's medical status, a complete health history is always recommended when making final decisions regarding the need for antibiotic prophylaxis.

Clinical reasoning for the recommendation

1. There is evidence that dental procedures are not associated with prosthetic joint implant infections.
2. There is evidence that antibiotics provided before oral care do not prevent prosthetic joint implant infections.
3. There are potential harms of antibiotics, including risk for anaphylaxis, antibiotic resistance, and opportunistic infections like *Clostridium difficile*.
4. The benefits of antibiotic prophylaxis may not exceed the harms for most patients.
5. The individual patient's circumstances and preferences should be considered when deciding whether to prescribe prophylactic antibiotics prior to dental procedures.

Source: AAOMS, 2017/American Association of Oral and Maxillofacial Surgeons.

In patients preparing to have HCT (or other organ transplants), the following recommendation is made (Table 23.5):

"When feasible, the most effective approach to management of oral infections is prevention. With respect to odontogenic infections and risk of bacteremia in patients undergoing HCT, all potential oral sources of infection should be eliminated before the initiation of conditioning therapy. This requires a comprehensive pre-HCT oral evaluation that can efficiently and conveniently be completed off-site by a patient's local dentist who is guided by detailed written instructions from the oncology (or other treating service) service. Treatment ideally should be completed at least 2 weeks before admission for HCT" [15].

Systemic Prophylactic Agents for Immunocompromised Patients

In 2009 the American Society for Blood and Marrow Transplantation reported thorough guidelines on the prevention of infectious complications in HCT recipients.

Third Molars/Extractions

There is no consensus statement to date that supports the perioperative use of antibiotic prophylaxis for third molar extractions. The evidence regarding this subject is often conflicting, and for this reason it is particularly important to know the data supporting your clinical decision. There are many clinical trials that are readily available to the surgeon. These individual clinical trials are great examples of how separate studies – each carried out in a double-blind, randomized fashion, with appropriate exclusion criteria and similar evaluation parameters – can have different outcomes. Table 23.6 summarizes the results of several of these randomized clinical trials as well as two comprehensive systematic reviews and metaanalyses.

Many studies have returned contradictory data on this topic over the past decades. However, there has been such an immense amount of research conducted on this single topic that a general consensus can be reached. Antibiotics are effective in reducing infection, but third molar extraction in an otherwise healthy patient population does not present with enough postoperative infections and dry socket to warrant prescription of antibiotics to every patient.

The effectiveness of prophylactic antibiotics seems to rely on administration before incision, so that adequate systemic concentrations are achieved before inoculation of the wound and bloodstream with microorganisms. In procedures that seem particularly contaminated or difficult, or in patients susceptible to infection, antibiotics may be the prudent and wise choice.

Orthognathic Surgery

It is a widely accepted practice to prescribe antibiotics to reduce the incidence of postoperative infections before and after orthognathic surgery. A search of the primary and composite data, however, reveals a general lack of consensus in antibiotic administration along with contradictions of data and results (Table 23.7). The latter is attributed to the overall research sample size relating to orthognathic surgery. In addition, there is no consensus on the timing,

Table 23.5 Prophylactic Antimicrobial Agents for Patients Undergoing Hematopoietic Cell Transplantation (HCT).

First line			Alternative	
Antibacterial agents[a]				
Levofloxacin		500 mg PO qd		
			Azithromycin	250 mg qd
Ciprofloxacin		500 mg PO qd		
Antiviral agents				
HSV[b]	Aciclovir	400-800 mg PO bid	Valaciclovir	500 mg PO bid
VZV[c]	VZV Ig (postexposure)	5 vials (125 units each)	Valaciclovir[d]	1 g PO tid
	Aciclovir (reactivation)	800 mg BID for 1 year	Valaciclovir	500 mg PO bid for 1 year
	Monitoring			
	CMV-DNA Polymerase chain reaction			
	CMV pp65 antigenemia			
	Preemptive treatment			
	CMV[e]	Ganciclovir (prophylaxis)	5 mg/kg/dose IV bid For 7–14 days then qd until indicator test is negative	Foscarnet (cidofovir or valganciclovir can be used if necessary)
Antifungal agents[f]				
Fluconazole		400 mg PO qd 400 mg IV qd	Fluconazole	200 mg PO/IV qd
			Itraconazole	200 mg oral solution bid
			Micafungin	50 mg IV qd
			Voriconazole	4 mg/kg IV bid or 200 mg PO bid
			Posaconazole	200 mg PO tid

a) Adults anticipated to be neutropenic for 7 days or more, started at day 0 and continued until recovery from neutropenia.
b) Starting from the beginning of conditioning therapy and continued until engraftment or until mucositis resolves.
c) If exposed to varicella or zoster then postexposure prophylaxis should be initiated if the patient is not more than 2 years out of transplant or if they are on immunosuppressive therapy or have chronic GVHD. If a patient receiving conditioning therapy is exposed to a vaccinee who has developed signs of primary disease, they should receive postexposure prophylaxis. If the patient has signs or symptoms of reactivation then initiate prophylaxis of disease reactivation.
d) Day 3–22 after exposure.
e) Prophylaxis or preemptive strategies can be used. In preemptive strategy, treatment is initiated if monitoring tests are positive for CMV. These strategies can be combined in seropositive patients receiving cord blood transplant. Prophylaxis strategy is generally used in seronegative recipients independent of donor status. In addition to this, those at increased risk for CMV disease undergo preemptive strategy until immunocompetent but that is beyond the scope of this chapter.
f) From the start of conditioning until engraftment [15]. *Source:* Palmason et al., 2011/With permission of Elsevier.

Table 23.6 Study Outcomes and Conclusions – Third Molars and Extractions.

Main author/year	Study type	Regimen/conclusion
Halpern/2007 [16]	RCT: 118 subjects 59 experimental – 0 infections 59 control – 5 infections	IV abx vs IV saline prior to surgery significantly reduces infections
Arteagoitia/2015 [17]	RCT: 118 subjects 58 experimental – 2 infections 60 control – 5 infections	2 g amox/125 mg clavulanate pre- and postop Routine use not recommended
Arora/2014 [18]	RCT: 48 subjects 24 experimental 24 control	All received preop abx. Postop abx variable. Postop abx not recommended for routine use
Poeschl/2005 [19]	RCT: 288 subjects Three groups	Variable postoperative course No significant difference Routine postoperative abx not justified
Arteagoitia/2016 [20]	Systematic review Metaanalysis	Amoxicillin not significantly effective Amox/clavulanate does significantly reduce the risk of infection Routine use not justified
Ramos/2016 [21]	Systematic review Metaanalysis	Prophylactic use of abx does significantly reduce the risk of infection

abx, antibiotics; IV, intravenous; RCT, randomized controlled trial.

type, use of, and dosing of antibiotic medications because of the diversity of study results and conclusions. Several systematic reviews seemed to provide engaging discussions with well-considered recommendations even if without evidence-based results.

Most studies compared preoperative and perioperative antibiotic prophylaxis with or without continuous postoperative administration. Among the weaknesses of the included studies were incorrect handling of withdrawals and dropouts along with little to no description of inclusion and exclusion criteria. Many of the studies investigating the advantages of antibiotic prophylaxis are of poor quality and are not placebo controlled.

Table 23.7 Current Antibiotic Prophylaxis Recommendations in Orthognathic Surgery.

Main author/year	Study type	Conclusion
Lindeboom/2003 [22]	RCT	Postop abx not supported
Tan/2011 [23]	RCT	Postop abx not significant
Brignardello/2015 [24]	Systematic review	Postop abx supported
Tan/2011 [25]	Systematic review	Postop abx no benefit

abx, antibiotics; RCT, randomized controlled trial.

Two complex systematic reviews were found to have a low to moderate risk of bias [24, 25]. Although both studies concluded that the use of antibiotics in orthognathic surgery was beneficial, Tan et al. concluded that extending antibiotic coverage offered no further benefit and Brignardello-Petersen suggested the opposite. A number of primary studies were searched. Lindeboom et al. [22] found no statistically significant difference between single-dose antibiotics given presurgically compared to the same dose followed by a postoperative administration in sagittal split osteotomies. In the well-designed clinical study done by Tan et al. [23], there was no significant difference in the infection rate in the groups with or without a postoperative intravenous antibiotic regimen.

Based on the available evidence, preoperative antibiotic prophylaxis appears to be effective in reducing the postoperative infection rate in orthognathic surgery. However, there is no evidence for the effectiveness of prescribing additional continuous postoperative antibiotics. More trials with a low risk of bias are needed to produce evidence-based recommendations and establish guidelines.

Cleft lip and palate

There are no consensus evidence-based guidelines about the use of antibiotic prophylaxis in repair of cleft lip and palate. Several fairly large studies have shown that generally, preoperative antibiotics are justified but evidence for

Table 23.8 Cleft lip and palate repair and antibiotic prophylaxis.

Author/year	Study type	Results/conclusions
Chuo/2005 [26]	Retrospective review 91 cultures showing *S. aureus* and B hemolytic strep	Recommend use of prophylactic abx
Aznar/2015 [27]	RCT 518 patients received preop abx Experimental with postop abx Control without postop abx	Postop abx reduced complication rates
Schonmeyr/2015 [28]	Retrospective review 3108 cases received preop abx Experimental with postop abx Control without postop abx	Evidence does not support postop abx
Roode/2017 [29]	Cohort study of microorganisms and complication rates	Supports preop cultures to guide abx selection to reduce complications

abx, antibiotics; RCT, randomized controlled trial.

the use of postoperative antibiotics was mixed (Table 23.8). Preoperative swabs and cultures were recommended to support antibiotic choice decisions [30].

Wound infection in cleft lip and repair can have morbid results, including hemorrhage, fistulas, affected speech, and further surgery. The general consensus is that preoperative antibiotic administration is supported by the literature and postoperative antibiotics may be prudent. Although there is little evidence to support prophylactic antibiotics, the consequences of a wound infection are so catastrophic that surgeons often feel their use is warranted.

Dental Implants

Implant surgery represents an area of oral and maxillofacial surgery in which the patient often expects exceptional outcomes without complications. Treatment planning and management of these cases will greatly reflect on the success of this aspect of oral and maxillofacial surgery – both to the patient and referring dentists. The use of prophylactic antibiotics is widely accepted yet the high-level evidence-based data remains inconclusive.

A literature review by Surapaneni et al. [31] evaluated the data of many studies to determine the indication – or lack thereof – for peri- and postoperative prophylactic antibiotic prescription. Their data showed that prophylactic preoperative antibiotics significantly reduced the failure rate (1.5%) compared with the group receiving no antibiotics (4.0%). The study also summarized similar findings from multiple other studies. The authors concluded that preoperative and/or perioperative prophylactic antibiotics significantly reduce the rate of infection, but that long-term antibiotics >7 days were not indicated.

A 2015 systematic review by Lund et al. [32] explored numerous primary studies and systematic reviews with the goal of providing antibiotic guidelines backed by scientific evidence. After extensive searching and critical elimination, the authors were left with seven systematic reviews and 10 primary studies. After a metaanalysis, the authors determined that the scientific evidence for antibiotic prophylaxis with dental implants is limited. Based on the information retrieved, the authors concluded that prophylactic antibiotics reduce implant failure rate by approximately 2%. With this information, the group recommends against prophylactic antibiotics in the healthy patient and does not expand upon recommendations for more complicated cases.

A Cochrane review completed in 2013 by Esposito et al. [33] also investigated the potential benefit of prophylactic antibiotics. The study looked for an RCT with a minimum 3-month follow-up. Participants included patients undergoing dental implant placement. Interventions included a single antibiotic therapy against a control group, or administration of different antibiotics, different doses, or different durations. The data was filtered similarly to the Lund review, with review authors determining relevance based on title, then abstract, and finally the full articles. A metaanalysis was completed of the remaining studies. The authors of this review feel it is reasonable to prescribe a routine single dose of amoxicillin 2 g before implant placement.

Table 23.9 Current Recommendations for Implant and Bone Grafting Prophylaxis.

Author/year	Study type	Conclusions
Surapaneni/2016 [31]	Systematic review and metaanalysis	Preoperative and/or perioperative antibiotics significantly reduces the infection rate
Lund/2015 [32]	Metaanalysis of seven systematic reviews and 10 primary studies	Recommends against the routine use of prophylactic antibiotics in the healthy patient
Eposito/2013 [33]	Systematic review and metaanalysis	One preoperative dose is supported by the evidence (i.e., amoxicillin 2 g)

Table 23.9 summarizes the results of these three high-quality, comprehensive systematic reviews with metaanalysis. It is apparent that even with comprehensive systematic reviews and metaanalyses, the authors have reached significantly different conclusions. Based on the evidence provided, prophylactic antibiotics reduce the implant failure rate by anywhere from 2% to 4%. It is generally accepted that the benefit of saving 2–4 of every 100 implants placed outweighs the risk of a single prophylactic dose of antibiotic.

Sinus Lift Bone Grafting

Sinus augmentation is both safe and rarely compromised by surgical complications. Schneiderian membrane perforation occurs in approximately 7–44% of procedures. Sinus infection, barrier membrane or graft exposure are less common. A study by Barone et al. [34] aimed to determine the rate of complications and the effect these complications had on treatment. There is little evidence-based data regarding the efficacy of preoperative prophylactic antibiotics. There is also no consensus on the dosage, timing or specific antibiotics used.

In the study, 70 patients with the need for sinus lifting and grafting in the face of maxillary bone atrophy with residual maxillary sinus floor less than 3 mm were selected. The patients were systemically healthy. It should be noted that 21 patients were smokers and 49 were not. A total of 124 maxillary sinus lifts were performed, 16 unilateral and 54 bilateral. The cases were completed under general anesthesia. All patients received 2 g cephalosporin and 8 g dexamethasone preoperatively. It was found that smoking and onlay bone grafting significantly increased the chances of acute infection.

A retrospective study was completed on the effects of membrane perforation on sinus augmentation outcome by Oh et al. [35]. The augmentations were completed using intravenous sedation. The graft material used was a porous hydroxyapatite, which was hydrated with platelet-rich plasma. All patients received 20 mg of dexamethasone and 2 g of ampicillin unless allergies dictated otherwise. A total of 175 sinus augmentations were completed among 128 patients, with 60 perforations and four sinus infections. Three of the four sinus infections occurred in patients with perforations. All infections resolved with culture and sensitivity and appropriate antibiotic treatment. In these 175 sinus augmentations, 438 dental implants were placed and a total of five implants failed. Four of these five implants occurred in perforated sinuses.

There is no research concerned specifically with the most appropriate antibiotic regimen for sinus augmentation. Most data is concerned with the rate of sinus perforation and its effects on sinus augmentation outcome. It is apparent that sinus grafting and implant placement success have a significant inverse correlation with sinus perforation. Given that there is a relatively high rate of perforation, and that these perforations can have serious consequences, a prophylactic or intraoperative dose of antibiotics seems warranted. In addition, should there be a sinus perforation, a course of antibiotics known to cover the oral and nasal flora (i.e., augmentin) should be prescribed.

Trauma

The management of facial fractures is a vital aspect of oral and maxillofacial surgery. It is imperative to know not only when surgical intervention is indicated, but also when antibiotics are necessary. Numerous studies exist in the literature that evaluate not only the timing of antibiotic administration but also which antibiotics to use.

A three-part study by Zix et al. [36] of facial fractures examined the difference between a 5-day and 1-day course of antibiotics on postoperative infections. The study examined orbital floor, mandibular and midface fractures, including both LeFort and zygomatic fractures. The patients' fractures were surgically corrected and followed by a 1-day course of 1.2 g intravenous amoxicillin/

Table 23.10 The Role of Postoperative Prophylactic Antibiotics in the Treatment of Facial Fractures.

Preoperative antibiotics: all patients	
Postoperative antibiotics, first day: all patients – amoxicillin/clavulanate 1.3 g q8h	
Postoperative antibiotics, after first day: experimental group; as above for 4 days; control group; placebo	
Part 1 Orbital fractures: 62 patients	No significant difference in infection rates
Part 2 Mandibular fractures: 59 patients	Postoperative antibiotics not indicated based on findings
Part 3 LeFort and zygomatic fractures: 94 patients	

Source: Based on [36].

clavulanic acid every 8 hours. This was followed with either 625 mg amoxicillin/clavulanic acid or placebo, each administered every 8 hours for the next 4 days. The results are depicted in Table 23.10.

A systematic review and metaanalysis completed by Habib et al. [37] used 13 studies to determine if the timing of antibiotic therapy affected the infection rate. They found that there is no difference between groups receiving preoperative, perioperative or postoperative antibiotics. No reduction was found in infection rates with antibiotics. Previous systematic reviews also failed to show significant reduction in infection rate with antibiotic prophylaxis. The study concludes that growing evidence shows routine postoperative antibiotic prophylaxis is unnecessary in maxillofacial fractures.

When taken together as a cumulative work, it appears that there are a few takeaway points. Perioperative antibiotics are often the gold standard and mandated by hospital policy. Beyond this immediate perioperative dosing, the only fractures that may warrant antibiotic prophylaxis in the pre- and postoperative period are open mandible fractures in the dentate region (Table 23.10).

The surgeon should still assess the likelihood for postinjury and postoperative infection based on common risk factors such as a contaminated injury, BMI >30, diabetes, tobacco use, immunodeficiency, etc. When faced with a setting involving one or more of these factors, the surgeon should consider extended use of antibiotics.

Conclusion

The prophylactic use of antibiotics in oral and maxillofacial surgery remains controversial. For most uses, there is little or no evidence for routine antibiotic prophylaxis based on randomized clinical trials. The use of prophylactic antibiotics is not without potential adverse consequences for the patient. On a global scale, the overuse of antibiotics has created an increasing crisis of resistant organisms. Certainly, there are classes of patients, such as the immunocompromised or those with specific conditions, for which the risk of infection far outweighs the risk of reactions to the antibiotic. When an evidence-based decision is made to give prophylactic antibiotics, their administration should be based on sound principles (see Table 23.2).

References

1 Flynn, T. (2011). What are the antibiotics of choice for odontogenic infections, and how long should the treatment course last? *Oral Maxillofac. Surg. Clin.* 23 (4): 519–536.

2 Forner, L., Larsen, T., Kilian, M. et al. (2006). Incidence of bacteremia after chewing, toothbrushing and scaling in individuals with periodontal inflammation. *J. Clin. Periodontol.* 33: 401–407.

3 Geerts, S.O., Nys, M., De, M.P. et al. (2002). Systemic release of endotoxins induced by gentle mastication: association with periodontitis severity. *J. Periodontol.* 73: 73–78. https://doi.org/10.1902/jop.2002.73.1.73.

4 Hossaini-zadeh, M. (2016). Current concepts of prophylactic antibiotics for dental patients. *Dent. Clin. North Am.* 60 (2): 473–482.

5 Havard, D.B. and Ray, J.M. (2011). How can we as dentists minimize our contribution to the problem of antibiotic resistance? *Oral Maxillofac. Surg. Clin. North Am.* 23: 551–555.

6 Shamo, R. and Shafer, D. (2017). Prophylatic and perioperative antibiotics. In: *Anesthesia Considerations for Oral and Maxillofacial Surgeons* (ed. M. Mizukawa, S. McKenna and L. Vega), 49–62. Chicago, IL: Quintessence Publishing.

7 Bratzler, D.W., Dellinger, E.P., Olson, K.M. et al. (2013). Clinical practice guidelines for antimicrobial prophylaxis in surgery. *Am. J. Health* 70: 195–283.

8 Lee Ventola, C. (2015). The antibiotic resistance crisis: part 1: causes and threats. *Pharm. Ther.* 40 (4): 277–283.

9 Thornhill, M.H., Dayer, M., Prendergast, B. et al. (2015). Incidence and nature of adverse reactions to antibiotics used as endocarditis prophylaxis. *J. Antimicrob. Chemother.* 70 (8): 2382–2388.

10 Ray, J.M. and Triplett, G. (2011). What is the role of biofilms in severe head and neck infections? *Oral Maxillofac. Surg. Clin.* 23 (4): 497–505.

11 American Dental Association (2017). Oral Health Topics. www.ada.org/en/member-center/oral-health-topics/antibiotic-prophylaxis.

12 AAOMS (2017). Parameters of Care. Appendix 4. www.aaoms.org/practice-resources/anesthesia/anesthesia-resources/anesthesia-parameters-of-care.

13 Wilson, W., Taubert, K.A., Gewitz, M., Lockhart, A.D.A. Antibiotic prophylaxis prior to dental procedures. www.ada.org/en/member-center.

14 AAOMS (2017). Parameters of Care. Appendix 5. www.aaoms.org/practice-resources/anesthesia/anesthesia-resources/anesthesia-parameters-of-care.

15 Palmason, S., Marty, F.M., and Treister, N.S. (2011). How do we manage oral infections in allogeneic stem cell transplantation and other severely. immunocompromised patients? *Oral Maxillofac. Surg. Clin.* 23 (4): 579–599.

16 Halpern, L.R. and Dodson, T.B. (2007). Does prophylactic administration of systemic antibiotics prevent postoperative inflammatory complications after third molar surgery? *J. Oral Maxillofac. Surg.* 65 (2): 177–185.

17 Arteagoitia, I., Ramos, E., Santamaria, G. et al. (2015). Amoxicillin/clavulanic acid 2000/125mg to prevent complications due to infection following completely bony-impacted third molar removal: a clinical trial. *Oral Surg Oral Med Oral Pathol Oral Radiol* 119 (1): 8–16.

18 Arora, A., Roychoudhury, A., Bhutia, O. et al. (2014). Antibiotics in third molar extraction; are they really necessary: a non-inferiority randomized controlled trial. *Natl. J. Maxillofac. Surg.* 5 (2): 166–171.

19 Poeschle, P., Eckel, D., and Poeschl, E. (2005). Postoperative prophylactic antibiotic treatment in third molar surgery – a necessity? *J. Oral Maxillofac. Surg.* 62 (1): 3–8.

20 Arteagoitia, M.I., Barbier, L., Santamaría, J. et al. (2016). Efficacy of amoxicillin and amoxicillin/clavulanic acid in the prevention of infection and dry socket after third molar extraction. A systematic review and meta-analysis. *Med. Oral Patol. Oral Cir. Bucal.* 21 (4): e494–e504.

21 Ramos, E., Santamaria, J., Santamaria, G. et al. (2016). Do systemic antibiotics prevent dry socket and infection after third molar extraction? A systematic review and meta-analysis. *Oral Surg. Oral Med. Oral Pathol. Oral Radiol.* 22 (4): 403–425.

22 Lindeboom, J.A., Baas, E.M., and Kroon, F.H. (2003). Prophylactic single-dose administration of 600 mg clindamycin versus 4-time administration of 600 mg clindamycin in orthognathic surgery: a prospective randomized study in bilateral mandibular sagittal ramus osteotomies. *Oral Surg. Oral Med. Oral Pathol. Oral Endod.* 95 (2): 145–149.

23 Tan, S.K., Lo, J., and Zwahlen, R.A. (2011). Are postoperative intravenous antibiotics necessary after bimaxillary orthognathic surgery? A prospective, randomized, double-blinded, placebo-controlled clinical trial. *Int. J. Oral Maxillofac. Surg.* 40 (12): 1363–1368.

24 Brignardello-Petersen, R., Carrasco-Labra, A., Araya, I. et al. (2015). Antibiotic prophylaxis for preventing infectious complications in orthognathic surgery. *Cochrane Database Syst. Rev.* 1: CD010266.

25 Tan, S.K., Lo, J., and Zwahlen, R.A. (2011). Perioperative antibiotic prophylaxis in orthognathic surgery: a systematic review and meta-analysis of clinical trials. *Oral Surg. Oral Med. Oral Pathol. Oral Radiol. Endod.* 112 (1): 19–27.

26 Chuo, C.B. and Timmons, M.J. (2005). The bacteriology of children before primary cleft lip and palate surgery. *Cleft Palate Craniofac. J.* 42 (3): 272–276.

27 Aznar, M.L., Schönmeyr, B., Echaniz, G. et al. (2015). Role of postoperative antimicrobials in cleft palate surgery: prospective, double-blind, randomized, placebo-controlled clinical study in India. *Plast. Reconstr. Surg.* 136 (1): 59e–66e.

28 Schönmeyr, B., Wendby, L., and Campbell, A. (2015). Early surgical complications after primary cleft lip repair: a report of 3108 consecutive cases. *Cleft Palate Craniofac. J.* 52 (6): 706–710.

29 Roode, G.J., Bütow, K.W., and Naidoo, S. (2017). Preoperative evaluation of micro-organisms in non-operated cleft in soft palate: impact on use of antibiotics. *Br. J. Oral Maxillofac. Surg.* 55 (2): 127–131.

30 Smyth, A.G. and Knepil, G.J. (2008). Prophylactic antibiotics and surgery for primary clefts. *Br. J. Oral Maxillofac. Surg.* 46 (2): 107–109.

31 Surapaneni, H., Yalamanchili, P.S., Basha, H. et al. (2016). Antibiotics in dental implants: a review of literature. *J. Pharm. Bioallied Sci.* 8 (Suppl 1): S28–S31.

32 Lund, B., Hultin, M., Tranaeus, S. et al. (2015). Complex systematic review – perioperative antibiotics in conjunction with dental implant placement. *Clin. Oral Implants Res.* 26 (Suppl 11): 1–14.

33 Esposito, M., Grusovin, M.G., and Worthington, H.V. (2013). Interventions for replacing missing teeth: antibiotics at dental implant placement to prevent complications. *Cochrane Database Syst. Rev.* 31 (7): 1–39.

34 Barone, A., Santini, S., Sbordone, L. et al. (2006). A clinical study of the outcomes and complications associated with maxillary sinus augmentation. *Int. J. Oral Maxillofac. Implants* 21 (1): 81–85.

35 Oh, E. and Kraut, R.A. (2011). Effect of sinus membrane perforation on dental implant integration: a retrospective study on 128 patients. *Implant. Dent.* 20 (1): 13–19.

36 Zix, J., Schaller, B., Iizuka, T., and Lieger, O. (2013). The role of postoperative prophylactic antibiotics in the treatment of facial fractures: a randomized, double-blind, placebo-controlled pilot clinical study: part 1: orbital fractures in 62 patients. *Br. J. Oral Maxillofac. Surg.* 51: 329–333.

37 Habib, A.M., Wong, A.D., Schreiner, G.C. et al. (2018, 2019). Postoperative prophylactic antibiotics for facial fractures: a systematic review and meta-analysis. *Laryngoscope* 129 (1): 82–95.

38 Wilson, W., Taubert, K.A., Gewitz, M. et al. (2021). Prevention of Viridans Group Streptococcal Infective Endocarditis: A Scientific Statement from the American Heart Association. *Circulation* 143: e963–e978.

24

Management of Patients on Anticoagulation

Earl Clarkson and Vivian Lim

Introduction

Routine dental procedures are generally low-risk procedures in which there is little chance of adverse outcomes under normal circumstances. For the population of patients with acquired bleeding disorders such as those on anticoagulation, however, careful attention should be given to the assessment of bleeding risk as appropriate dental management can help to avoid catastrophic adverse outcomes.

Anticoagulants, which are agents that hinder the formation of blood clots, are the mainstay of treatment for many thromboembolic disorders, including stroke from atrial fibrillation, deep vein thrombosis, and pulmonary embolism. An estimated 30 million prescriptions are written annually in the United States for the anticoagulant warfarin alone [1]. As all dental providers will no doubt encounter patients in this large subset, this chapter will review anticoagulants and their management concerns in the dental setting.

The general algorithm for managing patients on anticoagulation is to first determine the bleeding risk of the procedure that is planned as that will dictate whether or not anticoagulation will pose a significant risk. Routine dental procedures such as localized periodontal scaling or single tooth extraction are considered low risk and anticoagulation should not be interrupted if the level of anticoagulation is appropriate [2]. As the complexity of the procedure and surgical time increase, so does the potential for hemorrhage. For elective procedures, one might consider staging procedures to decrease risk (i.e., limiting the number of extractions per visit, conservative flap design, etc.). In general, the risk of thromboembolism increases transiently as anticoagulants are discontinued, so careful planning of elective procedures will benefit the patient.

If, however, a significant risk of procedural bleeding remains, careful assessment of the anticoagulant is essential. Anticoagulants fall into three major categories: vitamin K antagonists, heparins, and direct anticoagulants (direct thrombin inhibitors/direct factor Xa inhibitors). The anticoagulant that requires the most attention with regard to outpatient dental procedures is warfarin, a vitamin K antagonist, as it is the most widely prescribed and requires close monitoring. However, newer anticoagulants such as the direct thrombin inhibitors are gaining attention due to their broad therapeutic window.

Vitamin K Antagonists

The management of patients on warfarin is challenging due to the need for frequent monitoring as the dosing can be labile depending on the patient's genetics, diet, acute illness, and drug interactions. Warfarin (Coumadin®, Bristol-Meyers Squibb) blocks the function of the vitamin K epoxide reductase complex in the liver. This inhibits the action of vitamin K-dependent factors II, VII, IX, and X and proteins C and S. The therapeutic window is narrow for warfarin, which requires frequent testing via INR. INR, which stands for international normalized ratio, is used to standardize PT or prothrombin time as this test can vary widely among laboratories [3].

The normal INR for a patient not on anticoagulation ranges from approximately 0.8 to 1.4. In general, the target INR for a patient requiring anticoagulation is 2.5, ranging from 2 to 3, but some conditions such as the presence of an artificial heart valve require a higher target INR of 3 (range 2.5–3.5). Additionally, for post-myocardial infarction (MI) patients with high risk of thromboembolism, low-dose antiplatelet medication in addition to

Oral and Maxillofacial Surgery, Medicine, and Pathology for the Clinician, First Edition. Edited by Harry Dym, Leslie R. Halpern, and Orrett E. Ogle.

warfarin is recommended. These patients on high-intensity anticoagulation have a fivefold greater risk for bleeding compared to those on low-intensity anticoagulation.

As a general rule, anticoagulation should not be discontinued prior to low-risk procedures, such as a simple dental extraction, if the INR on the day of surgery is within the therapeutic range, or less than 3.5. The half-life of warfarin is approximately 36–42 hours and therefore after discontinuing warfarin, it takes approximately 2–3 days for the INR to fall below 2. INR should be measured within 24 hours of surgery or within 72 hours for an INR-stable patient.

If the INR is above 3.5, then low-risk procedures are contraindicated as significant bleeding can occur [2].

The American College of Chest Physicians (ACCP) recommends the perioperative administration of an oral prohemostatic agent (e.g., 5 mL tranexamic acid rinse 5–10 minutes before surgery and 3–4 times daily for the next 1–2 days), which is associated with a low risk (<5%) of a major bleeding event [4].

Discontinuing anticoagulation medication should always be done in conjunction with the patient's primary care provider. When appropriate, warfarin is generally stopped 5 days prior to the intended procedure and the INR is drawn 1 day prior to surgery. If it is still greater than 1.5, then low-dose vitamin K can be administered (1–2 mg). INR is then rechecked on the day of surgery to ensure that it is normal or less than 1.4. Postoperatively, warfarin can usually be restarted 12–24 hours following the procedure as long as the risk of significant postoperative hemorrhage has passed. Since warfarin takes approximately 5–10 days to reach therapeutic levels, patients with high risk of thromboembolism might require bridging therapy in which an anticoagulant with a shorter onset and offset is used perioperatively [5].

Heparins

While heparin is not of much interest in an outpatient setting as it needs to be administered IV or subcutaneously, unfractionated heparin is often indicated as a bridging therapy (in the event that warfarin needs to be stopped) or as an inpatient anticoagulation for thromboembolism, because the onset is immediate. Heparin binds to an enzyme inhibitor, antithrombin III, which inactivates thrombin, factor Xa, and other proteases. Laboratory monitoring of heparin efficacy is through partial thromboplastin time (PTT) and the target is approximately 1.5–2.5 times the pretreatment PTT.

One word of caution is that platelet function should be monitored as well, since heparin-induced thrombocytopenia (HIT) can occur. This is caused by antibodies that activate platelets in the presence of heparin. Type I HIT is a nonimmunologic-mediated response that usually appears within the first 2–3 days after the initiation of heparin treatment. It typically causes a mild and transient thrombocytopenia (rarely <100 000/mm^3), which occurs due to a direct interaction with platelets and heparin that causes clumping and is not associated with an increased risk of thrombosis. HIT type II, however, is associated with an immunologic response and does have an increased risk of thrombosis and can be detected via laboratory testing (heparin-induced platelet aggregation [HIPA] and the serotonin release assay). The treatment is immediate cessation of heparin therapy and monitoring until thrombocytopenia resolves [6].

Prior to major surgery, low molecular weight heparin (enoxaparin) should be discontinued 24 hours in advance and unfractionated heparin can be stopped 4–5 hours before as these agents have a relatively short half-life [2].

Direct Thrombin Inhibitors, Direct Xa Inhibitors

In recent years, newer anticoagulants have gained popularity over direct vitamin K antagonists because of their more predictable anticoagulation. Direct thrombin inhibitors have broad therapeutic windows, allow fixed dosing, and lack interaction with cytochrome P450 enzymes which eliminates the need for frequent monitoring. In fact, laboratory testing does not adequately determine the level of anticoagulation. Dabigatran (Pradaxa®, Boehringer-Ingelheim) is currently the only widely available oral direct thrombin inhibitor, but parenteral drugs in this class are available and include lepirudin, desirudin, bivalirudin, and argratroban. They are currently approved for use in the prevention of venous thromboembolism and stroke in nonvalvular atrial fibrillation.

Direct thrombin inhibitors prevent thrombin from cleaving fibrinogen to fibrin, which is involved in the formation of clots. This effect is exerted on both the soluble and fibrin-bound forms of thrombin. Additionally, thrombin activates factors V, VIII, XI, and XIII, and binds to thrombomodulin and activating protein C [7].

Studies show that the risk of bleeding associated with the direct thrombin inhibitors is similar to that of warfarin. The incidence of major perioperative bleeding was estimated at 4.6% with warfarin, 3.8% with dabigatran 110 mg, and 5.1% with dabigatran 150 mg [8]. Despite the similar risk profile, one area of concern is the lack of reversibility and monitoring for direct thrombin inhibitors. Since these medications do not affect common laboratory test results

(INR, PT, aPTT, or clotting time) and therefore cannot be monitored easily, it is important to preoperatively assess the risk of bleeding associated with surgical procedures and proceed cautiously.

When on direct thrombin inhibitors, the risk of hemorrhage is comparable to anticoagulation with warfarin, with an INR of 2.0–3.0. When the risk of hemorrhage is significant and anticoagulation needs to be discontinued, renal function should be considered as 80% of the drug is excreted unchanged in urine and therefore a patient with reduced creatinine clearance will require a longer drug hiatus prior to surgery [8].

For low risk of bleeding, dabigatran can be held for 24 hours prior to surgery. For high risk of bleeding, it can be held 48–72 hours or longer if renal function is diminished. Postoperatively, due to its fast onset, dabigatran can be restarted once hemostasis is achieved or within 24 hours after low-risk procedures and 48–72 hours if high risk [9].

The direct Xa inhibitors include rivaroxaban (Xarelto®, Janssen Pharmaceuticals), apixaban (Eliquis®, Pfizer), and typically end in "xaban." Direct Xa inhibitors and thrombin inhibitors are grouped together because, unlike other anticoagulants, they antagonize the activity of a single step in coagulation. These agents prevent factor Xa from cleaving prothrombin to thrombin, which is needed to activate platelets and produce fibrin for clot formation. The inhibition of factor Xa is important and provides a robust response because one molecule of factor Xa can cleave approximately 1000 molecules of prothrombin to thrombin. Additionally, factor Xa exists in both circulating and clot-bound forms and direct Xa inhibitors are able to act on both. Similar to the direct thrombin inhibitors, direct Xa inhibitors should be managed in a similar fashion [7].

Rivaroxaban should be discontinued 48 hours in advance of a high-risk procedure and restarted as soon as hemostasis has been achieved (or in 48–72 hours if there is high risk of postoperative bleeding). For lower risk bleeding procedures, rivaroxaban can be stopped as little as 1 day prior if renal function is normal.

Due to limited data currently available on the management of apixaban (Eliquis) in the perioperative period, each case should be managed individually. Apixaban is recommended to be discontinued 2–3 days in advance of a high-risk procedure in those with normal renal function. In low-risk procedures such as dental extractions (excluding multiple tooth extraction), apixaban can be continued [9].

It is important to note that the direct Xa inhibitors lack a reversal agent and therefore local measures are extremely important. For patients who experience minor bleeding, consider local hemostatic measures (suturing, placement of gelatin sponge, and tranexamic acid rinse). In moderate-to-severe bleeding, mechanical compression, fluid replacement, hemodynamic support, oral charcoal (if recent ingestion <2 hours to remove the prodrug from the gastrointestinal tract) or hemodialysis may be appropriate. In situations where there is major life-threatening bleeding, administration of a four-factor prothrombin complex concentrate (PCC) (factors II, VII, IX, X) is recommended [8, 10].

Two classes of medications, antiplatelet agents and nonsteroidal antiinflammatory drugs (NSAIDs), cause alterations in hemostasis and should be mentioned as the former is often taken in conjunction with anticoagulants and the latter is often recommended for postoperative pain control. Although their potential to cause bleeding is generally minor, these medications should be avoided if possible in patients who are already on anticoagulation.

Antiplatelet Agents

Aspirin is often prescribed to prevent cardiovascular disease events and, as noted earlier, is sometimes used in conjunction with warfarin in those patients who are at high risk for thromboembolic events. It is recommended in men to reduce the incidence of MI and in women for ischemic stroke. Aspirin interferes with platelet function as it acts as a platelet cyclooxygenase inhibitor (COX-1 and COX-2) by covalent acetylation. For simple dental procedures, there is no need to discontinue aspirin prior to surgery. However, for more invasive noncardiac surgery, the recommendation is to discontinue aspirin 5–10 days prior to surgery and resume when the risk of major bleeding has resolved.

Nonsteroidal Antiinflammatory Drugs

Nonsteroidal antiinflammatory drugs are frequently recommended for postoperative pain management in the dental setting. They inhibit COX-1, leading to decreased production of thromboxane A2. Thromboxane A2 is released by platelets to aid in platelet aggregation. It is recommended that NSAIDs be avoided for postoperative pain in patients who are on anticoagulants as this can increase the risk of postoperative hemorrhage and gastrointestinal (GI) bleeding [11] (Table 24.1).

Local Hemostatic Measures

Often, for simple procedures, localized tamponade with gauze will be enough to provide hemostasis. Caution should be exercised as even though the patient might be

Table 24.1 Summary of anticoagulant recommendations.

Medications altering hemostasis	Laboratory testing	Clinical management
Anticoagulants Vitamin K antagonists – warfarin (Coumadin)	INR	INR <24 h of procedure, up to 72 h if INR stable For low-risk procedure, INR <3.5 Caution increase of INR with antibiotics (amoxicillin) Reversal with low-dose vitamin K or for rapid INR correction, fresh frozen plasma (FFP) or prothrombin complex concentrates
Unfractionated heparin	PTT CBC (platelet monitoring for HIT) Seratonin assay if HIT suspected	PTT within 1.5–2.5 normal Protamine sulfate for rapid reversal
Direct thrombin inhibitors	None	No reversal agent except for dabigatran (idarucizumab)
Dabigatran (oral; Pradaxa), bivalirudin, lepiruden, agatroban		Low risk: hold 24 h prior High risk: hold 2–3 days prior (consider renal function) Restarting postoperatively: low risk: 24 h high risk: 48–72 h (consider bridging therapy)
Direct Xa inhibitors	None	
Rivaroxaban (Xarelto)		Low risk: hold 24 h prior High risk: hold 2 days prior (consider renal function) Restart after hemostasis is achieved or in 48–72 h for high-risk bleeding
Apixaban (Eliquis)		Low risk: continue preoperatively High risk: hold 1–2 days prior (consider renal function)
Medications disrupting platelet function		
Aspirin	Increases bleeding time, but no effect on PT or PTT	Continue for low-risk surgery, discontinue 5–10 days if high risk Local hemostatic measures Platelet transfusion for uncontrolled bleeding
NSAIDs		Avoid for use as pain control in patients already on anticoagulation

CBC, complete blood count; HIT, heparin-induced thrombocytopenia; INR, international normalized ratio; NSAID, nonsteroidal antiinflammatory drug; PT, prothrombin time; PTT, partial thromboplastin time.

Table 24.2 Summary of local hemostatic agents.

Hemostatic agent	Description	Recommended use	Notes
Gelatin matrix (Gelfoam®, Surgifoam®)	Sterile compressed absorbable gelatin sponge, porcine origin	Mechanical hemostasis, absorbing up to 45× weight of whole blood; use by manually applying to bleeding site with pressure until hemostasis occurs	Completely absorbed in 4–6 weeks, neutral pH
Bone wax	Nonresorbable mixture of beeswax, paraffin, and isopropyl palmitate	Bleeding from within bony vascular channels; inexpensive	Nonresorbable and can inhibit osteogenesis, therefore should not be used in areas where bone regeneration is desired, i.e., future implant site
Microfibrillar collagen (Avitene™)	Made from bovine collagen; promotes platelet adherence and activation	Can be used for extraction and graft sites	Proteolytic resorption in 8 weeks;, limited use if thrombocytopenia
Oxidized cellulose (Surgicel®)	From oxidized wood pulp cellulose; causes red cell lysis and formation of a pseudoclot	Conforms well to surgical sites, acidic pH, antimicrobial	Small amounts absorbed in 8 weeks; larger amounts will take longer; acidic pH delays resorption, additionally should not be used near nerve tissue as acidic pH can cause nerve damage
Topical thrombin	Factor II (thrombin) from bovine origin; initiates cleavage of fibrinogen to fibrin	Indicated for oozing and minor bleeding from small venules	Can be sprayed topically, followed by pressure with damp sponge
Tranexamic acid	Competitively inhibits multiple plasminogen binding sites, decreasing plasmin formation	Multiple formulations as mouthwash and intravenous form	Can be used perioperatively as irrigant, then as mouthwash

hemostatic upon leaving the office, they often have secondary bleeding if the clot is disrupted later in the day during eating, speaking, or unadvised spitting. Local measures are tremendously important and should be undertaken regardless of hemostasis immediately after surgery. The routine use of hemostatic measures will undoubtedly prevent some patients from ending up in the emergency room after a simple tooth extraction due to slow but persistent bleeding following surgery [12] (Table 24.2).

Conclusion

As this chapter covers basic principles for the management of patients on anticoagulation, each clinical situation is different and will require the utmost attention to patient history, appropriate laboratory testing, and sound clinical judgment. If any hiatus in anticoagulation is necessary, it is important to carry this out under the guidance of the patient's primary physician [13].

References

1 Wysowski, D.K., Nourjah, P., and Swartz, L. (2007). Bleeding complications with warfarin use: a prevalent adverse effect resulting in regulatory action. *Arch. Intern. Med.* 167 (13): 1414–1419.

2 Douketis J, Lip, G. (2017). Perioperative management of patients receiving anticoagulants. Www.uptodate.com/contents/perioperative-management-of-patients-receiving-anticoagulants?Search=anticoagulation%20and%20surgery&source=search_result&selectedtitle=1~150&usage_type=default&display_rank=1#H6446132

3 Wigle, P., Bloomfield, H., Tubb, M. et al. (2013). Updated guidelines on outpatient anticoagulation. *Am. Fam. Physician* 87 (8): 556–566.

4 Douketis, J.D., Spyropoulos, A.C., Spencer, F.A. et al. (2012, 2012). Perioperative management of antithrombotic therapy: antithrombotic therapy and prevention of thrombosis, 9th ed: American College of Chest Physicians Evidence-Based Clinical Practice Guidelines. *Chest* 141 (2 Suppl): e326S–e3250S.

5 Cushman, M., Lim, W., and Zakai, N. (2011). Clinical practice guide on anticoagulant dosing and management of anticoagulant associated bleeding. *Am. Soc. Hematol.* 8: 1–3.

6 Ahmed, I., Majeed, A., and Powell, R. (2007). Heparin induced thrombocytopenia: diagnosis and management update. *Postgrad. Med. J.* 83 (983): 575–582.

7 Leung L., Mannuccio, P., Tirnaur, J. (2017). Direct oral anticoagulants and parenteral direct thrombin inhibitors: dosing and adverse effects. www.uptodate.com/contents/direct-oral-anticoagulants-and-parenteral-direct-thrombin-inhibitors-dosing-and-adverse-effects?search=Direct%20oral%20anticoagulants%20and%20parenteral%20direc&source=search_result&selectedTitle=1~150&usage_type=default&display_rank=1

8 Davis, C., Robertson, C., Shivakumar, S., and Lee, M. (2013). Implications of dabigatran, a direct thrombin inhibitor, for oral surgery practice. *J. Can. Dent. Assoc.* 79: d74.

9 Sunkara, T., Ofori, E., Zarubin, V. et al. (2016). Perioperative management of direct oral anticoagulants (DOACs): a systemic review. *Health Serv. Insights* 9 (Suppl 1): 25–36.

10 Garcia, D. and Crowther, M. (2017). Management of bleeding in patients receiving direct oral anticoagulants. www.uptodate.com/contents/management-of-bleeding-in-patients-receiving-direct-oral-anticoagulants?source=see_link

11 Scottish Dental Clinical Effectiveness Programme (2015). Management of dental patients taking anticoagulants or antiplatelet drugs. www.sdcep.org.uk/in-development/anticoagulants-and-antiplatelets/

12 Mingarro de Leon, A., Chaveli Lopez, B., and Gavalda, E.C. (2014). Dental management of patients receiving anticoagulant and/or antiplatelet treatment. *J. Clin. Exp. Dent.* 6 (2): 155–161.

13 American Dental Association (2015). Anticoagulant and antiplatelet medications and dental procedures. www.ada.org/en/member-center/oral-health-topics/anticoagulant-antiplatelet-medications-and-dental-

25

Burning Mouth Syndrome

Orrett E. Ogle and Arvind Babu Rajendra Santosh

Introduction

Burning mouth syndrome (BMS) is characterized by a chronic intraoral burning sensation that has no readily identifiable causes. The condition has also been referred to as glossodynia (painful tongue), glossopyrosis (burning sensation of tongue), oral dysesthesia (burning pain over entire oral cavity) or stomatodynia (burning sensation of mouth) [1]. Lamey and Lamb described burning mouth syndrome as being characterized by a burning, painful sensation of the oral cavity in the absence of significant mucosal abnormalities [2]. The syndrome is often times multifactorial, and the etiology could range from simple local causes to more complex systemic conditions. Often times, it is difficult to make a definitive diagnosis because there are no universally accepted diagnostic criteria available for the condition.

Local factors that have been proposed as initiating burning mouth syndrome include physical trauma to oral tissues, bruxism, tongue thrusting, cheek biting, teeth clenching, geographic tongue, ill-fitting dentures, parafunctional activity of lip pressure, lip licking, lip sucking, and mouth breathing. Other suggested conditions that may predispose to a burning sensation of mouth are microbial infections (bacteria such as *Helicobacter pylori*, *Enterobacter*, fusospirochetal, *Klebsiella*, fungal organism such as *Candida* or viral pathogen herpes group) in normal-appearing oral mucosa; allergies to mouth rinses, toothpastes, mint, chewing gum, dental restorative materials; and lichenoid mucosities.

The principal clinical characteristic of burning mouth syndrome is a continuous weak to intense burning sensation of oral tissues, often bilaterally or symmetrically presented. The burning sensation is usually not present during sleep but other symptoms such as dysgeusia, xerostomia, and thirst may be observed.

Epidemiology

Many authors have rightly pointed out that it has not been possible to arrive at any precise prevalence rates of BMS because there is no universally accepted definition, and published epidemiologic studies have used different diagnostic clinical criteria to define BMS (Table 25.1). Prevalence varies from 21% in a cross-sectional study of 150 psychiatric patients at a single hospital in India [3] to between 0.7% and 2.6% in a dental publication [4]. Sardella and Lodi found a prevalence of BMS in the general population of 0.5–5% [5]. A study of over 1000 patients randomly selected from the Swedish public dental service records revealed that 3.7% subjects were diagnosed with BMS [6]. A retrospective metastudy comprising over 3000 patients referred to an oral pathology service in Brazil reported a prevalence of about 1% [6]. Interestingly, a study by Tammiala-Salonen et al. found that after organic causes for burning mouth symptoms were treated, the suspected BMS prevalence rate decreased from 15% to 1% [7]. Therefore, many cases reported as BMS may actually not be so. Generally, the prevalence of reported BMS is somewhere between 0.5% and 5%.

Burning mouth syndrome is highly associated with both advanced age and female sex; 75–87% of patients with BMS are women [8, 9]. In men, BMS is not generally found before 40–49 years [9]. The median age of all patients is 62 years old, with a range between 40 and 85 years old [10]. No racial or ethnic differences have been reported.

Oral and Maxillofacial Surgery, Medicine, and Pathology for the Clinician, First Edition. Edited by Harry Dym, Leslie R. Halpern, and Orrett E. Ogle.

Table 25.1 Epidemiologic studies of burning mouth syndrome: US reports.

Location	Prevalence %	Study method
Olmsted County, Minnesota	0.13	Population-based retrospective review from Jan 1 2000 to Dec 31 2010[a]
Pittsburgh, Pennsylvania	2.1	Cross-sectional study of 216 volunteers[b]
North Florida	1.7	Telephone survey of 1636 volunteers from age >65 y/o[c]

[a] Kohorst JL, Bruce AJ, Torgerson RR, et al. A population-based study of the incidence of burning mouth syndrome. Mayo Clin. Proc. 2014;89(11):1545–1552.
[b] Moore PA, Guggenheimer J, Orchard T. Burning mouth syndrome and peripheral neuropathy in patients with type 1 diabetes mellitus. J Diabetes Complications 2007;21(6):397–402.
[c] Riley JL 3rd, Gilbert GH, Heft MW. Orofacial pain symptom prevalence: selective sex differences in the elderly? Pain 1998;76(1–2):97–104.

Etiology and Risk Factors

The etiology of BMS is not known but due to the vast variations in symptoms, the complex clinical picture and possible association with systemic diseases, a number of etiologies have been proposed. What is definitely clear from clinical experience and epidemiologic reports is that BMS has a clear predisposition related to sex, age, and menopause. The female-to-male ratio is 7:1 with a peak age of 62. Approximately 90% of the women in studies of the syndrome have been postmenopausal, with the greatest frequency of onset reported to be from 3 years before to 12 years after menopause [3, 11].

Hypoestrogenemia is considered to be an important factor in burning mouth syndrome, but hormone replacement therapy has not been an effective treatment in postmenopausal women with the disorder [12]. Decrease in estrogen and progesterone levels can result in dryness of mucosal membranes which may cause BMS. It is believed that the fall in neuroprotective gonadal and adrenal steroids during menopause leads to a concomitant decrease in neuroactive steroids, which causes degeneration of oral mucosal small nerve fibers and affects brain areas involved in oral somatic sensations. These changes can become irreversible, resulting in burning neuropathic type pain and other associated symptoms [13].

Xerostomia is a common finding in patients with BMS, being reported in 35–39% of affected patients [14]. One report has even reported 60% [15]. Because of a prevalence ranging between 35% and 60%, xerostomia has been considered to be an etiologic factor. However, decreased estrogen (salivary glands have estrogen receptors), diabetes, medications, and other factors may account for the dry mouth, making the xerostomia merely a symptom of another disease and not an etiologic factor. Salivary flow rate studies in affected patients have not been conclusive and some studies have not shown any significant decrease in unstimulated or stimulated salivary flow [16]. Alterations in salivary components of mucin, IgA, phosphates, pH, and electrical resistance have, however, been reported [16], but the relationship to BMS has not been determined.

Diabetes can cause peripheral neuropathy in the mouth which may manifest as burning or pain, and may also cause metabolic changes in the oral mucosa which can generate, among other disturbances, hypofunction of the salivary glands with secondary reduction of saliva [17].

Evidence in the literature has linked BMS to a peripheral neuropathy. Some studies suggest that BMS is a specific form of cranial neuropathy, based on the pattern of sensorial findings (hypoesthesia) and reduction of nociceptive threshold, as well as on neurophysiologic findings which are suggestive of trigeminal small-fiber sensory neuropathy or axonopathy [18, 19]. Many other factors have been reported as etiologic causes for BMS. Table 25.2 lists some of these factors from various sources.

Primary and Secondary Burning Mouth Syndrome

The two routinely recognized forms of BMS are primary and secondary types. The primary type or essential/idiopathic BMS is when no local and/or systemic pathologies are identifiable. Secondary BMS is when local and/or systemic pathologies can be identified. The secondary form of BMS alerts the clinician to formulate etiology-directed therapy. The distinction of BMS subtypes may further guide physicians and dental clinicians to systematic approaches in patient management.

Primary burning mouth syndrome (P-BMS) represents a small subgroup where the etiology is not clearly identified and is therefore difficult to manage. Primary BMS is diagnosed based on the exclusion of cause, and hence the diagnosis of primary BMS must be made by excluding systemic, infectious or associated oral and/or dermatologic condition(s). The relevance of concomitant psychologic factors is still unclear [20, 21].

The majority of BMS cases fall into the secondary group. Secondary BMS (S-BMS) is diagnosed when the burning sensation is associated with local and/or systemic pathologic conditions. A wide range of concurrent local and

Table 25.2 Etiologic factors of burning mouth syndrome.

Factors	Diseases and defects
Neurologic	Neuropathic pain, neurodysregulation of afferent pain stimuli, hyperesthesia/neuroma following trauma to lingual or mandibular nerves after oral surgery, idiopathic neuralgia
Psychologic	Depression, anxiety, personality disorders, stress
Nutritional	Vitamin B deficiency, iron deficiency anemia, low levels of zinc
Hyposalivation disorders	Sjögren/sicca syndrome, radiation therapy, medication related – ACE inhibitors, beta-blockers, diuretics, antihyperglycemics, antihistamines, sodium lauryl sulfate in toothpaste
GI disorders	GERD, dysgeusia
Endocrine disorders	Menopause, diabetes, hypothyroidism, alteration of gonadal, adrenal, and neuroactive steroid levels
Oral mucosal lesions	Lichen planus, geographic tongue
Immunologic	Contact allergy to dental materials, food antigens like acids, thyroid type immunologic disease, Sjogren syndrome, systemic lupus erythematosus
Infections	Candidiasis, viral infections, *Helicobacter pylori*
Unknown	Nevirapine and efavirenz have been reported to cause BMS via an unknown mechanism; levodopa

ACE, angiotensin-converting enzyme; GI, gastrointestinal; GERD, gastroesophageal reflux disease.

systemic pathologic conditions are associated with secondary BMS.

Based on the intensity of pain, Lamey and Lewis [22] classified BMS into three types.

- Type 1 is when the patient experiences a burning sensation every day; it is absent on waking but develops during the day and is maximal in the evening. Type 1 is linked with systemic disorders, nutritional deficiencies, and endocrine disorders.
- Type 2 is when patient experiences a burning sensation every day; it is present on awakening and often makes sleep difficult at nights. Type 2 BMS patients experience mood changes, alterations in eating habits, and reduced socialization.
- Type 3 is an intermittent burning sensation identified on some days but not on a regular basis. The burning sensation is reported to be in the floor of the mouth, buccal mucosa, and throat. Type 3 patients often have allergic reactions to food additives and suffer from anxiety disorder.

Clinical Presentation

The clinical characteristics of BMS are varied but widely categorized as monosymptomatic (oral burning pain) and polysymptomatic (oral burning pain and other mucosal pathologies). Gorsky et al. [23] presented two clinical forms: (i) "symptomatic triad," which includes unremitting oral burning pain, dysgeusia, and xerostomia; and (ii) "no signs," which includes oral mucosal pain with no other detectable change(s) of oral mucosa.

In general, the symptoms of BMS will involve four features: (i) oral mucosal pain (burning, scalding, tingling, numbness); (ii) dysgeusia (persistent altered taste perception); (iii) xerostomia (dry mouth); and (4) others (thirst, headache, temporomandibular joint [TMJ] pain and discomfort, tenderness or pain in masticatory, neck, shoulder or suprahyoid muscles) [23]. The pain is usually described as bilateral and symmetric burning, which is episodic to continuous and is weak. It is not paroxysmal and is not usually experienced during sleep [24].

Further, electrophysiologic examination reveals an abnormal blink reflex in BMS which is similar to disorders such as Parkinson disease and facial dyskinesias [25]. The abnormal reflex in BMS patients is due to decreased dopaminergic inhibition and is suggestive of nigrostriatal dopaminergic system disorders that primarily affect the regulation of nociception of the trigeminal system and cause loss of sensory inhibition [26].

Diagnosis

Diagnosis will focus largely on primary BMS. Thorough oral examination plays a critical role in the correct diagnosis of BMS. Patients exhibiting oral burning sensation with concurrent oral mucosal abnormalities such as atrophied mucosa, erythema, erthyematous or ulcerated lesions, geographic tongue, lichen planus, lichenoid reaction, atrophic candidiaisis or other miscellaneous lesions should not be initially diagnosed as BMS. Patients exhibiting oral burning sensation without signs of other oral mucosal disease(s) or pathology can be initially diagnosed as BMS [27].

A systematic approach to examining a patient with burning mouth sensation should include standard clinical examination of oral tissues, salivary flow rate, sialochemistry, taste perception evaluation, general hematologic investigations, estrogen/progesterone levels, blood glucose levels, gastroenterology control, and psychiatric assessment [28]. No specific laboratory tests are available to diagnose BMS, though decreased brain activation to heat stimuli, as seen in neuropathic pain, has been demonstrated with fMRI in BMS patients [29]. These functional imaging studies, however, will not generally be available to the dental clinician. The history and examination of oral cavity may indicate the need for laboratory tests. A thorough and complete history is the most important factor.

Scala et al. [27] proposed inclusion diagnostic criteria for BMS and stated that a chief complaint of burning oral pain represents the principal "inclusion symptom criterion" but that other common complaints in BMS should also be considered as additional "inclusion symptomatic criteria" (Table 25.3). Individuals experiencing a burning pain pattern as stated in the "inclusion symptomatic criteria" must be screened for oral mucosal status. Such individuals who exhibit well-defined sign(s) and/or symptom(s) of white lesion, erythematous lesion, erosion, atrophy, and ulcer should be diagnosed as stomatitis, whereas individuals experiencing a burning pain pattern without any oral mucosal pathologies should be diagnosed as BMS [30].

Most patients with primary BMS suffer from subclinical neuropathic pain. Lesions at several levels of the neuraxis can give rise to clinical symptoms of a burning mouth. Three distinct subclasses of BMS have been neurophysiologically characterized: (i) peripheral small-fiber neuropathy; (ii) subclinical major trigeminal neuropathy; and (iii) central pain that may be related to deficient dopaminergic top-down inhibition.

It has been postulated that the clinical diagnosis of primary BMS encompasses at least three distinct, subclinical neuropathic pain states that may overlap in individual patients. The first subgroup (50–65%) is characterized by peripheral small-fiber neuropathy of intraoral mucosa. The second subgroup (20–25%) consists of patients with subclinical lingual, mandibular, or trigeminal system pathology that can be detected with careful neurophysiologic examination but is clinically indistinguishable from the other two subgroups. The third subgroup (20–40%) fits the concept of central pain that may be related to hypofunction of dopaminergic neurons in the basal ganglia [31].

Table 25.3 Inclusion symptom criteria for burning mouth syndrome.

Inclusion symptom criteria (main complaint, i.e., burning pain)	Inclusion symptomatic criteria (other additional complaint)
(1) Is experienced deep within oral mucosa (2) Is unremitting for at least 4–6 months (3) Is continuous throughout all or almost all the day (4) Seldom interferes with sleep and (5) Never worsens, but may be relieved by eating and drinking	(6) The occurrence of other oral symptoms, such as dysgeusia and/or xerostomia (7) The presence of sensory/chemosensory anomalies (8) The presence of mood changes and/or specific disruption(s) in patient personality traits

Source: Data from Scala et al. [27].

Diagnosis of Secondary BMS

Differentiation of P-BMS and S-BMS should be done specifically to recognize local and/or systemic factors which will suggest specific treatment. Both clinical and laboratory tests are helpful in differentiating P-BMS and S-BMS (Figure 25.1). The clinical tests should focus on evaluation of the masticatory system that includes examination of masticatory muscles, TMJ apparatus, occlusal disturbances from premature contact, denture design, restorations, parafunctional habits, and objective evaluation of taste sensation [32]. Laboratory tests such as salivary tests can evaluate the changes in salivary flow (i.e., identification of hyposalivation or xerostomia) and sialochemistry (i.e., identification of specific alterations in salivary composition) [33] (Table 25.4). If systemic disease involvement is suspected then appropriate laboratory tests should be done. Appropriate biochemical laboratory tests must be done to rule out nutritional deficiency, diabetes mellitus, hormonal imbalance, thyroid conditions, adrenal insufficiency, menopausal problems or gastrointestinal problems [27].

Biopsy procedures should be done when conditions such as lichen planus, lichenoid reaction, oral submucus fibrosis or erythroplakia are suspected. Cytology or biopsy should be done when candidiasis or viral infection of oral cavity is suspected. Oral patch test, sialochemistry or biopsy may be conducted when allergic oral diseases are suspected [34]. Benzoyl peroxide, cobalt chloride, mercury, methylmethacrylate monomer, nickel sulfate, and petrolatum cadmium sulfate are frequently reported dental materials associated with BMS. Food allergens include chestnuts, nicotinic acid, octyl allate, peanuts, propylene glycol, and sorbic acid [27]. When the results of these diagnostic tests show one or more positive report for local and/or systemic factors, then the patient must be considered as S-BMS.

Treatment

Because there is no specific etiology for BMS, the clinician must recognize that this is a complex pain disorder and that no specific treatment will be effective for all people. It

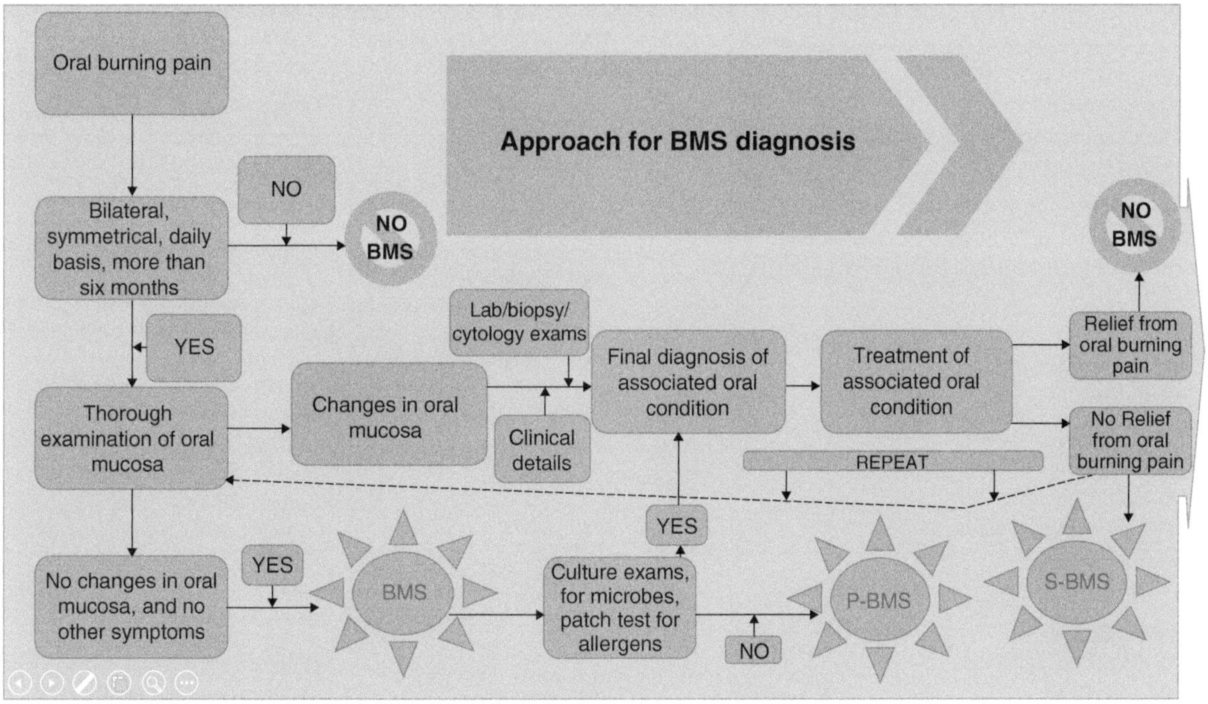

Figure 25.1 Approach to the diagnosis of burning mouth syndrome.

will be necessary, therefore, to design individualized treatment options for each patient. In general, the treatment of BMS is directed at its symptoms.

Secondary Burning Mouth Syndrome

The symptoms of secondary BMS will improve when an identifiable underlying medical condition, such as diabetes, gastroesopheal reflux disease or candidiasis, is treated. The goal, therefore, should be directed at treating the causative systemic disease, withdrawing offending medications if possible, and addressing local factors. The treatment of some specific underlying medical conditions that contribute to secondary BMS is shown in Table 25.5. Methods of managing the symptoms of secondary BMS are presented in Box 25.1.

Primary Burning Mouth Syndrome

When underlying factors cannot be identified and corrected, the therapeutic options for BMS are limited and many patients become refractory to standard pain management. Neurophysiologic, neuropathologic, and functional imaging studies have revealed that several neuropathic mechanisms, mostly subclinical, act at different levels of the neuraxis and contribute to the pathophysiology of primary BMS [31]. This may suggest that pain management should follow the general guidelines for treating neuropathic pain: first-line treatments including certain antidepressants (i.e., tricyclic antidepressants and dual reuptake inhibitors of both serotonin and norepinephrine), calcium channel alpha-2-delta ligands (i.e., gabapentin and pregabalin), and topical lidocaine [35]. Opioid analgesics should be avoided.

Many pain treatment regimens have been tried with variable success. Several drugs have been recommended over the years but their long-term effectiveness has not been consistent. Some of the more popular ones include alpha-lipoic acid (an antioxidant used in diabetic neuropathy), amisulpiride (a second-generation neuroleptic that in low dosages presents dopaminergic activity), topical clonazepam, and gabapentin. In a review of the pharmacologic treatments used in a 10-year span from 1996 to 2006 to reduce the symptoms of BMS, Mínguez Serra et al. [36] found the following.

- Capsaicin and clonazepam, administered systemically via the oral route, can be discarded as a viable option because of their adverse reactions.
- Gabapentin did not show efficacy in alleviation of BMS pain while alpha-lipoic acid appeared useful, but loses its efficacy over time.
- Benzidamine and trazodone were not found to be better than placebo in the treatment of BMS.
- With amisulpiride, paroxetine, sertraline, and sucralfate, the patients reported improvement but the study designs were deficient.

Table 25.4 Chairside, laboratory, and imaging tests in BMS.

Evaluation of masticatory system
1) Muscles of mastication
2) Temporomandibular joint examination
3) Occlusal examination

Evaluation of dental procedures
1) Dental restorations
2) Prosthesis – partial/complete dentures, fixed and implant prostheses

Salivary test
1) Salivary flow rate
2) Sialochemistry
3) Salivary proteins

Test for systemic pathologic conditions
1) Nutritional deficiencies
2) Blood glucose levels in diabetes
3) Hormonal evaluation
4) Gastric reflux examination

Diagnostic imaging
1) Head and neck malignancies
2) Thyroid enlargements
3) Systemic sclerosis

Biopsy examination
1) Lichen planus
2) Oral lichenoid reaction
3) Erythroplakia
4) Oral submucus fibrosis

Bacterial/viral/fungal examinations
1) Candidiasis
2) Fusospirochetal
3) *Klebsiella*
4) Herpes virus
5) *Helicobacter pylori*
6) *Enterobacter*

Allergic test
Oral patch test/patch test

Gustatory evaluation

- Topical clonazepam currently seems to be the best option, with improvement reported in almost half of all patients (40%) [36, 37].

Grushka et al. [38, 39] proposed a regimen consisting of a combination of clonazepam, gabapentin, and baclofen as the best treatment for the syndrome (Table 25.6).

The American Academy of Oral Medicine suggests the use of clonazepam either as a mouthrinse or in dissolvable wafer or pill form along with amitriptyline, nortriptyline, doxepin, and gabapentin as needed [40] (Table 25.7).

Mock and Chugh found that psychologic factors, though unlikely to be the primary cause, are often operative in BMS, and they suggested the combination of cognitive behavioral therapy, alpha-lipoic acid, and/or clonazepam as a very promising approach for the treatment of BMS [41].

Table 25.5 Possible causes of secondary burning mouth syndrome and management.

Primary condition	Management
Nutritional: deficiencies in vitamins B1, B2, B6, B12, C, folic acid, iron, zinc	Oral supplementation
Hyposalivation: secondary to drugs, following chemotherapy or radiation therapy, altered salivary content, Sjögren syndrome	Modify medication intake, limit caffeine intake, stop smoking, limit alcohol use, suck on ice cubes, sip cold water, boost saliva production (pilocarpine or cevimeline), artificial saliva or moisturizing sprays or rinses
Gastroesophageal reflux disease	Antacids (Maalox, Mylanta®, Rolaids®, Tums®, etc.); proton pump inhibitors (Prevacid®, Prilosec®); H2-receptor blockers (Tagamet®, Pepcid®, Zantac®)
Menopause	Hormone replacement therapy if otherwise indicated
Diabetes	Control of diabetes by physician
Oral mucosal lesions: lichen planus, pemphigus, pemphigoid	Establish diagnosis and treat mucosal condition – usually prednisone
Candidiasis	Topical nystatin rinses, ingested fluconazole

Based on the majority of studies that have reported on the use of laser, laser treatment appears to be capable of reducing pain in BMS and should be considered [42].

Conclusion

Burning mouth syndrome is a chronic, multifactorial pain syndrome and patients must be made aware that it may take months or years before the pain is at a manageable level and that attempting combinations of therapies may be necessary. In the clinical picture, BMS is no different to other idiopathic chronic pain syndromes and the treating clinician must recognize that treatment should be individualized based on symptoms. Clonazepam either as a mouthrinse or in dissolvable wafer or pill form should be tried first, as presently it seems to be the best option, with healing of almost half of all patients (40%). If this does not give adequate relief then combinations suggested by Grushka would be the follow-up option. Psychologic conditions should also be considered.

Box 25.1 Localized treatment of xerostomia

- Sip a cold water or suck on ice chips when there is pain.
- Avoid smoking even after underlying medical condition is controlled.
- Never use chewing tobacco since more nicotine is absorbed through the oral mucosa by chewing tobacco than by smoking a cigarette.
- Avoid alcohol or products containing alcohol, such as mouthwashes with high alcohol content.
- Avoid drinking or eating products high in acid, such as citrus fruits and juices, pineapples, blue plums, grapes, etc.
- Avoid spicy foods,
- Decrease the temperature of beverages like coffee or tea,
- Swish and spit with diphenhydramine, Kaopectate®, Maalox®, etc. to coat dry mucosa.
- Lidocaine viscous rinses and sucking lozenges with benzocaine may offer short-term relief.

Table 25.6 Drugs used for treating burning mouth syndrome.

Medication	Classification	Dosage range
Amitriptyline (Elavil®)	Tricyclic antidepressant	10–150 mg per day
Nortriptyline (Pamelor®)	Tricyclic antidepressant	75–150 mg per day
Chlordiazepoxide (Librium®)	Benzodiazepine	10–30 mg per day
Clonazepam (Klonopin®)	Benzodiazepine	0.25–2 mg per day
Gabapentin (Neurontin®)	Anticonvulsant	300–1600 mg per day
Lidocaine transoral delivery system (DentiPatch®)	Local anesthetic	Apply to buccal mucosa; 46.1 mg lidocaine
Lidocaine viscous 2%	Local anesthetic	Maximum dose is 15 mL per dose q3h. Should not exceed 8 doses in a 24-hour period
Capsaicin liquid	Topical analgesic	Rinse mouth with one teaspoon of a 1:2 dilution 3 or 4 times daily

Source: Data from Medications for Burning Mouth Syndrome (Glossopyrosis). www.drugs.com/condition/burning-mouth-syndrome.html

Table 25.7 Suggested regimen for management of burning mouth syndrome.

Drug	Management
Amitriptyline	10 mg at bedtime. Increase dosage by 10 mg weekly until oral burning is relieved. Maximum dose 150 mg
Nortriptyline	Start with 25 mg at bedtime; increase by 25 mg weekly up to 150 mg as needed
Chlordiazepoxide	0.5–2 mg at bedtime. 0.5–1 mg dissolved on tongue three times daily
Clonazepam	0.25 mg at bedtime; increase dosage by 0.25 mg every 4–7 days until oral burning is relieved. Maximum dose 4 mg
Gabapentin	100 mg at about 5 pm in the evening or at bedtime; increase dosage by 100 mg weekly up to 3600 mg until oral burning is relieved or side-effects occur

References

1 Drage, L.A. and Rogers, R.S. (2003). Burning mouth syndrome. *Dermatol. Clin.* 21 (1): 135–145.

2 Lamey, P.J. and Lamb, A.B. (1988). Prospective study of etiological factors in burning mouth syndrome. *Br. Med. J.* 296 (6631): 1243–1246.

3 Dangore-Khasbage, S., Khairkar, P.H., Degwekar, S.S. et al. (2012). Prevalence of oral mucosal disorders in institutionalized and non-institutionalized psychiatric patients: a study from AVBR hospital in Central India. *J. Oral Sci.* 54 (1): 85–91.

4 Klausner, J.J. (1994). Epidemiology of chronic facial pain: diagnostic usefulness in patient care. *J. Am. Dent. Assoc.* 125 (12): 1604–1611.

5 Sardella, A. and Lodi, G. (2013). Acupuncture and burning mouth syndrome: a pilot study. *Pain Pract.* 13 (8): 627–632.

6 Gurvits, G.E. and Tan, A. (2013). Burning mouth syndrome. *J. Gastroenterol.* 19 (5): 665–672.
7 Tammiala-Salonen, T., Hiidenkari, T., and Parvinen, T. (1993). Burning mouth in a Finnish adult population. *Community Dent. Oral Epidemiol.* 21 (2): 67–71.
8 Gao, J., Chen, L., Zhou, J., and Peng, J. (2009). A case-control study on etiological factors involved in patients with burning mouth syndrome. *J. Oral Pathol. Med.* 38 (1): 24–28.
9 Bergdahl, M. and Bergdahl, J. (1999). Burning mouth syndrome: prevalence and associated factors. *J. Oral Pathol. Med.* 28 (8): 350–354.
10 Coculescu, E.C., Ţovaru, S., and Coculescu, B.I. (2014). Epidemiological and etiological aspects of burning mouth syndrome. *J. Med. Life* 7 (3): 305–309.
11 Grushka, M. (1987). Clinical features of burning mouth syndrome. *Oral Surg. Oral Med. Oral Pathol.* 63 (1): 30–36.
12 Forabosco, A., Criscuolo, M., Coukos, G. et al. (1992). Efficacy of hormone replacement therapy in postmenopausal women with oral discomfort. *Oral Surg. Oral Med. Oral Pathol.* 73 (5): 570–574.
13 Woda, A., Dao, T., and Gremeau-Richard, C. (2009). Steroid dysregulation and stomatodynia (burning mouth syndrome). *J. Orofac. Pain* 23 (3): 202–210.
14 Aggarwal, A. and Panat, S.R. (2012). Burning mouth syndrome: a diagnostic and therapeutic dilemma. *J Clin Exp Dent* 4 (3): 180–185.
15 Grushka, M. and Epstein, J.B. (2003). Burning mouth syndrome and other oral sensory disorders: a unifying hypothesis. *Pain Res. Manag.* 8 (3): 133–135.
16 Ship, J.A., Grushka, M., Lipton, J.A. et al. (1995). Burning mouth syndrome: an update. *J. Am. Dent. Assoc.* 126 (7): 842–853.
17 Minor, J.S. and Epstein, J.B. (2011). Burning mouth syndrome and secondary oral burning. *Otolaryngol. Clin. North Am.* 44 (1): 205–219.
18 Stuginski-Barbosa, J., Rodrigues, G.G., Bigal, M.E. et al. (2008). Burning mouth syndrome responsive to pramipexol. *J. Headache Pain* 9 (1): 43–45.
19 Lauria, G., Majorana, A., Borgna, M. et al. (2005). Trigeminal small-fiber sensory neuropathy causes burning mouth syndrome. *Pain* 115 (3): 332–337.
20 Pokupec-Gruden, J.S., Cekic-Arambasin, A., and Gruden, V. (2000). Psychogenic factors in the aetiology of stomatopyrosis. *Coll. Antropol.* 24 (Suppl 1): 119–126.
21 Grushka, M., Sessle, B.J., and Howley, T.P. (1987). Psychophysical assessment of tactile, pain and thermal sensory functions in burning mouth syndrome. *Pain* 28 (2): 169–184.
22 Lamey, P.J. and Lewis, M.A. (1989). Oral medicine in practice: burning mouth syndrome. *Br. Dent. J.* 167 (6): 197–200.
23 Gorsky, M., Silverman, S. Jr., and Chinn, H. (1991). Clinical characteristics and management outcome in the burning mouth syndrome. An open study of 130 patients. *Oral Surg. Oral Med. Oral Pathol.* 72 (2): 192–195.
24 Woda, A. and Pionchon, P. A unified concept of idiopathic orofacial pain: clinical features. *J. Orofac. Pain* 13: 172–184. discussion:185-195;1999.
25 Jaaskelainen, S.K., Forssell, H., and Tenovuo, O. (1997). Abnormalities of the blink reflex in burning mouth syndrome. *Pain* 73 (3): 455–460.
26 Jaaskelainen, S.K., Rinne, J.O., Forssell, H. et al. (2001). Role of the dopaminergic system in chronic pain – a fluorodopa-PET study. *Pain* 90 (3): 257–260.
27 Scala, A., Checchi, L., Montevecchi, M. et al. (2003). Update on burning mouth syndrome: overview and patient management. *Crit. Rev. Oral Biol. Med.* 14 (4): 275–291.
28 Coculescu, E., Radu, A., and Coculescu, B. (2014). Burning mouth syndrome: a review on diagnosis and treatment. *J. Med. Life* 7 (4): 512–515.
29 Albuquerque, R.J.C., de Leeuw, R., Carlson, C.R. et al. (2006). Cerebral activation during thermal stimulation of patients who have burning mouth disorder: an fMRI study. *Pain* 122 (3): 223–234.
30 International Association for the Study of Pain. Burning mouth syndrome. www.orofacialpain.org.uk/education/burning-mouth-syndrome 2017
31 Jääskeläinen, S.K. (2012). Pathophysiology of primary burning mouth syndrome. *Clin. Neurophysiol.* 123 (1): 71–77.
32 McNeill, C. (e.) (1997). Objective basis of treatment. In: *Science and Practice of Occlusion*, 306–324. Chicago, IL.: Quintessence Publishing.
33 Tammiala-Salonen, T. and Söderling, E. (1993). Protein composition, adhesion, and agglutination properties of saliva in burning mouth syndrome. *Scand. J. Dent. Res.* 101 (4): 215–218.
34 Minciullo, P.L., Paolino, G., Vacca, M. et al. (2016). Unmet diagnostic needs in contact oral mucosal allergies. *Clin. Mol. Allergy* 14 (1): 10.
35 Dworkin, R., O'Connor, A., Audette, J. et al. (2017). Recommendations for the pharmacological management of neuropathic pain. *Mayo Clin. Proc* 85: S3–S14.
36 Mínguez Serra, M.P., Salort Llorca, C., and Silvestre Donat, F.J. (2007). Pharmacological treatment of burning mouth syndrome: a review and update. *Med. Oral Patol. Oral Cir. Bucal.* 12 (4): E299–E304.

37 Dahiya, P., Kamal, R., Kumar, M. et al. (2013). Burning mouth syndrome and menopause. *Int. J. Prev. Med.* 4 (1): 15–20.

38 Grushka, M., Ching, V., and Epstein, J. (2006). Burning mouth syndrome. *Adv. Otorhinolaryngol.* 63: 278–287.

39 Grushka, M., Epstein, J.B., and Gorsky, M. (2002). Burning mouth syndrome. *Am. Fam. Physician* 65 (4): 615–621.

40 Burning mouth syndrome. American Academy of Oral Medicine. (2015) https://maaom.memberclicks.net/index.php?option=com_content&view=article&id=81:burning-mouth-syndrome&catid=22:patient-condition-information&Itemid=120

41 Mock, D. and Chugh, D. (2010). Burning mouth syndrome. *Int. J. Oral Sci.* 2 (1): 1–4.

42 Al-Maweri, S.A., Javed, F., Kalakonda, B. et al. (2017). Efficacy of low level laser therapy in the treatment of burning mouth syndrome: a systematic review. *Photodiagn. Photodyn. Ther.* 17: 188–193.

Index

Oral and Maxillofacial Surgery, Medicine, and Pathology for the Clinician, First Edition. Edited by Harry Dym, Leslie R. Halpern, and Orrett E. Ogle.